Diets for Sick Children

DOROTHY E. M. FRANCIS
SRD
Group Chief Dietitian
The Hospitals for Sick Children
Great Ormond Street, London, and
Queen Elizabeth Hospital for Children
Hackney Road, London

FOREWORD BY

BARBARA E. CLAYTON
CBE MD PhD Hon DSc FRCP FRCPE FRCPath
Honorary Fellow of the British Dietetic Association
Dean of the Faculty of Medicine and
Professor of Chemical Pathology and Human Metabolism
University of Southampton

FOURTH EDITION

BLACKWELL SCIENTIFIC PUBLICATIONS

OXFORD LONDON EDINBURGH

BOSTON PALO ALTO MELBOURNE

© 1965, 1970, 1974, 1987 by
Blackwell Scientific Publications
Editorial offices:
Osney Mead, Oxford OX2 0EL
8 John Street, London WC1N 2ES
23 Ainslie Place, Edinburgh EH3 6AJ
52 Beacon Street, Boston
  Massachusetts 02108, USA
667 Lytton Avenue, Palo Alto
  California 94301, USA
107 Barry Street, Carlton
  Victoria 3053, Australia

First published 1965
Second edition 1970
Third edition 1974
Fourth edition 1987

Set, printed and bound in Great Britain by Butler &
Tanner Ltd, Frome, Somerset, and London

DISTRIBUTORS

USA
  Year Book Medical Publishers
  35 East Wacker Drive
  Chicago, Illinois 60601

Canada
Blackwell Mosby Book Distributors
  120 Melford Drive, Scarborough
  Ontario M1B 2X4

Australia
  Blackwell Scientific Publications
    (Australia) Pty Ltd
  107 Barry Street
  Carlton, Victoria 3053

British Library Cataloguing in Publication Data

Francis, Dorothy E. M.
    Diets for sick children. —— 4th ed.
    1. Children —— Nutrition   2. Metabolism,
Disorders of
    I. Title
    618.92′390654   RJ206
    ISBN 0–632–00505–X

Diets for Sick Children

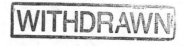

This book is dedicated to the children and their parents with whom I have had the honour to share the many experiences of life during 25 years dietetic paediatric practice.

Contents

Foreword to fourth edition

It is both a privilege and a pleasure to write a fore-word to the Fourth Edition of *Diets for Sick Children*. It is now 12 years since the Third Edition was published and the intervening years have seen remarkable progress in the treatment of sick children with therapeutic diets.

Much of this progress has been due to Miss Francis' enthusiasm, skill and originality and I know that this new edition has been eagerly awaited by dietitians and paediatricians alike. In 17 chapters she has covered diets for a wide variety of disorders, both common and rare. The newer topics of food intolerances and allergy and dietary fibre are all included. As always, she brings to the subject a fund of knowledge, sound commonsense and a practical approach which we all find so invaluable.

I congratulate Miss Francis most warmly on her achievement in undertaking this monumental task of producing a book whilst carrying an enormous day-to-day clinical load. Once again she has made an outstanding contribution to the care of sick children to whom she is devoted.

Barbara E. Clayton

Preface

At the Hospitals for Sick Children, Great Ormond Street, and Queen Elizabeth Hospital for Children, Hackney Road, London, we receive many requests for help with specialized therapeutic diets for children. The object of this book is to meet such needs. It is intended to give practical assistance to paediatricians, general practitioners, health visitors, dietitians, nurses and others who may be required to advise on, or provide, these diets. It is not meant for parents of children on special diets, as the diets should be adjusted to suit the individual by appropriate professionals.

The previous edition of *Diets for Sick Children* (Blackwell Scientific Publications, 1974) has been widely used, but there has been a further expansion in the field of paediatric dietetics, associated mainly with food allergy and metabolic disorders. In this completely revised and rewritten edition of *Diets for Sick Children*, the dietary information has been brought up to date in conjunction with new analytical data* and with regard to today's scientific knowledge, foods and changing meal patterns. The special dietary treatment of various metabolic disorders comprises a large section of the book. Also included is a normal range of therapeutic diets which have been adapted to children's requirements, based on the requirements and nutritional needs of children by Francis (1986) in *Nutrition for Children*. It is my intention that these two books should complement one another and this book should be used in conjunction with the principles and requirements detailed in *Nutrition for Children*.

Prescribed therapeutic diets must satisfy all the nutritional needs for growth and the doctor must monitor the amount of any restricted nutrient in the light of clinical biochemical findings as described in *Paediatric Chemical Pathology* (Clayton B.E., Jenkins P. & Round J. N. [1980] Oxford: Blackwell Scientific Publications). The child must be kept under strict and constant surveillance. Growth retardation should be avoided and follow-up is essential. Written details of special dietary regimens are essential. Diets should be revised, updated or abandoned as necessary; at least an annual review is advised.

A number of specially prepared products for therapeutic diets are available, some of which are classified by the Advisory Committee on Borderline Substances as drugs and are available at NHS expense for specific well-defined conditions (*see* Appendix I).

A list of products and the manufacturer's or distributor's address in the U.K. is included—Chapter 17. The composition and ingredients of such products change from time to time and may vary from country to country, or the varieties made for export may be different from the products of the same name on sale in a different country. *Before using any product the latest and appropriate information must be obtained from the manufacturer.*

The variety permitted in many diets can be expanded by inclusion of a number of commercially available convenience foods, provided such products exclude forbidden ingredients, e.g. sources of gluten or milk, and when the composition is suitable for inclusion in the diet. It is not practical to give detailed lists of such products in the text. A number of lists are available to dietitians through their professional association.

Although the latest product data have been checked during the preparation of this edition of *Diets for Sick Children*, no responsibility can be taken for any product quoted, or for changes in ingredients or composition. Only examples of products are quoted and in many instances alternative products of similar composition may be equally suitable.

---

* *McCance & Widdowson's The Composition of Food*, 4th Edition (1978) by Paul A. A. and Southgate D. A. T. and MRC Special Report No. 297 (London: HMSO) have been used for the calculation of foods and menus in the text examples.

Acknowledgements

Obviously, a work of this kind has involved the assistance of a number of people, whose help I gratefully acknowledge. Firstly, I must thank Professor Barbara Clayton for all the help, encouragement and advice she has given at each stage and every section of the book. I am also grateful for advice from the following consultant medical staff at The Hospitals for Sick Children, London (unless otherwise stated).

T. M. Barratt MB BChir FRCP, Professor of Paediatric Nephrology.

I. W. Booth MSc MB BS MRCP DObst RCOG DCH, Lecturer in Child Health, Birmingham.

R. Dinwiddie MB ChB FRCP DCH, Senior Lecturer (honorary).

D. G. Grant MD FRCP DCH, Consultant Paediatric Endocrinologist.

The Late J. T. Harries MD MSc FRCP DCH, Professor of Paediatric Gastroenterology.

V. F. Larcher BA MB BChir MRCP, Consultant Paediatrician, Queen Elizabeth Hospital for Children.

J. V. Leonard MA PhD MB BChir FRCP, Senior Lecturer in Child Health.

P. Milla MSc MB BS MRCP, Senior Lecturer in Child Health.

Joan Slack DM FRCP, Department of Clinical Genetics, Royal Free Hospital, London.

Isabel Smith MB Bsc BS FRCP DCH, Lecturer in Child Health (honorary).

J. F. Soothill MA MD BChir FRCP FRCPath, Professor of Immunology (retired).

J. A. Walker-Smith MD FRCP FRACP, Professor in Paediatric Gastroenterology, Queen Elizabeth Hospital for Children.

J. Wilson PhD FRCP, Consultant Neurologist.

I am also indebted to the dietetic staff for their support and help throughout the preparation of this manuscript, particularly Susan Allman BSc SRD, and to the Board of Governors of The Hospitals for Sick Children. I gratefully acknowledge the co-operation of all the manufacturers who have supplied the valuable information on their products. Finally, I wish to acknowledge the invaluable secretarial help of Sheila Button, Rebecca Knowles and Elisabeth Moore in compiling this manuscript.

Gastrointestinal disorders

PHYSIOLOGY OF THE SMALL INTESTINE

An understanding of the development and the normal physiology of digestion and absorption is essential for the ultimate provision of appropriate regimes for the treatment of the different gastrointestinal disorders. The development of the human gastrointestinal tract is characterized by the integrated maturation of its digestive and absorptive capacity, and has been reviewed by Grand *et al.* 1976, CIBA 1979, and Harries 1982a, b. The survival of the pre-term infant is largely dependent on its ability to adapt successfully from intrauterine to extrauterine life. Nutrition is a critical factor and largely depends on the state of maturation of gastrointestinal function. For example, glucose absorption capacity is dependent on nutritional status and length of gestation (McNeish *et al.* 1979) and continues to increase after birth and throughout infancy (Younoszai 1974). Animal studies suggest that amino acid and dipeptide transport mature similarly. Digestion of lactose has some limitation, and monosaccharide absorption is immature, but most pre-term infants cope with the carbohydrate of human milk without difficulty. Pancreatic amylase activity is relatively low in the newborn, and does not reach adult levels for several months, however human milk contains some amylase. Lipid absorption even in the full-term infant is limited by defects of pancreatic lipolysis and bile salt solubilization (CIBA 1979, Friedman & Nyland 1980), and may be severely impaired in the pre-term. Lingual, and particularly human milk, lipase are important in the newborn for optimal fat absorption (Harries 1982b). The absorption of other nutrients frequently relies on specific carrier ligands, which may be present in breast milk and so enhance absorption before the endogenous ligands appear.

The normal physiology of digestion of the mature gastrointestinal tract is summarized in Table 1.1.

GASTROENTERITIS: ACUTE DIARRHOEA

Acute gastroenteritis is the clinical syndrome of diarrhoea and/or vomiting of acute onset, often accompanied by fever and constitutional disturbance, which is of infective origin and not secondary to some primary disease process outside the alimentary tract (Walker-Smith 1979). Loss of body water and electrolytes, acidosis, shock and death can result. Severe dehydration occurs more readily in infants, as a result of their higher basal fluid requirements compared with adults, their inability to get easy access to water, immaturity of renal tubular reabsorption processes and the misconception that fluid should be withheld in infants with diarrhoea (Booth *et al.* 1984).

Acute diarrhoea is the commonest worldwide problem of fluid–electrolyte malnutrition and claims the lives of approximately 5 to 18 million children annually, mostly under five years of age, in Asia, Africa and Latin America. It is now probably the largest single cause of death in the world (Walsh & Warren 1979). Although 99% of such deaths occur in developing countries, acute diarrhoea in children remains a major health problem. In the U.K. over 400 children (0 to 4 years) per 100 000 required admission to hospitals in 1977 (Wharton 1981), and in the under-two-years group acute diarrhoea is an important preventable cause of death (Oakley *et al.* 1969). There is a peak prevalence in the second year in developing countries, and in the U.K. in the latter half of the first year.

In addition to producing such prodigious mortality worldwide, diarrhoeal disease is a major contributory factor to malnutrition, particularly in those with pre-existing protein–energy malnutrition (PEM). This probably occurs as a result of anorexia, withdrawal of nutrition during illness, stress-induced negative nitrogen balance and secondary carbohydrate intolerance, particularly to lactose (Booth & Harries 1982a). Also, malnutrition predisposes to diarrhoea, particularly during and after the weaning period.

Table 1.1 Physiology of absorption of the major foodstuffs (adapted from Lloyd 1970).

Food	Intraluminal phase		Mucosal cell	Extracellular transport
Fat (largely triglyceride)				
(a) Long-chain triglycerides* (LCT)	Emulsification (chyme)	Mechanical churning Bile salts Biliary lecithin Monoglycerides Lingual lipase	Resynthesis of triglyceride Chylomicron formation	As chylomicrons via intestinal lymphatics and thoracic duct to systemic bloodstream. (Some long-chain fatty acids can be transported in portal bloodstream.)
	Lipolysis to free fatty acids, 2-monoglycerides, diglycerides	Lipases†, lingual and pancreatic, pH dependent Colipase Phospholipase A Bile salts		
	Solubilization	Bile salts Micelles		
(b) Medium-chain triglycerides* (MCT)	Appreciably water-soluble and therefore less dependent on bile salts for emulsification or solubilization. Lipolysis by lipase more rapid than for LCT; intact triglycerides can also be absorbed.		Intact triglycerides hydrolysed No resynthesis of triglyceride No chylomicron formation	As fatty acids in portal blood-stream

Carbohydrate

(a) Starch amylopectin (80–90%)
  α-1–4 links ⎫ In glucose
  α-1–6 links ⎭ residue
  → Hydrolysis to maltose, maltotriose and α-limit dextrin
  → Salivary and pancreatic amylase†
  → Membrane digestion by maltases and sucrase–isomaltase to glucose
  → Active absorption of glucose

(b) Disaccharides
  Lactose
  → Membrane digestion by lactase to glucose and galactose
  → Active absorption of glucose and galactose by 'carriers'.
  Sucrose
  → Membrane digestion by sucrase to glucose and fructose
  → Absorption of fructose transported by carrier media.

(c) Monosaccharides Glucose, fructose, galactose
  → Absorption as above.

  → As monosaccharides in portal bloodstream.

Protein

  Gastric pepsin
  Pancreatic proteolysis—trypsin, chymotrypsin, elastase and carboxypeptidases as inactive precursors (zymogens)
  → Digestion to small peptides and amino acids
  → Enterokinase activates trypsinogen. Trypsin then activates other proteolytic enzymes
  → Active absorption of amino acids by 'carriers' specific for different amino acid groups. Absorption of intact dipeptides.

  → As amino acids and dipeptides in portal bloodstream.

* Long-chain triglycerides, which comprise the majority of ordinary dietary fat, contain fatty acids with more than 10 carbon atoms; medium-chain triglycerides contain fatty acids with 8 or 10 carbon atoms.

† Human milk contains lipase and some amylase.

Irreversible arrest of intellectual development and
subsequent intellectual deficit can occur as a result of
the severe degree of malnutrition caused by diarrhoeal disease.

Breast-feeding provides major protection against
gastroenteritis and infection (Narayanan *et al.* 1982,
Holmes *et al.* 1983) due to both its relative cleanli-
ness and the provision of a number of antimicrobial
factors, including antigens, lactoferrin, macrophages
and neutrophils, together with the encouragement of
a 'normal' gut flora (Soothill 1976). This protection,
although not complete (Kingston 1973), is more
effective when the infant is exclusively breast-fed.
Feeds, both bottles and solids, which are heavily contaminated with microbial organisms greatly increase
the risk of gastroenteritis (Jelliffe & Jelliffe 1978).

The soluble content of the feeding regimen and fluid
intake at the commencement of diarrhoea largely determines the type of dehydration and risk of hypernatraemia. Breast-feeding, or low-solute feeds such as
those now recommended as modified infant feeds
(DHSS 1980) and made up in the correct dilution, is
important to the clinical outcome of gastroenteritis
when it does occur. Both hypernatraemia accompanying dehydration and gastroenteritis in young infants are far less common in the United Kingdom
since the DHSS 1974 recommendation that infants
should be breast-fed or given modified milks until at
least six months of age (Walker-Smith 1979). Exclusive demand breast-feeding of infants should be encouraged worldwide, and practical advice should be
given to achieve its success (*see* Francis 1986), to
provide adequate nutrition for normal growth and to
reduce the incidence of diarrhoeal disease with its
catastrophic consequences.

Rotaviruses are now known to be the most important viral cause of acute infectious diarrhoea in
young children between six months and two years,
and account for about 50% of episodes in temperate
climates, but the incidence in the tropics is more variable. There is a male predominance. Outbreaks are
seasonal, occurring in the winter months in the
United Kingdom (Booth & Harries 1982a). Adeno-
viruses are the next most common viral cause and
coronaviruses are associated with outbreaks of enteri-
tis in older age groups. *Escherichia coli* accounts for
approximately 60% of diarrhoeal episodes in people
over two years old. Cholera, *E. coli*, *Salmonella*, *Shi-
gella* and other bacteria and viruses cause diarrhoea
by a number of different mechanisms (Booth *et al.*
1984). Many, like the cholera toxin, cause acute profuse secretory diarrhoea with severe fluid and electrolyte losses. Others, particularly those of parasitic ori-

gin, e.g. amoebic dysentery, cause chronic diarrhoea
(Ebrahim 1977). Oral rehydration therapy is effective, irrespective of the mechanism and cause.

ORAL REHYDRATION THERAPY

Life-saving oral rehydration therapy (ORT) represents
one of the most important advances in modern medicine since the introduction of antibiotics. It should
be initiated as soon as diarrhoea starts, in order to
prevent or correct dehydration. If hypovolaemia and
shock accompany severe dehydration, intravenous
resuscitation is essential to reduce the high risk of
mortality. In other patients with diarrhoea oral rehydration with an appropriate carbohydrate–electrolyte solution has been shown to be as successful and
safer than intravenous rehydration (Santosham *et al.*
1982, Pizarro *et al.* 1983).

The scientific basis of ORT arose from the fundamental observation that sodium transport was en-
hanced by concurrent glucose transport in the small
intestine. Historically, glucose was added as a source
of energy, and the high carbohydrate content of the
early formulae, and indeed of some currently available (*see* Table 1.2), may result in increased stool
volume due to an osmotic effect (Booth *et al.* 1984).

The World Health Organization has proposed a
'universal' oral rehydration solution (WHO 1976)
based largely on experience with cholera patients.

Concern was initially expressed by paediatricians
in the western world regarding the high sodium content (9 mmol sodium/100 ml) of the WHO solution
(Finberg 1980, Tripp & Harries 1980). Subsequently,
controlled studies (Santosham *et al.* 1982, Pizarro *et
al.* 1983) have shown that such a solution, if correctly prescribed, is equally appropriate for oral rehydration in well-nourished children as for those in
developing countries. There is further evidence that
it is safe and effective treatment of out-patients as
well as in-patients (Santosham *et al.* 1983).

The arguments regarding the optimal composition
of oral rehydration solution (ORS) are discussed by
Booth *et al.* (1984) who conclude that 'solutions containing 9 mmol sodium per 100 ml are safe and effective in the management of overt dehydration (5% or
greater) in well-nourished bottle-fed children in industrial countries irrespective of the serum sodium
concentration at presentation. In fact, in the presence
of hypernatraemic dehydration, ORT with such a solution may be safer than intravenous rehydration'.
However, 'water should be administered in addition
to the WHO-ORS (containing 9 mmol sodium per
100 ml) in a ratio of WHO-ORS 2:water 1, except

Table 1.2 Oral rehydration solutions: composition per 100 ml reconstituted.

	WHO	Dextrolyte (Cow & Gate)	Dioralyte (Armour)	Electrolyte Mixture QEH formula	Lytren (Mead Johnson, USA)	Oral Rehydration Solution (Wyeth, USA)	Pedialyte (Ross USA)	Rehidrat (Searle)
Sodium mmol/100 ml	9	3·5	3·5	2·4	3·0	3·0	3·0	5·0
Potassium mmol/100 ml	2	1·3	2·0	2·8	2·5	2·0	2·0	2·0
Bicarbonate mmol/100 ml	3		1·8					2·0
Lactate mmol/100 ml		1·8						
Citrate mmol/100 ml				1·0	3·6	2·3	2·8	0·9
Phosphate mmol/100 ml				0·5	0·5	0·5		
Chloride mmol/100 ml	8	3·1	3·7	1·6	2·5	3·0	3·0	5·0
Calcium mEq/100 ml					0·4	0·4	0·4	
Magnesium mEq/100 ml					0·4	0·4	0·4	
Sulphate mEq/100 ml					0·4			
Carbohydrate total (g)	2	3·6	4	As added	8·1	7·5	5·0	4·9
glucose (g)	2	3·6	4		7·2	7·5	5·0	1·6
sucrose (g)								3·2
glucose polymer (g)					0·9			
fructose (g)								0·03
Osmolality mmol/l	N/S	297	310	N/S	N/S	N/S	N/S	336

Footnote

1 g glucose per 100 ml is approximately equivalent to 56 mmol/l.
2 g glucose per 100 ml is approximately equivalent to 111 mmol/l.
3 g glucose per 100 ml is approximately equivalent to 167 mmol/l.
N/S Not specified.

perhaps in those patients who are severely hyponatraemic'. It is also imperative to differentiate between the use of ORS to rehydrate overt dehydration in children (5 to 10% acute loss of body weight) and the use of ORS in the maintenance phase after rehydration or in the prevention of dehydration early in the course of diarrhoea. In the latter instances an equal quantity of water should be administered along with WHO-ORS. Alternatively, and ideally, a second solution containing 4 to 5 mmol sodium/100 ml should be available for maintenance and prevention of dehydration (Booth *et al.* 1984).

Oral rehydration solutions should contain both sodium and carbohydrate to enhance water absorption, together with potassium to replace stool losses, and bicarbonate, acetate, lactate or citrate to correct electrolyte and acid–base balance. Overconcentrated carbohydrate and hyperosmolar solutions should not be used as they are poorly absorbed and can lead to hypernatraemia and further dehydration. Glucose is the carbohydrate chosen historically and by WHO. Sucrose is an effective alternative (Rahilly *et al.* 1976). Sucrose, due to its lower osmolality, easy and cheap availability and palatability, may be preferable to glucose (Tripp & Harries 1980). Starch, particularly rice powder, has been used (Patra *et al.* 1982), and has the advantage of providing a small amount (7 to 10%) of protein, which is a source of nitrogen for the malnourished child and, due to its constituent amino acids, notably glycine, enhances sodium and water absorption (Nalin *et al.* 1970). Where available on a local basis it has practical advantages over glucose and is equally effective for oral rehydration therapy.

In the treatment of moderate and moderately severe dehydration in developing countries WHO-ORS is currently administered to infants in a volume of 100 ml/kg body weight over four hours followed by 50 ml/kg of water (or breast milk *ad lib.*) over the next two hours (WHO 1976). After the six-hour course of therapy, the infant should be re-examined (clinically and by weight gain). If complete rehydration has been achieved the infant enters the maintenance phase of therapy. If dehydration is now mild (about 5%), WHO-ORS is continued for six more hours with half the volume ORS being offered (50 ml/kg), as for the moderately dehydrated state. This regimen is successful in 50% of children in six hours, in 65% by 12 hours and in 95% by 18–24 hours. Following rehydration, WHO-ORS is given in maintenance amounts of 100 ml/kg over 24 hours. In addition, oral nutrition should be recommenced in the form of breast-feeding *ad lib.* or a half-strength milk formula (120 ml/kg per day), both of which provide free water with which to handle the sodium load given during the maintenance period of rehydration. Plain water or an alternative low-solute fluid should also be offered during this phase, to provide more free water if necessary. The child is regraded back onto a normal diet as soon as dehydration is corrected and vomiting has stopped. In the malnourished child this should be supplemented with locally available high energy density foods (Booth *et al.* 1984).

In areas of the world where the provision of pre-packed sugar and electrolyte mixtures is not available the adoption of a home-made simple sugar and salt solution is recommended. Safe concentrations of sugar and salt can be obtained by the use of double-ended plastic spoons or a 5-ml teaspoon and 1-litre bottle (Hendrath 1978). Rates of rehydration and correction of acidosis with such a solution compared to WHO-ORS are satisfactory (Clements *et al.* 1981), but vomiting and hypokalaemia were a greater problem with the simple sugar and salt solution. A locally available source of potassium, such as bananas, is now recommended with such regimens. In the U.K. it should be unnecessary to use a home-made solution.

Commercially available ORS in U.K. have a lower sodium content than the WHO-ORS (Table 1.2). These therefore do not require the addition of water recommended when using the WHO-ORS. The ORS are largely under-utilized by primary health care teams in the U.K. (Morrison & Little 1981), and clearly much remains to be done to deliver ORS to children with diarrhoea. An adequate volume of ORS should be given initially every 1 to 2 hours to prevent or correct dehydration. Fluid intake should keep pace with faecal fluid losses and be at least 20% higher than normal recommended intakes. Table 1.3 gives fluid intake suggestions for different groups. ORS contribute insignificant dietary nutrients apart from electrolytes and fluid, and should not be used alone for long periods. Breast-feeding should usually continue during rehydration, whereas bottle-fed infants may need up to 24 hours during which ORS alone is given and milk formula omitted temporarily.

Table 1.3 Theoretical fluid intake suggested for different age groups (adapted from Walker-Smith 1979).

Age	Volume/kg per day
0–6 months	150 to 200 ml
6–9 months	120 to 150 ml
12 months	90 to 100 ml
2 years	80 to 90 ml
4 years	70 to 80 ml
8 years	60 to 70 ml
12 years	50 to 60 ml

Additional fluid will be needed to meet faecal fluid losses in gastroenteritis.

There is no good scientific basis for regrading compared to return to full-strength feeds immediately after rehydration (Booth *et al.* 1984), but it has a lower relapse rate in the author's experience, though this is a matter of opinion.

Traditionally after rehydration and vomiting has been resolved regrading is made in increments over 2 to 4 days as follows:

$\frac{1}{4}$ milk formula + $\frac{3}{4}$ oral rehydration solution
$\frac{1}{2}$ milk formula + $\frac{1}{2}$ oral rehydration solution
$\frac{3}{4}$ milk formula + $\frac{1}{4}$ oral rehydration solution
then full-strength milk formula

Once the infant is on full-strength feeds, appropriate solids for age should be reintroduced. Loose stools may persist for several days after gastroenteritis, and weight gain may be poor for a week or two. A maintenance intake of ORS in addition to feeds may be appropriate during this period to prevent dehydration recurring. Some nutrients are always absorbed and are important to normal bowel function; prolonged periods without food are inappropriate. This is particularly important in malnourished children, in whom adequate energy and nutrition is vital to prevent the vicious cycle of diarrhoea, malnutrition leading to further infection, PEM and death. Rapid reintroduction of full-strength feeds after diarrhoea has stopped results in less weight loss and is not associated with longer periods of hospitalization with mild diarrhoea (Dugdale *et al.* 1982), but further evaluation of this practice is needed in patients who have been more severely dehydrated.

In the majority of infants, regrading onto a cow's milk-based modified infant formula is tolerated well, and only a small number require a therapeutic milk protein-free and/or lactose-free regimen.

Delayed recovery following acute diarrhoea is more prevalent in those in the youngest age group (under three months), and those whose weight, corrected for dehydration, is below the third percentile (Gribbins *et al.* 1973). Significant diarrhoea and failure to gain weight following acute diarrhoea requires further investigation. An underlying primary cause such as coeliac disease or cystic fibrosis must be excluded. Delayed recovery may be due to either carbohydrate intolerance (usually lactose) and/or milk protein intolerance (Kilby *et al.* 1976) or similar enteropathy due to other proteins such as soya (Ament & Rubin 1972), fish, chicken or rice (Vitoria *et al.* 1982).

The post-enteritis enteropathy with mucosal abnormality (demonstrated by jejunal biopsy findings) occurs in only some children, mostly those under two years old with prolonged diarrhoea and those with the most severe illness. In those in whom it occurs milk protein and other relevant proteins such as soya and/or gluten should be excluded for a temporary period of about 3 to 6 months, before reintroduction of a normal diet ultimately. Human milk or a hydrolysed protein formula, such as Pregestimil or Pepdite 0–2 in infants and Nutramigen or a Pepdite formula for those over three months, is appropriate to replace milk and soya formulae. The prophylactic use of an appropriate formula may prevent post-enteritis enteropathy. Manuel *et al.* (1980) and Manuel and Walker-Smith (1981) have compared three infant formulae for the prevention of delayed recovery after infantile gastroenteritis and found advantages in using Pregestimil. The length of time such a formula would need to be used and the cost of such recommendations must be considered. A less sensitizing highly heated cow's milk formula (McLaughlin *et al.* 1981), such as the evaporated formula if available, is a cheaper, practical alternative. Further controlled trials are needed to evaluate the benefit of such regimens.

ANTIDIARRHOEAL AGENTS

Numerous clinical studies have shown that in general children with diarrhoea can be managed with ORS without antibiotics, except in cholera and dysentery. Sugar–electrolyte solutions, while highly effective in combating dehydration and its consequences, do not diminish the rate or volume of diarrhoeal stools: stool volume may in fact be increased with such therapy, though the net balance is greatly on the side of absorption (Editorial 1983). A pharmaceutical agent that would rapidly and effectively control the diarrhoea has been sought. Many drugs have been reported to have antisecretory properties, but few have been tested by controlled trials in man. As yet it is not possible to recommend the use of any such agents as an adjunct to ORT in the routine management of acute diarrhoea in children. In the U.K., however, the inappropriate prescription of drugs for the symptomatic relief of diarrhoea in children is widespread (Morrison & Little 1981, Catford 1980). Several reports suggest that oral rehydration can be modified to enhance intestinal absorption, so decreasing faecal losses. Glucose and glycine both enhance water and electrolyte absorption. Thus ORS containing both glucose and glycine are superior to standard ORS (Editorial 1983). Phenylalanine acts similarly to glycine. As already mentioned, rice powder provides both carbohydrates and amino acids, which also enhance water and electrolyte absorption. In the future it should be possible to produce 'super OR solutions' that enhance intestinal absorption so potently that they almost turn off diarrhoeal stool losses of body water and electrolytes (Editorial 1983).

CARBOHYDRATE INTOLERANCE

Carbohydrates are an important constituent of diets throughout the world, and after intestinal hydrolysis and absorption (*see* Table 1.1) provide a critical source of metabolic energy. The major carbohydrates ingested by man are starch, lactose and sucrose. Defects in hydrolysis and absorption result in retention of residues within the intestinal tract, and gastrointestinal symptoms result, i.e. carbohydrate 'intolerance'. This is a common clinical problem and may have serious consequences, particularly when it occurs in young children (Harries 1982a).

Only minute quantities of oligosaccharides are absorbed intact. Prior to absorption of the monosaccharides across the brush border membrane of the enterocyte, the disaccharides formed by the action of pancreatic and salivary amylase on starch, maltose, maltotriose, and α-limit dextrin, plus sucrose and lactose, have to be hydrolysed by the relevant disaccharidases to form glucose, galactose and fructose. The enzymes lactase, maltase and sucrase–isomaltase catalyse this hydrolysis, which is an extremely rapid and efficient process. These enzymes are largely glycoproteins, which work at an optimum pH of approximately 6, with their active sites oriented towards the intestinal lumen. Peak oligosaccharidase activities are found in the proximal jejunum and are much lower in the duodenum and distal ileum. Three distinct lactases (β-galactosidases) have been identified, but only the brush border enzyme is physiologically important. As much as 75% of mucosal maltase activity can be accounted for by sucrase. Sucrase–isomaltase is a hybrid molecule made up of two non-identical sub-units joined by one or more disulphide bonds. Sucrase and isomaltase may act in concert in the hydrolysis of α-limit dextrin to glucose, sucrase by hydrolysing the α-1–4 bonds and isomaltase cleaving the α-1–6 links of the molecule. It has been postulated that the oligosaccharidases are situated immediately adjacent to the brush border membrane monosaccharide carriers (Harries 1982a).

Glucose and galactose share the same sodium-coupled, energy-dependent transport system which is electrogenic.

Fructose absorption is carrier-mediated, but that transport is independent of sodium and energy (Harries 1982a).

Primary disorders of carbohydrate absorption

Familial disorders of carbohydrate absorption are well-recognized; all are rare with the exception of the non-Caucasian variety of lactase deficiency. These are:

1 Familial lactose intolerance.
2 Lactase deficiency
   (a) Congenital lactase deficiency,
   (b) Acquired lactase deficiency (adult-type hypolactasia).
3 Sucrase–isomaltase deficiency.
4 Trehalase deficiency.
5 Congenital glucose–galactose malabsorption.

1   Familial lactose intolerance

This condition is characterized by vomiting, severe failure to thrive, disacchariduria and aminoaciduria from early infancy. It was first clearly described by Durand (1958). Mental retardation and hiatus hernia (Moncrieff & Wilkinson 1954) and hepatic dysfunction (Hoskova *et al.* 1980) occur in some patients. Small intestinal lactase activity is normal. However, symptoms disappear on exclusion of lactose from the diet, suggesting that the primary problem is increased absorption of lactose. It is a transient disorder and children recover their tolerance to lactose between 12 and 18 months of age (Harries 1982a). Although familial it is not known whether the condition is genetically determined.

2   Lactase deficiency

(a) Congenital type.   This condition, first described by Holzel *et al.* (1959), presents with profuse watery diarrhoea soon after the introduction of milk feeds. Unless an early diagnosis is made and lactose excluded the condition is fatal. Lactase activity is absent or deficient (Levin *et al.* 1970). It is inherited probably as an autosomal recessive trait.

(b) Acquired lactase deficiency (adult-type hypolactasia).   Most human adults have hypolactasia, as lactase activity reaches a peak in the perinatal period, declining during weaning to the low levels found in the adult, which are only 10% of the maximal level. In non-Caucasian races the prevalence of hypolactasia is extremely high (50 to 90%), whereas in Caucasians the prevalence is only 2 to 30% (Gray 1975). The ability to digest lactose in some adults is unusual, and acquired lactose intolerance is common, but gastrointestinal symptoms are relatively mild and appear usually between the ages of one and five years, but sometimes later (McNeish & Harran 1980). Frequently it is asymptomatic and many tolerate up to 250 ml milk/day quite happily (Habte *et al.* 1973, Walker-Smith 1979). A genetic basis is now generally accepted for the difference in adult lactase levels, high levels being inherited as an autosomal dominant, and reduced levels as an autosomal recessive, trait (Johnson *et al.* 1977), and there is convincing evidence that human lactase activity is independent of lactose intake.

3   Sucrase–isomaltase deficiency

This congenital condition, inherited in an autosomal recessive fashion, was first described by Weijers *et al.* (1961), and although believed to be rare it may occur in as many as 0·2% of North Americans and 10% of Greenland Eskimos. There is a wide spectrum of symptoms, from severe diarrhoea in infancy to intermittent bothersome symptoms in the older child (Antonowicz *et al.* 1972, Ament & Perera 1973). The diagnosis may be missed or attributed to 'irritable colon' or 'maternal anxiety'. A definite diagnosis requires the demonstration of deficiency of sucrase–isomaltase activity, and maltase activity is also reduced. Removal of sucrose from the diet results in symptomatic improvement and clinical tolerance improves with age.

4 Trehalase deficiency
This condition has only been documented once, by Madzarovova-Nohejlova (1973). Trehalose is a non-reducing disaccharide in lower plants such as young mushrooms.

5 Congenital glucose–galactose malabsorption
This condition is thought to be due to a brush border translocation defect resulting in glucose and galactose malabsorption. However, the precise defect has not yet been defined (Harries 1982a). First described by Lindquist *et al.* (1962) it causes severe gastrointestinal symptoms following the ingestion of carbohydrate-containing feeds (dextrose or milk) in the neonatal period, and unless glucose and galactose are withdrawn from the diet the condition can be fatal. Fructose is absorbed normally and when it replaces all other dietary carbohydrates the diarrhoea resolves automatically. Renal tubular reabsorption of glucose may also be affected, with resultant glucosuria. Hydrolysis of disaccharides is normal, as the disaccharidases are present. Although the glucose transport defect persists (Ament *et al.* 1973), clinical tolerance of the offending carbohydrates improves with age, making some dietary relaxation possible in the older child.

Secondary carbohydrate intolerance

The secondary carbohydrate intolerances (primarily lactose) can occur as a complication of other conditions, such as gastroenteritis, protein enteropathies, PEM and surgery on the intestine, which affect the intestinal mucosa and suppress the disaccharidase activity. The resultant unabsorbed sugars cause gastrointestinal symptoms. Treatment of the primary condition is of paramount importance. Temporary omission of the offending sugar(s) is advised when clinical symptoms related to their inclusion occur.

Lactose intolerance is by far the commonest (Clayton *et al.* 1966, Harries & Francis 1968, Anderson 1970, Desjeux *et al.* 1973, Harrison 1974, Walker-Smith 1979, Hansen *et al.* 1982) of the secondary intolerances.

Sucrase–isomaltase deficiency as a secondary phenomenon rarely causes clinical intolerance warranting dietary exclusion of sucrose for more than perhaps a few days.

A secondary temporary glucose–galactose intolerance occurs usually as a complication of severe gastroenteritis, but is much rarer than disaccharide intolerance (Burke & Anderson 1966, Walker-Smith 1979). In glucose–galactose intolerance, fructose is tolerated.

A temporary and complete monosaccharide intolerance can occur, affecting absorption of all monosaccharides, including glucose, galactose and fructose (Burke & Anderson 1966, Harries & Francis 1968), and requires withdrawal of all oral carbohydrate. The risk of hypoglycaemia when all oral carbohydrate is removed from the diet is greatly increased, even when intravenous carbohydrate is given (Lifshitz *et al.* 1970), and this affects the ultimate prognosis of this condition. In infants with secondary monosaccharide intolerance of glucose, fructose and galactose, the resultant hypoglycaemia which frequently occurs appears to be multifactorial, including glycogen reserves being depleted, poor gluconeogenesis, and the stimulatory effect of protein on insulin production. Prevention is by continuous adequate intravenous carbohydrate, avoidance of hypothermia, and a frequent feeding schedule, as most of these infants cannot withstand even a four-hour fast. Blood sugar monitoring is essential as hypoglycaemia can go undetected, although hypothermia is an 'occult' sign and should alert those responsible to the imminent danger of hypoglycaemia.

Complete monosaccharide intolerance appears to be temporary, particularly accompanying kwashiorkor, PEM or the acute stage of gastroenteritis, or following intestinal surgery. Carbohydrate-free diets have been used as early as 1937 by von Chwalibogowski and more recently as reported by Harries and Francis (1968), but these are not without hazard, as described above; a temporary oral regimen based on the module Comminuted Chicken regimen can be devised (*see* p. 34). The use of parenteral nutrition (Booth & Harries 1982b) can be life-saving in these patients.

Symptoms and diagnosis
The infant or young child with carbohydrate intolerance presents with severe watery diarrhoea with a low pH due to the osmotic effect of the unabsorbed carbohydrate(s). The acidity of the stools is due to bacterial action on the undigested carbohydrate(s)

which produce volatile short-chain organic acids such as acetic, butyric, propionic, and lactic acid, together with carbon dioxide and hydrogen. Severe dehydration, abdominal pain and distension, perianal excoriation, vomiting and electrolyte imbalance may occur. Poor growth and failure to thrive may result, due to the accompanying malabsorption, unless corrected by the appropriate diet.

A *fresh* specimen of stool contains excess amounts of sugars, which can be confirmed by stool chromatography. The bedside Clinitest stool test to identify the presence of sugars was described by Kerry and Anderson (1964). It is important to test the fluid part of a fresh specimen of stool. Sucrose is not a reducing substance and will give a false-negative test unless the specimen is first hydrolysed with acid. Drugs and the sugar in medicine can give a false-positive test. Lactulose, formed during the manufacture of liquid milk formulae ('ready-to-feed', and evaporated milks), can also cause diarrhoea (Walker-Smith 1979). A knowledge of the dietary carbohydrate intake is essential to interpret the results. Normal neonates may have up to 0·75% reducing substances in stools (Walker-Smith 1976) which disappear rapidly in the full-term neonate, but may continue for some time in the pre-term infant. Dietary manipulation is only required when clinical intolerance is causing symptoms.

Sugar chromatography will identify specific sugars in stool (or urine) (Menzies & Seakins 1976). Oral loading tests may prove dangerous in the acutely ill child, but are useful in the older child. Two gram per kilogram of the carbohydrate concerned is given to the fasting child, and blood sugars and stools analysed. A rise of less than 30 mg/100 ml blood is suggestive of carbohydrate malabsorption.

The hydrogen breath test has proved somewhat disappointing in diagnosing childhood carbohydrate intolerance (Gardiner *et al.* 1981a, b). Mucosal enzymes can be measured in a jejunal biopsy specimen, but are not helpful in assessing the clinical importance of carbohydrate intolerance in secondary malabsorption. Absence, or low levels, of mucosal enzymes is diagnostic of congenital deficiency when histology is normal. The congenital glucose–galactose transport defect requires *in vitro* jejunal mucosal studies and confirmation of normal gut histology and disaccharidases to confirm the diagnosis.

Sometimes an exact diagnosis can be made immediately, and the correct dietary treatment prescribed. Frequently clinical response to dietary elimination and retrospective diagnosis may be all that is possible.

Treatment of carbohydrate intolerance

Treatment of carbohydrate intolerance is by removal of the offending sugar(s). In the primary sugar intolerances, the diet must be continued, although symptoms are less severe after infancy and some relaxation of the diet is usually possible. The length of time for which dietary treatment is required in the secondary conditions depends on clinical response and on the primary underlying condition, and recovery usually correlates with the recovery of the small intestinal mucosa. Intolerance can be very transient, as seen in PEM and kwashiorkor (Hanson *et al.* 1982), and in most patients with secondary intolerance reintroduction can be attempted within two to three months for lactose, and sooner for glucose (and starch), and even within days for sucrose if exclusion is required at all. Symptomatic relapse after reintroduction of a specific carbohydrate on several occasions, e.g. sucrose (and starch), or lactose, or glucose and galactose, in a clinically well child suggests the possibility of a primary carbohydrate intolerance, which should be appropriately investigated by jejunal biopsy studies.

Enzyme replacement therapy for primary sugar intolerance in conjunction with a modified diet has been used. Lactase, e.g. Kerulac, Maxilact (Gist-Brocades), or β-galactosidase (BDH Pharmaceuticals Ltd) has been used to split the lactose of milk to galactose and glucose for patients with lactose intolerance (Clayton *et al.* 1966). However, it is difficult to remove adequate lactose by this method to provide a satisfactory 'milk' for treating the acutely ill patient, but it may be satisfactory for the older patients with hypolactasia or acquired lactase deficiency in whom additional 'milk' would be beneficial.

Various diets for the different carbohydrate intolerances have been devised, and details are given under each carbohydrate. The more common carbohydrates present in foods, from which information the diets have been devised, are given by Cornblath and Schwartz (1976) and Southgate *et al.* (1978).

LACTOSE

Lactose is the carbohydrate of all the mammalian milks (human, cow, goat, ewe) commonly ingested by man. These milks are contraindicated in patients with lactose intolerance, which appears to be the most widespread sugar intolerance (Walker-Smith 1979).

Milk is a major source of nutrients, at least in the diet of infants and young children. Five-hundred ml of cow's milk supplies a two-year-old with 100% calcium, 50% protein, 24% energy and 100% riboflavin compared to the recommended daily intakes. A nutritional replacement of milk is essential for infants and pre-school age children to ensure adequate intake of all the nutrients necessary for normal growth and development.

For infants under six months the lactose-free substitute chosen should meet the nutritional guidelines of *Artificial Feeds for the Young Infant* (DHSS 1980), have a low osmolality, and be clinically suitable for the individual, e.g. Pregestimil, Pepdite 0–2 and MCT Pepdite 0–2 are suitable hydrolysed protein-based formulae, or the soya formulae, Prosobee, Soya S formula and Wysoy, are suitable for infants. Nutramigen is suitable for those over 3 to 4 months and Pepdite 2 + or MCT Pepdite 2 + is suitable for patients over two years old (Table 1.4).

A further group of lactose-free milk substitutes containing casein is given in Table 1.5. These are suitable for patients over six months old who tolerate casein. Currently some need major modification and/or supplementation if used as the sole source of nutrition in the young child. Some contain medium-chain triglycerides (MCT) as an energy replacement of part or all of the fat content. A more complex module diet, based on Comminuted Chicken, can be devised to meet the nutritional needs of the patient. Details of how to devise such a diet are given later on p. 34 and in Table 1.18. The composition of the various supplements and ingredients used in module diets are given in Table 1.6. For older children a lactose-free calcium supplement alone may suffice (400 mg elemental calcium/day), provided adequate protein, energy, vitamins and minerals are taken from a variety of conventional foods, and/or a social replacement of milk (Table 1.7) may be all that is required.

Some of the milk substitutes are unpalatable, especially for older children, and are therefore difficult to incorporate into recipes, custards, or for use on cereals in the diet. Flavouring, e.g. milk-shake syrups and chocolate essences, cocoa or coffee powder, selected appropriately for the required dietary regime, are useful but may increase the osmolality of the product considerably, which may precipitate diarrhoea in some patients. Children will take the milk substitutes more readily if given in a baby bottle, teacher beaker or from a straw, which overcome the problem of the unusual smell. Others are better served either chilled or hot.

The MCT-containing lactose-free 'milk' substitutes may need to be introduced slowly, because of the osmotic effect of MCT, e.g. use a $\frac{1}{4}$ strength, $\frac{1}{2}$ strength, $\frac{3}{4}$ strength then full-strength formula, over 2 to 4 days.

Some of the low-lactose milk substitutes do not have added vitamins or trace minerals. At least the normal requirement of all known vitamins and at least the major trace minerals should be given. These can be given medicinally and the vitamins should not normally be incorporated into the feed, where they can be rejected if all the feed is not consumed or deteriorate on standing or during terminal pasteurization. A comprehensive vitamin and mineral supplement can be given as the Cow & Gate Supplementary Vitamin Tablets (6 to 12 daily according to age) plus a source of vitamins A and D equivalent to 10 μg/day (400 i.u.). Although the Cow & Gate vitamin and mineral supplement tables contain traces of sucrose (70 mg/tablet), this is usually unimportant clinically. A complete range of carbohydrate-free vitamins can be given as Ketovite Tablets (1 × t.d.s.) plus 5 ml Ketovite Liquid daily. Since the latter do not contain trace minerals or iron, medicinal zinc and iron should be prescribed, or a comprehensive trace mineral mixture given, unless other dietary sources provide adequate intake. The recommended supplement required for use with each product is listed in Tables 1.4 and 1.5 and a review is given by Francis (1986).

Infants and children with profuse diarrhoea lose a large quantity of electrolytes and fluid in the stools. Care should be taken to ensure that electrolyte and fluid intake is adequate to cover losses. Dietary sodium intake can be calculated, and serum electrolytes monitored. Either a maintenance intake of oral rehydration solution (Table 1.2) or prescribed supplements of normal saline (15·4 mmol sodium/100 ml) and potassium chloride can be used, with appropriate caution and supervision, to replace part of the water used to reconstitute the feed. Such feeds should be monitored for osmolality and rejected if over 500 mmol/l. The renal solute load can also be calculated from the feed: mmol/100 mol of sodium + potassium + chloride + (protein [g] × 4) = mmol/100 ml solute. A renal solute in excess of 15 mmol/100 ml should be used with caution or avoided in young children to prevent overload on the kidneys.

Minimal lactose diet
Treatment of the ill child or infant, after initial rehydration, is with a suitable lactose-free, and unless a firm diagnosis has been made a milk protein-free, 'milk' substitute (Table 1.4).

Table 1.4 Milk substitutes: milk protein- and lactose-free. Suitable for infants and young children (manufacturers' data 1984).

Product	Company and recommended dilution	100 ml normal reconstituted value				
		Protein (g)	Carbohydrate (g)	Fat (g)	kcal	kJ
Human milk mature*		1·3	7·2	4·1	69	289
(a) Hydrolysed protein formulae						
Pregestimil	Mead Johnson ≃ 15% solution	Enzyme hydrolysed casein (charcoal-treated) +L-tyrosine +L-cystine +L-tryptophan	Corn syrup solids and tapioca starch	Corn oil, MCT, soy, lecithin		
		1·9	9·1	2·7	67	287
Pepdite 0–2	SHS 15% solution	Hydrolysed meat and soya. Peptides and amino acids	Maltodextrin corn origin	Vegetable and animal fats		
		2·1	8·4	3·5	70	300
MCT Pedite 0–2	SHS 15% solution	Hydrolysed meat and soya. Peptides and amino acids	Maltodextrin corn origin	Vegetable oils and MCT		
		2·1	9·4	2·8	67	280
Pepdite 2 +	SHS 20% solution	Hydrolysed meat and soya. Peptides and amino acids	Maltodextrin corn oil	Vegetable oils		
		2·8	12·6	3·6	90	376
MCT Pepdite 2 +	SHS 20% solution	Hydrolysed meat and soya. Peptides and amino acids	Maltodextrin corn oil	Vegetable oils and MCT		
		2·8	12·5	3·8	92	386
Alfaré Semi-Elemental formula	Nestlé 15% solution	Hydrolysed whey protein	Glucose polymer, starch, trace lactose	MCT, milk fat and corn oil		
		2·5	7·8	3·6	72	301
Nutramigen (not recommended for infants under 3 months)	Mead Johnson 15% solution	Hydrolysed casein	Sucrose and tapioca starch	Corn oil		
		2·3	8·9	2·7	69	290
(b) Modified soya milks						
Formula S Soya (1986 revision)	Cow & Gate 12·7% solution	Soy isolate and L-methionine	Glucose syrup	Vegetable oils		
		1·8	6·7	3·6	67	280
Prosobee (also available as liquid concentrate)	Mead Johnson 13% solution	Soy isolate and L-methionine	Corn syrup solids	Coconut and corn oil		
		2·0	6·7	3·6	67	281
Wysoy (also available as Ready to Feed)	Wyeth Labs. 13·5% solution	Soy isolate and L-methionine	Sucrose and corn syrup solids	Oleic (beef fat), corn and coconut oils		
		2·1	6·9	3·6	67	280

*Paul and Southgate (1978).

Notes:

(a) All contain a range of vitamins. Some enteral and elemental diet formulae are also lactose and/or milk protein-free (*see* Table 2.9 and Francis 1986).

(b) Renal solute load is the sum of (protein[g] × 4) + mmol Na$^+$ + mmol K$^+$ + mmol Cl$^-$ per 100 ml.

(c) Zinc phytate molar ratio 1 : 9.

Osmolality (mmol/kg)	Renal solute (mmol/100 ml)	100 ml reconstituted value								
		Na+ (mmol)	K+ (mmol)	Ca²+ (mmol)	P− (mmol)	Mg+ (mmol)	Fe+ (μmol)	Cu+ (μmol)	Zn+ (μmol)	·Cl− (mmol)
264 to 300	8·5	0·6	1·5	0·9	0·1	0·2	1·3	0·6	4·3	1·2
338	12·5	1·4	1·9	1·6	1·4	0·3	23	0·9	6·0	1·6
195	12·3	1·3	1·5	1·1	1·1	0·2	14·3	0·9	9·2	1·1
337	13·0	2·0	1·5	1·1	1·1	0·2	14·3	0·9	9·2	1·1
288	16·6	1·8	2·6	1·0	1·4	0·6	17·2	1·5	14·7	1·0
360	17·5	2·7	2·6	1·0	1·4	0·6	17·2	1·5	14·7	1·0
220	16·3	1·9	2·3	1·5	1·2	0·4	16·1	0·6	8·3	2·1
443	13·8	1·4	1·8	1·6	1·6	0·3	23	1·0	6·6	1·4
218	12·8	1·3	1·6	1·4	1·3	0·2	11·0	0·6	5·7 (c)	1·1
160	11·7	1·1	1·5	1·5	1·3	0·3	21·5	0·9	7·6 (c)	1·1
242	12·2	0·9	1·9	1·6	1·4	0·3	12·1	0·8	5·7 (c)	1·0

Table 1.5 Lactose-free milk substitutes: contain casein and/or milk protein.

| Product | Company and recommended dilution | 100 ml normal reconstituted value | | | | | | Supplements and precautions required when used as the sole source of nutrients or for young children |
		Protein (g)	Carbohydrate (g)	Fat (g)	kcal	kJ	Osmolality (mmol/kg)	
MCT 1 milk formula (to be reformulated 1986 as a complete formula. MCT 2)	Cow & Gate 12½% solution 1 scoop to 1 oz water	Partially washed casein 3·2	Liquid glucose 5·1	MCT oil of C8 and C10 fatty acids. Contains no essential fatty acids. 3·5	63	265	146/1	The present formula is *not a modified formula*. Very low in cystine. *Contains no essential fatty acids*. Very low in zinc and trace minerals. Trace mineral and complete vitamin supplements are essential. *Rarely used, except in minimal fat diets.*
Portagen	Mead Johnson 15·2% solution 1 scoop to 2 oz water	Sodium caseinate 2·5	Corn syrup and sucrose 8·2	MCT and corn oil 3·4	70	296	236	Not a modified formula. Has added vitamins and minerals. Contains essential fatty acids. Can be adapted for an adult enteral feed by using a 20% solution.

	Manufacturer	Preparation	Protein source		Carbohydrate source		Fat source					Comments
Triosorbon	Merck	1 sachet plus 400 ml water	Whey, casein and L-cystine	4·0	Mono-, oligo- and polysaccharide. Maltodextrin.	11·9	MCT and sunflower oil	4·0	106	446	238	Not a modified formula. Does contain added cystine, vitamins and minerals and essential fatty acids.
Galactomin No. 17 (to be reformulated in 1986 as a complete formula)	Cow & Gate	12½% solution. Approximately 1 scoop to 1 oz water	Partially demineralized (washed) casein	2·8	Liquid glucose	6·3	Coconut and maize oil	2·8	60	250	178/1	*The present formula is not a modified formula and is not ideal for infants under six months.* It is high in protein, low in cystine. Sodium intake is quite low and may need to be supplemented. *Rarely used.* Low in zinc, iron and trace minerals. Trace mineral and complete vitamins supplements essential.
Galactomin Fructose Formula 19 (to be reformulated 1987)	Cow & Gate 12½% solution			2·8		7·3		1·8	55	228	N/S	As Galactomin 17 present formula

Table 1.6 Products used in module feeds*

	Product	Company	Composition per 100 g
I	*Proteins and peptides*		
	Maxipro HBV	Scientific Hospital Supplies Ltd	Not a complete feed: carbohydrate-free. 88 g whey protein 4 g fat 10 mmol sodium 11·5 mmol potassium 7·5 mmol calcium 12·5 mmol phosphorus Trace lactose only
	Casilan	Farley Glaxo	Washed casein. Not a complete feed: carbohydrate-free. 90 g protein 1·8 g fat ≤ 4 mmol sodium 30 mmol calcium Trace lactose only
	Comminuted Chicken	Cow & Gate	Finely puréed chicken meat in water. Not a complete feed: carbohydrate-free. 7 to 8 g protein 2·5 to 4 g fat 250 kJ 60 kcal
	Albumaid Hydrolysate Complete	Scientific Hospital Supplies Ltd	Beef serum hydrolysate with some minerals and vitamins. Carbohydrate- and fat-free. 89·4 g amino acids 43·5 mmol sodium 5·1 mmol potassium 7·5 mmol calcium 32·3 mmol phosphorus
II	*Glucose polymers*		
	Caloreen	Roussel Laboratories	96 g carbohydrate < 1·8 mmol sodium < 0·3 mmol potassium 1606 kJ 384 kcal
	Maxijul	Scientific Hospital Supplies Ltd	96 g carbohydrate 2 mmol sodium 0·1 mmol potassium 1670 kJ 400 kcal

Table 1.6 *continued*

Product	Company	Composition per 100 g
LE Maxijul (low-electrolyte)	Scientific Hospital Supplies Ltd	96 g carbohydrate 0·01 mmol sodium 0·01 mmol potassium 1670 kJ 400 kcal
Polycal	Cow & Gate	96 g carbohydrate 2·2 mmol sodium 1·3 mmol potassium 1610 kJ 380 kcal

III *Oils and emulsions*

Product	Company	Composition per 100 g
Prosparol (50% arachis oil emulsion)	Duncan Flockhart	50 g fat 26 g EFA/polyunsaturated fat 0·7 mmol sodium 1900 kJ 450 kcal
Calogen (50% arachis oil emulsion)	Scientific Hospital Supplies Ltd	50 g fat 11·5 g EFA/polyunsaturated fat 0·9 mmol sodium 0·5 mmol potassium 1880 kJ 450 kcal
Liquigen (52% medium-chain triglyceride emulsion)	Scientific Hospital Supplies Ltd	52 g fat (MCT) 1·7 mmol sodium 0·7 mmol potassium 1700 kJ 400 kcal
Safflower, sunflower, corn and soy oils		Various oils rich in essential fatty acids can be made into an emulsion with gum acacia. 100 ml ≃ 100 g fat; 3700 kJ; 900 kcal
MCT (medium-chain triglyceride) oils	Mead Johnson Cow & Gate Scientific Hospital Supplies Ltd Lovelock Alembicol D	Mainly C8 and C10 fatty acids (saturated). Source of energy in low-fat diets; free of EFA and cannot be metabolized to EFA. 100 ml ≃ 100 g fat; 3500 kJ; 830 kcal

*Not used as sole source of nutrition unless in conjunction with one another calculated to provide appropriate nutrition with vitamin and mineral supplements—*see* Chapter 3, Francis 1986.

An appropriate total volume per day (Table 1.3) (total volume of fluid may be elevated due to faecal losses) is introduced as clinically tolerated, as full-strength feeds, or by regrading over 2 to 4 days (*see* p. 6). A frequent feeding schedule may be required initially.

Nutritional supplement and solids are introduced appropriately for the child's age and clinical condition.

Nutritionally inadequate regimens for more than a few days should be avoided wherever possible, and if the clinical condition indicates long-term inadequacy is likely, e.g. in protracted diarrhoea or post-gastrointestinal surgery, parenteral nutrition should be instigated and oral nutrition can be introduced more slowly. The feed concentration and quantity can be increased as the child's clinical condition improves, and then the number of feeds per day reduced to normal for age and weight. The electrolyte intake

Table 1.7   Social replacements of milk.

(a) *Lactose-free*

Plamil	Plantmilk Ltd	Plant food very low in carbohydrate and calcium. Soya-based. Not a complete feed. A carbohydrate-free Plamil formula is also available.
Granogen	Granose	Soya food powder. Not a complete feed.
Soya Bean Milk	Itona	Soya food powder. Not a complete feed.
Soya Milk	Granose	Liquid soya milk. Not a complete feed.
Pareve-mate (kosher)	Carnation via Eliko Foods Ltd	Jewish Coffee-mate which is milk-free. Of no nutritional value but convenient for drinks and cereals.

(b *Milk protein-free, lactose-containing milks from other mammals; sometimes tolerated by patients who are intolerant to cow's milk*

	Protein (g)	Carbohydrate (g)	Fat (g)	kcal	kJ	
Goat's milk (100 ml)	3·3	4·6	4·5	71	296	Not recommended for infants under six months. It is recommended that goat's milk be pasteurized or boiled before use. Vitamins A, D, C and a source of folic acid and vitamin B_{12} are recommended, e.g. three Ketovite Tablets and 5 ml Ketovite Liquid when goat's milk provides a major proportion of nutrients in the diet. Some powdered goat's milk products are now available but reconstitute to whole goat's milk.
Ewe's (sheep) milk (100 ml)	5·3	4·9 lactose	6·3	100	420	Not recommended for infants under one-year old or young children as sole source of nutrition. It is recommended that ewe's milk is diluted and either pasteurized or boiled before use. Appropriate vitamin supplements, e.g. three Ketovite Tablets and 5 ml Ketovite Liquid, are recommended when ewe's milk provides a major proportion of nutrients in the diet.

should be re-assessed continually whilst diarrhoea continues. Gradually energy and nutrient intake is increased until the child starts to gain weight, and may need to be 50% or 100% higher than normal requirement for actual weight in malnourished patients during the catch-up growth period. The energy of the feed can be fortified by gradual increments to the feeds, e.g. of 1 to 3% glucose polymer and/or 2 to 5% fat emulsion, but overconcentration must be avoided, as increased osmolarity may cause osmotic diarrhoea. If the clinical condition deteriorates at any stage, recent changes in diet should be scrutinized, feed osmolality checked, stool and urinary sugars assessed, and other factors such as secondary infection considered, e.g. if sucrose has either recently been added in food, or given coincidentally in medicine, and the child's stools deteriorate, or contain sucrose, secondary sucrose intolerance should be considered. Medicines in tablet form frequently contain an inert filler of lactose. Antibiotics frequently precipitate diarrhoea irrespective of their carbohydrate content.

Frequently both milk protein and lactose have to be excluded, either because a differential diagnosis is not possible initially, or because milk protein intolerance is the primary cause of the lactose intolerance.

In this case the washed and whole casein-based milk substitutes (Table 1.5), e.g. Galactomin, MCT 1 and Portagen, are contraindicated. The hydrolysed casein products, e.g. Pregestimil, the Pepdite range, Nutramigen or soya 'milks', are the milk substitutes of choice (Table 1.4).

The minimal lactose diet must exclude all lactose and milk products: whey, casein, caseinate, milk hydrolysate. For example, infant cereals and weaning foods often contain milk solids, and lactose is frequently the filler in retail monosodium glutamate and some sugar substitutes, e.g. Sweet 'n' Low and Canderel powder, as well as in tablets. The diet should contain adequate amounts of meat, fish, egg, milk-free cereal and bread, a suitable 'milk-free' margarine, fruit and vegetables. Patients who are clinically well should have the appropriate diet for age, selected from Table 1.8.

Although there are minor differences between a minimum lactose and a milk protein-free diet, they are unimportant, at least in the first instance. Later, items such as butter and hard cheeses containing only traces of lactose can be introduced if tolerated. However, by this stage many patients with secondary lactose intolerance may have adequate lactase activity for reintroduction of a normal or near-normal diet.

Patients with hypolactasia and the non-Caucasian acquired type of lactose intolerance often require only omission of visible milk, the major source of lactose, for long-term treatment. During acute illness or gastroenteritis, a minimal lactose milk-free diet may be indicated, and in the event of the need for enteral feeding a lactose-free formula should be selected. Recent work suggests that many patients with this type of lactose intolerance may also have cow's milk protein intolerance, demonstrated by mucosal changes (Walker-Smith 1979).

SECONDARY DISACCHARIDE INTOLERANCE

Patients with secondary disaccharide intolerance may occasionally, though rarely, need a minimal lactose and sucrose diet (Table 1.9) with an appropriately selected milk substitute (Table 1.4 or 1.5). Milk protein may or may not also need to be avoided. By the time initial clinical improvement is observed, sucrose is usually tolerated. Naturally occurring sucrose-containing foods, e.g. unsweetened fruit and fruit juices, cereals and savoury foods, are the first items to be introduced. Later, foods containing added sugar are permitted if the above are tolerated. A formal sucrose load is not necessary unless initial introduction of these foods causes further diarrhoea, when primary sucrose–isomaltose intolerance should be considered. Lactose reintroduction may then be considered the appropriate next step.

SUCROSE

When sucrose intolerance occurs, a low-sucrose diet is required, and this is frequently all that is needed in the treatment of primary sucrase–isomaltase deficiency.

Sucrose is used extensively in the normal diet in the form of cane and beet sugar, in syrups, including those carrying medicines, and in sweets, chocolate, candy, biscuits, cakes, jams, and manufactured foods. Fruit and many vegetables contain natural sucrose and initially should be excluded from the diet. Sucrose can be replaced with glucose, glucose polymer or fructose. A suitable source of sucrose-free vitamin C, e.g. tomatoes or unsweetened tomato juice, should be included in the diet as given in Table 1.10. Infants can have one of a wide range of the modified milk formulae, provided there is no added sugar (sucrose). Children's vitamin A, D, C drops, at least in under-two-year-olds should be given as a source of vitamins. Selected home-prepared sucrose-free weaning foods can be introduced as suggested in the weaning minimal sucrose diet, but many commercial baby foods are unsuitable, including some of those entitled low-sugar rusks and cereals.

Following successful introduction of this diet many patients can tolerate naturally occurring unsweetened fruits and vegetables, at least in small quantities, which makes the diet much more practical. Even in patients with primary sucrase–isomaltase deficiency small quantities of sucrose may cause no ill-effect in the older patient, though large quantities of sucrose may still cause diarrhoea, Table 1.11 gives the sucrose content of common fruits.

STARCH

Some difficulty in digesting starch is found in cystic fibrosis and Shwachman's syndrome due to pancreatic amylase deficiency, but is treated with pancreatic enzyme replacement (*see* Chapter 6).

In sucrase–isomaltase deficiency, even though dietary sucrose needs to be eliminated or restricted, exclusion of starch is virtually never required because of the small percentage of α-1–6 linkages needing isomaltase for the digestion of the amylopectin in starch (Walker-Smith 1979).

Table 1.8 Minimal lactose and cow's milk protein-free diet.

(a) Allowed and forbidden foods.

Foods allowed	Foods forbidden
Milk substitute selected from Table 1.4, 1.5 or 1.7 as appropriate.	Milk, cream, cheese, yoghurt, butter, ordinary margarine, ice-cream. Casilan, Compliment, Coffee-mate, 'filled' milks, Fast Pints, Five Pints and similar products. Products containing casein, whey, milk solids, caseinate, etc. Lactose and milk sugar.
Eggs	

Meat
    Beef, lamb, pork, veal, ham, bacon
Offal
    Liver, kidney
Poultry
    Chicken, turkey
Fresh fish
	Sausages unless milk-free, Fish fingers and fish in batter unless milk-free. Tinned meat, ham, fish, etc. unless brand and ingredients are checked. Savoury foods containing milk or cheese. Meats cured in brine containing milk solids.

Milk-free margarine and low-fat spreads. Vegetable oils, pure fats, lard.	Outline spread and products with whey or milk solids.

Cereals
    Wheat, rye, barley, oats, rice, maize, flour (self-raising and plain), semolina, sago (cooked without milk or with milk substitute)
Macaroni, spaghetti, baking powder
Breakfast cereals
    Rice Krispies, Shreddies, bran, All Bran, Weetabix
Baby cereals
    e.g. Robinson's Baby Rice, Milupa Plain Rice Cereal, Farley's Original Rusk, Farex Weaning Food
	Milk puddings, e.g. custard, creamed rice. 'Non-milk fat' products. Instant custard mix. Egg noodles, macaroni cheese, tinned spaghetti with cheese, e.g. Spaghetti Hoops, Italian spaghetti. Instant Whip, Angel Delight. Baby cereals fortified with milk solids, Special K, Swiss-type cereals and muesli. Farley's Low Sugar Rusk, Liga Low Sugar Rusk.

Sugar, jam, honey, jelly, syrup Marmite, Bovril, Oxo, Bisto Salt and pepper, herbs, spices, essences	Monosodium glutamate retail powder with lactose filler. Sugar substitutes containing lactose, e.g. Sweet 'n' Low, Canderel sweetener. Hydrolysed milk sugar.
Bread e.g. Wholemeal, Hovis, plain white milk-free, Vit Be, granary breads Cakes and biscuits known to be free of milk	Milk breads, Procea Cakes and biscuits containing milk
Salad cream, mayonnaise (check ingredients)	
Tea, coffee, cocoa, drinking chocolate	Horlicks, Ovaltine, Bournvita, Milo
Boiled sweets, lollies, pastilles, gums, Terry's Bitter Chocolate	Fudge, toffee. All types of ice-cream (including non-milk fat types). Milk chocolate. Many dark and diabetic chocolates, e.g. Bournville Chocolate, Terry's Dark Chocolate. Opal Fruits, etc.
Fruits, all varieties	
Vegetables without butter or milk products. Potatoes. Plain crisps. Pulses.	Instant potato containing milk and/or butter. Mashed potato containing milk and/or butter. Potato salad. Flavoured crisps, e.g. salt and vinegar, etc. Vegetable salad.
Fruit juices and squash, fizzy pop, Coke, Pepsi, Lucozade.	
Tinned or processed foods known to be free of milk products, etc. Check every label before use.	Manufactured and processed food unless checked to be free of milk, cream, casein, caseinate, whey, milk solids, hydrolysed milk, butter, cheese, lactose, etc. Cream, tinned and packet soups. Tablets containing lactose.

Table 1.8 (a) *continued*

(b) Minimal lactose, cow's milk protein-free diet: sample menu.

Breakfast	Weetabix, cornflakes or porridge
	Sugar
	Milk substitute
	Bacon and tomato or egg
	Milk-free bread or toast
	Milk-free margarine or low-fat spread
	Marmalade, jam, honey, Marmite, Bovril
	Milk substitute flavoured with tea or coffee or cocoa
Mid-morning	Fruit juice or milk substitute
Lunch	Meat, chicken, fish, egg ⎫
	Potato—roast, boiled, chips ⎬ Cooked without milk or butter
	Vegetables ⎪
	Fruit, jelly ⎭
	Special custard made with milk substitute and suitable custard powder
	Suitable fruit pie, tart (made without milk, butter)
Tea	Suitable milk-free biscuit or cake
	Milk substitute
Supper	Meat, chicken, fish, egg (milk-free recipe) ⎫
	Salad or vegetables ⎬ Cooked without milk or butter
	Chips or plain crisps ⎪
	Milk-free bread ⎭
	Milk-free margarine or milk-free, low-fat spread
	Marmite, jam, honey
	Milk-free biscuit or cake
	Fruit
	Milk substitute flavoured with tea or coffee
Bedtime	Milk substitute
	Fruit

Vitamin supplement as appropriate

(c) Weaning diet: sample menu. (Use in conjunction with a nutritionally adequate modified milk substitute feed as appropriate for age, e.g. Cow & Gate S Formula or Pregestimil, Table 1.4.)

Breakfast	Farex Weaning Food, Robinson's Baby Rice, Farley's Original Rusk, Milupa Rice Cereal Mix with milk substitute feed as prescribed
Lunch	Sieved or minced meat or milk-free scrambled or boiled egg
	Sieved vegetables
	Special custard made with milk substitute and suitable custard powder
	or Strained baby food known to be free of milk (check ingredients on every tin or packet)
Tea	Fruit purée and suitable custard as lunch
	or Strained baby food, free of milk, as lunch (check ingredients on every tin or packet)

Manufactured products. A list of suitable products is prepared and revised periodically for the use of dietitians by the British Dietitic Association.

Recipes. Many recipes from ordinary cook-books can be selected provided ingredients are suitable or appropriate substitutes chosen, e.g. milk-free margarine in place of butter, milk substitute in place of milk, cheese omitted, etc.

Table 1.9 Minimal lactose and sucrose diet.

(a) Allowed and forbidden foods.
   1 Lactose is the sugar in milk, therefore all milk and milk products must be excluded from the diet.
   2 Sucrose is cane and beet sugar, and castor, icing and brown sugar, so all food containing sugar must be excluded from the diet. Sucrose also occurs in other naturally occurring foods like fruit and some vegetables.

Foods allowed	Foods forbidden
Milk substitute selected from Table 1.4, 1.5 or 1.7 as appropriate.	Milk, cream, cheese, yoghurt, ice-cream. Milk substitutes containing sucrose. Products containing casein, whey, milk solids, caseinate, etc. *Casilan, *Compliment, *Coffee-mate, 'filled' milks, Fast Pints, Five Pints, and similar products. Nutramigen, Wysoy, Granolac Infant, etc. containing sucrose.
Egg	
Meat: beef, lamb, pork, veal, ham, bacon. Offal: liver, kidney. Poultry: chicken, turkey. (Casseroles and stews—omit carrot, etc. and use tomato, celery, onion only.)	Tinned meat, meat and fish pastes, sausages and fish fingers unless milk-free. Meat with milk or sugar brine, e.g. Tendersweet bacon and ham. Meats cured in brine containing milk solids. Savoury dishes including milk, cheese, or vegetables not permitted.
Fresh fish	
Milk-free margarine, Tomor margarine, Telma margarine. Milk-free low-fat spreads. Lard, salad oil, pure fat and oil.	Butter, ordinary and vegetable margarines. Outline, etc. containing whey solids.
Cereals Wheat, rye, rice, barley, oats, maize. Custard powder, †flour (self-raising and plain), cornflour, semolina, sago (cooked without milk or with milk substitute and glucose). Pasta, macaroni, spaghetti. Baking powder.	Milk puddings. 'Non-milk fat' products. Blanchmange powder, Instant Whip and custard mixes. Ordinary custard, creamed cereals made with milk. Jelly, jelly creams, junket. Caramel. Tinned spaghetti containing cheese. Macaroni cheese.
†Breakfast cereals Puffed Wheat, Shredded Wheat, Grapenuts, porridge oats, Ready Brek (plain). Baby cereals Robinson's Baby Rice, Milupa Plain Rice Cereal, Farex Weaning Food.	Adult breakfast cereals, baby cereals and rusks containing milk and/or sugar. Most commercial baby foods including savouries. Special K, flavoured Ready Brek, muesli, etc. low-sugar rusks.
†Bread: e.g. Wholemeal, Hovis, plain white milk-free, VitBe, granary bread. †Lactose- sucrose-free biscuits and cakes (home-made), water biscuits, matzos, cream crackers, †Ryvita, †Vita-Wheat, †wheat crisp-breads. Glucose meringues (home-made). Aminex biscuits.	Milk breads, Procea, sweetened buns, cakes, biscuits, pastry, rusks, containing milk and/or sugar. Meringues, other crispbreads.
Glucose, Glucodin, galactose, fructose, glucose polymers, e.g. Calonutrin, Caloreen, Maxijul. Liquid glucose, e.g. Hycal, Lucozade. †Pure fresh honey (check sucrose-free).	Sugar and lactose in all forms. Artificial powdered sweeteners, e.g. Sweet 'n' Low. Sweets, chocolates, lollies. Nuts, jelly, syrup, jam. Pastes and sandwich spread.
Marmite, Bovril, Bisto, Oxo, salt, pepper, herbs, spices, essences. Salad cream, mayonnaise (check ingredients), gelatine.	Soups, sauces, pickles, chutney, salad cream containing sucrose and/or lactose. Gravy browning and gravy mixes with caramel. Monosodium glutamate retail powder with lactose filler.
Tea, coffee, cocoa powder. †Dietetic squash with no added sugar, e.g. Boots, Roses. Soda water, sugarless drinks, e.g. diet lemonade, Diet Pepsi, OneCal, Tab, Slimline drinks, etc.	Drinking chocolate, milk-shake syrups and powder. Horlicks, Ovaltine, Bournvita, malted milks. Sweetened squashes, all fruit juices. Fizzy drinks and sweetened drinks. Jelly.

Table 1.9 (a)   *continued*

Foods allowed	Foods forbidden
Sugarless pastilles	Sweets. Diabetic and slimming chocolate. Glucose sweets. Caramel, etc.
†Fruit: fresh blackberries, cherries, figs, grapes, lemons, rhubarb. †Tinned cherries in water (Dietade). †Bottled or canned grapefruit juice.	All other fruit, dried, tinned and fresh. Glacé cherries.
Vegetables: only aubergine, ackee, asparagus, beanshoots, broccoli, cabbage, cauliflower, celery, chicory, cress, cucumber, French and runner beans, greens, leeks, lettuce, marrow, mushrooms, okra, onions, peas frozen boiled, peppers, spinach, sprouts, tomato, turnip, unsweetened tomato juice.	Pulses. Canned, dried and raw frozen peas, butter and red kidney and baked beans, lentils. Root vegetables: beetroot, swede, carrot, parsnip. Sweetcorn, plantain. Vegetables not listed should be checked for sucrose content. Instant potato containing milk powder. Tomato paste. Vegetable salad.
Potato, chips, plain crisps and salted only.	Flavoured crisps, e.g. salt and vinegar.
Tinned or processed foods known to be free of lactose, milk and sugar (sucrose) or other forbidden foods.	Medicines, tablets and syrups containing lactose and sucrose (and sorbitol). Check all medicines with chemist before use.

* Casilan and Coffee-mate are lactose-free but contain milk casein(ate) protein.
† Contain traces of sucrose but in insignificant amounts for older patients with carbohydrate intolerance.

(b)   Minimal lactose and sucrose, milk-free diet: sample menu.

Breakfast	Puffed Wheat, Shredded Wheat, porridge oats or plain Ready Brek
	Milk substitute
	Glucose
	Eggs, bacon, fish (without milk or butter)
	Bread or toast (milk-free)
	Milk-free margarine or low-fat spread
	Marmite, Bovril, honey
	Milk substitute may be flavoured with tea, coffee, cocoa and glucose if desired
Mid-morning	Dietetic low-calorie squash or milk substitute
Dinner	Meat, poultry, offal, fish
	Potatoes—roast or boiled or chips ⎫ Cooked without
	Greens, tomato, cauliflower, marrow ⎬ milk or butter
	or vegetables from permitted list ⎭
	Home-made gravy
	Pudding made with milk substitute and glucose, e.g. custard, rice, semolina or egg
or	Sponge pudding made with glucose (no milk or butter)
Tea	Milk-free bread and milk-free margarine or low-fat spread
	Tomato, Marmite, Bovril, honey
	Home-made low-lactose, low-sucrose biscuits, cake, cream crackers, matzos
	Dietetic squash or milk substitute, or bottled/canned grapefruit juice
Supper	Meat, fish, egg, poultry, ham (without milk or butter)
	Salad or potato and vegetables from permitted list
	Sucrose-free jelly made with gelatine and glucose, and/or low-lactose, low-sucrose pudding or cake or biscuit.
	Fresh grapes or cherries
Bedtime	Milk substitute and low-lactose, low-sucrose biscuit

Table 1.9 (c)   *continued*

(c)   Minimal lactose and sucrose, milk-free weaning diet: sample menu. (Use in conjunction with suitable milk substitute feeds appropriate for the child's age.)

a.m.	Farex weaning food, Robinson's Baby Rice, Lyon's plain Ready Brek
	Milk substitute
Noon	Sieved or minced meat, fish, egg
	Home-made gravy
	Milk-free boiled or mashed potato
	Sieved greens, tomato, cauliflower or vegetable from permitted list
	Low-lactose, low-sucrose custard, rice, semolina
	or Egg pudding made with glucose and milk substitute
Mid-afternoon	Crust of milk-free bread or low-lactose, low-sucrose biscuits or Aminex biscuit
p.m.	Custard made with milk substitute and glucose
	or Cereal and milk substitute as at breakfast
	or Boiled egg and milk-free bread and milk-free margarine or low-fat spread
	or Sucrose-free jelly made from gelatine and glucose

Table 1.10   Minimal sucrose diet.

(a) Allowed and forbidden foods.

Sucrose is the sugar from beet and cane and is added to many products and recipes. It also occurs naturally in fruit and many vegetables which may or may not be permitted. Most medicines in liquid form also contain sucrose. Added sugar can be replaced with glucose, glucose polymers (or fructose) if necessary.

Allowed foods	Forbidden foods
Infant milk formulae without sugar, e.g. Aptamil, Osterfeed, Premium, SMA. Milk, skimmed milk, cream, butter, cheese. Goat's milk, butter milk. Unsweetened evaporated milk. Natural yoghurt, Coffee-mate, Compliment, 'filled' milks, Five Pints, Fast Pints, etc.	Sweetened condensed milk. Milk formulae and milk substitutes with sugar (sucrose), e.g. Wysoy, Granolac Infant, Nutramigen.
Meat, fish, egg, offal, poultry, ham, bacon. (Casseroles and stews should omit carrot, etc. and use onion, tomato, celery.)	Tinned meat, meat and fish pastes. Meat prepared in sugar brine e.g. Tendersweet ham and bacon. Savoury dishes with sugar or containing forbidden vegetables. Most baby foods in cans, jars and powder.
Butter, margarine, oils, lard, pure fat and low-fat spreads.	Imitation and non-dairy creams containing sugar, e.g. Sainsbury's.
Cereals:† wheat, rice, barley, oats. Custard powder (unsweetened). †Flour wholemeal and white (self-raising or plain), cornflour, semolina, tapioca, sago, arrowroot. Macaroni, spaghetti, baking powder.	Blancmange powder, Instant Whip and custard mixes. Jelly, junket tablets and powders. Table creams. Caramel flavouring.† Soya flour. Tinned spaghetti, baked beans.
Breakfast cereals containing less than 2% sucrose*: porridge, plain Ready Brek, Shredded Wheat, Puffed Wheat, Grapenuts. Baby cereals: Robinson's Baby Rice, Farex Weaning Food, Aminex biscuits. Milupa Plain Rice Cereal. †Bread: wholemeal, wheatmeal, white, brown, rolls (except sweetened loaves). Matzos, oatcakes, chapati, Water biscuits, cream crackers, crispbread, Ryvita, Vitawheat. Sucrose-free biscuits (home-made). Glucose meringues (home-made).	Adult breakfast cereals, muesli, Rice Krispies. Baby cereals unless checked to be free of sucrose. Low-sugar rusks. All sweetened breads, biscuits, cakes, pastries, pies, buns, puddings, meringues.

Table 1.10 (a) *Continued*

Allowed foods	Forbidden foods
Glucose, glucodin, fructose, lactose, galactose. Glucose polymers, e.g. Caloreen, Maxijul, Calonutrin. Liquid glucose, Hycal, saccharine, aspartame, Nutrasweet-type sweeteners. †Pure fresh honey (check sucrose content).	Sugar: all forms, castor, icing, brown, demerara, white. golden syrup, jam, marmalade, treacle. Jelly. Sucron and similar powder sweetening agents. Ice-cream, lollies, sweets, toffee, candy, caramel. Chocolates. Nuts. Glucose sweets, diabetic jam. Pastes and sandwich spreads. Hundreds-and-thousands, sugar strands and cake decorations.
Marmite, Bovril, Oxo, Bisto. Salt, pepper, herbs, spices, monosodium glutamate, pickles, e.g. piccalilli.	Gravy browning and instant gravies with added caramel. Soups, sauces, sweetened pickles and chutneys and salad creams containing sugar (sucrose).
Tea, coffee, cocoa (unsweetened), Lucozade. Diabetic squash with no added sugar, e.g. Boots, Roses. Soda water, sugarless lemonade, e.g. Slimline, OneCal, Diet Pepsi, Tab. Essences and food colourings. Gelatine. Rennet. Diabetic sugarless jelly.	Drinking chocolate, milk-shake syrup and powder, malted milks, Bournvita. All fruit juices and squash. Fizzy pop. Sweetened drinks, e.g. sweetened coffee essence. Jelly
Sugarless pastilles. Diabetic chocolate plain and milk	Sweets, chocolates, glucose sweets, caramel, toffee. Filled and nut diabetic chocolate.
Fruit containing less than 1% sucrose: grapes, avocado pear, blackberries, cherries, lemons, loganberries, rhubarb. Bottled or canned grapefruit juice.	Other fruit, dried, tinned, fresh. Fresh grapefruit. Glacé cherries.
Vegetables containing less than 1% sucrose: ackee (canned), onion, aubergine, runner beans, haricot beans, beanshoots, broccoli tops, Brussels sprouts, cabbage, cauliflower, celery, cucumber, laver bread, leeks, lettuce, marrow, mushroom, mustard and cress, okra, frozen boiled peas, parsley, peppers, potatoes, pumpkin, radish, seakale, spinach, spring greens, tomato, turnip, watercress, yam	Other vegetables and pulses, e.g., red kidney beans, baked beans, root vegetables, carrot, parsnip, swede. Raw and frozen peas, garden peas, etc. Tomato paste and puree. Tomato soup. Vegetable soup. Vegetable salad.
Potato, chips, plain salted crisps	Flavoured crisps
Tinned or processed foods known to be free of sucrose and forbidden ingredients. Check all labels and ingredients.	Manufactured foods containing sugar and with doubtful ingredients. Medicines in syrup, some tablets: check all medicines with your chemist before use. Children's toothpaste containing sugar.

† Contain traces of sucrose, but in insignificant amounts for older patients with carbohydrate intolerance.

(b) Minimal sucrose diet: sample menu.

Breakfast	Shredded Wheat, plain Ready Brek or porridge—sweeten with glucose Milk Bacon and/or egg Tomatoes if desired Bread or toast and butter or margarine Marmite or Bovril or honey Milk, tea, coffee or cocoa, sweetened with glucose if desired.
Mid-morning	Milk or dietetic squash or bottled/canned grapefruit juice or lemon juice sweetened with glucose or unsweetened tomato juice

Table 1.10 (b)   *continued*

Dinner or evening meal	Meat or fish or liver or poultry
	Home-made gravy or white sauce
	Potatoes, roast, boiled, mashed, jacket, chips
	Permitted vegetables, e.g. cabbage, sprouts, cauliflower, runner beans, tomatoes, lettuce, watercress,
	Home-made milk pudding sweetened with glucose
	Home-made sponge pudding sweetened with glucose or milk jelly or ice-cream (*see* Recipes)
Tea/snacks/bedtime	Bread and margarine or butter, cheese, Marmite or honey
	Crispbread or cream crackers and butter or margarine
	Crisps (plain or salted)
	Milk or dietetic squash or tea sweetened with glucose if desired or sugarless drink, e.g. Diet Pepsi or Lucozade
Evening meal or	Egg, ham, fish, cheese or meat
school dinner	Potatoes or home-cooked spaghetti or macaroni
	Permitted vegetables or salad
	Bread and margarine or butter, crisps (plain or salt & vinegar)
	Permitted fruit, e.g. grapes, rhubarb sweetened with glucose
	Home-made pudding or cake sweetened with glucose
	Milk or cocoa sweetened with glucose

(c) Minimal sucrose weaning diet: sample menu. Use in conjunction with a modified infant milk formula appropriate for age, e.g. Gold Cap SMA, Premium, Osterfeed, Aptamil, etc.

a.m.	Farex Weaning Food or Robinson's Baby Rice or other permitted cereal.
	Mix with infant milk feed
Lunch	Liquidized, sieved or minced meat, fish, home-made gravy
	Potato and sieved permitted vegetables, tomato, cauliflower, cabbage
'Snack'	Crust of bread or Aminex biscuit
p.m.	Mashed hard-boiled egg or grated cheese or mashed sardines and bread and butter or margarine
	or Custard made with infant milk feed
	or Permitted cereal and infant milk feed and sweetened with glucose
	Purée of minced meat, potato and permitted vegetables

Starch intolerance from other causes is extremely rare. When it does occur in children and adults, restriction of starch, and/or enzyme replacement therapy, is adequate. Soya flour has much less starch (15%) than other flours and cereals (65 to 80%), and can be useful to incorporate into the diet as a substitute for other flours (*see* Recipes, p. 48). A basic low-starch diet is given in Table 1.12, and an example of a minimal sucrose, low-starch diet menu in Table 1.13. Restricted quantities of starch can be introduced as tolerated; Table 1.14 gives a list of foods containing 10 g starch. Limited quantities of sucrose may also be permitted; *see* Table 1.11.

A starch-restricted diet requires thiamine (vitamin B_1) supplements, and dietary fibre from vegetables and/or bran should be included. A general vitamin supplement, e.g. Abidec, 0·6 ml/day, containing thiamine, or a more comprehensive supplement such as Ketovite Tablets (3/day) plus Ketovite Liquid (5 ml/day), is usually recommended.

GLUCOSE–GALACTOSE

Glucose and galactose and the poly- and disaccharides from which they are derived by enzymic action are widely distributed in food and milk, necessitating their elimination from the diet in glucose–galactose intolerance. All dietary carbohydrate must be supplied as fructose (laevosan or laevulose). The only milk substitute formula which contains fructose as the sole carbohydrate is Galactomin Fructose Formula 19 (Cow & Gate), or a module-based feed must

Table 1.11 Sucrose content of some fruits (adapted from Southgate *et al.* 1978).

Fruit	% Sucrose
Apples, eating	3
Apricot, fresh	5·8
Banana	6·6
Grapefruit	2·1
Cantaloupe melon	3·3
Yellow melon	1·4
Water melon	2·4
Oranges	3·7
Peaches	6·6
Pears, eating	1·3
Pears, cooking	1·1
Pineapple	7·9
Plums, eating	4·9
Raspberries, fresh	2·0
Strawberries, fresh	1·1

be devised for the infant and young child, based on Comminuted Chicken, or Maxipro HBV, to which fructose, a source of fat, complete minerals and vitamins must be added (Table 1.15). Internationally, some carbohydrate-free formulae are available from Nestlé, Mead Johnson, Abbotts and Syntex to which fructose can be added. Galactomin Fructose Formula 19 is currently not a complete formula, but reformulation is planned; meanwhile, vitamin and trace mineral supplements are essential.

Initially for the ill child or infant, the milk substitute may need to be introduced as a dilute, but frequent, feeding schedule in an appropriate total volume per day (total fluid requirement is elevated with diarrhoea). Oral rehydration solution without glucose, or specially prepared with fructose as the carbohydrate, may be required, or appropriate electrolyte supplements of sodium, potassium and bicarbonate may be given, as requirements may be elevated due to faecal losses. Fructose is added to the module and carbohydrate-free formula initially at a rate of 5 g/100 ml of feed, unless intravenous carbohydrate is given. The feed is increased quickly to full strength, unless the child is given parenteral nutrition, to avoid further malnutrition. As fructose is a monosaccharide, feeds containing it are relatively high in osmolality, compared to those containing glucose polymers. Gradually the total nutritional intake is increased until the child starts to gain weight; nutrient requirements may need to be 50% or 100% higher than normal requirement for actual weight, to allow for catch-up growth. The energy of the regimen can be increased by adding increments of fat

emulsion and/or fructose to the feed (Table 1.15). The quantity of fat in the feed should not exceed the carbohydrate content unless intravenous carbohydrate is provided.

As this diet severely restricts food intake, especially in infants and young children, the importance of all essential nutrients must be stressed, and supplements including the minor vitamins and trace minerals should be prescribed. Complete vitamin supplements such as Ketovite Tablets (1 × t.d.s.) plus 5 ml Ketovite Liquid daily are carbohydrate-free and can be given with this diet. Trace elements or complete mineral supplements according to the milk substitute selected are also recommended in young children (*see* Francis 1986).

In the older child or in infants, as the clinical state improves suitable carbohydrate-free solids (Table 1.16) can be added to the diet to increase energy, variety and bulk. A milk substitute such as Galactomin Fructose Formula 19 or recipe (c) in Table 1.15 is appropriate for the child over two years old. Care must be taken to ensure adequate fructose intake continues, even beyond infancy, or ketosis may occur.

All medicines should be carbohydrate- and sorbitol-free; tablets frequently contain lactose, and syrups sucrose or sorbitol. There is often as much as 3 g sucrose in a 5 ml dose of syrup medicines.

Great caution must be taken in reintroducing glucose to patients with temporary intolerance of glucose–galactose. It is suggested that initially $\frac{1}{2}$ g glucose per feed or 0·5% glucose should be given in the first instance. Immediate withdrawal of the glucose should be made if any ill effect is noted. If 0·5% glucose is tolerated the glucose should slowly be increased, over 5 to 10 days, as a replacement of part or all of the fructose, then other carbohydrates, e.g. starch, can be introduced, and later the disaccharides. Failure to tolerate glucose introduction on several occasions, once the child is clinically well, warrants investigation of possible congenital glucose–galactose intolerance.

PROTRACTED OR INTRACTABLE DIARRHOEA OF INFANCY

Protracted diarrhoea has been defined as diarrhoea persisting for more than two weeks with four or more loose stools/day, accompanied by failure to thrive or actual weight loss (Larcher *et al.* 1977). It usually occurs in infants of less than six months old. A variety of disorders can cause this syndrome, but often

Table 1.12 Basic low-starch diet.

(a) Starch-free, starch-containing and possible starch-containing foods

Starch-free foods	Starch-containing and possible starch-containing foods
Modified milks for infants with lactose as carbohydrate. Milk, cheese, butter, cream, yoghurt. Margarine, fats, oils.	Arrowroot, cornflour, Bengers. Milk substitutes and soya milks containing starch, and/or glucose polymers, e.g. Ostermilk Complete, Pregestimil, Galactomin.
Meat, fish, poultry, eggs	Sausages, tinned meats with cereal filler. Textured vegetable protein.
*Soya biscuits and soya flour	Bread, cakes, biscuits, pastries. Wheat, flour, oats, rye, rice, barley, sago, semolina, tapioca, cornflour, custard power, blancmange, spaghetti, macaroni and other pasta. Baby cereals, breakfast cereals.
Ripe fruit	Unripe fruit
Vegetables not listed as containing starch	Pulses: beans, lentils. Potatoes, parsnip, sweetcorn. Nuts and some seeds.
Tea, coffee, Marmite, Bovril	Gravy mix, Bisto.
Boiled sweets, fruit squashes and juices. Sugar, jam, jelly, honey.	Liquid glucose, glucose polymers, dextrins, maltose, malt, corn syrup solids. Ice-cream (check ingredients).
Home-made clear soups and broths Salt, pepper, vinegar, herbs, spices Essences, food colourings Rennet, gelatine, jelly, ice-lollies	Thickened soups
Tinned or processed foods known to be free of starch (ingredients on manufactured foods should be scrutinized carefully)	

* Soya flour contains only 15% starch which is much less than any other cereal. Biscuits made from soya flour may be useful to reduce starch intake (see Recipes).

(b) Low-starch diet: sample menu.

Breakfast	Bacon or egg or ham or fish Fruit, fresh, tinned, stewed *Special soya biscuits (see recipe) Butter, margarine Marmite, Bovril or jam or honey Milk or milky tea to drink
Mid-morning	Milk or fresh fruit juice or Marmite or Bovril as a drink
Dinner	Meat or fish or poultry or liver (cooked without flour or breadcrumbs) Permitted green vegetables Egg custard or home-made milk jelly or fruit—fresh, tinned, dried or stewed
Tea	Milk or milky tea or fresh fruit juice *Special soya biscuits (see recipe) Butter, margarine Marmite, Bovril or cheese or ham or jam or honey
Supper	Meat or fish or cheese or egg dish Green vegetables or salad or tomato Home-made ice-cream, jelly or fruit Milk to drink

* Permitted quantities of cereals, bread, etc. should be determined individually.

Table 1.13

(a)   Minimal sucrose and low-starch diet: sample menu.

Breakfast	Egg, bacon, ham, fish Special *soya biscuits (savoury) Butter or margarine Marmite, Bovril, honey Milk, tea, coffee, cocoa sweetened with glucose if desired
Mid-morning	Milk or dietetic squash sweetened with glucose
Dinner	Meat, fish, cheese, egg Vegetables permitted (*see* Table 1.10†) Butter or margarine Unthickened gravy or meat juices Egg custard sweetened with glucose Home-made sucrose-free jelly or ice-cream
Tea	Special *soya biscuits made with glucose Butter or margarine Marmite, Bovril, honey Milk or dietetic squash sweetened with glucose
Supper	Egg, ham, cheese, meat, fish Salad, fruit or vegetables permitted (*see* Table 1.10†) Special *soya biscuits (savoury) Home-made sucrose-free jelly or ice-cream, grapes or cherries Milk or tea sweetened with glucose if desired

(b) Minimal sucrose, minimal starch weaning diet: sample menu.
   This should be used in conjunction with an appropriate modified sucrose/starch-free infant feed, e.g. Aptamil, Gold Cap SMA, Premium, Osterfeed, etc.

a.m.	Milk feed Egg-yolk or scrambled egg
Noon	Homogenized or minced meat or fish Purée vegetables from permitted list (Table 1.10†) Butter or margarine Egg custard sweetened with glucose
Mid-afternoon	Special *soya biscuit as a rusk 5% dextrose or milk feed
p.m.	Homogenized or minced meat, fish, egg Purée vegetable from permitted list (Table 1.10†) Sucrose-free jelly

See Recipes (p. 50).
†Omit those containing starch, such as potatoes and pulses.

Table 1.14   Starch exchanges = 10 g starch.

20 g (⅔ oz) bread (½ slice of large sliced loaf)
15 g (½ oz) cereal, e.g. oats, Ready Brek, Robinson's Baby Rice, Shredded Wheat, Puffed Wheat
15 g (½ oz) flour
50 g (2 oz) potato (1 small)
10 only special *soya biscuits, recipe page 50.

no cause can be firmly established (Larcher *et al.* 1977). Diagnosis of an underlying primary condition should be sought, and treated vigorously once identified. Such conditions include surgical causes, post-surgery on the intestine and gut resection, post-gastroenteritis, cow's milk protein intolerance, other dietary protein enteropathies (soya, egg, wheat,

Table 1.15 Examples of glucose-free formulae.

	Protein (g)	Carbohydrate (g)	Fat (g)	Energy kJ	Energy kcal	Calcium (mmol)	Sodium (mmol)	Potassium (mmol)
Suitable for infants								
(a) Using Comminuted Chicken (Cow & Gate)								
30 g Comminuted Chicken	2·25	Nil	1·0	75	18	Trace	0·12	0·4
5 to 10 g fructose	Nil	5 to 10	Nil	80 to 160	20 to 40		—	—
8 ml Prosparol/Calogen*	Nil	Nil	4·0	148	36		—	—
1 g Aminogran/Metabolic Mineral Mixture†						2·1	1·74	2·0
Complete vitamin supplement medicinally‡								
Water to 100 ml								
100 ml *total*	2·25	5 to 10	5·0	303 to 383	74 to 94	2·1	1·86	2·4
(b) Using Casilan or Maxipro HBV§								
2 g Casilan or Maxipro HBV§	1·8	—	Trace	31	7·5	0·6	Trace	Trace
5 to 10 g fructose	Nil	5 to 10	Nil	80 to 160	20 to 40	—	—	—
10 ml Prosparol/Calogen*	Nil	Nil	5·0	185	45	—	—	—
1 g Aminogran/Metabolic Mineral Mixture†						2·1	1·74	2·0
Complete vitamin supplement medicinally‡								
Water to 100 ml								
100 ml *total*	1·8	5 to 10	5·0	296 to 376	73 to 93	2·7	1·74	2·0
(c) Galactomin Fructose Formula 19 (Cow & Gate) (*see* Table 1.5) plus vitamins‡								
(d) *Children over 2 years old* ‖								
4 g Casilan or Maxipro HBV§	3·6	—	Trace	63	15	1·2	0·2	Trace
10 g fructose	Nil	10	Nil	160	40	—	—	—
10 ml Calogen/Prosparol*	Nil	Nil	5	185	45	—	—	—
Water to 100 ml								
100 ml *total*	3·6	10	5	408	100	1·2	0·2	Trace

* Prosparol (Duncan Flockhart) and Calogen (SHS) are 50% oil emulsions. If steatorrhoea also occurs, part of the quantity can be replaced with Liquigen (SHS), a 52% MCT emulsion, provided an adequate alternative source of essential fatty acid is provided.
† Complete mineral mixture dose 1°5 g/kg per day to total 8 g daily. Aminogran Mineral Mixture (Allen & Hanburys), Metabolic Mineral Mixture (SHS).
‡ 3 Ketovite Tablets and 5 ml Ketovite Liquid (Paines & Byrne) daily.
§ Casilan is low in cystine and contains milk protein. Maxipro is a high biological whey protein.
‖ For the older child, vitamin mineral supplements will depend on total dietary intake or supplement as in † and ‡ above.

chicken, rice, etc.), disaccharide or monosaccharide intolerance, immune deficiency states, lymphangiectasia, cystic fibrosis, necrotizing enterocolitis, congenital chloridorrhoea, acrodermatitis enteropathica and the recently described lethal familial protracted diarrhoea (Candy *et al.* 1981). An enteropathy is a common albeit not a universal finding in these children (Shwachman *et al.* 1973). An immune abnormality may play an important part in the pathogenesis of such an enteropathy, which may be due to hypersensitivity to antigens, including food proteins. Disaccharide and/or monosaccharide intolerances are relatively common. Although some improvement in mortality has occurred with modern management it is still unacceptably high, especially in those in whom no primary diagnosis can be made (Larcher *et al.* 1977).

Table 1.16 Minimal glucose–galactose diet‡.

Only the following are allowed: no other foods should be used unless checked and found to be glucose-free.

*Milk substitute containing fructose as the sole
   carbohydrate (Table 1.15). Casilan, Maxipro HBV
Meat
   All types—beef, lamb, poultry, mutton, veal, pork
Eggs
Fish
   All types fresh and frozen, smoked fish
†Fruit
   Only avocado pear, lemon juice
Fructose, laevulose
†Vegetables
   Only ackee (tinned), runner and French beans,
   beansprouts, broccoli tops, Brussels sprouts, cauliflower,
   celery, laverbread, lettuce, boiled and frozen peas,
   spinach
Pure gelatine
Marmite, Bovril, stock cubes
Milk-free 'kosher' margarine, Telma margarine, milk-free
   low-fat spreads
Pure white fat, lard, salad and cooking oils. Prosparol,
   Calogen, Liquigen. MCT oil
Salt, pepper
Vinegar, herbs, spices, essences, colouring
Sugarless pastilles
Tea, coffee, sugarless drinks, e.g. Diet Pepsi, Tab, OneCal,
   Slimline drinks. Cocoa powder (unsweetened) may be
   used in limited quantities in the older child.

---

* Supplements. This restricted diet requires complete
  supplementation with vitamins, Ketovite Tablets, 1 × t.d.s.,
  plus 5 ml Ketovite Liquid (Paines & Byrne Ltd), in all
  patients and a source of trace elements, including iron
  and zinc and possibly calcium or a complete mineral
  mixture.
† Contain less than 1% glucose and ½% sucrose (Southgate
  et al. 1978).
‡ Care must be taken to include sufficient fructose to avoid
  ketosis.

LETHAL FAMILIAL PROTRACTED DIARRHOEA

A highly lethal form of protracted diarrhoea in 24 patients from 10 families has been reported by Candy *et al.* (1981). None of the established genetically determined causes of protracted diarrhoea was diagnosed. The familial pattern, however, suggested a genetic basis for the diarrhoea, probably by an autosomal recessive mode, although there may have been more than one recessive condition present in the group as a whole. Onset of diarrhoea was within the first three weeks of life in 22 of the 24 patients, and the diarrhoea was cholera-like. In the two patients in whom steady-state perfusion studies were performed, there was secretory diarrhoea with loss of water. Glucose absorption was markedly reduced, and in one patient fructose absorption was also reduced. Dietary exclusion of disaccharides, monosaccharides, cow's milk, soya protein or gluten had no effect on the diarrhoea and therefore parenteral nutrition was essential for management. The two patients who recovered appeared to do so spontaneously.

MANAGEMENT OF PROTRACTED DIARRHOEA

This is one of the most difficult problems of paediatric gastroenterology. The first step is to correct dehydration and any electrolyte or acid–base imbalance with intravenous fluids. The temporary withdrawal of oral intake allows observation as to whether the diarrhoea persists without oral intake (Larcher *et al.* 1977, Candy *et al.* 1981). If this is the case a period of total parenteral nutrition (TPN), described by Booth & Harries 1982b, Grotte *et al.* 1982, is almost invariably necessary and it can be life-saving in these infants.

Appropriate oral nutrition can be introduced gradually in conjunction with parenteral nutrition. Some food is always absorbed, long fasts are contraindicated. Even with parenteral nutrition it is the author's practice, wherever possible, to offer small quantities of enteral nutrition to maintain oral habits and avoid the risk of atrophic changes in the gut and pancreas with the concurrent impairment of function seen in experimental animals when luminal nutrients were excluded during TPN (Hughes & Dowling 1980, Hughes *et al.* 1980). Intraluminal nutrients are also important in preventing liver disease with TPN, and also in the adaptation of intestinal function following extensive gut resection, and possibly in the promotion of post-natal gut development and maturation. These trophic effects on the intestinal mucosa may be direct and/or mediated by gastrointestinal hormones (*see* details given by Booth & Harries 1982b), and the liver disease may be related to deficiency of various nutrients, such as taurine, from TPN regimens (Cooper *et al.* 1984).

After initial rehydration, those infants not requiring parenteral nutrition are graded onto oral feeds. Human milk, if tolerated, is the ideal feed for the young sick infant and may have a therapeutic value in some instances (MacFarlane & Miller 1984 and Lucas 1984). It can be supplied by the infant's own mother or donated from human milk banks. Unpasteurized human milk has immunological advantages (Narayanan *et al.* 1982), but must be monitored microbiologically to reduce the risk of contamination being transmitted to the sick infant (DHSS 1981). Expressed human milk is higher in energy than 'drip' human milk which constitutes much of the 'bank' milk in this country. Bolus feeding reduces the risk of coincidentally feeding low-fat human milk, due to the fat clinging to tubing and drip chambers of nasogastric tube feeding equipment (Narayanan et al. 1983, Stocks et al. 1985). Only very rarely is human milk protein not tolerated, and even lactose when given in human milk may be tolerated. However, if lactose intolerance is a problem lactase enzyme preparations (Kerulac by Gist Brocades or β-galactosidase by BDH) could be used to hydrolyse the lactose to galactose and glucose. With the choice of alternative commercial lactose-free formulae now available, the latter is rarely used these days.

Alternatively, a nutritionally adequate milk protein-, disaccharide- and soya-free formula with a low osmolality should be selected (Table 1.4). A previous history or suspicion of monosaccharide intolerance will necessitate cautious introduction of the feed and careful consideration regarding the carbohydrate content. If steatorrhoea is present, a low-fat formula containing MCT to provide adequate energy may be indicated. Pregestimil and the Pepdite formulae are the most appropriate commercial formulae for infants and young children, as they contain hydrolysed protein and amino acids, glucose polymers and/or starch, vegetable oils and/or MCT and comprehensive ranges of vitamins and minerals (see Table 1.4).

In some patients with protracted diarrhoea, starch as well as lactose and sucrose cannot be hydrolysed to the respective monosaccharides glucose, galactose and fructose. Occasionally, even the glucose polymers and maltodextrins are not tolerated, in which case Pregestimil, the Pepdite formulae, Galactomin Formula 17, etc. are all contraindicated, and glucose polymers must be replaced with glucose and/or fructose in a module oral-feeding regimen. When the transport of glucose and galactose is affected, fructose is the carbohydrate of choice, but where complete monosaccharide intolerance exists a carbohydrate-free oral feed must be devised and intravenous carbohydrate must be supplied, together with careful observation of the patient to prevent and correct any hypothermia and hypoglycaemia.

A module diet gives more scope to introduce nutrients singly and to tailor the feed to the nutritional requirement of the individual. It can be used as the sole source of nutrition or in conjunction with parenteral nutrition. In the author's experience a feed based on chicken protein, glucose polymer, an oil emulsion and vitamins and minerals using Comminuted Chicken (Table 1.6) is most appropriate (Larcher et al. 1977). Full details of the Comminuted Chicken regimen are given on pp. 34–37. In the rare circumstances of chicken not being tolerated, a module diet based on peptides or amino acids can be devised.

Initially a dilute, frequent feeding schedule is given orally, or by nasogastric tube administered by bolus or continuously by paediatric enteral pump. As Comminuted Chicken is a suspension and not a solution it cannot be given as a continuous feed, but can be given by nasogastric tube as bolus feeds or from a large-holed feeding bottle. The feed is introduced in planned increments as clinically tolerated: $\frac{1}{4}$, $\frac{1}{2}$, $\frac{3}{4}$ full-strength feed with 5% added carbohydrate then 1% increments, fat in 0·5% increments (i.e. 1 ml of 50% oil emulsion to each 100 ml feed). See Tables 1.18 and 1.19.

Close monitoring of stools for consistency, volume and reducing substances, and of daily weight gain, and electrolytes and nutrient intake, is essential. A team approach, including ideally a paediatric gastroenterologist and nursing and dietetic staff, is essential. Long periods of inadequate nutrition must be avoided.

It is essential to calculate all feed changes and the actual consumed intake, especially of multi-ingredient feed regimens, whether administered parenterally or enterally, at least for protein, energy, carbohydrate, fat, sodium, potassium, calcium and, from time to time, zinc, copper, iron and vitamins. The feed osmolality should also be measured.

Catabolic and marasmic patients, and patients with malabsorption, have increased nutrient requirements for energy, fluid and electrolytes and also, particularly if catch-up growth is to be achieved, for protein, vitamins and some minerals. Table 1.17 summarizes the increased requirements needed by infants, and Francis (1986) has details regarding catabolism in children.

When selecting diets and formulae for patients with malabsorption, factors affecting absorption and bioavailability of nutrients should be considered.

1 Osmolality

High osmolar solutions draw water into the gut and can cause diarrhoea. Infant feeds, enteral feeds and milk substitutes, especially those used in paediatrics, should not exceed an osmolality of 500 mmol/l. The osmolality of various feeds is given in Table 1.4 and Table 1.5.

Table 1.17 A guide to nutrient intake for malnourished and catabolic infants.

Protein		⎱
0–6 months	3 to 4 (maximum 6*)	
6–12 months	3 to 6 (maximum 10*)	
Energy		
High	540 to 630 kJ (130–150 kcal)	Per kg actual weight per day
Very high	630 to 900 kJ (150–220 kcal)	
Sodium ⎱ High	2·5 mmol ⎱ Or as indicated biochemically	
Potassium ⎰ Very high	3·0 mmol ⎰ and to meet faecal losses	
Fluid (oral without i.v.)	200 (maximum 300) ml	⎰
Calcium	At least 1·25 to 1·8 mmol/kg per day to 15 mmol per day	
	0·75 to 3 mmol/100 ml feed	
Phosphorus	0·5 to 1·9 mmol/100 ml feed	
Calcium : phosphorus ratio	1·2 : 1 and not more than 2·2 : 1	
Magnesium	0·12 to 0·5 mmol/100 ml feed	
Iron†	0·18 mmol/day	
Zinc†		
0–6 months	46 μmol/day	
6–12 months	75 μmol/day	
Copper†		
0–6 months	7·9 to 11 μmol/day	
6–12 months	11 to 15·7 μmol/day	

Vitamins, at least normal requirement including:

Thiamine	0·3 mg	⎱
Riboflavin	0·4 mg	
Nicotinic acid equivalent	5 mg	
Total folate	50 μg	
Ascorbic acid	20 mg	Minimum per day
Vitamin A retinol equi-valent	450 μg	
Vitamin D cholecalciferol	7·5 μg	⎰

* Such high protein intakes will be partially used for energy, and elevated blood urea or blood amino acids can occur; biochemical monitoring and adjustment of the intake is essential.

† Full details of trace mineral requirements and interactions are given by Aggett and Davies (1983) and in Francis (1986). Higher intakes may be needed to compensate losses in malabsorption.

The following should be considered:

(a) *Carbohydrates.* Monosaccharides have a higher osmolality for the same percentage solution than disaccharides or glucose polymers and starch. The amount of carbohydrate (g) in each 100 ml feed (% solution) is a guide to tolerance. A 5% carbohydrate solution is usually tolerated even as monosaccharides. A 7% carbohydrate solution, present in modified infant feeds, is usually tolerated. A 10% carbohydrate solution may be tolerated, especially if partially in the form of glucose polymer and/or starch. A 12% carbohydrate solution is rarely tolerated by infants with malabsorption, but may be tolerated by children; 15 to 20% carbohydrate solutions are usually only tolerated by those without malabsorption and if given in the form of glucose polymers and/or starch.

An occasional patient cannot split glucose polymers; in such patients monosaccharides have to be given. A mixture of glucose and fructose is often better absorbed than the total carbohydrate content given as a single monosaccharide. Honey contains a mixture of glucose and fructose and can be useful if monosaccharides are not easily available; 7 g honey $\simeq$ 5 g carbohydrate. Some batches of honey have been reported to have microbial contamination. Also, as it contains a number of sensitizing allergens, depending on the source of pollen from which it is made, it is not recommended in patients at risk of atopic disease.

(*b*) *Protein.*   Amino acids have a higher osmolality than peptides or protein for the same percentage solution. Dipeptides are more rapidly absorbed than amino acids (Matthews 1971, 1975).

The biological value of protein should be high, and for infant feeds should mimic the amino acid profile of human milk, e.g. whey-based cow's milk formulae have a higher biological value protein with a reduced methionine and phenylalanine, but increased cystine and arginine, content compared to cow's milk. Added methionine is usual in soya-based feeds to improve the protein quality. Vivonex, which contains no cystine or taurine and has an unacceptably high osmolality and carbohydrate content, is unsuitable for infants or as the sole source of nutrition in children. The casein-based formulae, Galactomin, MCT 1, Portagen, and to a lesser extent Nutramigen, are high in protein but low in cystine. Galactomin and MCT 1, which in the past have been nutritionally inadequate in all vitamins and trace elements, are being reformulated.

(*c*) *Fat.*   Medium-chain triglycerides are not a source of essential fatty acids, nor can they be metabolized to essential fatty acid (EFA). They have a higher osmolality than long-chain fat for the same percentage solution. MCT is therefore only recommended as a supplementary source of energy when steatorrhoea is present. It should be introduced slowly and with caution.

(*d*) *Bioavailability.*   Requirements differ from one individual to another by as much as ±15% in healthy individuals, and change with alteration in the composition and nature of the diet, because such alterations may affect the efficiency with which nutrients are absorbed and utilized as a result of their bioavailability. A number of factors affecting vitamin and mineral uptake are discussed by Francis (1986).

2   Age
Infants are less able to handle high osmolar and concentrated feeds than children; and young children are less able than adults. The young infant cannot handle a high renal solute load due to the immature kidney being unable to concentrate urine, or high protein intakes because of immature liver enzymes for their degradation (*see* Francis 1986; also Chapters 8 and 10).

3   Clinical condition
Marasmic and/or catabolic patients frequently have diarrhoea, food intolerances, malabsorption and occasionally steatorrhoea. Antibiotics and other medicines may increase malabsorption and the sorbitol or lactose filler in which they are given may encourage loose stools. Catabolism increases nutrient requirements.

4   Administration of feed
Small frequent feeds are more easily absorbed than larger volume, infrequent 'bolus' feeds. One- to two-hourly feeds are preferable to three- to four-hourly in the sick infant (by nasogastric tube when the patient is asleep), in which case a larger total volume of feed may be tolerated and therefore better nutrient intake achieved. Nasogastric or nasojejunal continuous feeds can be given via a fine-bore tube but require careful positioning and supervision of the feeding tube and frequent, accurate monitoring of volume, e.g. by syringe pump in infants or paediatric enteral pump in children with a burette giving-set to avoid fluid overload with subsequent risk of vomiting and feed inhalation.

5   Sterility of feed
An aseptic delivery technique and feed preparation is essential for bottle, bolus and nasogastric or nasojejunal enteral feeds. Terminal pasteurization of hospital feeds is recommended, e.g. 63°C for 30 minutes or 67·5°C for four minutes. Terminal sterilization is not suitable as it causes loss of vitamins (C, B_6), protein denaturation and lysine loss due to the Maillard reaction and caramelization of carbohydrates and lactulose formation (from lactose), with subsequent diarrhoea in the patient and loss of nutrients. Even carefully monitored ready-to-feed and evaporated commercial liquid formulae containing lactose also contain some lactulose which can cause diarrhoea.

Practical details of Comminuted Chicken-based module feed for infants

This is a module diet which, like parenteral nutrition, must be calculated individually. The oral intake should not be overconcentrated. Regrading onto a suitable oral feed of complete nutrition varies from 4 to 40 days, according to the patient's clinical condition and whether or not the regimen is used in conjunction with parenteral nutrition. The feed is normally introduced in hospital, and only those patients who do not tolerate, or who are suspected of not tolerating, a simpler nutritionally adequate formula require this regimen.

Comminuted Chicken is sterilized purée chicken in water made by Cow & Gate which provides the protein, and some fat, including essential fatty acids, and some minerals in a complex feed. It should never be used as the sole source of nutrition. Suitable carbohydrate (orally or i.v.) must be provided, as the infants who require this regimen are very prone to hypoglycaemia and hypothermia. A glucose polymer is the most appropriate oral carbohydrate, but it can be replaced with glucose, glucose plus fructose, fructose alone and/or sucrose as necessary. Complete minerals, including trace elements, complete vitamins and additional fat are also essential. The proportions of the different nutrients can be adjusted to meet the individual's requirements. All module feeds should be monitored for osmolality and to ensure the nutritional adequacy of the regimen. These feeds are often used in conjunction with parenteral nutrition, in which case the initial oral nutrient intake may be negligible. Thereafter the combined intake of both the enteral and parenteral nutrition must be considered and care taken not to overconcentrate the feed. Vitamins are given medicinally as one Ketovite Tablet t.d.s. plus 5 ml Ketovite Liquid, unless the complete range of vitamins are given parenterally.

The Comminuted Chicken must be diluted with additional water, even to make a full-strength feed for infants and young children. The feed is normally

Table 1.18 Composition and nutrient content of Comminuted Chicken meat feeds.

		$\frac{1}{4}$ Strength	$\frac{1}{2}$ Strength	$\frac{3}{4}$ Strength	Full-protein, low-energy feed	Full-protein, normal-energy feed	Full-protein, high-energy feed
Ingredients per 100 ml							
Comminuted Chicken meat	g	7·5	15	22·5	30	30	30
Glucose polymer	g	5·0	5·0	5·0	5·0	10	10
50% vegetable oil emulsion*	ml	Nil	Nil	Nil	Nil	3	6
Mineral mixture†	g	0·2	0·4	0·6	0·8	0·8	1·0
Water (previously boiled)		to 100 ml	to 100 ml	to 100 ml	to 100 ml	to 100 ml	to 100 ml
Composition per 100 ml							
Protein	g	0·6	1·1	1·7	2·25	2·25	2·25
Carbohydrate	g	5·0	5·0	5·0	5·0	10	10
Fat	g	0·2	0·5	0·7	1·0	2·5	4·0
Energy	kcal	23	28	32	37	69	83
	kJ	98	117	135	155	291	346
Calcium	mmol (mg)	0·4(17)	0·9(34)	1·3(51)	1·7(68)	1·7(68)	2·1(85)
Sodium	mmol (mg)	0·4(9)	0·7(17)	1·1(26)	1·5(35)	1·5(35)	1·9(43)
Potassium	mmol (mg)	0·5(20)	1·1(41)	1·6(61)	2·1(81)	2·1(81)	2·5(98)
Renal solute load	mmol/100 ml	3	7	10	13	13	14
Osmolality	mmol/kg	78	106	134	159	221	247

* Prosparol (Duncan Flockhart), Calogen or Liquigen (SHS).
† Aminogran Mineral Mixture (Allen & Hanburys) or Metabolic Mineral Mixture (SHS).
Notes:
1 The progression from $\frac{1}{4}$ strength feeds to full-protein, high-energy feeds may take several weeks depending upon individual tolerance.
2 Glucose and/or fructose may be used if glucose polymer is not acceptable.
3 Higher levels of calcium may be obtained by the addition of calcium gluconate.
4 Proximate compositional data have been calculated by using the mid-range values for Cow & Gate Comminuted Chicken Meat.
5 Osmolality values refer to feeds prepared with glucose polymer and a fat source of 50% arachis oil dispersion in water.
6 Ketovite Tablets plus 5 ml Ketovite Liquid (Paines & Byrne) are essential as a comprehensive vitamin supplement.

introduced by grading onto a dilute frequent feeding regimen (Table 1.18). Providing i.v. fluid is not being given a volume of 200 ml/kg actual weight per day is recommended. During grading and introduction of oral feeds specific attention regarding the fluid and electrolyte intake must be given, and stool losses replaced to prevent dehydration and electrolyte depletion. All medicines should initially be carbohydrate- and sorbitol-free. Weaning solids are discontinued temporarily. The feed is increased in planned increments until an adequate nutrient oral intake is derived. Table 1.18 provides recipes for different strength feeds and three energy levels in the full-protein feed. Parenteral nutrition is proportionally decreased as the oral intake increases.

The feed should be fed from a large-holed infant feeding-bottle. The bottle should be shaken at intervals to ensure the chicken muscle fibres and minerals (which are present as a suspension and not a solution) are consumed. Although this feed can be given as a bolus enteral tube feed, as the chicken muscle fibres and minerals are in suspension, it cannot successfully be given as a continuous enteral feed.

Once the infant is established on the Comminuted Chicken-based feed a less frequent feeding schedule can be instigated and suitable solids for age introduced. Initially, weaning solids which are milk-free, lactose-free and sucrose-free (unless a specific diagnosis has been established) are selected. When coeliac disease is suspected, or cannot initially be differentiated from milk protein intolerance, gluten should also be avoided. Milk protein and gluten are introduced separately at a later date. Each new food should be introduced singly, and if tolerated given in the diet regularly thereafter.

Suitable solids include

1   Rice cereal mixed with water, 5% dextrose or the feed, e.g. Farex Weaning Cereal, Robinson's Baby Rice, Milupa *Plain* Rice Cereal.
2   Boiled potato (mashed milk-free) moistened with a suitable gravy, or a little Comminuted Chicken.
3   Vegetable purée (low-sucrose greens, e.g. runner beans, cauliflower, tomato, cabbage).
4   Purée meats cooked in their own juices.
5   Hard-boiled egg-yolk once the infant is over six months of age; then, if tolerated, milk-free scrambled egg can be given.
6   Most commercial baby foods are unsuitable as they contain milk and/or lactose. However, selected varieties can be introduced if appropriate.

Caution should be taken when introducing new foods in patients with atopic disease or those suspected to have multiple food sensitivities and food allergy.

Once the child is tolerating the feed well, small quantities of sucrose are usually tolerated and a selection of savoury milk-free, lactose-free and/or gluten-free baby foods may be introduced. Natural low-sucrose foods such as puréed unsweetened fruit and fruit juices could also be introduced. The feed intake should be adjusted to meet the infant's changing nutritional requirements and some infants can be transferred to a simpler formula before discharge.

Discharge arrangements for patients on Comminuted Chicken-based feeds

This regimen needs to be taught to the parents over several sessions before the feed can be made safely at home. The practical arrangements for home and teaching should be discussed well in advance of the patient's discharge, so ingredients can be measured appropriately in calibrated scoops, night feeds omitted and items on prescription arranged.

Follow-up is essential on this regimen and is best done where dietetic expertise is available. Once catch-up growth has occurred, the total energy and nutrient intake is gradually decreased to appetite and normal requirements; occasionally, secondary temporary obesity occurs. After a period of six weeks to six months, as is appropriate for the clinical circumstances, disaccharides, milk protein and finally a normal diet for age can usually be reintroduced.

Module feeds are difficult to prepare due to the multiple ingredients having to be measured and the risks involved should an error in preparation occur, e.g. hyperosmolality, hypoglycaemia, ketosis, electrolyte imbalance, nutritional inadequacy. This is particularly relevant in the home or where the facilities of a centralized milk kitchen are not available.

Variations of the Comminuted Chicken-based feed

Thickening.   Some infants benefit from a thickened feed, which helps slow down transit time and allows increased absorption. Patients who have had a gut resection or surgery on the intestine particularly benefit from a thickened feed, as do those with a hiatus hernia. The Comminuted Chicken-based feed can be thickened by the addition of starch, e.g. 2 to 4 g cornflour or arrowroot to each 100 ml feed, either in addition to, or as a replacement of, part of the carbohydrate. The starch must be cooked by boiling for two minutes in part of the water used for the feed preparation. The other ingredients are then carefully blended into the cooked starch mixture. Alternatively, the feed could be thickened with a hemicellulose preparation, Nestargel or Instant Carobel, 0.3 to 1 g per 100 ml of feed. These have no nutritional value, increase stool bulk and possibly interfere with absorption. It is preferable that the ingredients of the feed should not be cooked and hence are blended into the thickened water after cooking.

Glucose polymer and starch intolerance. Immature and very ill infants occasionally cannot hydrolyse and absorb these carbohydrates. They can be replaced with glucose and/or fructose. Because the latter increase the osmolality of the feed only 5%, to a maximum of 10%, carbohydrate should be added.

Glucose–galactose intolerance. The feed carbohydrate can be replaced with fructose as the added carbohydrate. A starch thickener is contraindicated, and a hemicellulose is the thickener of choice, should this be necessary. Alternative feeds are given in Table 1.15.

Steatorrhoea. Fat malabsorption in conjunction with multiple malabsorption can occur as a result of many of the causes of diarrhoea already described, due to liver disease, bile salt abnormalities and pancreatic enzyme deficiency, e.g. cystic fibrosis and Shwachman syndrome (Muller 1982). Where clinically indicated the fat content of the diet can be reduced by omitting the oil emulsion (Prosparol, Calogen) from the Comminuted Chicken-based feed and medium-chain triglycerides emulsion (Liquigen) can replace the energy deficit. Alternatively, an appropriate feed, Pregestimil, MCT Pepdite, Portagen or Flexical (Table 1.4), can be selected.

Alternative ingredients for module diets
The composition of various commercial products currently available in the United Kingdom is given in Table 1.6 from which various module diets can be devised. Alternative ingredients (Table 1.19) can be used; many are cheaper and readily available. However, precautions must be taken in preparing such ingredients, as bacterial contamination, particularly of frozen chicken and other meat, necessitates careful thawing, cooking and aseptic preparation of purées. Home-prepared purée meat mixtures are difficult to get through an infant feeding-bottle teat due to the muscle fibre size; chicken and rabbit have the finest muscle fibres. Chicken and turkey are higher in essential fatty acids than other meats, but lamb and beef are higher in fat quantity. Although pure honey is a useful alternative to glucose and fructose it can be contaminated with bacteria and contains various antigens, dependent on the pollen source. Egg is an excellent protein but is a common antigen and requires cooking, which helps to increase its absorption and destroys the antivitamin factor avidin.

New module products are continually coming onto the market (e.g. Cow & Gate, Nutricia, SHS) and must be assessed carefully for nutritional adequacy, particularly of trace nutrients, in the light of the latest

Table 1.19 Alternative ingredients for the Comminuted Chicken module feed.

Protein	30 g Comminuted Chicken (Cow & Gate) can be replaced with: 10 g cooked weight lean (minced) chicken, turkey breast or rabbit meat *or* 10 g cooked weight lean (minced) beef or lamb
Protein and fat	30 g Comminuted Chicken plus 2 ml oil emulsion (50%) can be replaced with: 20 g cooked egg (yolk and white)
Carbohydrate	10 g glucose polymer (Caloreen/Maxijul LE/Calonutrin) can be replaced with: 10 g glucose or fructose or sucrose *or* 14 g honey *or* 12 g starch (cornflour/arrowroot/rice powder)—must be cooked
Fat	8 ml 50% oil emulsion (Prosparol/Calogen/Liquigen) can be replaced with: 4 ml vegetable oil *or* 8 ml home-made 50% oil emulsion*

*   50 ml vegetable edible oil
     50 ml water (cold boiled)
     1 to 2 g edible gum, e.g. gum acacia

Liquidize to form a white stable emulsion. Make freshly every 2 to 3 days. Refrigerate until used.

knowledge regarding nutritional requirements and nutrient compatability, toxicity and bioavailability, particularly regarding trace elements.

Peptide- and amino acid-based module feeds

A feed based on hydrolysed proteins (Albumaid Complete), or newer peptide or L-amino acid modules can be devised similarly to the Comminuted Chicken-based feed and have proved useful in one or two children with multiple food intolerances.

Matthews (1971, 1975) has suggested that peptides may be more readily absorbed than L-amino acids in certain circumstances, and some peptides are absorbed intact. Ideally, preparations used should contain free amino acids and short-chain peptides of less than six amino acids, if whole protein is not tolerated. The biological value and the amino acid profile of the 'protein' should be compared to human milk when being considered for use in young infants. Albumaid Complete is a beef serum hydrolysate which does not have an optimal amino acid profile for growth in infancy.

These regimes should contain at least part of the fat intake as a vegetable oil emulsion such as Prosparol or Calogen to ensure provision of the essential fatty acid requirement, the basic requirement of which is provided by Comminuted Chicken in that regimen.

The Comminuted Chicken also contributes trace nutrients (e.g. zinc) which are absent in synthetic peptide amino acid mixtures (Lawson *et al.* 1977, Thorn *et al.* 1978) which therefore have to rely totally on commercial mineral and vitamin supplementation (*see* Francis 1986).

Complete carbohydrate or monosaccharide intolerance

A few infants have a temporary intolerance to all carbohydrates, including glucose, galactose and fructose, due usually to acute gastroenteritis and occasionally to gut resection or protracted diarrhoea. In these patients parenteral nutrition is recommended or at least intravenous carbohydrate should be given. A carbohydrate-free oral regimen can be used for a limited period of a few days.

If intravenous carbohydrate is not given the infant must be kept under observation, as hypoglycaemia, hypothermia and ketosis are serious risks (Lifshitz 1970). Frequent, e.g. four-hourly, blood sugar and electrolyte estimations should be made while the infant is on this regimen, and abnormalities imme-

diately corrected by suitable oral or intravenous supplements.

The above described feeds based on Comminuted Chicken (Tables 1.15, 1.18 and 1.19) or amino acid/peptide module feeds from which carbohydrate is temporarily omitted provide the basis of oral nutrition. Alternatively, CF1 (Nestlé International) or CHO Free (Syntex USA) can be used if available, but they contain cow's milk protein and, in the author's opinion, are less appropriate. Adequate energy cannot readily be given orally while the feed is carbohydrate-free. The total fat should not normally exceed the protein (and carbohydrate) content of any feed because of the risk of ketosis; medium-chain triglycerides are more ketogenic than dietary fats and oils.

As soon as clinical improvement occurs, or if intravenous carbohydrate cannot be maintained, glucose, glucose polymer or fructose should be reintroduced. An oral feed containing 0·5 to 1% carbohydrate should be tried initially in one or two feeds, then quickly increased to 5% and withdrawn immediately if there is ill effect. From the history and clinical evidence available glucose, glucose polymer or fructose may be chosen as the initial carbohydrate to introduce. Glucose polymers have the advantage of a lower osmolality than the monosaccharides. If there is no ill effect from the initial carbohydrate introduced, it can be increased cautiously, until the feed contains 5 to 10 g carbohydrate per 100 ml (5 to 10%) as tolerated clinically. A mixture of carbohydrates (e.g. half as glucose or glucose polymer and half as fructose) may be better tolerated in some patients. Once glucose and/or fructose is tolerated other carbohydrates can gradually be introduced, or a simpler feed tried, e.g. Pregestimil, Pepdite, in readiness for discharge.

Differential diagnosis between milk protein intolerance and lactose intolerance

The most important differential diagnosis for cow's milk protein intolerance is to distinguish this condition from lactose malabsorption. Usually this is impossible at the time of initial presentation as both may co-exist. Secondary lactose intolerance as a result of lactase deficiency can be caused by cow's milk protein intolerance (Harrison *et al.* 1976), particularly when it has occurred as a sequel to acute gastroenteritis. At the time of milk challenge it is practical and important to distinguish these two conditions. Visakorpi (1970) has described cow's milk protein intolerance as a transient accompaniment of coeliac disease, and transient gluten intolerance can accompany cow's milk intolerance, (Visakorpi 1970) or both can co-exist (Watt *et al.* 1983).

Cow's milk protein intolerance and lactose intolerance associated with gastroenteritis are nearly always temporary, although there is little documented information concerning the precise duration of these conditions (Walker-Smith 1979). On clinical grounds most children over two years, apart from those who have food allergic disease, are able to tolerate cow's milk without any untoward sequelae. Patients with secondary disaccharide intolerance recover more rapidly and a normal diet can be reintroduced as soon as clinically indicated. The majority can safely be challenged and graded onto a normal diet 2 to 3 months after the child starts to thrive and regain any previous weight loss. The timing of challenge with lactose and then cow's milk is arbitrary and varies from paediatrician to paediatrician. Secondary sucrose intolerance is even more transient, rarely necessitating treatment beyond days, or at most a few weeks.

Until recently the only satisfactory way to make the diagnosis of food intolerance was by clinical observation with repeated withdrawal and challenge with the offending foods associated with clinical remission and relapse (Goldman *et al.* 1963). This is still necessary for the diagnosis of other forms of food allergy and intolerance (*see* Chapter 4). These criteria have obvious drawbacks because (i) patients are reluctant to have repeated potentially hazardous challenges especially after one positive challenge, (ii) clinical relapse can be misleading, e.g. intercurrent infections can lead to misinterpretation of results, (iii) patients can take longer than 48 hours to relapse after a food challenge, and (iv) a positive challenge may not always have the same onset, duration and clinical features.

Serial small intestinal biopsies permit a firm diagnosis of cow's milk protein intolerance and similar enteropathies associated with foods (*see* Chapter 3 regarding coeliac disease). A variety of different proteins have been reported to cause mucosal damage (Vitoria *et al.* 1982), but cow's milk protein is the commonest cause, particularly in under-two-year-olds following gastroenteritis. A small intestinal biopsy is taken at the time of presentation at the first suspicion that symptoms are related to milk, after clinical response to milk withdrawal and after the return of symptoms following a milk challenge. If there is an abnormal mucosa in the first biopsy and clinical improvement on withdrawal of milk, a provisional diagnosis of cow's milk protein intolerance

can be made. The final diagnosis is confirmed by the return of a normal mucosa on milk withdrawal and relapse on milk challenge. However, at least some patients will have recovered spontaneously before the milk challenge and therefore the provisional diagnosis cannot be confirmed. Alternatively, some patients with a normal mucosa on milk challenge have clinical relapse and symptoms, in which case another cause of these symptoms must be sought, such as an intercurrent infection. Occasionally no other cause can be identified and cow's milk intolerance or allergy must be considered a possible diagnosis, particularly if clinical symptoms respond again to milk withdrawal.

In patients with atopic symptoms or other forms of food allergic disease, challenge with the offending item is essential to rule out placebo effect of the diet and to establish the subsequent maintenance diet needed. These patients may require long-term treatment on the appropriately devised maintenance diet, excluding foods which provoke symptoms on challenge. Such diets must be nutritionally adequate, monitored and modified continually. Rechallenge should be considered approximately yearly, and the need for diet reviewed, as many of these patients grow out of the need for diet after a period of time.

Various schemes are possible for the reintroduction of lactose, milk and sucrose. If lactose is tolerated, sucrose is usually tolerated, as sucrase is an extremely efficient enzyme, and a formal sucrose challenge is unnecessary. If lactose and milk intolerance are to be differentiated, each must be challenged separately.

Lactose reintroduction

The child should be clinically well at the time of challenge and intercurrent infections excluded.

(a) Replace part of the feed carbohydrate with lactose: initially replace 1%, then if there is no relapse of symptoms 3%, 5%, 7% in planned daily increments is replaced. This is difficult if the child is on a complete formula such as Pregestimil or Pepdite.

Or

(b) The child is fasted overnight and weighed, then given a lactose load of 2 g/kg to a maximum of 24 g lactose in 200 ml water. The patient is kept under observation, stools tested for sugars and all reactions recorded. No sooner than one hour after the lactose load, suitable milk-free solids may be given and the child allowed to drink a 7% lactose solution, with or without electrolyte supplements as appropriate, for 24 hours. Vomiting, diarrhoea and excessive stool sugars indicate lactose is not yet tolerated. Failure to reintroduce lactose on several occasions may suggest primary lactase deficiency, in which case traces of lactose are usually tolerated after infancy but must be assessed individually. Patients who have no adverse reaction to lactose can then have a milk challenge.

Cow's milk challenge and reintroduction
The procedure varies according to previous history (*see* above and Chapter 4) and no standard procedure has been devised. The following guidelines have proved useful in the author's experience:

1   *Patients who have had a previous anaphylactic reaction (collapse, hypotension, loss of consciousness) or respiratory obstruction.*   All such children should be admitted to hospital at least as a day case on a medical ward for challenge with the specific food that previously provoked or was suspected of causing such a reaction. It is suggested that at least a year should elapse before such reintroduction is attempted, and 'blind' challenge is contraindicated. The precaution of an intravenous infusion set up before the challenge may be advisable. Resuscitation equipment, adrenaline and an anaesthetist should be available, and the patient should be under observation. It is suggested that a skin prick test should be done first; a very severe reaction may indicate special caution and perhaps deferring the challenge. If there is no, or only a mild, skin reaction, initially 1 ml of 1:20 dilution of milk is given orally. If a reaction such as swelling, itching, redness, pain occurs, or of course if anaphylaxis occurs, no further milk is given. The patient and his parents should be advised to exclude *all* sources of milk protein from the diet, an appropriate milk substitute should be prescribed, and the parents should be instructed on how to interpret food labels. If anaphylaxis has occurred the parents should be supplied with adrenaline for home use and instructed in its administration in the case of an accidental ingestion of milk or milk-containing food.

If no reaction occurs from the initial test dose of milk within 20 to 30 minutes, anaphylaxis is unlikely, though not entirely ruled out (David 1984), and a severe reaction can still occur later. A further test dose after one hour of 1 ml full-strength milk is administered and the patient kept under observation. Thereafter, frequent, rapidly increasing doses are given, reaching the normal quantity by approxi-

mately the fourth day, e.g. $\frac{1}{4}$, $\frac{1}{2}$, $\frac{3}{4}$, full-strength feeds in daily increments, provided no abnormal reaction occurs. In infants, after the first few test doses a modified infant formula can be used, decreasing other milk substitute feeds accordingly.

After successful reintroduction the patient should take milk as part of his regular diet. Some patients may develop symptoms, e.g. vomiting, diarrhoea, or skin rash, in hours or days after reintroduction of milk; withdrawal may then be necessary. Other causes of these symptoms should be excluded. If gastrointestinal symptoms occur a further jejunal biopsy is useful, and if the previously normal mucosa is now abnormal a firm diagnosis of cow's milk protein intolerance is made and a milk-free diet reinstigated.

2   *Those who have had other reactions to milk, e.g. diarrhoea, vomiting, eczema, etc.*   If the previous reaction was severe the first dose of milk should be at the hospital under supervision of medical and nursing staff, and resuscitation equipment should be available. A period of dietary elimination of a food allergen may heighten the severity of a reaction on its subsequent reintroduction (David 1984). If a milk challenge is planned at home it is advisable that two adults are present for the first few hours and are instructed regarding appropriate action in the case of a severe reaction occurring. It is wise to inform the family doctor before the milk is given. Initially administer 5 ml undiluted milk orally. If no reaction occurs within 20 to 30 minutes a marked reaction is unlikely, though subsequent reaction may occur, and if so milk should again be withdrawn. If no reaction occurs a second test dose is given after one hour and thereafter frequent, rapidly increasing, quantities of milk or modified infant feed are given, reaching the normal quantity in approximately four days, e.g. $\frac{1}{4}$, $\frac{1}{2}$, $\frac{3}{4}$, full-strength milk in daily increments. If the introduction is successful milk should then be included in the diet regularly. If a reaction occurs once other causes of the reaction such as intercurrent infections have been ruled out, withdrawal of milk may again be necessary. If there is doubt regarding the interpretation of symptoms a double-blind challenge can be used to confirm the diagnosis.

3   *Other children at risk, e.g. children who have not had a food allergic reaction but who have been on milk elimination diets, e.g. those on special feeds such as Pregestimil or soya formula post-surgery or post-gastroenteritis.*   The mother could introduce milk at home. A test dose of 5 ml (1 teaspoon) of milk is given

initially. Thereafter the quantity of milk or infant formula is gradually increased over a four-day period, provided no adverse reaction occurs. It is wise to inform the family doctor before the milk is given and for two adults to be present for the first few hours after the test dose. If the introduction is successful milk should then be included in the diet regularly.

Other food challenges
Reintroduction is carried out similarly for the same three categories described for cow's milk, but with test doses of 1 to 5 c.c. of the respective food, gradually increasing to a normal size serve for the child's age.

Sucrose reintroduction
Sucrose occurs naturally in many basic foods, such as fruit and vegetables. It is introduced to the diet in this form, e.g. fruit purée and juice, etc. Added sugar can then be permitted. If lactose is tolerated then invariably sucrose will also be tolerated, since secondary lactose intolerance persists longer than secondary sucrose intolerance. Failure to tolerate sucrose on several occasions may suggest primary sucrase–isomaltase deficiency (*see* p. 8).

Gluten reintroduction
It is essential to reintroduce gluten, usually as normal wheat-containing food, after a period of exclusion in order to confirm the diagnosis of coeliac disease, wheat allergy or transient intolerance. Pre- and post-challenge jejunal biopsies to distinguish milk intolerance and coeliac disease may be indicated. However, not all patients with milk intolerance or wheat allergy have mucosal changes, e.g. those with atopic eczema, asthma. In coeliacs diagnosed by an initial jejunal biopsy, confirmation by rechallenge of gluten- or wheat-containing food with pre- and post-jejunal biopsy is necessary to establish the diagnosis of the life-long condition (*see* Chapter 3). The optimal age for challenge is a matter of opinion, as is the time of the post-challenge biopsy.

Follow-up. This is essential for a period of time after reintroduction of a normal diet in case of relapse or subsequent poor growth. The diet of children who fail to tolerate one or other of the above challenges should be assessed and simplified, and follow-up planned accordingly, and primary intolerance or food allergic disease should be considered.

TODDLER DIARRHOEA AND FUNCTIONAL BOWEL DISEASE

Toddler diarrhoea, variously known as non-specific diarrhoea or irritable colon syndrome (Davidson & Wasserman 1966), has been recently reviewed by Walker-Smith (1980) and Fenton *et al.* (1983). It usually presents between 6 and 20 months of age and before three years, and has intermittent gastrointestinal symptoms of abdominal pain and diarrhoea, without growth failure, for which no obvious cause is found. Boys are more frequently affected than girls. Symptoms are often attributed to emotional disturbance and treated by behavioural therapy (Howarth 1977).

Symptoms only tend to occur during waking hours and are intermittent. The stools are loose and/or watery and contain mucus and undigested food remnants, but the child's growth is not affected. A past history of infantile colic and a family history of bowel disorders is common.

Tripp *et al.* (1978) have found evidence of an increased enzyme activity for adenyl cyclase and Na^+, K^+-ATPase in small intestinal biopsy, though the intestinal mucosa morphology was normal.

Dietary regimens which have been claimed to be effective include addition of dietary fat (Lloyd-Still 1979), removal of different carbohydrate(s), or increased dietary fibre (Burman *et al.* 1982) to keep the stools soft, together with encouragement of normal bowel habits and behavioural therapy. Some workers have suspected food allergic disease, especially when recurrent abdominal pain is a feature (Letters 1973). Most recommendations for treatment concentrate on support for the family and warn of the dangers of overinvestigation and unnecessary diets (Walker-Smith 1979, Fenton *et al.* 1983).

INFLAMMATORY BOWEL DISEASE (IBD)— CROHN'S AND COLITIS

Children and infants with IBD differ from adults with these conditions, primarily because they are growing and therefore produce differing symptoms and management problems (Booth & Harries 1984). The more important causes of IBD in children are similar to those in adults, with the exception of food allergy, which is an important and underestimated cause of colitis in infancy (*see* p. 44).

There is evidence that there has been a recent increase in the incidence of Crohn's disease. This increase has occurred in all ages, and in the U.K., in contrast to ulcerative colitis, has been associated with a growing mortality rate (Booth & Harries 1984). No single environmental factor has been implicated for this increased incidence (Sacher *et al.* 1980).

In contrast to Crohn's disease the incidence of ulcerative colitis has not changed. Although the incidence of both is currently somewhat similar, there is a difference between ulcerative colitis and Crohn's disease in the distribution of age at presentation, such that more Crohn's disease is seen in paediatrics (Booth & Harries 1984).

Crohn's disease

Crohn's disease is a chronic inflammatory disorder that may affect any part of the alimentary tract with a characteristic pattern of clinical and pathological features (Lennard Jones 1970). Involvement of the jejunum and ileum is often extensive and this is more common in children than adults (Walker-Smith 1979). The lesions are discontinuous along the alimentary tract with so-called 'skip' areas; fistulas and anal lesions are common.

Clinical features of Crohn's disease classically include pain, fever, diarrhoea, growth reduction, anorexia and anaemia (O'Donaghue & Dawson 1977). The abrupt onset of symptoms usually leads to an immediate and correct diagnosis. However, the onset is often insidious and the correct diagnosis may be delayed for months or years (O'Donaghue & Dawson 1977), and considerable growth retardation may have occurred as a result of both an inadequate nutritional intake and the nutrient losses associated with the condition. Growth failure occurs in 30% of children with Crohn's disease (Kelts *et al.* 1979) and weight is usually appropriate for height.

Diagnosis is made by macro- and microscopic examination of the colon, currently by colonoscopy which should be performed in children by a skilled paediatric endoscopist.

MANAGEMENT OF CROHN'S DISEASE AND COLITIS

The aim of treatment is to induce and maintain remission in both conditions. This is more easily achieved in ulcerative colitis than Crohn's disease. Nutritional measures are extremely important in both diseases, but particularly in Crohn's disease, where the growth failure may respond favourably to the introduction of nutritional repletion (Kirschner *et al.* 1981) and remission may be induced (O'Morain *et al.* 1982).

Surgery is reserved for patients with complications such as obstruction, toxic megacolon, fistulae and abscesses, together with those whose symptoms do not respond to medical treatment, particularly if associated with growth failure (Booth & Harries 1984).

Short-term corticosteroid therapy is appropriate in children with severe Crohn's disease. However, long-term corticosteroids carry a serious risk of iatrogenic growth retardation, although this may be reduced by alternate-day treatment without losing remission. Sulphasalazine is used in patients with colonic involvement, and immunosuppressive therapy with azathioprine in children with symptomatic Crohn's disease has proved useful (Booth & Harries 1984).

NUTRITION

Nutritional support is important in two respects. Increased intakes of nitrogen and energy, enterally or parenterally if necessary, may have a specific role in the management of not only the inflammatory process, but also growth failure. Nutritional measures also play an important part in the restoration of specific nutritional deficits commonly seen in Crohn's disease (Booth & Harries 1984).

1 The poor nutritional status of children with Crohn's disease is due to:

(a) Decreased intake. Kirschner *et al.* (1981) found the mean energy intake to be only 56% of recommended intakes for age and height, whereas the protein intakes were within the recommended range, and Kelts *et al.* (1979) reported energy intakes of 82% compared to recommended intakes. Reduced intake may be due to anorexia, nausea, bolus pain following food, or in some cases zinc deficiency producing a loss of taste sensation (McClain *et al.* 1980).

(b) Impaired absorption as a result of a widespread mucosal abnormality, stagnant loops, fistulae, disordered motility or gut resection.

(c) Increased losses of blood and intestinal protein are common. Faecal nitrogen excretion is raised, but is not increased following dietary supplementation, suggesting the abnormality is due to mucosal losses and not protein malabsorption (Motil *et al.* 1982). Catabolism during corticosteroid treatment also causes increased nitrogen losses.

2 Enteral or parenteral nutrition improves nutritional status in IBD, and in adults parenteral nutri-

tion can induce remission of symptoms in 80% of patients (Driscoll & Rosenberg 1978) but the remission may be short-lived. Parenteral nutrition in 17 paediatric patients (Strobel *et al.* 1979) with severe symptomatic Crohn's disease treated at home showed symptomatic improvement and weight gain, and 10 had catch-up growth in height. Remission occurred in 12 patients and this was long-term in four patients after the first course of parenteral nutrition. Enteric protein loss was high following treatment in those who had early relapse, whereas it became normal in those who had long-term remission, suggesting this investigation is a useful predictor of possible outcome (Booth & Harries 1984).

Elemental diets (*see* Chapter 2) have also received a considerable amount of attention in the management of IBD (Navarro *et al.* 1977), but most reported series are uncontrolled trials. Remission can be induced, and malnutrition, anaemia and hypoalbuminaemia corrected. There is no good evidence that nitrogen retention is less with whole-protein diets with the same energy value than with elemental diets (Moriarty *et al.* 1981). There is preliminary evidence to suggest that nutritional restitution, using an elemental diet, in patients with Crohn's disease in relapse is equally as effective in inducing remission as prednisolone treatment (O'Morain *et al.* 1982). Thus, elemental diets, despite being unpalatable and in some patients precipitating diarrhoea, provide a convenient method of achieving improved nutritional status and may also represent a means of inducing remission without the hazards of steroid therapy (Booth & Harries 1984).

Growth can be improved in children with Crohn's disease by a period of either parenteral nutrition (Kelts *et al.* 1979) or enteral feeding (Kirschner *et al.* 1981). An extended period, over one year, of improved growth followed only an eight-week period of parenteral nutrition (Kelts *et al.* 1979). Artificial supplementation is, however, not essential. Kirschner and colleagues used an elemental diet for 12 months in seven children, six of whom thereafter received only conventional foods. During a follow-up period of four years the energy intake was boosted from 56% to 91% of the recommended intake for height, and five of the children had improved growth, such that their height came within 5% of their pre-illness height centile.

Adequate nutritional support is therefore essential in children with Crohn's disease. We reserve parenteral nutrition for patients with severe malnutrition, patients in whom medical treatment has failed and are unsuitable for surgery, or to improve nutrition pre- and post-surgery. In our patients we have mostly used an enteral low-antigen hydrolysate formula which is nutritionally adequate, e.g., in the past, Pregestimil and/or Flexical, but some of the newer more palatable formulae, such as the Pepdite range, are now being evaluated. A suitable product is selected (Table 2.9) depending on the child's age and individual nutritional needs. Nutritional supplements are added as necessary. The feed is usually administered as a continuous nasogastric or nasojejunal feed with an enteral pump. The Viomedex paediatric equipment is useful, and the battery-operated portable shoulder carrying pack allows patient mobility.

We currently select a low-antigen formula in preference to a milk-based feed because of the theoretical increased risk of these patients having or acquiring intolerance or allergy (Jones *et al.* 1985). After a period of total enteral feeding, conventional foods (initially low-antigen, e.g. milk- and egg-free) are permitted and the enteral feed is gradually reduced to an overnight supplement, once oral intake is adequate to meet the nutritional requirements. Some patients will take these formulae orally from either an infant feeding-bottle, or teacher beaker or with a straw, appropriately flavoured according to individual preference. It should be remembered that some flavourings will increase the feed osmolality to unacceptable levels, and others contain various antigens (e.g. tartrazine) which may be contraindicated for these patients.

The regimen can be continued at home once the child is in remission, and supplements are discontinued only once adequate conventional foodstuff is being taken to permit catch-up growth.

3 Specific deficiencies. Iron deficiency is occasionally seen due to a poor intake, malabsorption and/or intestinal loss. It should be differentiated from the normochromic anaemia seen in patients with chronic inflammatory disorders. Sulphasalazine therapy, together with malabsorption, can cause folate deficiency. Vitamin B_{12} absorption is impaired, as a result of terminal ileal disease, in 50% of children with Crohn's disease, although serum B_{12} level are rarely low. Appropriate supplements should be administered.

Zinc deficiency in Crohn's disease is probably common and is associated with depressed taste sensation (McClain *et al.* 1980). Cell-mediated immunity is impaired in association with zinc deficiency and characteristic eczematous rashes have been described in some adult patients with Crohn's disease. However, the relationship between zinc deficiency, impaired taste sensation and growth failure in Crohn's disease has not been clearly defined. Measurement of plasma zinc and alkaline phosphatase activity (which is depressed in zinc deficiency) should be performed in all patients, and zinc supplements administered in those in whom these parameters are low (Aggett & Harries 1979).

Ulcerative colitis

Fulminating colitis, possibly with toxic megacolon, is the presenting feature in approximately 10% of children. However, ulcerative colitis most frequently presents with an insidious onset of mild diarrhoea, with or without bleeding. Severity of the acute disease depends on the anatomical extent of the inflammation and the depth of the ulceration. The inflammation may affect only the rectum or any proportion of the rectum and colon. Growth failure, although a major problem in children with ulcerative colitis, is less common than in Crohn's disease.

Liver disease may be the sole presenting feature of IBD in children and therefore liver disease of unknown aetiology should be investigated with respect to possible IBD (Booth & Harries 1984).

MANAGEMENT OF ULCERATIVE COLITIS

Medical treatment is aimed at inducing and maintaining a remission. Nutritional support is necessary if there is growth failure. Topical and systemic steroids, together with sulphasalazine, are used in children in the same manner as in adults, but children are more likely to have active and more extensive disease than adults. Long-term corticosteroids administered on alternate days may lessen growth suppression, but a child requiring a dose sufficiently high to produce side-effects usually benefits from a colectomy. A colectomy is curative, but the optimal timing and the possible psychological effects of an ileostomy must be balanced with the dangers of long-term ill health and cumulative effects of treatment (Booth & Harries 1984).

The severity of fulminating colitis in childhood is easily underestimated, and as a result referral to an experienced centre is delayed (Booth & Harries 1984). All require intravenous fluids and electrolytes, and many require blood transfusion and frequent albumin infusion. The majority come to surgery sooner rather than later (Werlin & Grand 1977). The severest complication is toxic megacolon and the experience of Booth and Harries (1984) shows that all children with this complication require surgery.

Allergic colitis in infants

In contrast to colitis occurring in adults and older children, food allergy appears to play an important role in colitis in infancy and accounts for what previously appeared to be an increased incidence of ulcerative colitis in the first year of life. Jenkins *et al.* (1982) reported eight such infants who were seen at the Hospitals for Sick Children, London, in three years. The infants presented with bloody diarrhoea after the introduction of artificial feeds. Six of the eight infants were under four months of age at presentation and prompt remission of symptoms occurred when a low-antigen elimination diet was introduced. Cow's milk protein was the most common offending antigen, but sensitivity to beef and soya was also demonstrated. There was a strong family history of atopy and the presence of IgE anticow's milk antibody and eosinophilia. Colonoscopy macroscopic appearance of the colon was indistinguishable from ulcerative colitis, but there was a marked increase in eosinophils in the lamina propria. Differential diagnosis is important, and provided the condition is recognized and appropriately treated with an exclusion diet and a milk substitute such as Pregestimil the prognosis appears to be excellent (Booth & Harries 1984). Further details regarding food allergy are given in Chapter 4.

PATIENT SUPPORT GROUP

The National Association for Colitis and Crohn's disease, 3 Thorpefield Close, Marshalswick, St. Albans, Herts., provides information on these diseases and parent/patient support.

REFERENCES
AGGETT P.J. & DAVIES N.T. (1983) Some nutritional aspects of trace metals. *J. Inherited Metabolic Disease* 6, Suppl. I, 22–30.
AGGETT P.J. & HARRIES J.T. (1979) Current status of zinc in health and disease. *Arch. Dis. Childh.* 54, 909–17.
AMENT M.E. & PERERA D.R. (1973) Sucrase–isomaltase deficiency—a frequently misdiagnosed disease. *J. Pediat.* 83, 721.
AMENT M.E. & RUBIN C.E. (1972) Soy protein—another cause of the flat intestinal lesion. *Gastroenterology* 62, 227–34.
ANDERSON C.M. (1970) Malabsorption in childhood. In *Modern Trends in Paediatrics*, 3rd Edition (ed. Apley J.), p. 216. London: Butterworths.
ANDERSON C.M., KERRY K.R. & TOWNLEY R.R. (1965) An inborn defect in intestinal absorption of certain monosaccharides. *Arch. Dis. Childh.* 40, 1–6.

ANTONOWICZ I., LLOYD-STILL J.D., KHAW K.T. & SHWACHMAN H. (1972) Congenital sucrase–isomaltase deficiency. Observations over a period of six years. *Pediatrics* 49, 847–53.

AURICCHIO S., DAHLQUIST A., MURSET G. & PARKER A. (1963) Isomaltose intolerance causing decreased ability to utilize dietary starch. *J. Pediat.* 62, 165–76.

BARTROP R.W. & HULL D. (1973) Transient lactose intolerance in infancy. *Arch. Dis. Childh.* 48, 963.

BOOTH I.W. & HARRIES J.T. (1982a) Oral rehydration therapy: an issue of growing controversy. *J. trop. Pediat.* 28 (No. 3), 116–23.

BOOTH I.W. & HARRIES J.T. (1982b) Parenteral nutrition in young children. *Brit. J. Intravenous Therapy* 3, 31–40.

BOOTH I.W. & HARRIES J.T. (1984) Inflammatory bowel disease in childhood—progress report. *Gut* 25 (No. 2), 188–202.

BOOTH I.W., LEVINE M.M. & HARRIES J.T. (1984) Oral rehydration therapy in acute diarrhoea: medical progress. *J. pediat. Gastoenterol. Nutr.* 3, 491–9.

BURKE V. & ANDERSON C.M. (1966) Sugar intolerance as a cause of protracted diarrhoea following surgery of the gastrointestinal tract in neonates. *Aust. Paediat. J.* 2, 114.

BURMAN D., PERHAM T.G.M. & CLOTHIER C. (1982) Nutrition in systemic disease. In *Textbook of Paediatric Nutrition*, 2nd Edition (eds. McLaren D.S. & Burman D.), p. 353. Edinburgh: Churchill Livingstone.

CANDY D.C., LARCHER V.F., CAMERON D.J.S., NORMAN A.P., TRIPP J.H., MILLA P.J., PINCOTT J.R. & HARRIES J.T. (1981) Lethal familial protracted diarrhoea. *Arch. Dis. Childh.* 56, 15–26.

CATFORD J.C. (1980) Quality of prescribing for children in general practice. *Brit. med. J.* 280, 1435–7.

CIBA FOUNDATION SYMPOSIUM 70 (1979) *Development of Mammalian Absorption Processes.* Amsterdam: Excerpta Medica.

CLAYTON B.E., ARTHUR A.B. & FRANCIS D.E. (1966) Early dietary management of sugar intolerance in infancy. *Brit. med. J.* 2, 679–82.

CLEMENTS M.L., LEVINE M.M., CLEAVES F., HUGHES T.P., CACERES M., ALEMAN E., BLACK R.E. & RUST J. (1981) Comparison of simple sugar/salt versus glucose/electrolyte oral rehydration solution in infant diarrhoea. *J. trop. Med. Hyg.* 84, 189–94.

COOMBS R.R.A. Chairman (1980) Clinical manifestations workshop summary. *Proceedings of the First Food Allergy Workshop*, p. 45. Medical Education Services Ltd.

COOPER A., BETTS J.M., PEREIRA G.R. & ZIEGLER M.M. (1984) Taurine deficiency in the severe hepatic dysfunction complicating total parenteral nutrition. *J. pediat. Surg.* 19, 462–5.

CORNBLATH M. & SCHWARTZ R. (1976) Disorders of carbohydrate metabolism in infancy. In *Major Problems in Clinical Paediatrics*, Vol. III. 2nd Edition (ed. Shaffer A.). Philadelphia: W.B. Saunders.

COUNAHAN R. & WALKER-SMITH J.A. (1976) Stool and urinary sugars in normal neonate. *Arch. Dis. Childh.* 51, 517–20.

DAVID T.J. (1984) Anaphylactic shock during elimination diets for severe atopic eczema. *Arch. Dis. Childh.* 59, 983–6.

DAVIDSON M., KUGLER M.M. & BAUER C. (1963) Diagnosis and management in children with severe and protracted constipation and obstipation. *J. Pediat.* 62, 261–75.

DESJEUX J.F., SASSIER P., TICHET J., SARRUT S. & LESTRADET H. (1973) Sugar absorption in flat jejunal mucosa. *Acta. paediat. scand.* 62, 531.

DHSS (1974) *Present day practice in infant feeding.* London: HMSO.

DHSS (1980) *Artificial feeds for the young infant*, Report No. 20. London: HMSO.

DHSS (1981) *The collection and storage of human milk*, Report No. 22. London: HMSO.

DHSS (1983 revision) *Present day practice in infant feeding*, Report No. 18 (1980). London: HMSO.

DRISCOLL R.H. & ROSENBERG I.H. (1978) Total parenteral nutrition in inflammatory bowel disease. *Med. Clin. N. Amer.* 62, 185–201.

DUGDALE A., LOVELL S., GIBBS V. & BALL D. (1982) Refeeding after acute gastroenteritis: a controlled study. *Arch. Dis. Childh.* 57, 76–8.

DURAND P. (1958) Lattosuria idiopatica in una paziente con diarrea cronica ed acidosi. *Minerva Pediat.* 10, 706.

EBRAHIM G.J. (1977) Parasitic infections. In *Essentials of Paediatric Gastroenterology* (ed. Harries J.T.). Edinburgh: Churchill Livingstone.

EDITORIAL (1983) Management of acute diarrhoea. *Lancet* 1, 623–5.

FENTON T.R., HARRIES J.T. & MILLA P.J. (1983) Disordered small intestinal motility: a rational basis for toddler diarrhoea. *Gut* 24, 897–903.

FINBERG L. (1980) The role of oral electrolyte solutions in hydration of children: international and domestic aspects. *J. Pediat.* 96, 51–4.

FRANCIS D.E.M. (1978) Treatment of multiple malabsorption syndrome of infancy. *J. hum. Nutr.* 32, 270–8.

FRANCIS D.E.M. (1986) *Nutrition for Children.* Oxford: Blackwell Scientific Publications.

FRIEDMAN H.I. & NYLAND B. (1980) Intestinal fat digestion, absorption and transport: a review. *Amer. J. clin. Nutr.* 33, 1108–39.

GARDINER A.J., TARLOW M.J., SYMONDS J. & HUTCHINSON J.G. (1981a) Failure of hydrogen breath test to detect primary sugar inabsorption. *Arch. Dis. Childh.* 56, 368.

GARDINER A.J., TARLOW M.J., SUTHERLAND I.T. & SAMMONS H.G. (1981b) Lactose malabsorbtion during gastroenteritis assessed by hydrogen breath test. *Arch. Dis. Childh.* 56, 364–7.

GOLDMAN A.S., ANDERSON D.W., SELLERS W., SAPERSTEIN S., KNIKER W.T. & HALPERN S.R. (1963) Milk allergy. *Pediatrics* 32, 425.

GRAND R.J., WATKINS J.B. & TORTI F.M. (1976) Development of the human gastrointestinal tract: a review. *Gastroenterology* 70, 790–810.

GRAY G.M. (1975) Carbohydrate digestion and absorption. *New Engl. J. Med.* 292, 1225.

GRIBBINS M., WALKER-SMITH J.A. & WOOD C.R.S (1973)

Delayed recovery following acute gastroenteritis. *Acta. paediat. belg.* **29**, 167.

GROTTE G., MEURLING S. & WRESTLIND A. (1982) Parenteral nutrition. In *Textbook of Paediatric Nutrition*, 2nd Edition (eds. McLaren D.S. & Burman D.), pp. 228–58. Edinburgh: Churchill Livingstone.

HABTE D., STERK G.C. & HJALMARSSON B. (1973) Lactose malabsorption in Ethiopian children. *Acta paediat. scand.* **62**, 649.

HANSON J.D.L., BUCHANAN N. & PETTIFOR J. (1982) Protein energy malnutrition. In *Textbook of Paediatric Nutrition*, 2nd Edition (eds. McLaren D.S. & Burman D.), pp. 114–42. Edinburgh: Churchill Livingstone.

HARRIES J.T. (ed.) (1977) *Essentials of Paediatric Gastroenterology*. Edinburgh: Churchill Livingstone.

HARRIES J.T. (ed). (1982a) *Clinics in Gastroenterology*. Philadelphia: W.B. Saunders.

HARRIES J.T. (1982b) Fat absorption in the new born. *Acta paediat. scand.* **299**, 17–23.

HARRIES J.T. & FRANCIS D.E.M. (1968) Temporary monosaccharide intolerance. *Acta paediat. scand.* **57**, 6, 505.

HARRIES J.T. & MULLER D.R.R. (1980) Basic causes of carbohydrate malabsorption. In *Inherited Disorders of Carbohydrate Metabolism* (eds. Burman D., Holten J.B. & Pennock C.A.). Lancaster: MPT Press.

HARRISON B.M., KILBY A., WALKER-SMITH J.A., FRANCE N.E. & WOOD C.B.S. (1976) Cow's milk protein intolerance: a possible association with gastroenteritis, lactose intolerance and IgA deficiency. *Brit. med. J.* **1**, 1501.

HARRISON M. (1974) Sugar malabsorption in cow's milk protein intolerance. *Lancet* **1**, 360.

HENDRATH L. (1978) Spoons for making glucose–salt solution. *Lancet* **1**, 612.

HOLMES G.E., HASSANEIN K.M. & MILLER H.C. (1983) Factors associated with infections among breast fed babies and babies fed proprietary milks. *Pediatrics* **72**, 300–6.

HOLZEL A., SCHWARTZ V.. & SUTCLIFFE K.W. (1959) Defective lactose absorption causing malnutrition in infancy. *Lancet* **1**, 1126.

HOSKOVA A., SABACKY J., MRSKOS A. & POSPISIL R. (1980) Severe lactose intolerance with lactosuria and vomiting. *Arch. Dis. Childh.* **55**, 304–16.

HOWARTH R.V. (1977) Gastrointestinal symptoms related to psychological disturbances. In *Essentials of Paediatric Gastroenterology* (ed. Harries J.T.), pp. 235–47. Edinburgh: Churchill Livingstone.

HUGHES C.A. & DOWLING R.H. (1980) Speed of onset of adaptive mucosal hypoplasia and hypofunction in the intestine of parenterally fed rats. *Clin. Sci.* **59**, 317–27.

HUGHES C.A., PRINCE A. & DOWLING R.H. (1980) Speed of change of pancreatic mass and intestinal bacteriology of parenterally fed rats. *Clin. Sci.* **59**, 329–36.

JELLIFFE D.R. & JELLIFFE E.F. (1978) The weanling dilemma. *Lancet* **1**, 611.

JENKINS H.R., MILLA P.J., PINCOTT J.R., SOOTHILL J.F. & HARRIES J.T. (1982) Food allergy: the major cause of infantile colitis? *Gut* **23**, A924.

JOHNSON J.D., SIMOONS F.J., HURWITZ R., GRANGE A., MITCHELL C.H., SINATRA F.R., SURCHIN P., ROBERTSON W.V., BENNETT P.H. & KRETCHMER N. (1977) Lactose malabsorption among the Pima Indians of Arizona. *Gastroenterology* **73**, 1299–1304.

JONES R.H.T. (1964) Disaccharide intolerance and mucoviscidosis. *Lancet* **2**, 120–1.

JONES V.A., WORKMAN E., FREEMAN A.H., DICKINSON R.J., WILSON A.J. & HUNTER J.O. (1985) Crohn's disease. Maintenance of remission by diet. *Lancet* **2**, 177–80.

KELTS D.G., GRAND R.J., SHEN G., WATKINS J.B., WERLIN S.L. & BOEHME C. (1979) Nutritional basis of growth failure in children and adolescents with Crohn's disease. *Gastroenterology* **76**, 720–7.

KERRY K.R. & ANDERSON C.M. (1964) A ward test for sugar in faeces. *Lancet* **1**, 981.

KINGSTON M.E. (1973) Biochemical disturbances in breast fed infants with gastroenteritis and dehydration. *J. Pediat.* **82**, 1073.

KILBY A., WALKER-SMITH J.A. & WOOD C.B.S. (1976) Studies on the immunoglobin containing cells and intraepithelial lymphocytes in the small intestinal mucosa of infants with post-gastroenteritis syndrome. *Aust. paediat. J.* **12**, 241.

KIRSCHNER B.S., KLICH J.R., KALMAN S.S., DE FAVARO M.V. & ROSENBERG I.H. (1981) Reversal of growth retardation in Crohn's disease with therapy emphasising oral nutrition restitution. *Gastroenterology* **80**, 10–15.

KRAFT S.C. (1979) Inflammatory bowel disease (ulcerative colitis and Crohn's disease). In *Immunity of the Gastrointestinal Tract* (ed. Asquith P.), p. 95. Edinburgh: Churchill Livingstone.

LARCHER V.F., SHEPHERD R., FRANCIS D.E.M. & HARRIES J.T. (1977) Protracted diarrhoea in infancy—analysis of 82 cases with particular reference to diagnosis and management. *Arch. Dis. Childh.* **52**, 597–605.

LAWSON M.S., CLAYTON B.E. & DELVES H.T. (1977) Evaluation of new mineral and trace metal supplement for use with synthetic diets. *Arch. Dis. Childh.* **52**, 62–7.

LENNARD JONES J.E. (1970) Crohn's disease. In *Modern Trends in Gastroenterology* (eds. Card W.C. & Creamer B.) London: Butterworth.

LETTERS (1973) Recurrent abdominal pain. Recurrent controversy. *Pediatrics* **51**, 307 and **52**, 144.

LEVIN B., ABRAHAM J.M., BURGESS E.A. & WALLIS P.G. (1970) Congenital lactose malabsorption. *Arch. Dis. Childh.* **45**, 173.

LIFSHITZ F., COELLO-RAMIREZ P. & GUTIÉRREZ-TOPETE G. (1970) Monosaccharide intolerance and hypoglycaemia in infants with diarrhoea I and II *J. Pediat.* **77**(4), 595–603 and 604–12.

LINDOUIST B.. MEEUWISSE G.W. & MELIN K. (1962) Glucose–galactose malabsorption. *Lancet* **2**, 666.

LLOYD J.K. (1970) *Nutrition* **24**, 162.

LLOYD STILL J.D. (1979) Chronic diarrhoea in childhood and misuse of elimination diets. *J. Pediat.* **95**, 10–13.

LUCAS A. (1984) Hormones, nutrition and the gut. In *Neonatal Gastroenterology: Contemporary Issues* (eds. Tanner M.S. & Stocks R.J.). Newcastle upon Tyne: Intercept.

McClain C., Souter C. & Zieve L. (1980) Zinc deficiency: a complication of Crohn's disease. *Gastroenterology* 78, 272–9.

McLaughlin P., Anderson K.J., Widdowson E.M. & Coombs R.R.A. (1981) Effect of heat on the anaphylactic-sensitising capacity of cow's milk, goat's milk, and various infant formulae fed to guinea pigs. *Arch. Dis. Childh.* 56, 165–171.

McNeish A.S. & Harran M.J. (1980) Clinical aspects of disordered carbohydrate absorption. In *Inherited Disorders of Carbohydrate Metabolism.* (eds Burman D., Holten J.B. & Pennock C.A.), pp 39–57. Lancaster: MTP Press.

McNeish A.H., Ducker D.A., Warren I.F., Davies D.T., Harran M.J. & Hugh C.A. (1979) The influence of gestational age and size on the absorption of D-xylose and D-glucose from the small intestine of the human neonate. In *CIBA Foundation Symposium 70, Development of Mammalian Absorption Processes.* Amsterdam: Excerpta Medica.

MacFarlane P.I. & Miller V. (1984) Human milk in the management of protracted diarrhoea in infancy. *Arch. Dis. Childh.* 59, 260–5.

Madzarovova-Nohejlova J. (1973) Trehalase deficiency in a family. *Gastroenterology* 65, 130.

Manuel P.D., Walker-Smith J.A. & Suoeparto P. (1980) Cow's milk sensitive enteropathy in Indonesian infants (letter). *Lancet* 2, 1365–6.

Manuel P.D. & Walker-Smith J.A. (1981) A comparison of three infant feeding formulae for the prevention of delayed recovery after infantile gastroenteritis. *Acta paediat. belg.* 34, 13–20.

Marshall W.C., Lloyd-Still J. & Seakins J.W. (1967) Congenital sucrase and isomaltase deficiency with temporary lactose intolerance. *Acta paediat. scand.* 56, 211–15.

Matthews D.M. (1971) Protein absorption. *J. clin. Pathol.* 5, (suppl. 24) 29–40.

Matthews D.M. (1975) Intestinal absorption of peptides. *Physiol. Rev.* 55, 537.

Menzies I.S. & Seakins J.W.T. (1976) Sugars. In *Chromatographic and Electrophorectic Techniques*, Vol. 15 4th Edition (eds. Smith I. & Seakins J.W.T.), pp. 183–217. London: Heinemann.

Moncrieff A. & Wilkinson R.H. (1954) Sucrosuria with mental defect and hiatus hernia. *Acta paediat. scand.* (Suppl. 100), 495–516.

Moriarty K.J., Hegarty J.E., Clarke M., Fairclough P.D. & Dawson A.M. (1981) A comparison of the relative nitrogen-sparing properties of whole protein, protein hydrolysate, and the equivalent amino acid mixture in man. *Gastroenterology* 80, 1234.

Morrison P.S. & Little T.M. (1981) How is gastroenteritis treated? *Brit. med. J.* 283, 1300.

Motil K.J., Grand R.J., Matthews D.E., Bier D.M. & Maletskos C.J. & Young V.R. (1982) Whole body leucine metabolism in adolescents with Crohn's disease and growth failure during nutritional supplementation. *Gastroenterology* 82, 1359–68.

Muller D.P.R. (1982) Disorders of fat absorption. In *Clinics in Gastroenterology* (ed. Harries J.J.). Philadelphia: W.B. Saunders.

Nalin D.R., Cash R.A., Rahman M. & Yunus M. (1970) Effect of glycine and glucose on sodium and water absorption in patients with cholera *Gut* 11, 768–72.

Narayanan I., Praskash K., Prabhakar A.K. & Gujral V.V. (1982) A planned prospective evaluation of the anti-infective property of varying quantities of expressed human milk. *Acta. paediat. scand.* 71, 441–5.

Narayanan I., Singh B. & Harvey D. (1984) Fat loss during feeding of human milk. *Arch. Dis. Childh.* 59, 475–7.

Navarro J., Ricour C., Mougenot J.F. & Duhamel J.F. (1977) Constant rate enteral alimentation in Crohn's disease (at hospital and at home). *Acta. paediat. belg.* 30, 195.

Oakley J.R., McWeeney P.M., Hayes–Allen M. & Emery J.L. (1969) Possibly avoidable deaths in hospital in the age group one week to two years. *Lancet* 2, 113–4.

O'Donoghue D.A. & Dawson A.W. (1977) Crohn's disease in children. *Arch. Dis. Childh.* 52, 627.

O'Morain C.A., Segal A.W. & Levi A.J. (1982) Elemental diets in the treatment of acute Crohn's disease: a controlled study. *Gut* 23, 891.

Patra F.C., Mahalanbis D., Jalan K.N., Sen A. & Banerjee P. (1982) Can acetate replace bicarbonate in oral rehydration solution for infantile diarrhoea? *Arch. Dis. Childh.* 57, 625–37.

Paul A.A. & Southgate D.A.T. (1978) *McCance & Widdowson's The Composition of Foods*, 4th Edition. London: HMSO.

Pizarro D., Posada G., Villacencio N., Mohs E. & Levine M.M. (1983) Routine treatment of hypernatraemia and hyponatraemia diarrheal dehydration in infants using an oral glucose electrolyte solution containing 90 mmol/l sodium. *Amer. J. Dis. Child.* 137, 730–4.

Prinsloo J.C., Wittmann W., Pretorius P.J. & Kruger H. (1969) Effect of different sugars on diarrhoea of kwashiorkor. *Arch. Dis. Childh.* 44, 593.

Rahilly P.M., Shepherd R., Challis D., Walker-Smith J.A. & Manly J. (1976) Clinical comparison between glucose and sucrose additions to a basic electrolyte mixture in the outpatient management of acute gastroenteritis in children. *Arch. Dis. Childh.* 51, 152–4.

Sachar D.B., Auslander M.O. & Walfish J.S. (1980) Aetiological theories of inflammatory bowel disease. *Clinics in Gastroenterology* 9 (no. 2), 231–57.

Santosham M., Daum R.S., Dillman L., Rodriquez J.L., Luque S., Russel R., Kourany M., Ryder R.W., Bartlett A.V., Rosenberg A., Benenson A.S. & Sack R.B. (1982) Oral rehydration therapy of infantile diarrhoea: a controlled study of well-nourished children hospitalized in the US and Panama. *New Engl. J. Med.* 306, 1070–6.

Santosham M., Carnera E. & Sack R.B. (1983) Oral rehydration therapy in well nourished ambulatory patients. *Amer. J. trop. Med. Hyg.* 32, 804–8.

Shepherd R.W., Truslow S., Walker-Smith J.A. *et al.* (1975). Infantile gastroenteritis—a clinical study of reovirus-like agent infection. *Lancet* 2, 1082–4.

Shwachman H., Lloyd-Still J.D., Khaw K.T. & Antonowicz I. (1973) Protracted diarrhoea of infancy treated by intravenous alimentation. II. Studies of small intestine biopsy results. *Amer. J. Dis. Child.* **125**, 360.

SOOTHILL J.F. (1976) Breastfeeding: the immunological argument. *Brit. med. J.* **1**, 1466.

SOUTHGATE D.A.T., PAUL A.A., DEAN A.C. & CHRISTIE A.A. (1978) Free sugars in foods. *J. hum. Nutr.* **32**, 335–47.

STOCKS R.J., DAVIES D.P., ALLEN F. & SEWELL D. (1985) Loss of breast milk nutrients during tube feeding. *Arch. Dis. Childh.*, Vol. **60**, No. 2, 164.

STROBEL C.T., BYRNE W.J. & AMENT M.E. (1979) Home parenteral nutrition in children with Crohn's disease: an effective management alternative. *Gastroenterology* **77**, 272–9.

THORN J.M., AGGETT P.J., DELVES H.T. & CLAYTON B.E. (1978) Mineral and trace metal supplements for use with synthetic diets based on comminuted chicken. *Arch. Dis. Childh.* **53** (no. 12), 931–8.

TRIPP J.H. & HARRIES J.T. (1980) Letter. UNICEF/WHO glucose electrolyte solution not always appropriate. *Lancet* **2**, 793.

TRIPP J.H., MANNING J.A., MULLER D.P.R., WALKER-SMITH J.A., O'DONAGHUE D.P., KUMAR P.J. & HARRIES J.T. (1978) Mucosal adenylate cyclase and sodium–potassium stimulated adenosine triphosphatase in jejunal biopsies of adults and children with coeliac disease. In *Perspectives in Coeliac Disease—3rd International Coeliac Symposium* (eds. McNicol B., McCarthy C.F. & Fottrell P.F.), p. 461. Lancaster: MTP Press.

VISAKORPI J.K. (1970) An international enquiry concerning the diagnostic criteria of coeliac disease. *Acta. paediat. scand.* **59**, 463.

VITORIA J.C., CAMERERO C., SOJO A., RUIZ A. & RODRIQUEZ-SORIANO J. (1982) Enteropathy related to fish, rice and chicken. *Arch. Dis. Childh.* **57**, 44–8.

VON CHWALIBOGOWSKI A. (1937) *Acta paediat.* **2**, 110.

WALKER-SMITH J.A. (1975) Cow's milk protein intolerance. *Arch. Dis. Childh.* **50**, 347–50.

WALKER-SMITH J.A. (1979) *Diseases of the Small Intestine in Childhood*, 2nd Edition. London: Pitman Medical.

WALKER-SMITH J.A. (1980) Toddler diarrhoea. *Arch. Dis. Childh.* **55**, 329–30.

WALSH J.A. & WARREN K.S. (1979) Selective primary health care: an interim strategy for disease control in developing countries. *New Engl. J. Med.* **301**, 967–74.

WATT J., PINCOTT J.R. & HARRIES J.T. (1983) Combined cow's milk protein and gluten-induced enteropathy: common or rare? *Gut* **24**, 165–70.

WEIJERS H.A., VAN DE KAMER J.H., DICKE W.K. & IJSSELING J. (1961) Diarrhoea caused by deficiency of sugar splitting enzymes. I. *Acta. paediat.* (*Uppsala*) **50**, 55.

WERLIN S.L. & GRAND R.J. (1977) Severe colitis in children and adolescents: diagnosis, course and treatment. *Gastroenterology* **73**, 828–32.

WHARTON B.A. (1981) Gastroenteritis in Britain: management at home. *Brit. med. J.* **283**, 1277–8.

WHO (1976) *Treatment and Prevention of Diarrhoeal Disease: a Guide for use at the Primary Level.* Geneva: World Health Organization.

WRIGHT R. & TRUELOVE S.R. (1965) A controlled therapeutic trial of various diets in ulcerative colitis. *Brit. med. J.* **2**, 138.

YOUNOSZAI M.K. (1974) Jejunal absorption of hexose in infants and children. *J. Pediat.* **85**, 446–8.

Recipes

MINIMAL LACTOSE, MINIMAL SUCROSE RECIPES

Custard

15 g ($\frac{1}{2}$ oz) milk substitute powder, e.g. Cow & Gate S Formula
1 to 2 tsp unsweetened custard powder
1 tsp glucose to sweeten
Water to 100 ml ($3\frac{1}{2}$ oz)

Whisk powders into water. Bring to the boil in a saucepan stirring all the time until thickened.
Variation. Freeze till just thickening, beat with a rotary beater to aerate then re-freeze until set. Food colouring may be added.

Sucrose-free jelly

7 g ($\frac{1}{4}$ oz) gelatine
15 g ($\frac{1}{2}$ oz) glucose and/or fructose and/or glucose polymer
Dietetic squash to flavour
Water to 300 ml ($\frac{1}{2}$ pint)

Dissolve gelatine in a little hot water. Add to remaining ingredients and stir. Allow to set in a cool place.
Variation. Freeze to make ice-lolly substitute.

Milk substitute jelly

7 g ($\frac{1}{4}$ oz) gelatine
35 g ($1\frac{1}{4}$ oz) milk substitute powder, e.g. Prosobee

Glucose to sweeten
Food colouring and/or essence to flavour
Water to 300 ml ($\frac{1}{2}$ pint)

Dissolve gelatine in a little hot water.
Dissolve milk substitute powder, glucose
and flavouring essence in the remaining
water. Slowly pour the dissolved gelatine
into the milk substitute mixture. Stir well, or
whisk to prevent curdling. Allow to set in a
cool place.
Variations.
   1   Whisk to aerate with a rotary beater
when just beginning to set.
   2   Make two or three different flavours
and colours and set in layers. Add an egg-
yolk to the milk substitute mixture just
before adding the dissolved gelatine.
Allow to just begin to set.
   3   Beat-egg white until stiff. Whisk jelly
mixture, then fold egg-white into the jelly
mixture. Allow to set.
   4   The aerated mixtures of (1) and (3)
can be frozen to make an ice-cream
substitute.

Biscuits

170 g (6 oz) flour
85 g (3 oz) kosher margarine
45 g (1$\frac{1}{2}$ oz) glucose
$\frac{1}{2}$ egg or 1 egg-yolk

Rub fat into dry ingredients. Mix to a dough
with the egg and a little water if necessary.
Roll out on a well-floured board. Cut into
shapes. Or add an extra 1 tablespoon hot
water and pipe into shapes on a baking tray
greased with oil. Cook at 180°C (350°F),
regulo 3, for 10 minutes.
Variation.   Add vanilla, cocoa or essence or
food colouring. Vary shapes. 'Ice' with
glucose icing.

Sponge cake or pudding

3 eggs
115 g (4 oz) glucose
2 tbsp hot water

115 g (4 oz) self-raising flour
Vanilla essence and/or food colouring

Grease two sandwich tins with oil and dust
with a little flour. Beat eggs to a foam, add
glucose and beat until dissolved. Add water,
essence, then fold in sifted flour very lightly
with a tablespoon. Pour into greased tins.
Bake 15 to 20 minutes at 180°C (350°F),
regulo 3. Cool. Ice with a mixture of glucose
and Tomor margarine icing.
Variation.   Place spoonfuls in cup cases.
Cook for 10 minutes only.
Or pudding—steam for 40 minutes in a
basin over boiling water.
Or add honey in place of half the glucose.

Melting moments

170 g (6 oz) flour
170 g (6 oz) kosher margarine
   60 g (2 oz) cornflour
   60 g (2 oz) glucose

Work margarine into sifted ingredients and
knead into dough. Make into small balls and
place, well-spaced, on a greased baking
tray. Flatten balls with a fork to also give a
pattern. Bake in a slow oven 150°C (300°F),
regulo 1$\frac{1}{2}$ for 10 minutes.
Variation.   Add 1 tablespoon hot water to
soften dough, then pipe biscuit shapes with
a forcing biscuit bag.

Glucose icing

60 g (2 oz) glucose
30 g (1 oz) kosher margarine
Water to mix

Cream magarine and add in all glucose to a
stiff dough. Add water, drop by drop, to
give a creamy icing. Colour with food
colouring and/or essence and/or cocoa if
desired. Spread and smooth on cakes and
biscuits with a knife dipped in hot water.

Oatmeal biscuits

115 g (4 oz) flour
$\frac{1}{2}$ tsp baking powder

¼ tsp salt
85 g (3 oz) kosher margarine
85 g (3 oz) glucose
85 g (3 oz) oatmeal
1 egg

Sift flour, baking powder and salt. Beat egg.
Rub fat into flour mixture. Add oatmeal,
then glucose. Mix to a stiff dough with egg.
Knead on a floured board. Roll out thinly.
Cut into shapes. Bake on a greased tray for
10 to 15 minutes at 180°C (350°F), regulo
3.

Glucose meringues

2 egg-whites
60 g (2 oz) glucose and/or glucose polymer

Beat egg-white until very stiff. Slowly add
glucose and continue beating after each
addition until approximately half is added.
Fold remaining glucose into the mixture.
Place spoonfuls onto an oiled greaseproof
paper. Place in a cool oven 100 to 120°C
(200 to 250°F), regulo ½ to 1 until set and
just brown. Store in an airtight tin; as
glucose absorbs water from the air these
meringues will go sticky with keeping.
Variation. Use fructose instead of glucose
for fructose meringues. These absorb water
very rapidly and therefore will not keep more
than a few days.

Other recipes can be devised using an
ordinary cookery book, replacing butter with
kosher margarine, sugar, icing sugar, etc.
with glucose, syrup with honey, and milk
with water or the milk substitute.
    Omit or do not use recipes including
forbidden ingredients such as jam, fruit,
carrot, cream, etc.

RECIPES FOR LOW-STARCH DIET

Sweet biscuits

120 g (4 oz) soya flour
  60 g (2 oz) butter or margarine
  60 g (2 oz) sugar or glucose as appropriate

Cream butter and sugar. Work in soya flour,
adding a little water if necessary. Roll out,
cut into shapes and bake in moderate oven
for 15 minutes. Makes 16 biscuits; each
biscuit contains 1 g starch.

Savoury biscuits

120 g (4 oz) soya flour
  60 g (2 oz) butter or margarine
1 egg-yolk
Salt to taste

Work soya flour into the butter. Add egg-
yolk. Roll out, cut into 16 biscuits and bake
in a moderate oven for 15 minutes. Each
biscuit contains 1 g starch.

MINIMAL GLUCOSE–GALACTOSE RECIPES

Egg custard

5 g Casilan
1 egg
150 ml (5 oz) water
Vanilla essence
Fructose to sweeten if desired, or salt and
    pepper for savoury custard

Beat egg and Casilan in the water, add
vanilla and fructose. Place in a double
saucepan over boiling water and stir until
thickened.
Or place mixture in a greased dish. Bake in a
slow oven in a dish of water until set.

Fructose meringues

2 egg-whites
60 g (2 oz) fructose

Beat egg-white, gradually beat in the
fructose. Place in spoonfuls on greaseproof
paper. Place in a cool oven, 100 to 120°C
(200 to 250°F), until set and just brown.
These meringues tend to go sticky, as
fructose is hydroscopic, and will only keep
for 1 to 2 days.

Fructose toffee

115 g (4 oz) fructose
  30 ml (1 oz) water
1 knob margarine

Heat slowly until fructose dissolves. Boil the mixture until just golden brown. Pour onto greased foil. Cool. Break into small pieces. These toffees tend to go sticky, as fructose is hydroscopic, and will only keep for 1 to 2 days.

Fructose jelly

  15 g ($\frac{1}{2}$ oz) gelatine
  60 g (2 oz) fructose
300 ml (10 oz) water
2 to 3 drops food colouring, e.g. red
2 drops strawberry or other essence

Boil water and add gelatine and fructose. Colour and flavour. Allow to set in a cool place.

Scrambled egg

1 egg
Kosher margarine
1 tbsp water
Salt

Cook in the usual way.

MINIMAL SUCROSE RECIPES

Most home-made household recipes are suitable if glucose is substituted for sugar. Omit jam, syrup, dried fruit, and fruits which are not permitted.

Milk jelly

15 g ($\frac{1}{2}$ oz) gelatine
150 ml (5 oz) hot water
360 ml (12 oz) milk
30 g (1 oz) glucose
Essence and colouring, e.g. vanilla, almond
  essence or cocoa powder, coffee, etc.

Dissolve gelatine in hot water. Add glucose; carefully add the milk. Flavour with essences, add colouring. Pour into mould and allow to set. Freeze to make into a 'mousse'.

Ice-cream

420 ml (14 oz tin) unsweetened evaporated
  milk
45 g (1$\frac{1}{2}$ oz) glucose
Vanilla essence or other permitted flavouring

Chill evaporated milk, whisk with rotary whisk until very stiff. Add glucose and vanilla essence. Put in ice-tray in freezing compartment of refrigerator until frozen.

Jelly

15 g ($\frac{1}{2}$ oz) gelatine
60 ml (2 oz) sugar-free squash*
Water to 560 ml (1 pint)

or bottle or canned grapefruit juice plus
  water to 560 ml (1 pint)

or lemon juice plus glucose plus water to
  560 ml (1 pint)

Permitted fruit, e.g. grapes, for decoration if desired

Dissolve gelatine in a little hot water. Add dietetic squash or fruit juice and water. Refrigerate until set. Permitted fruit may be added or used to decorate.
* Unsweetened fruit juices may be used if permitted in the diet.

Toffee

120 g (4 oz) glucose
  30 g (1 oz) water
Knob of butter or margarine

Place glucose, water and butter in a small solid-base saucepan. Heat slowly until glucose dissolves. Boil until mixture just changes colour. Pour at once into paper cases or onto greased baking tin. Cool. Keep in an airtight dry tin. Break 'lumps' into bite-size pieces as necessary.

CHAPTER 2

Dietary fibre: high- and low-fibre diets

DIETARY FIBRE

Dietary fibre is composed of plant polysaccharides including cellulose, hemicellulose, pectins and lignins, which are not digested by human hydrolytic enzymes and so contribute to faecal matter. These compoumds are bound with gums, waxes, cutins and certain trace elements. Cereal fibre, mostly as bran, increases faecal weight; vegetable fibre and pectins have a similar but lesser effect (Bingham 1979). The increase in faecal weight associated with an increased dietary fibre is at least partially due to the affinity for water of dietary fibre, and therefore reduced water absorption by the colon, increased peristalsis and reduced transit time. However, dietary fibre and bile salts are fermented by bacteria in the gut to form unconjugated bile salts and volatile fatty acids which have a cathartic effect in the large intestine (Cummings 1978). Increased dietary fibre changes the gut flora, softens the stools, and increases bulk and frequency of defaecation (Stephen & Cummings 1979, 1980, Bingham 1979, Burman *et al.* 1982).

The diet of modern society is relatively low in fibre due to the extensive use of refined cereals and lack of fruit and vegetables intake. The fibre is removed in modern processing of flour and cereals, the bran frequently being discarded. Table 2.1 compares the fibre content of various flours, breads and cereals. The British adult diet contains approximately 20 g of dietary fibre per day, whereas vegetarian diets and many national diets in the developing world have a higher fibre content. Vegans are reported to have 100 to 200% higher dietary fibre intakes, and ovolacto vegetarians a 50% increase, compared to omnivore controls (Sanders 1978). Some workers have recommended an increase in dietary fibre in the national diet (James 1983) to 30 g per day for adults.

Lack of dietary fibre intake has been proposed in the aetiology of a number of diseases of modern society (Burkitt 1973), such as chronic constipation

Table 2.1 Fibre content of various breads and flour.

100 g	Fibre (g)
Bread	
Brown	5·1
Hovis	4·6
Sunblest Hi Bran	11·1+
Vitbe Wheatgerm	4·8+
White	2·7
Wholemeal	8·5
Bran	
Wheat	44
Flour	
White	3 to 3·7
Wholemeal	9·6
Chapatis	3·7
Crispbread	
Rye	11·7
Starch-reduced	4·9
Cereals	
All Bran	26·7
Cornflakes	11·0
Muesli	7·0
Oatmeal, raw	7·0
Ready Brek	7·6
Rice Krispies	4·5
Rice, white boiled	0·8
Shredded Wheat	12·3
Sugar Puffs	6·1
Weetabix	12·7

in both children and adults, a common disorder in which there is difficulty or delay in the passage of stools. Other diseases in adults may be associated with a lack of fibre and include diverticulitis (Painter 1975), irritable colon (Davidson & Wasserman 1966), bowel cancer and possibly diseases of affluence such as obesity or those associated with cholesterol metabolism (Burkitt 1973).

There are many factors which are involved in the development of diseases associated with modern society. Dietary fibre is only one such factor. A change of diet should be initiated early in life because these are long-term effects, and also because it is easier to bring about a change in the eating pattern of population groups from childhood (Burkitt *et al*, 1980). An increase in natural fibre intake by the use of wholemeal bread and wholegrain cereals should be encouraged in the British diet, largely as a replacement of sucrose and refined carbohydrates.

Clearly, a balance between a low-energy density, high-fibre, but inadequate diet and a high-energy density, low-fibre diet must be achieved in order to provide optimal nutrition (Francis 1984). Many fibre-containing foods also contain phytate, which inhibits the availability of a number of trace minerals (*see* Francis 1986, Andersson *et al.* 1983, Wise 1983), and an excess intake, especially in conjunction with a marginal intake of these minerals such as zinc, may result in a negative balance and growth failure. To avoid the dangers of mineral imbalance, raw bran should be avoided. A better source of fibre is wholemeal bread, where the action of phytase in yeast will reduce the mineral-binding capacity of phytate during fermentation. Alternatively, the dephytinized bran products which are now becoming available should be used (Andersson *et al.* 1983) and/or naturally low-phytate cereals such as oats encouraged.

Use of wholemeal bread and wholegrain cereals is advised for all age groups beyond infancy in place of refined cereals. Wholemeal bread and unrefined cooked cereals are appropriate during the weaning of infants, from the age of introducing finger foods at about 8 to 10 months. Suitable wholegrain cereals for infants include crushed Weetabix, baby muesli and Ready Brek; later a rusk of wholemeal bread can be given. Fruit and vegetables also contribute fibre as well as other important nutrients to the diet, and should be encouraged.

Increased dietary fibre is obviously indicated in constipation to soften faecal matter, retain water and ease defaecation. In diarrhoea it can provide faecal mass, and a more normal appearance of stool results (Burman *et al.* 1982), but whether it decreases faecal loss and malabsorption, or simply alters the appearance of the stools, is uncertain. Clinical improvement with an increased fibre intake has been shown in some patients with diverticulitis (Painter *et al.* 1972, Taylor & Duthie 1976) Chronic ulcerative colitis (*see* Chapter 1) and irritable colon may also benefit from an increased fibre intake (Harvey *et al.* 1973).

DISADVANTAGES OF DIETARY FIBRE

High-fibre diets are not without disadvantages, as they may inhibit nutrient availability and are low in energy density (Burkitt *et al.* 1980). An energy deficit can result, particularly in the young child (Francis 1984), and this is now considered to be a major cause of the almost universal undernutrition seen in the developing world. This is in contrast to the higher energy density, lower fibre diet of industrialized society. The use of a higher energy density, lower fibre diet largely correlates with the improved nutritional state now found in young children (Burkitt *et al.* 1980).

Whole-wheat flour contains appreciable amounts of calcium, iron and zinc, but this is largely not available due to binding with phytate (Wise 1983). Refined cereals lose much of these minerals and phytate (Davidson *et al.* 1979). A high phytate intake, especially in conjunction with a suboptimal mineral intake, can lead to potential deficiency (*see* Francis 1986). Calcium deficiency is unlikely, provided the intake of vitamin D is adequate. James *et al.* (1978) have shown that calcium absorption increases slowly after a change to a high-fibre diet. Zinc absorption is reduced by phytate (Reinhold 1976, Andersson *et al.* 1983, Wise 1983, Reilly 1978). The reduced bioavailability of minerals observed with high-fibre diets is related to their phytate content, with the possible exception of iron (Andersson *et al.* 1983). Zinc deficiency can cause growth failure (FAO 1974). The fermentation process used during bread-making largely destroys phytic acid, due to the action of the enzyme phytase present in yeast. Thus wholemeal bread is an ideal source of dietary fibre, as are cereals such as oats, rather than soya and wheat which more easily inhibit mineral uptake. Macrobiotic, soya and cereal-based diets are of greatest concern with respect to the availability of minerals including calcium, iron and zinc. Adding unprocessed (raw) bran to the diet, especially those based on refined cereal, is not recommended, as it is less satisfactory nutritionally than a diet based on wholemeal bread and wholegrain cereals. Meat should normally be included in diets, as it is an excellent source of available zinc, as well as iron, protein and other nutrients.

Constipation and soiling

Bowel problems in children are common, but often difficult to manage, and the boundary between physical and emotional factors is often blurred. The rectum and anal canal have two tasks, to store faeces temporarily and to evacuate at a socially convenient time.

The breast-fed baby varies from passing a stool every feed to one stool in 7 to 10 days, but this stool is of soft consistency. Bottle-fed infants often pass dry hard faeces with difficulty, and even traces of fresh blood may be present. Attention to fluid intake (extra water or natural fruit juice) is usually sufficient to correct this problem. The temporary addition of small amounts of brown sugar to solids or drinks can be helpful, but should not be used routinely because of the long-term risks of dental caries, 'sweet tooth' syndrome and obesity. Cereal, fruit and vegetable purées should be introduced with other appropriate solids during weaning. Persistent constipation at this age, especially when present from birth, requires further investigation. Straining is very marked in the newborn and often convinces the mother that her baby is constipated, whereas it is usually just his exaggerated response to the 'desire to defaecate' sensation. It is therefore essential to ensure that the mother correctly describes the symptoms of constipation (Clayden 1976). Physiological causes of constipation must be ruled out.

Potty training may bring problems, particularly if the parents are overanxious and persuasive and the child is not old enough to control his bowel movements. Reassurance of the parents to remove anxiety usually overcomes the problem.

Acute constipation in children requires medicinal treatment as described by Clayden (1976). If the child is prone to constipation a higher fibre diet should be recommended subsequently.

Chronic constipation is defined as persistent delay and difficulty in defaecating, often associated with soiling. Delay may be as long as three weeks (and occasionally longer), after which a large stool is passed, but fluid stool soiling occurs between evacuation. The faecal mass needs to be moved initially by medicinal means; physical, environmental and emotional causes should be investigated. Adequate time, and privacy, for defaecation should be allowed in the day's routine. For example, outside, cold, wet, unlockable toilets at school may result in the child avoiding defaecation; pain from a previous fissure may cause reluctance to defaecate. Use should be made of the gastrocolonic response to the overnight fast followed by food and fluid (breakfast), and time allowed for the child to use the toilet after the meal. After faecal clearance, and/or anal dilation as appropriate (Clayden & Lawson 1976), prolonged use of added bulk is recommended in order to obtain a daily stool. For example, methylcellulose (Cologel, Cellucon or Calevac), lactulose or dephytinized bran products, along with a stimulant like Senokot, may be necessary for a few months. A high-fibre diet should be advised in order to produce an adequate bulk of soft matter and prevent recurrence of constipation. Adequate fluids should be included to avoid as far as possible hard dry stools.

High-fibre diet

The commonest use of a high-fibre diet in paediatrics is for constipation or soiling. Such a diet should incorporate wholemeal bread, wholegrain cereals, e.g. 'brown' rice and 'brown' pasta made from the whole grain, wholemeal cakes and biscuits, e.g. muesli bars in place of 'white' refined alternatives, and muesli, Weetabix and Cornflakes rather than Rice Krispies (Table 2.1). Snacks, especially of refined carbohydrates, 'candy and Coke', should be replaced with fruit, dried fruit and nuts. Whole nuts are only recommended from four years old, due to the high risk of inhalation, but peanut butter is a useful alternative at any age once the child is weaned.

Fruit, especially dried apricots or prunes, and vegetables should be encouraged, even though they have a less-specific effect on faecal mass than cereal fibre; they are notoriously rejected by children with constipation. Almost all vegetables can be eaten raw and are often accepted better and are more nutritious than 'overcooked greens'. They can be included in a variety of salad dishes. The parents' acceptance, particularly father's, will most easily ensure that the children accept diet changes or modification.

High-fibre foods are listed in Table 2.2 and a sample menu is given in Table 2.3. Adequate fibre should be included in the diet to ensure 1 to 3 soft stools per day. If the above measures are inadequate, it is preferable that dephytinized bran be used to increase the dietary fibre, rather than unprocessed (raw) bran which inhibits mineral absorption. A number of children find bran dry, unpalatable and difficult to take. A small quantity should be started initially and increased gradually, and excess is not recommended. Bran supplements are inappropriate in young children, especially those under two years old.

If bran products are necessary, they can be given mixed with milk, sprinkled on cereals, or simply

Table 2.2 Foods to encourage on a high-fibre diet.

Bread. Select a high-fibre type from Table 2.1, e.g. wholemeal bread, Hi Bran and bran breads. Rye bread, especially pumpernickel (dark rye bread).

Wholemeal flour, brown wholemeal pasta.

Wholegrain cereals, e.g. oats, brown rice, muesli, barley, All Bran, Bran Flakes, Cornflakes, Shredded Wheat, Weetabix.

Wholegrain crispbread and biscuits, rye crispbread, oatcakes, digestive biscuits, muesli bars, wholewheat crisps.

Dried fruits, apricots, raisins, sultanas.

Nuts as crunchy peanut butter, nutmeats, or as whole nuts which are suitable in over-4-year-olds, marzipan.

Vegetables. Lightly cooked 'Chinese-style', salads, raw vegetables such as coleslaw, grated carrot.

Fruit should be washed, but apples, pears, etc. should not be peeled.

Coarse marmalade rather than jelly marmalade.

---

mixed with honey, syrup or fruit juice, or taken with a drink or incorporated into home-baked products. An increasing number of bran-enriched cereals, bread and biscuits are now available, e.g. All Bran (Kelloggs), Hi-Bran bread (Sunblest), Bran Loaf (St Michael), wholewheat crisps, fruit and bran biscuits, muesli bars, etc. Wholemeal flour and dried fruits with or without bran can be made into a variety of palatable cookies, cakes and tea-loaves.

Initially flatulence and abdominal pain may occur when the dietary fibre intake is increased, and therefore the fibre content should be increased gradually and patients warned of this temporary effect.

Low-fibre (residue) diets

Faecal matter consists of water (70 to 76%), bacteria, endogenous losses and undigested food. The confusion over terminology of fibre, residue and roughage has been highlighted by Adamson *et al.* (1973) and Bingham (1979). Fibre has a major role in faecal weight and colonic contents. Other nutrients have little effect, except possibly for protein and milk (Bingham 1979), and fat in patients with steatorrhoea. Specific foods such as prune juice, cabbage, baked beans (Kramer *et al.* 1962), dates, raisins,

Table 2.3 Sample menu of a high-fibre diet.

On waking	Natural fruit juice
Breakfast	Wholegrain cereal, e.g. oats, All Bran, Bran Flakes or Weetabix
	Egg or bacon or ham or fish (optional)
	Wholemeal bread or toast, and butter or margarine
	Coarse marmalade or crunchy peanut butter
	Milk, with tea or coffee if desired
Lunch/supper	Vegetable soup if desired
	Meat, liver or poultry including casseroles and stews
	Jacket potatoes if possible, and butter or margarine
	Large helpings of green and root vegetables or salad
	Fresh or stewed fruit, nuts or dried fruit, or pudding made with wholemeal flour
School dinner/ tea/supper	Wholemeal bread as sandwiches including appropriate fillings
	Meat, fish, cheese, egg, baked beans or fish fingers
	Salad or green vegetables or winter salad, coleslaw, shredded cabbage, grated carrot and dried fruit, nuts
	Lemon juice or salad dressing
	Wholemeal crisps
	Wholemeal bread and butter or margarine
	Oatcake, wholemeal cake, fruit cake, digestive biscuit or bran crispbread
	Fruit—fresh, dried, stewed; nuts for over-4-year-olds
Bedtime	Milk or tea or water to drink
	Fruit or digestive biscuit or bran crispbread and butter

This diet includes the foods recommended in Tables 2.1 and 2.2. Adequate intake of fluid is also important in patients with constipation.

peaches, apricots, banana and strawberries are reported to increase ileostomy output (Kramer 1964).

Elemental diets reduce faecal weight, but this appears to be directly related to their non-fibre content, as other non-elemental isonitrogenous fibre-free regimens, e.g. enteral feeds, give similar results unless small bowel absorption is impaired (Bingham 1979). Changes in the bacterial population of the gut are reported with enteral feeds, including elemental diets

(Winitz *et al.* 1970, Attebury *et al.* 1972), and are important to the changes observed in faecal output.

For practical purposes a low-fibre diet is adequate for most clinical situations requiring faecal reduction, and such a diet can be scientifically devised with the data on fibre that are now available (Southgate *et al.* 1976). Low-fibre diets are rarely required, except as a temporary measure pre- and post-operatively for procedures in the large bowel (Russell 1975, Burman *et al.* 1982), in acute ulcerative colitis and enterocolitis, and for rectal prolapse. Children with cystic fibrosis should avoid excess fibre in conjunction with their high energy and protein diet and pancreatin supplements (*see* Chapter 6); rectal prolapse is more common in these children. There is no evidence that a low-fibre diet is beneficial in chronic ulcerative colitis (*see* Chapter 1) and the psychological disadvantage of such a diet should be remembered.

Non-fibre diet

One of the following can be selected: (i) an elemental diet, (ii) an enteral feed or a fluid diet based on milk, glucose polymer and cream or Calogen or Prosparol (*see* Francis 1986), or (iii) a diet based on non fibre-containing natural foods (Tables 2.4 and 2.5). The latter are more palatable, better accepted and contain more variety, and can be used in conjunction with supplements of milk or an enteral feed. The diet should also be easily digested by avoiding tough meats, gristle or skin and fatty or fried food, and should be readily absorbed by avoiding hyperosmolar feeds.

To reduce the faecal output to a minimum, milk and protein foods should be restricted to approximately 1 to 2 g protein/kg per day in children, mostly from tender meat, egg, and fish, and in infants as a whey-based modified milk. Additional energy from pure carbohydrate, sugar, glucose, or glucose polymer, and fats, oil, cream, Prosparol or Calogen, should be provided as drinks and appropriate made-up dishes. Such diets should only be used temporarily.

A minimal residue infant feed can be devised, such as the example in Table 2.6, but it should only be used for a few days as it will not be adequate for growth. Alternatively, Pregestimil or Pepdite 0–2 could be used as an elemental diet for this age group.

Low-fibre diet

The avoidance of high-fibre cereals, use of white bread and avoidance of dried fruits, nuts and pips and skins may suffice. Alternatively a more scientific

Table 2.4   Non-fibre foods.

Tender meat (omit gristle, skin, bone)*, egg*, fish (omit bone, skin)* (not fish fingers or batter).

Milk*, cheese*, natural yoghurt*.

Strained fruit juices (not prune juice), fruit squashes, carbonated beverages, Lucozade, Hycal.

Bovril, Marmite, consommé, tea, coffee.

White sugar, glucose polymers, honey, boiled sweets, jelly sweets—gelatine type—peppermints, Nesquik milk-shake powder† and similar synthetic flavourings†.

Jelly, gelatine, meringues (egg white-type).

Cream, butter, margarine, oil, Prosparol, Calogen.

Salt, mayonnaise, oil and vinegar dressing.

Sago, tapioca†, custard powder†, cornflour†, arrowroot†, baking powder†.

Vitamin supplement, e.g. 0·6 ml Abidec (Parke Davis).

* To reduce faecal output to a minimum, it is suggested that protein be restricted to approximately 1 g/kg per day and milk products be limited to the equivalent of 300 ml/day.
† Fibre figures not available.

approach is to use, in addition to the non-fibre foods listed in Table 2.4, appropriate quantities of low-fibre foods selected from Table 2.7. It is important to consider the nutritional value and variety in the diet. Protein and milk restriction is not required with such diets. If the diet is used for any length of time vitamin supplements of A, D, C plus B complex, such as Abidec (Parke Davis) 0·6 ml daily, are recommended, and iron and zinc supplements may be appropriate. A sample menu of a low-fibre diet is given in Table 2.8.

Elemental diets

An increasing number of chemically defined, synthetic, elemental fluid diets are available for oral and enteral use in adults, along with a more limited range for infants (Table 2.9). They are fibre-free, like most enteral feeds, but largely consist of predigested nutrients. The main use of elemental diets is in nasogastric feeding in patients who do not absorb more conventional enteral feeds, discussed by Francis (1986), or as a cheaper and safer alternative to parenteral nutrition.

Table 2.5 Sample menu for a non-fibre diet for a child, aimed to reduce faecal output.

		Approximate protein (g)
Daily	300 ml milk	10
	'Milk' shake ⎧ 50 ml double cream/Prosparol/Calogen ⎨ 50 g glucose polymer/sugar/Nesquik, etc. ⎩ water to 500 ml	1 to 0
Vitamins	0·6 ml Abidec (Parke Davis)	
Breakfast	Strained fruit juice, e.g. orange juice or blackcurrant juice, plus glucose polymer	
	Bacon, crisp grilled, or egg (boiled or scrambled in butter/margarine)	6
	Salt	
	'Milk' shake or tea/coffee or milk from allowance	
Snack	'Milk' shake or strained fruit juice or carbonated beverage	
	Meringue, cheese cubes	Trace to 10
Lunch and supper	Consommé (optional)	Trace
	20 g tender meat and gravy thickened with cornflour or fish (grilled, baked or steamed)	6
	No vegetables	
	Jelly, meringue, creamed sago/tapioca or lemon sago ⎫	6
	Egg custard or natural yoghurt (from milk allowance) ⎬	Trace to 6
	Cream and sugar/glucose polymer ⎭	
Bedtime	'Milk' shake or remaining milk allowance or cheese	
	Supper	6
	*Total**	28 to 38

*Protein and energy intake should be adjusted for age and weight. Such a diet should only be used temporarily.

Table 2.6 Example of minimal residue non-fibre feeds for an infant, aimed to reduce faecal output.

	Carbohydrate (g)	Fat (g)	Protein (g)	Energy kJ	Energy kcal
(a)* 60 ml reconstituted whey-based modified milk or hydrolysed protein formula, e.g. Gold Cap SMA	4·5	2·2	1·0	170	40
10 g glucose, sugar or glucose polymer†	10	—	—	160	40
10 ml Prosparol/Calogen†	—	5·0	—	185	45
Water to 150 ml					
Total	14·5	7·2	1·0	515	125
Per 100 ml	10	4·8	0·7	343	83
(b) 100 ml Pregestimil	9·1	2·7	1·9	287	69

*Use feed (a) for a limited period of time, e.g. up to five days, as this feed is not nutritionally adequate for growth. Offer approximately 150 ml/kg per day divided into feeds.
†May be replaced with appropriate fibre-free solids according to age.

Table 2.7 Low-fibre foods.

(a)   Foods containing less than 2% fibre.

Boiled white rice.

Biscuits made from white flour, such as semi-short, short-bread, semi-sweet, sandwich, wafer and ginger nuts.

Scones and pancakes made from white flour.

Cakes made from white flour such as gingerbread, Madeira, sponge-type, custard tarts, jam tarts, buns.

Sponge-type puddings, milk puddings, lemon meringue pie (made from white flour).

Jam, tomato sauce, plain or milk chocolate* (not nut or fruit types).

Potato (not baked jacket, canned or crisps). Chips may be permitted.

Asparagus tips, cauliflower, tomato (normally skins and pips are removed), celery (stem only), cucumber (flesh only), lettuce, radish, marrow, pumpkin, onion (flesh only and not spring onions), peppers.

Eating apples (peeled), cherries†, fruit salad (canned), grapes†, grapefruit, lychees, mandarins (canned), melon, oranges, peaches, pineapple, tangerines.

* Fibre figures not available.
† Skins, pips and seeds should be removed, e.g. by sieving, to remove fibre.

(b)   Foods containing more than 2% but less than 5% fibre.

White bread, flour, rolls, chapati, pasta (not brown/whole-meal types).

Rice Krispies.

Cream crackers, matzos, chocolate biscuits (not digestive).

Pastry and fruit pies (suitable fruit or filling) and white flour.

Canned cream-type or clear soups.

Aubergine, beans (not dried or baked beans), bean sprouts, beetroot, broccoli, Brussels sprouts, cabbage, carrot, leek, lentils (boiled), mushrooms, spring greens, turnip, cress (not stalk).

Cooked apple, apricot, banana, gooseberries†, guava†, nectar-ine, olives, pears, plums, rhubarb†, strawberries†.

† Skins and pips/seeds should be removed, e.g. by sieving, to minimize residue.

There is now evidence that nutritional repletion with an elemental diet in Crohn's disease may induce a remission. Whether this is related to an improved nutritional state or to the oligo-antigenic nature of these products is still unknown (Booth & Harries 1984 and see Chapter 1). Their predigested nature makes them particularly useful in certain malabsorptive states such as protracted diarrhoea and Crohn's disease. As they are based on hydrolysed protein (peptides and amino acids) or L-amino acids they can provide, either alone or together with other suitable foods, an oligo-antigenic diet which is nutritionally adequate during dietary elimination trials (see Chapter 4). A major disadvantage of elemental diets is their poor palatability and expense. Flavourings have been devised to disguise their taste, but even so much encouragement and perseverance is necessary to get a child to take them orally. This applies to both the commercially available formulae (Russell 1975) and those devised from module ingredients incorporating hydrolysates or amino acids (Yassa et al. 1978). Monotony of the regimen, even with flavour alternatives, is another disadvantage. Nasogastric or jejunal feeding, either as bolus feeds or as a continuous feeding regimen, overcomes this problem and should be recommended where appropriate. The new portable (Viomedex) enteral feed (battery-operated) pump allows mobility of the child for play and social activities. The psychological effect of a fluid-based diet and enteral feeding in children must not be overlooked, particularly if it is required for prolonged periods.

Like any synthetic diet based on hydrolysate protein, amino acids, monosaccharides and medium-chain triglycerides, the osmolality of elemental diets is high, though recent improvement in this aspect has been made by the replacement of mono-saccharides with glucose polymers, increased energy from fat in place of carbohydrate, and use of vegetable oils in place of some medium-chain triglyceride. The high osmolality can cause osmotic diarrhoea, as can the high carbohydrate content of some formulae. The latter can also cause hyperglycaemia and salt and water overload. Nausea, abdominal pain and vomiting can also result from the unpalatability, osmolar load and gastric retention. Other problems resulting from elemental diets include disturbance in water balance, such as overhydration, hypertonic dehydration in association with accompanying diarrhoea, and osmotic diuresis. Hyperosmolar feeds should always be introduced as a dilute, frequent feeding regime in the first instance; those with a lower osmolality or which are isotonic can be intro-

Table 2.8   Sample menu of a low-fibre diet.

Breakfast	Strained fruit juice
	Rice Krispies*
	Egg or crisp grilled bacon (optional)
	White bread/toast*
	Butter, margarine, honey, Marmite/ Bovril
	Milk, tea/coffee
Mid-morning	Milk or strained fruit juice
	Cheese cubes
	Permitted fruit*
Lunch	Egg, grilled fish, tender meat (omit gristle, skin and bone)
	Potato* and permitted vegetables*
	Gravy
	Milk pudding or sponge pudding* and custard
Afternoon tea	*White bread
	Butter/margarine
	Cheese or jam or honey or Marmite/ Bovril
	Permitted fruit*
	Meringues
	Milk or tea/coffee or strained fruit juice
Supper	Tender meat or grilled/baked/steamed fish (omit gristle, skin and bone) or macaroni cheese,* etc.
	Permitted vegetables and fruit*
	Meringues, egg custard or strained fruit juice
Bedtime	Milk
Vitamins	0·6 ml Abidec (Parke Davis) is recommended

* *See* Tables 2.1 and 2.7 for fibre content.

duced at normal dilution immediately provided the patient's clinical condition permits. This omits the delay in providing full nutrition from the beginning of treatment, (Keohane *et al.* 1984). Those with an osmolality above 500 mmol/kg are not ideal and an alternative should be selected if at all possible.

Vitamin and trace mineral deficiencies can occur due to the synthetic nature of the elemental diet whose adequacy can only be as good as current technology. Deficiencies can also occur when formulae designed for adult nutrition are used in children, who have different nutritional requirements, and in whom the full adult volume is inappropriate. The use of elemental formulae requires careful monitoring and scrutiny regarding dietary adequacy (Bunker & Clayton 1983). This also applies to enteral feeds and fluid regimes designed for adults. Young children, and particularly infants, require a higher ratio of protein (nitrogen), vitamins and minerals to energy, and a higher fluid intake for weight, than adults. Without special adaptation and provision of appropriate supplements, adult formulae replacement diets are not suitable for infants and young children under about five years. For example, Vivonex (Eaton Labs) contains no cystine or taurine, and Flexical (Mead Johnson) is relatively low in cystine which is a semi-essential amino acid in infants, and therefore these formulae are not recommended for this age group. Flexical and Vivonex have a high osmolality and therefore need dilution and supplementation if used in young children.

Pregestimil, Pepdite 0–2, Pepdite 2+ or the new neonatal elemental amino acid diets by Scientific Hospital Supplies have the most appropriate paediatric formulation for infants and young children. They have an excellent nitrogen:energy ratio and the protein hydrolysates are fortified with specific amino acids to improve the biological value for infant nutrition. The combination of Pregestimil and Flexical or the Pepdite formulae can meet the needs of many paediatric patients. A comparison of elemental formulae is given in Table 2.9. Alternatively, a synthetic module elemental diet can be devised using the principles discussed in Chapter 1 for module diets using the ingredients in Table 1.6. Hydrolysed protein or amino acid preparations can be used, together with glucose polymer, minerals, trace elements, complete range of vitamins, essential fatty acids and vegetable oil emulsion and/or MCT emulsion. The nutritional adequacy and osmolality of such formulae must be monitored. New products based on protein hydrolysates and amino acids are continually being developed (Neocate, Scientific Hospital Supplies).

A non-fibre fluid (enteral) diet can be devised from milk, with added carbohydrate and fat, or an enteral feed (*see* Francis 1986) can be used, which has the advantage of better palatability, lower osmolality and lower cost compared with elemental diets.

Because of as yet unknown nutritional factors and interactions, elemental and synthetic diets should be used with caution in paediatric patients.

Table 2.9 Elemental diet formulae.

Product	Company	Normal dilution (g/100 ml)	Type of protein	Amino acid or protein (g/100 g)	Amino acid or protein/ 100 ml dilution	Type of carbohydrate	Carbohydrate (g/100 g)	Carbohydrate (g/100 ml dilution)	Type of fat	Fat (g/100 g)	Fat (g/100 ml dilution)
Adult formulae											
Flexical	Mead Johnson	22.7	Enzyme hydrolysed protein, casein and amino acids	9.9	2.3	Corn syrup solids and starch	67.3	15.3	Soy oil and MCT	15	3.4
Nutranel	Roussel	25.3	Hydrolysed whey	15.8 protein	4.0	Maltodextrin and lactose	74.0	18.8	Corn oil and MCT	4.0	1.0
Peptisorbon	Merck	25	Lactalbumin hydrolysate	18.0	4.5	Maltodextrin and enzyme hydrolysate starch	70	17.5	MCT and sunflower seed oil	5.3	1.3
Vivonex	Eaton Laboratories	26.7	Amino acid free of cystine and taurine	7.7 amino acids	2.1	Glucose solids	86.3	23	Purified safflower oil	0.54	0.14
Vivonex HN	Eaton Laboratories	26.7		16.6 amino acids	4.3	Glucose solids	79.1	21	Purified safflower oil	0.33	0.09
Enteral 400	SHS	21.6	Whey protein isolate	13.3 protein	2.9	Glucose polymer	66.5	14.4	Arachis oil and MCT	18.1	3.9
Elementa 60 (unflavoured 028)	SHS	20	Amino acids	12 amino acids	2.4	Maltodextrin	77.8	15.6	Arachis oil	6.64	1.3
Paediatric formulae											
Pregestimil	Mead Johnson	14.8	Enzyme hydrolysed, casein and amino acids	12.8 protein	1.9	Corn syrup solids and starch	61.6	9.1	Corn oil and MCT	18.3	2.7
Peptide 0-2	SHS	15	Hydrolysed meat and soya peptides and amino acids	13.8	2.1	Maltodextrin (corn origin)	56	8.4	Vegetable and animal fats	23.5	3.5
MCT Peptide 0-2	SHS	15	Hydrolysed meat and soya peptides and amino acids	13.8	2.1	Maltodextrin (corn origin)	62.6	9.4	Vegetable oils	18.9	2.8
Pepdite 2+	SHS	20	Hydrolysed meat and soya peptides and amino acids	13.9	2.8	Maltodextrin (corn origin)	63	12.6	Vegetable oils	18.1	3.6
MCT Pepdite 2+	SHS	20	Hydrolysed meat and soya peptides and amino acids	13.9	2.8	Maltodextrin (corn origin)	62.4	12.5	Vegetable oils	18.8	3.8
Alfaré (semi-elemental formula)	Nestlé	15	Hydrolysed whey protein	16.5	2.5	Glucose polymer	51.7	7.8	MCT oil, milk fat and corn oil	24	3.6

Product	Energy per 100 g (kJ)	(kcal)	per 100 ml (kJ)	(kcal)	Osmolality/ osmolarity	Sodium (mmol)	Potassium (mmol)	Calcium (mmol)	Zinc (µmol)	Phosphorus (mmol)	Iron (µmol)	Vitamin D (µg)	Vitamin A (µg)	Vitamin C (mg)
Adult formulae														
Flexical	1850	441	420	100	550 mmol/kg	1·5	3·2	1·5	15·3	1·6	16·1	0·5	75	15
Nutranel	1663	396	420	100	410 mmol/l	2·0	3·6	1·2	10·7	1·2	17·9	0·5	75	5·5
Peptisorbon	1675	400	419	100	400 mmol/l	6·0	3·0	1·3	11·5	2·0	15	0·25	92·5	4·5
Vivonex	1570	375	419	100	550 mmol/l	3·7	3·0	1·4	12·2	1·8	17·9	0·6	83·4	3·3
Vivonex HN	1570	375	419	100	800 mmol/l	3·4	1·8	0·83	7·6	1·1	10·8	0·3	50	2·0
Enteral 400	1934	462	420	100	300 mmol/l	2·7	3·0	1·2	15·3	1·6	18·5	0·5	81·3	7·1
Elementa 60 (unflavoured O28)	1673	400	335	80	450 mmol/l	2·2	2·4	0·9	12·7	1·3	14·9	0·4	65	5·7
Paediatric formulae														
Pregestimil	1940	462	287	68	338 mmol/kg	1·4	1·9	1·6	6·5	1·4	22·6	1·1	63·3	5·5
Peptide 0–2	1985	475	300	70	195 mmol/kg	1·3	1·5	1·1	9·2	1·1	14·3	1·1	80	6·2
MCT Peptide 0–2	1870	450	280	67	337 mmol/kg	2·0	1·5	1·1	9·2	1·1	14·3	1·1	80	6·2
Peptide 2 +	1880	450	376	90	288 mmol/kg	1·8	2·6	1·0	14·7	1·4	17·2	0·4	75·6	6·6
MCT Peptide 2 +	1930	460	386	92	360 mmol/kg	2·7	2·6	1·0	14·7	1·35	17·2	0·4	75·6	6·6
Alfaré (semi-elemental formula)	2010	480	301	72	220 mmol/kg	1·9	2·3	1·5	8·3	1·2	16·1	1·1	72	5·8

* Range trace minerals included.

† Comprehensive range of vitamins included.

‡ Range of vitamins included.

§ Appropriate energy, vitamin and mineral supplements may be required in young children not taking the full adult recommended volume. The required intake should be calculated from protein needs, and additional energy, vitamin and mineral supplements calculated by comparing the difference between requirement and that provided.

Hyperosmolar elemental diets must be introduced initially as a dilute frequent feeding or continuous nasogastric drip feed.

REFERENCES

ADAMSON C.J., BROWN A.M. & TRUSWELL A.S. (1973) Survey of high and low residue (fibre) diets in British hospitals. *Nutrition* 27, 159.

ANDERSSON A., NÄVERT B., BINGHAM S.A., ENGLYST H.N. & CUMMINGS J.H. (1983) The effect of bread containing similar amounts of phytate but different amounts of wheat bran on calcium, zinc, and iron balance in man. *Brit. J. Nutr.* 50, 503–10.

ATTEBURY H.R., SUTTER V.L. & FINEGOLD S.M. (1972) Effect of a partially chemical defined diet on normal human fecal flora. *Amer. J. clin. Nutr.* 25, 1391.

BINGHAM S. (1979) Low residue diets: a reappraisal of their meaning and content. *J. hum. Nutr.* 33, 5–16.

BOOTH I.W. & HARRIES J.T. (1984) Inflammatory bowel disease in children. Progress report. *Gut* 25 (No. 2), 188–202.

BUNKER V.W. & CLAYTON B.C. (1983) Trace element content of commercial enteral feeds. *Lancet* 2, 426–8.

BURKITT D.P. (1973) Some diseases characteristic of modern western civilization. *Brit. med. J.* 1, 274.

BURKITT D., MORLEY D. & WALKER A. (1980) Dietary fibre in under and over nutrition. *Arch. Dis. Childh.* 55, 803–7.

BURMAN D., PERHAM T.G.M. & CLOTHIER C. (1982) Nutrition in systemic disease. In *Textbook of Paediatric Nutrition*, 2nd Edition (eds. McLaren D.S. & Burman D.), p. 351. Edinburgh: Churchill Livingstone.

CLAYDEN G.S. (1976) Constipation and soiling in childhood, *Brit. med. J.* 1, 515–17.

CLAYDEN G.S. & LAWSON J.O.N. (1976) Investigation and management of long-standing chronic constipation in childhood, *Arch. Dis. Childh.* 51, 918–23.

CUMMINGS J.H. (1978) Dietary fibre and colonic function, *J. roy. Soc. Med.* 71, 81.

DAVIDSON M. & WASSERMAN R. (1966) Irritable colon of childhood (chronic non-specific diarrhoea syndrome). *J. Pediat.* 69, 1027.

DAVIDSON SIR STANLEY, PASSMORE R., BROCK J.F. & TRUSWELL A.S. (eds.) (1979) *Human Nutrition and Dietetics*, 7th Edition, p. 168. Edinburgh: Churchill Livingstone.

FAO (1974) *Handbook on Human Nutritional Requirements*. Rome: FAO.

FRANCIS D.E.M. (1984) Should we be advising on low fat diets in U.K.? *Health Visitor* 57, 145–6.

FRANCIS D.E.M. (1986) *Nutrition for Children*. Oxford: Blackwell Scientific Publications.

HARVEY R.F., POMARE E.W. & HEATON K.W. (1973) Effect of increased dietary fibre on intestinal transit. *Lancet* 1, 1278.

JAMES W.P.T. Chairman (1983) *Proposals for Nutritional Guidelines for Health Education in Britain*. National Advisory Committee on Nutrition Education. Health Education Council.

JAMES W.P.T., BRANCH W.J. & SOUTHGATE D.A.T. (1978) Calcium binding of dietary fibre. *Lancet* 1, 638.

KEOHANE P.P., ATTRILL H., LOVE M., FROST P. & SILK D.B.A. (1984) Relation between osmolality of diet and gastrointestinal side effects in enteral nutrition. *Brit. med. J.* 288, 678–80.

KRAMER P. (1964) The meaning of high and low residue diets. *Gastroenterology* 47, 649.

KRAMER P., KEARNEY M.M. & INGELFINGER F.J. (1962) The effect of specific foods and water loading on the ileal excreta of ileostomised human subjects. *Gastroenterology* 42, 535.

ORNSTEIN M.H., MCLEAN BAIRD I., HOWARD A.N. & FOWLER J. (1982) Colon preparation prior to surgery using a new low residue diet. In *Recent Advances in Clinical Nutrition* 1 (eds. Howard A.N. & McLean Baird I.), pp. 153–5. London: John Libbey.

PAINTER N.S. (1975) *Diverticular Disease of the Colon*. London: Heinemann Medical.

PAINTER N.S., ALMEIDA A.Z. & COLEBOURNE K.W. (1972) Unprocessed bran in treatment of diverticular disease of the colon. *Brit. med. J.* 11, 137.

REILLY C. (1978) Zinc—the unassuming nutrient. In *Getting The Most out of Food*, 13th in a series of studies on the modern approach to feeding and nutrition, p. 45. Van den Berghs & Jurgens Ltd. Uckfield APR.

REINHOLD J.G. (1976) *Trace Elements in Human Health and Disease* (eds. Prasad A.S. & Oberleas O.), p. 163. New York: Academic Press..

RUSSELL R.I. (1975) Progress report: elemental diets. *Gut* 16, 68–79.

SANDERS T. (1978) Vegan diet—A remedy for diseases of affluence. In *Getting The Most Out Of Food*, 13th in a series of studies on the modern approach to feeding in nutrition, p. 103. Van den Berghs & Jurgens Ltd. Uckfield APR.

SOUTHGATE D.A.T., BAILEY B., COLLINSON E. & WALKER A.F. (1976) A guide to calculating intakes of dietary fibre. *J. hum. Nutr.* 30, 303.

STEPHEN A.M. & CUMMINGS J.H. (1979) Water-holding by dietary fibre *in vitro* and its relationship to faecal output in man. *Gut* 20, 722–9.

STEPHEN A.M. & CUMMINGS J.H. (1980) The microbial contribution to human faecal mass. *J. med. Microbiol.* 13, 1, 45–56.

TAYLOR I. & DUTHIE H.L. (1976) Bran tablets for diverticular disease. *Brit. med. J.* 1, 988.

WINITZ M., ADAMS R.F., SEEDMAN D.A., DAVIS P.N., JAYKO L.G. & Hamilton J.A. (1970) Studies in metabolic nutrition employing chemically defined diets. *Amer. J. clin. Nutr.* 23, 546.

WISE A. (1983) Dietary factors determining the biological activities of phytate. *Nutr. Abstr. Rev. in clin. Nutr.* Series A, Vol. 53, 9, 791–806.

WRIGHT R. & TRUSELOVE S.R. (1965) A controlled therapeutic trial of various diets in ulcerative colitis. *Brit. med. J.* 2, 138.

YASSA J.G., PROSSER R. & DODGE J.A. (1978) Effects of an artificial diet on growth of patients with cystic fibrosis. *Arch. Dis. Childh.* 53, 777–83.

CHAPTER 3

Gluten-free diet for coeliac disease

COELIAC DISEASE

'Coeliac disease is a disease of the proximal small intestine characterized by an abnormal small intestinal mucosa and associated with a permanent intolerance to gluten. Removal of gluten from the diet leads to a full clinical and pathological remission.' (Walker-Smith 1979).

Coeliac disease affects both children and adults, causing a range of symptoms related to malabsorption. Gluten, or more specifically the gliadin fraction of gluten, causes damage to the small intestinal mucosa (Walker-Smith 1979). Treatment is with a life-long gluten-free diet, except during a gluten challenge required to confirm the diagnosis. The majority of children presenting with gastrointestinal symptoms due to coeliac disease are under two years of age, and most are under five years of age at diagnosis. Symptoms frequently occur some 3 to 9 months after the introduction of gluten-containing solids. Occasionally symptoms occur immediately gluten is introduced (Walker-Smith & Kilby 1977). However, the diagnosis of children with short stature as the primary manifestation of coeliac disease may be delayed till late childhood or the teenage years. (Groll *et al.* 1980). Such delay may have important and permanent implications for psychological, physical, and sexual development. Recently there has been an increase in the number of adults diagnosed with coeliac disease.

Since the advent of a gluten-free diet, first described by Dicke in 1950, mortality in coeliac disease of childhood has been reduced almost to vanishing point (Sheldon 1969). However, it is incorrect to think of children with coeliac disease as cured, as relapse occurs with the reintroduction of gluten. In later life anaemia, a low serum folate and sometimes a low serum iron level are present if a normal diet is resumed. Sooner or later such individuals with coeliac disease show increasing clinical evidence of malabsorption and do relapse. Coeliac disease is a chronic and persistent disorder, and adult patients have an increased incidence of cancer of all sites and particularly lymphoma of the gut (Stokes & Holmes 1974, Holmes *et al.* 1976). Treatment with a gluten-free diet does not appear to protect against this complication (Holmes *et al.* 1976).

Incidence and heredity

Coeliac disease only occurs in areas of the world where gluten is ingested, and predominantly in populations of European origin (McNeish *et al.* 1974). The incidence of coeliac disease in the past has been thought to be 1 in 3000 in England, but recent work has shown that in the west of Ireland it is about 1 in 300 (Mylotte *et al.* 1973), and past assessments may have underestimated the incidence. Recently the number of children diagnosed with coeliac disease has decreased. Whether this is a true reduction of incidence or simply a delay in onset and diagnosis is unknown. This may be related to the now common practice of delaying the introduction of wheat-containing cereals in the first months of life, and to the fact that more infants are now breast-fed.

Relatives of patients with coeliac disease are found in 10 to 12% of cases to have an abnormal mucosa on small intestinal biopsy. Identical twins are not always affected (Walker-Smith 1979), even when the diagnosis is made on biopsy findings and environmental factors appear to be similar, e.g. age and type of weaning. However there appears to be a genetically determined susceptibility to coeliac disease related to the histocompatibility antigen (Editorial 1977).

There are two theories regarding the toxic effect of gliadin–gluten toxicity, (a) a specific enzyme deficiency and various dipeptidase deficiencies have been found, and (b) a disorder of immunology and a number of abnormalities have been demonstrated. Whether these phenomena are primary or secondary is not established, though these two theories are not mutually exclusive (Walker-Smith 1979).

Symptoms

Children with coeliac disease present with a wide range of symptoms; 70% have diarrhoea and malabsorption, which manifests particularly as pale, bulky, offensive stools, frequently with obvious fat globules present. Occasionally constipation may occur, but the faeces are usually pale. (Egan-Mitchell & McNicholl 1972). However, some 30% of children with active coeliac disease do not have steatorrhoea at the time of diagnosis on a gluten-containing diet with adequate amounts of fat (Walker-Smith 1979). 'Pot belly' is a common finding in children, as is a poor appetite (Walker-Smith & Kilby 1977). Reduced blood folate, associated haematological abnormalities and a reduced tolerance to xylose may be present.

Other features which may occur include vomiting, lethargy, floppiness, irritability and anaemia. Symptoms of malnutrition, including calcium depletion and bone changes, are most frequently found in adults with coeliac disease. Clinical rickets was seen in the past but less frequently now, as diagnosis is made at an earlier age, but post-treatment rickets can occur (Walker-Smith 1979) during the period of rapid catch-up growth.

Most children at the time of diagnosis are underweight or show evidence of failure to thrive, and wasting is apparent in many cases. Short stature may, however, be the only manifestation of coeliac disease, and therefore undiagnosed short stature, especially if the bone age is delayed by more than four years, is an indication for small intestinal biopsy; even in the absence of other symptoms (Groll et al. 1980). However, short stature is not an invariable finding, and therefore normal stature does not exclude coeliac disease.

Diagnosis

A small intestinal biopsy, first described by Sakula and Shiner (1957), is essential and should always be performed before starting treatment with a gluten-free diet. A biopsy is not always possible in a very ill infant with gross wasting, or in centres which are not experienced with the technique. Such infants are best referred to a special unit with experience in taking biopsies in such cases. An abnormal small intestinal mucosa is an essential finding for the diagnosis of coeliac disease.

It is essential that the diagnosis be confirmed following reintroduction of gluten at a later date (see Gluten challenge, p. 70).

An abnormal small intestinal mucosa, though most commonly due to coeliac disease (Walker-Smith 1979), can be due to a number of other conditions, particularly in children who are under the age of two years at the time of the first biopsy. Protein-induced enteropathies due to cow's milk, soya, chicken, fish and rice protein have all been described (Watt et al. 1983). Other causes include gastroenteritis, giardiasis, tropical sprue, and protein–energy malnutrition (Walker-Smith 1979).

The essential diagnosis of coeliac disease as laid down by the European Society of Paediatric Gastroenterology (Meeuwisse 1970) is summarized as follows:

1 It is a permanent condition.
2 Flat small intestinal mucosa demonstrated on a gluten-containing diet (biopsy 1).
3 Response to a gluten-free diet. (i) Relief of symptoms, and (ii) restoration of a normal intestinal mucosa (biopsy 2).
4 Reintroduction of gluten results in recurrence of an abnormal small intestinal mucosa (biopsy 3), even in the absence of clinical signs and symptoms.
5 Biochemical evidence of malabsorption, even though asymptomatic at the time of investigation.

The diagnostic criteria are given by Walker-Smith (1979) and are summarized in Fig. 3.1.

Patients with dermatitis herpetiformis are also treated with a gluten-free diet (Walker-Smith 1979).

Introduction of a gluten-free diet

As soon as coeliac disease or dermatitis herpetiformis is diagnosed the patient should be treated with a gluten-free diet appropriately modified for the clinical condition. The age at diagnosis varies and the clinical condition ranges from the severely ill to the apparently well child.

Considerable encouragement may be necessary to get the child to eat in the early stages of treatment when anorexia is common. However, as soon as the gluten-free diet is instigated the child becomes less irritable, a happy, pleasing disposition becomes evident and appetite returns to normal in response to treatment. Initially the child may need an increased intake of dietary nutrients to allow for catch-up growth, e.g. infants and toddlers may need 3 to 4 g protein/kg per day and 540 to 840 kJ (130 to 200 kcal)/kg per day with a generous intake of other nutrients. A general vitamin supplement including vitamin D and folic acid (e.g. three Ketovite Tablets plus 5 ml Ketovite Liquid), plus iron and possibly zinc supplements, is recommended during the first months

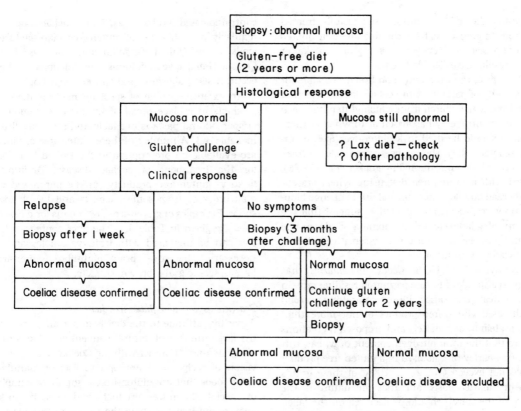

Fig. 3.1 Diagnostic criteria and investigation for coeliac disease. From Walker-Smith (1979) with permission.

of treatment. Once weight gain and growth are initiated a gluten-free diet suitable for the child's age and appetite should be given.

Gluten exclusion is highly successful and the intestinal mucosa returns to normal, even though the period of time varies with severity of the mucosal changes. In some children improvement has been found after only a week or two of treatment, in others it may take a year to return to normal (Anderson 1960). The initial response to treatment in children is often dramatic with a rapid clinical response and weight gain, though diarrhoea may persist for some time (Walker-Smith 1979).

The gluten-free diet

Gluten is a large complex molecule that has been divided chemically into four heterogeneous proteins: gliadins, glutenins, albumins and globulins. Gliadin is the fraction of gluten responsible for coeliac disease and is itself a complex protein consisting of 40 different components. Alpha-gliadin is particularly toxic, though the toxicity may be related to a small peptide. Beta-, gamma- and omega-gliadin are also toxic.

How the toxic fractions cause their effect is still unknown (Walker-Smith 1979). Alpha-gliadin is present in wheat protein except in a variant Chinese spring wheat (Kasarda *et al.* 1978) which awaits full evaluation before it can be used by patients with coeliac disease. Rye is also toxic to coeliacs (Walker-Smith 1979). However, controversy still exists over whether or not it is necessary to exclude oats and barley (Anderson *et al.* 1972). These cereals, particularly barley, are used less extensively in the United Kingdom diet than wheat. Dissanayake *et al.* (1974) concluded oats are harmless after administering 40–60 g oats per day to adult coeliacs for one month with no biopsy changes. Five children who had eaten oats regularly on a gluten-free diet had normal pre-challenge biopsies, and subsequently coeliac disease was proven in these children (Packer *et al.* 1978), which supports Dissanayake's conclusions. Oats contain the protein avenin, which is distinct from gluten. Barley, which contains the protein hordein, is reported to cause mucosal changes when given in highly artificial circumstances (Rubin *et al.* 1962), and most clinics now recommend that barley be omitted. Barley and oats have been permitted in the gluten-free diet of the author's successfully treated children, though except for the five children quoted above no scientific evidence of regular intake or biopsy results are available to date.

In the past, the only flour and bread available for the majority of patients with coeliac disease was that made from wheat starch from which gluten had been removed. Controversy has arisen as to whether these products should be used in a gluten-free diet, or indeed whether they should be termed 'gluten-free'. The author's patients, quoted by Packer *et al.* (1978), treated with a gluten-free diet using wheat starch-based bread and flour had normal pre-challenge biopsies. However, Ciclitira *et al.* (1985) suggest that the amount of gliadin found in nominally gluten-free products may be important in very sensitive patients. This awaits confirmation.

Recently, WHO (1979, *Codex Alimentarius*) has proposed a standard for the permitted residual protein in a wheat (or other gluten-containing cereal) starch-based gluten-free product of not more than 0.3% protein in dry matter, and proposed regulations require that the total nitrogen content of wheat, triticale, rye, barley or oats used in a gluten-free product should not exceed $0.05\,g$ per $100\,g$ of these grains on a dry matter basis, and that the nature of the source of the starch should be declared on the label. There is no evidence at present to suggest that products based on wheat starch which fulfil the *Codex Alimentarius* definition of a gluten-free product are unsuitable for use in the treatment of patients with coeliac disease. However, new technology is making possible a range of naturally gluten-free (i.e. wheat-free) flours and breads, which in time may totally replace those based on gluten-free wheat (and other gluten-containing cereal) starches.

Other cereals and all pulses are classified as naturally gluten-free and are not implicated; these include rice, maize, millet, buckwheat, soya and potato, all of which can be used as flour substitutes. Natural conventional foods such as milk, meat, egg, cheese, fruit, vegetables, butter, margarine, fats and oils are gluten-free (Table 3.1) but manufactured foods must be carefully scrutinized for sources of gluten from ingredients such as flour, farina, semolina, pasta or starch, including wheat starch, which does not meet the *Codex Alimentarius* gluten-free standard. Many convenience foods do not list the ingredients in an easily recognizable way, for example dry roast peanuts, 'MacDonald' type chips, flavoured crisps, and flavoured yoghurt can contain gluten. Some companies now use the gluten-free symbol ⓧ on appropriate products. Some medicines contain gluten and are

contraindicated (Table 3.2). The Coeliac Society* regularly publish a list of gluten-free manufactured foods in the United Kingdom and its news sheet, *Crossed Grain*, gives additions and deletions as they occur. It also publishes a gluten-free recipe book.

An extensive range of specially made gluten-free products to replace bread, flour, biscuits, semolina, crispbread and pasta is available and these are listed in Table 3.3. A number of these gluten-free products are available on prescription in the United Kingdom for the treatment of coeliac disease. Additional 'luxury' gluten-free products can be purchased on mail order or from some chemists and health food shops. Examples of gluten-free diet menus for different ages are given in Table 3.4. The fibre content of the diet can be increased with fruit, vegetables and, if necessary, the soya bran high-fibre gluten-free breads, whole grain 'brown' rice, etc.

Practical aspects of a gluten-free diet

A positive attitude to the diet is important, stressing the large number of natural conventional foods that are gluten-free. Contact with the Coeliac Society, provision of recipes and appropriate lists of manufactured foods that are gluten-free, a supply or samples of special gluten-free products and prescription of appropriate items all help the family to provide the correct diet during the early days of treatment. To integrate the patient on a gluten-free diet, the whole family should be encouraged to use the same type of menu, wherever possible. Stews, casseroles, gravy and custards can be thickened with cornflour (maize), and gluten-free brands of manufactured products can be used for everyone. Gluten-free substitutes can be made for many home-cooked dishes. Ordinary pasta can be replaced with gluten-free pasta or, on those occasions when the menu includes gluten-containing items, an alternative can be prepared for the coeliac, e.g. fruit, cheese and gluten-free crackers, or ice-cream or yoghurt (gluten-free brands) can replace puddings. A freezer can be used to store individual portions of gluten-free alternatives. Gluten-free bread can be sliced then frozen in convenient sized packs until required, or kept in the freezer compartment of an ordinary refrigerator for a short period. If a freezer is not available, gluten-free bread can be kept reasonably fresh by storing it in a plastic bag in a refrigerator. As it stales, toasting will make it acceptable. New pre-packed vacuum-packed gluten-free loaves are available with a longer shelf-life as an alternative

---

* The Coeliac Society, PO Box 220, High Wycombe, Bucks, HP11 4H7.

to the canned bread or home-made bread made from the gluten-free mixes or flours.

A strict gluten-free diet is essential. The patient with coeliac disease, from toddler age onwards, should be taught that certain foods will upset him, but acceptable alternatives are available. In all other respects the child should be treated normally. By school age the child should have a knowledge of which foods he can or cannot have on his diet. 'If in doubt leave it out' should be the motto. Occasional accidents may occur causing minor symptoms, but

Table 3.1 Gluten-free diet.

Gluten is a protein found in wheat and rye. Barley may also be implicated and is usually omitted. All foods made from or containing wheat, rye and barley must be omitted.

Oats are also excluded in some patients and therefore foods containing these items are marked*.

Proprietary products displaying the gluten-free symbol are guaranteed gluten-free.

(a) Basic foods which are *gluten-free* (provided no gluten-containing items are added in preparation).

Milk (fresh, tinned, powder), butter, margarine, cream, natural yoghurt.

Meat, fish, cheese, eggs.

Fruit, fresh, stewed, dried fruit, nuts. Canned or frozen fruit provided sugar only is added.

Vegetables, fresh or frozen, or tinned in water and salt only.

Potatoes.

Peas, lentils, dried beans and pulses.

Cereals

Maize (corn), cornflour, Cornflakes, corn-on-the-cob, sweetcorn.

Rice, rice flour, Rice Krispies, ground or flaked rice, baby rice, rice bran.

Tapioca and sago, arrowroot.

Special gluten-free flour—various brands (*see* Table 3.3).

Soya, soya flour, soya bran.

Potato flour.

Millet, buckwheat.

Soups and sauces made without wheat, rye, barley, oats, flour, etc.

Gravy made with cornflour and meat juices.

Bovril, Marmite.

Sugar, jam, honey, marmalade.

Salt, pepper, fresh herbs, vinegar.

Tea, coffee, cocoa, instant coffee.

Fruit juices, fizzy drinks and fruit squash.

Jelly, gelatine, rennet.

Oats*, porridge*, Ready Brek*.

(b) Foods which contain gluten unless specially prepared from gluten-free alternatives.

Wheat

Ordinary flour (wheat) used for baking, thickening, etc.

Bread, biscuits, cakes, pastry, wheatmeal, bran, rusks.

Crispbreads, starch-reduced bread, rolls, slimming rolls, ice-cream cones.

Weetabix, Puffed Wheat, Shredded Wheat, Grapenuts, Bemax, Sugar Puffs, Farley's babies' rusks, Farlene and similar baby foods.

Spaghetti, macaroni, noodles and all other pasta.

Semolina.

Ready-made dishes with breadcrumb coating, e.g. fish fingers.

Sausages, 'Bacon-Breakfast' slices.

Gravy made from flour, Bisto, etc.

Milk-shakes, Horlick's, malted milks, Benger's Food.

Any manufactured foods containing wheat or flour.

Rye

Rye bread, Ryvita, Rye crispbread.

Any manufactured foods containing rye.

Barley

Barley, barley bread, barley water and barley drinks, e.g. lemon barley. Any manufactured foods containing barley.

(c) Manufactured products likely to contain gluten which should be checked by brand in the list of gluten-free products published by the Coeliac Society.

The label should also be scrutinized for gluten-containing ingredients such as flour, farina, starch, etc.

Baby foods including cereals, dinners and desserts.

Sausages, beefburgers, tinned meat products, hamburgers, sausage meats.

Fish fingers, cod bites.

Coating on fish or meat, luncheon meat.

Thick soups, gravy, stock cubes, gravy mixes, Bisto, some spices and dried herbs.

Flavoured crisps, 'dry roast' peanuts.

Ready-to-eat meals, café and school dinners, e.g. 'MacDonald's' chips.

Sauces and ketchups.

Vegetables in sauce, e.g. baked beans, vegetable salad.

Pie fillings, yoghurt (some brands of fruit and flavoured types).

Many sweets and filled chocolates, e.g. seaside rock, boiled sweets, Smarties.

Ice cream, mousse.

Table 3.2 Examples of medicines which contain gluten.

Dimotane LA	Natirose
Dimotapp LA	Nulacin
Donatal LA	Saroten Tablets
Fybranta	Veracolate Tablets
Nardil Tablets	Pyridium
Benger's Food	Charcoal biscuits

Table 3.3 Proprietary products which are gluten-free.

Item	U.K. supplier
Bread	
*† Juvela Gluten-Free Loaf (Pre-baked)	GF Dietary Supplies
* Rite-Diet Gluten-Free Low-Protein Bread with or without salt (canned)	Welfare Foods Ltd
* Rite-Diet Gluten-Free Low-Protein Bread with Soya Bran (canned)	Welfare Foods Ltd
* Rite-Diet Gluten-Free Bread (Pre-baked) with or without fibre	Welfare Foods Ltd
Biscuits	
‡ Aglutella Azeta Low-Protein Gluten-Free Cream-Filled Wafers	GF Dietary Supplies
†‡ Aproten Biscuits	Ultrapharm (Carlo Erba) Ltd
*† Aproten Crispbread	Ultrapharm (Carlo Erba) Ltd
†‡ Bi-aglut Gluten-Free Biscuits	Ultrapharm (Carlo Erba) Ltd
‡ Chico San Inc. Rice Cakes	GF Dietary Supplies
†‡ Farley's Gluten-Free Biscuits	Farley Health Products Ltd
‡ GF Dietary Brand Gluten-Free Crackers	GF Dietary Supplies
†‡ GF Dietary Brand Gluten-Free Maize Biscuits with Chocolate	GF Dietary Supplies
†‡ GF Dietary Brand Gluten-Free Maize Biscuits with Hazelnuts	GF Dietary Supplies
‡ GF Dietary Brand Gluten-Free Thin Wafer Bread	GD Dietary Supplies
‡ Glutenex Biscuits (Liga)	Cow & Gate
‡ Hol-grain Natural Rice Waferets with or without salt	GF Dietary Supplies
‡ Rite-Diet Gluten-Free Biscuits (Sweet or Savoury)	Welfare Foods Ltd
†‡ Rite-Diet Gluten-Free Chocolate Biscuits Half-Coated	Welfare Foods Ltd
‡ Rite-Diet Gluten-Free Custard Creams	Welfare Foods Ltd
‡ Rite-Diet Gluten-Free Digestive Biscuits	Welfare Foods Ltd
‡ Rite-Diet Gluten-Free Sultana Biscuits	Welfare Foods Ltd
‡ Rite-Diet Low-Protein Gluten-Free Sweet Biscuits	Welfare Foods Ltd
‡ Rite-Diet Low-Protein Gluten-Free Vanilla Cream Wafers	Welfare Foods Ltd
†‡ Verkade Gluten-Free Biscuits	GF Dietary Supplies
Cake	
*† Rite-Diet Gluten-Free Rich Fruit Cake	Welfare Foods Ltd
Flour	
·* Aproten Gluten-Free Flour	Ultrapharm (Carlo Erba) Ltd
*† Juvela Gluten-Free Mix	GF Dietary Supplies
†‡ Juvela Gluten-Free Corn Mix	GF Dietary Supplies
* Juvela Low-Protein Mix	GF Dietary Supplies
†‡ Rite-Diet Gluten-Free Flour Mix	Welfare Foods Ltd
†‡ Rite-Diet Gluten-Free White Bread Mix	Welfare Foods Ltd
†‡ Rite-Diet Gluten-Free Brown Bread Mix	Welfare Foods Ltd
* Rite-Diet Low-Protein Gluten-Free Flour Mix	Welfare Foods Ltd
* Tritamyl Gluten-Free Flour	Procea Ltd
* Tritamyl PK Flour	Procea Ltd
‡ Trufree Special Dietary Flour	
‡ No. 1	Cantassium Co., Larkhall Labs
‡ No. 2 with rice bran	Cantassium Co., Larkhall Labs
‡ No. 3 for Cantabread } With yeast	Cantassium Co., Larkhall Labs
‡ No. 4 white	Cantassium Co., Larkhall Labs
‡ No. 5 brown	Cantassium Co., Larkhall Labs
‡ No. 6 plain	Cantassium Co., Larkhall Labs
‡ No. 7 self-raising	Cantassium Co., Larkhall Labs
Pasta	
‡ Aglutella Gentili gluten-free low-protein macaroni, semolina, spaghetti rings	GF Dietary Supplies
‡ Aproten Pasta ribbed macaroni, flat noodles, small pasta rings, spaghetti, small macaroni	Ultrapharm (Carlo Erba) Ltd
‡ Rite Diet Gluten-Free Low-Protein macaroni, spaghetti, rings	Welfare Foods Ltd
Miscellaneous	
‡ Ener-G Pure Rice Bran	GF Dietary Supplies
‡ Rite-Diet Gluten-Free Soya Bran	Welfare Foods Ltd
‡ Rite-Diet Gluten-Free Baking Powder	Welfare Foods Ltd
†‡ GF Brand Gluten-Free Pastry Mix	GF Dietary Supplies

* Contains gluten-free wheat starch which complies with *Codex Alimentarius* definition.
† Contains milk protein and/or lactose.
‡ Wheat- and gluten-free.
 Some items are classified as suitable for prescription for coeliacs at NHS expense.

Table 3.4 Gluten-free diet: sample menu.

Only gluten-free brands should be selected throughout and food items should be prepared without added flour or other gluten-containing items

(a)   Diet for the older child.

Breakfast	Permitted cereal, e.g. Rice Krispies, Cornflakes Milk and sugar Egg, bacon or cheese, or fish Gluten-free bread—may be toasted Butter or margarine Jam, honey, marmalade, Marmite if desired Milk, tea, coffee or cocoa to drink
Mid-morning	Fruit juice or milk
Dinner	Meat or fish, boiled, roast, steamed, poached, grilled or stewed (cooked with flour or breadcrumbs) Gluten-free gravy thickened with cornflour Potato or rice Vegetables Fruit Custard or suitable gluten-free pudding or jelly or junket
High tea or supper	Soup—homemade or suitable brand—optional Meat, fish, cheese, egg (cooked without flour or breadcrumbs) Vegetables and/or gluten-free bread, butter or margarine Fruit or milk pudding Gluten-free cakes or biscuits Milk, tea, coffee, cocoa to drink
Bedtime	Milk, fruit

(b)   Weaning diet.

	Modified infant feeds or milk as appropriate for age
a.m.	Farex Weaning Food, Baby Rice (Milupa or Robinsons) or suitable gluten-free cereal, with modified milk
Noon	Minced or homogenized meat, or fish or chicken Gluten-free gravy thickened with cornflour

	Potato and purée vegetable or gluten-free baby food Suitable gluten-free custard Purée fruit
Snack	Fruit juice, gluten-free rusk or gluten-free biscuit (Table 3.3)
p.m.	Gluten-free cereal, milk and sugar or suitable gluten-free custard
or	Egg and gluten-free bread and butter or margarine
or	Gluten-free baby food Purée fruit

these will usually pass in a few days, occasionally taking 2 to 3 weeks to completely clear. These episodes act as a warning against future dietary indiscretion. Older children may have no obvious symptoms on taking gluten and find it hard to see the need for the diet. Mucosal changes can occur even without symptoms; anaemia and growth failure may not be obvious in the short term.

Some practical problems arise in teenagers as a result of the need for a life-long gluten-free diet, especially in the current permissive society. Teenagers are usually in remission and find it hard to see why they should adhere to a rigid diet. Regular checks, especially of folate levels and for anaemia, should be made. Practical considerations and advice regarding the diet are helpful, including suitable snack foods, ideas for holidays, and social eating. A positive approach about what can be eaten is essential.

Social eating
Patients with coeliac disease should be encouraged to accept invitations to tea and parties, but with young children the hostess will need to be informed of the diet principles, menu suggestions given and appropriate special gluten-free foods supplied. The child should grow up to think it is 'normal' and socially acceptable to take along some gluten-free bread, biscuits or cake, when eating away from home. These items can be shared with friends. A light meal or snack before going out to waylay hunger is a help for the older child and teenager, in case there is limited gluten-free food available.

In restaurants and cafés simple foods such as grills, omelettes, egg and traditional chips, or cheese salad, and vegetables without dressing are the most suitable. Sauces, gravies and made-up dishes should be avoided. For snacks and parties for older children, teenagers and adults, most drinks are gluten-free and plain salted peanuts, cheese cubes, plain olives, sultanas, pineapple cubes and plain salted crisps are all suitable.

School lunches present a problem if the child cannot come home. A packed lunch (*see* Table 3.5) can be taken from home and a hot meal given in the evening. Alternatively, arrangements could be made with the headmaster and school meal organizer. In some areas, a gluten-free meal can be arranged. Schools can be supplied with a tin or pre-baked loaf of gluten-free bread, packet(s) of gluten-free biscuits and small tins of suitable brands of soup or baked beans to supplement meagre or unsuitable meals.

Table 3.5 Ideas for packed lunches for school (only gluten-free brands should be used).

Ham or cold meats
Permitted tinned meats
Chicken leg or portion (cooked)
Hard-boiled egg
Cheese, cottage cheese
Tinned salmon or tuna fish—pack in small airtight plastic containers or use ring-pull tins.
Sandwiches made from gluten-free bread
Gluten-free bread and butter/margarine
Gluten-free crispbread or gluten-free crackers and butter/ margarine
Salad packed in plastic box or foil or greaseproof paper
Fruit
Gluten-free biscuits
Gluten-free cake
Nuts and dried fruit
Chocolate or sweets or crisps for treats
Hot soup, coffee or tea, cocoa—in children's thermos or sent in a plastic container ready for the school to heat
Canned cold drinks or fruit juice in individual carton or in plastic container

Self-catering holidays with the occasional meal out present no problem. The Coeliac Society have a list of holiday hints for home and abroad. Adequate gluten-free supplies should be taken; the canned and/ or pre-baked gluten-free breads and crispbreads are particularly useful. Many hotels and even caravan site shops will permit gluten-free bread to be kept in the freezer. Children on scout and similar camps should take plenty of gluten-free products and menu substitutes (individual packets and tins of suitable brands of baked beans, cheese portions, soups and fish, e.g. sardines, to replace the unsuitable sausages

and beefburgers inevitably on the menu). Some extra pocket money to buy suitable snacks is a help.

DURATION OF TREATMENT

By definition, coeliac disease persists when diagnosed by the criteria of the European Society of Paediatric Gastroenterology. Even though symptoms may not be present, it is now strongly recommended that a gluten-free diet be continued for life (Walker-Smith 1979). It is hoped that this will avoid the development of chronic deficiencies and relapse with stress, and infertility may be avoided by the diet in adults with coeliac disease. There is uncertainty about whether a gluten-free diet from childhood will reduce the incidence of cancer seen in adults with coeliac disease in whom treatment with a gluten-free diet does not appear to protect against this complication.

Figure 3.1 indicates, however, that some patients who initially are treated with a gluten-free diet do not have coeliac disease. Such patients do not need continued treatment. Sequential biopsies before and after a gluten challenge are essential to determine which patients have coeliac disease necessitating life-long treatment.

Gluten challenge

Differing age groups and different dietary patterns result in a widely varying intake of wheat protein, and therefore gluten, on a normal diet. The encouragement to increase fibre and cereal intakes in the national diet will result in a higher wheat protein and gluten intake. Table 3.6 gives an estimate of the wheat protein content expected in the diet of different age groups on traditional United Kingdom diets.

Table 3.6 Assessed wheat protein intake of a normal diet in different aged children.

Age in years	Wheat protein (g/day)
Less than 1	Varies according to weaning intake
1 to 3	5 to 10
3 to 6	7 to 12
6 to 9	10 to 15
9 +	15 to 30

Natural foods containing wheat protein as the source of gluten have been found satisfactory, in the author's experience, during the gluten challenge. Usually a diet containing a minimum of 10 g protein from wheat is advised. Table 3.7 lists serves of food

Table 3.7 Foods which contain 2 to 3 g wheat protein when eaten in the amount stated.

Ordinary bread—1 small slice, 30 g = 2·2 g wheat protein
　　　　　　　　1 medium slice, 40 g = 3 g wheat protein
2 Farley Rusks (original or low-sugar)
1 Weetabix or Shredded Wheat
1 bowl Puffed Wheat
1 bowl Sugar Puffs
3 chipolata sausages
2 large sausages
3 fish fingers
3 medium-sized biscuits
1 slice cake = 30 g (1 oz)
1 portion sponge pudding
30 g (1 oz) portion pastry
30 g (1 oz) flour
4 tablespoons cooked or tinned spaghetti

---

containing 2 to 3 g of wheat protein, 4 to 5 serves of which can be incorporated into a gluten-containing 'challenge' diet.

Bread and cereals of wheat origin are more physiological then gluten powder (vital wheat protein, RMH and BDH). The latter is unpalatable and difficult to incorporate into the diet and the consistency makes it difficult to take as a medicine. In those patients in whom gluten powder is considered more appropriate, a dose of 10 to 15 g per day is advised in conjunction with a gluten-free diet.

Most children subsequently return to a gluten-free diet without undue difficulty though more problems are found in children under eight years old at the time of the gluten challenge than in older children (Packer *et al.* 1978). The optimal age of gluten challenge is controversial, though there is some advantage in confirming the need for a gluten-free diet before the child has to cope with social eating at school. The emotional stress of the biopsy and gluten challenge, to both parents and child, must be considered. Careful explanation of the procedure is essential, and the fear of so-called 'toxic' foods should not be overlooked, whether given as gluten powder or wheat-containing conventional foods. The optimal length of time for a gluten challenge has not been established (Packer *et al.* 1978, Walker-Smith 1979). If symptoms occur with the gluten challenge a biopsy may be taken after an interval of one week. Otherwise the routine in the author's hospital group is currently to take the second biopsy after three months on a 'challenge' diet containing at least 10 g wheat protein, that is approximately 4 to 5 items per day from Table 3.7. The rest of the diet can be either gluten-free or a 'free' diet as seems appropriate for

the individual and his family. If the biopsy is abnormal a diagnosis of coeliac disease is confirmed, and the child returned to a gluten-free diet. The opportunity is used to instruct the family about changes in products and new proprietary gluten-free items, recipes, etc. A normal small intestinal mucosa after three months on the 'challenge' gluten-containing diet necessitates a further biopsy when symptoms occur or after two years' exposure to gluten (Walker-Smith 1979). The precise timing is somewhat arbitrary and may be altered in the light of further experience.

Patients in whom the initial biopsy show a flat mucosa, but in whom subsequent 'challenge' biopsies are normal, should have a long-term follow-up in case of relapse, for example in adolescence or adulthood. This phenomenon is called transient gluten intolerance (Walker-Smith 1979). A gluten-free diet is indicated temporarily, but the optimal duration of treatment is still not determined (Walker-Smith 1979).

The dietitian has an important role in establishing the diagnosis by taking accurate dietary histories to assess gluten intake. An up-to-date knowledge of gluten-containing foods is essential, for example Farex Weaning Food (Farley) was a traditional source of gluten, but is now gluten-free; Farley's Rusks still contain gluten in both the original and new low-sugar variety. The wheat protein content of common foods is useful in determining intake, and the age at which the child is weaned and therefore is first exposed to gluten may be relevant in the initial diagnosis.

The dietitian is also important in assessing whether the gluten-free diet is truly gluten-free; that the school meal is appropriate and liberties at parties, etc. have not been taken; and that products are correctly scrutinized and selected for suitability for the gluten-free diet.

Complications of coeliac disease at the time of diagnosis which are of nutritional significance

Retarded growth
Some coeliacs are short for age and more frequently they are underweight (Verkasalo *et al.* 1978). Usually catch-up growth occurs once a gluten-free diet is instigated (Groll *et al.* 1980). Dietary intake of all nutrients, including trace vitamins and minerals, should be adequate. Dietary supplements may be necessary during the initial phase of treatment and young children should normally have a supplement of at least vitamins A, D and C.

Anaemia and haematological abnormalities

Anaemia is quite common and is usually the iron deficiency type, rather than megaloblastic anaemia, though blood folate levels are often reduced (Cook *et* *al.* 1970, Walker-Smith 1979). Iron and folic acid supplements are required to correct the deficiency. Zinc deficiency may also occur in some patients and can be corrected by supplements.

Table 3.8 Gluten-free milk protein-free, minimal lactose diet.

Gluten is a protein found in wheat and rye and therefore all wheat and rye products must be excluded from the diet. Barley may also be implicated and is usually omitted. Oats marked * are also excluded in some patients.
Milk protein is contained in all types of milk and products containing whey and/or casein; therefore milk and all such products must be excluded from the diet.
Lactose is the sugar in milk and is used as a filler in tablets and some powder flavourings.

Gluten-, milk-, lactose-free foods (provided no gluten-containing items are added in preparation)	Foods which contain or may contain gluten, milk, lactose
Suitable milk substitute, e.g. *soya*, Prosobee, Wysoy, Cow & Gate S Formula	Modified milks, cow's milk, dried and evaporated milks, cream, ice-cream, yoghurt
Hydrolysed casein, Pregestimil, Nutramigen	Filled milks, such as Five Pints, Coffee-mate and coffee creamers
Margarines, e.g. Tomor, Telma soft margarine, milk-free low-fat spreads (Safeway and Sainsbury) Cooking oils, lard	Butter, ordinary and polyunsaturated margarines, e.g. Stork, Flora, Outline, etc. All cheeses and cheese-spreads
Meat Poultry Eggs Fish	Tinned meats, pastes, sausages, beefburgers, hamburgers, sausage meats, meat or fish cooked in breadcrumbs or butter, e.g. rissoles, fish fingers, frozen made-up dishes, e.g. shepherd's pie, 'Bacon-Breakfast' slices
All fruit, fresh, tinned and frozen	Fruit pie fillings
All vegetables, fresh, tinned, frozen Potatoes, chips, plain crisps Peas, lentils, dried beans	Manufactured vegetable dishes, e.g. baked beans, potato salad, vegetable salad Flavoured crisps, 'MacDonald's' chips
Sugar, glucose, jam, honey, marmalade, golden syrup, treacle, plain boiled sweets, plain dark chocolate (check brand)	Chocolate, sweets, lactose Sugar substitute powders, which contain lactose, e.g. Sweet 'n' Low, hydrolysed milk sugar
Cereals Maize (corn), cornflour, Cornflakes, soya, soya flour, soya bran, rice, ground rice, rice flour, Rice Krispies, potato flour, Baby Rice, Farex Weaning Food, rice bran, tapioca, sago, arrowroot Oats*, porridge*, Ready Brek*	Wheat, e.g. Weetabix, Bemax. Rye, e.g. Ryvita, Ryking, rye breads, barley breads Flour, bread, biscuits, cakes Semolina, spaghetti, macaroni and all pastas made from wheat, muesli, baby foods containing milk solids and/or gluten Egg noodles, fresh spaghetti, Special K
Selected gluten-, milk-free flour, bread, biscuits (*see* Table 3.3), gluten-free baking powder Gluten-free custard powder, e.g. Bird's Jelly, gelatine, rennet	Instant Whip, Angel Delight, etc. Custard mix, jelly creams and made-up desserts Gluten-free products which contain milk
Bovril, Marmite. Home-made soups from permitted ingredients Salt, pepper, fresh herbs and spices, vinegar	Soups, sauces, gravies, Oxo, Bisto, ketchups, mayonnaise Manufactured and dried spices and herbs, monosodium glutamate retail powders
Fruit juices, tea, coffee, instant coffee, cocoa (made with milk substitute), fruit drinks and carbonated beverages, Pareve-mate	Bengers, malted milks, Ovaltine, Horlicks, barley drinks
	Lactose and medicines and tablets with lactose filler

* If permitted.

Hypothrombinaemia

This is due to vitamin K malabsorption and should be corrected by intramuscular vitamin K (1 mg) before taking the diagnostic biopsy (Walker-Smith 1979).

Coeliac crisis

The introduction of wheat at a later age during weaning, and the recognition and rapid diagnosis of active coeliac disease have resulted in fewer patients who are severely ill at diagnosis. The occasional

Table 3.9 Gluten-free, milk-free, minimal lactose diet: sample menu.

Only gluten and milk-free brands should be selected throughout and food should be prepared without flour, milk, etc.

(a) Diet for the older child.

Breakfast	Permitted cereal, e.g. Cornflakes, Rice Krispies
	Sugar
	Milk substitute
	Egg, bacon, ham or fish
	Gluten-, milk-, lactose-free bread (may be toasted)
	Tomor margarine, or milk-free, low-fat spread
	Jam, honey, marmalade or Marmite, Bovril
	Tea or coffee with milk substitute or fruit juice
Lunch	Meat, fish, egg (cooked without flour, breadcrumbs or milk)
	Gluten-free gravy thickened with cornflour
	Milk-free potato or rice
	Vegetables
	Fruit, custard or pudding made with milk substitute, custard powder, rice, egg, sago
	or Suitable gluten-, milk-, lactose-free pudding
High tea or supper	Meat, fish, eggs (no bread, flour or milk)
	Vegetables, or salad
	Gluten-, milk-, lactose-free bread and Tomor margarine
	Jelly, fruit or suitable pudding as at lunch
	Gluten-, milk-, lactose-free biscuits or cake made from suitable recipes or selected from Table 3.3 e.g. Glutenex biscuit or GF Brand gluten-free crackers

(b) Weaning diet.

	Milk substitute as appropriate for age
a.m.	Farex Weaning Food, Baby Rice, (Milupa or Robinson's), mix with milk substitute
	Egg-yolk may be included
Noon	Homogenized or minced meat, fish or chicken
	Gluten-free gravy thickened with cornflour
	Boiled potato or mashed milk-free potato
	Purée vegetables
	Purée fruit
Snack	Gluten-, milk-, lactose-free bread or biscuit (see Table 3.3)
	Fruit juice
p.m.	Custard or ground rice made with milk substitute and gluten-free custard powder and/or fruit purée
	Gluten-, milk-, lactose-free bread and Tomor margarine
	or Purée meat or fish, potato and vegetable
	or Cereal and milk substitute
	or Gluten-, milk-, lactose-free baby food

patient presents with severe dehydration and multiple malabsorption known as coeliac crisis. Initial rehydration and sequential introduction of an appropriate formula (e.g. Pregestimil) and gluten-free solids appropriate for the clinical conditions and child's age are indicated (see Chapter 1). A gluten-free milk protein-free, minimal lactose diet (Tables 3.8 and 3.9) may be needed as a temporary measure until the primary diagnosis is established by serial biopsies. It has been suggested that temporary use of corticosteroids may be useful in the severely sick infant (Lloyd-Still et al. 1972).

Milk protein enteropathy in association with coeliac disease

This has been well documented in one patient by Watt et al. (1983). The interesting feature of this case, now aged eight years, is the persistence of the milk protein intolerance which has generally been thought to resolve by two years of age. Others have reported both cow's milk and gluten as contributory factors to malabsorption in infants (Visakorpi & Immonen 1967, Kuitunen *et al.* 1975). This phenomenon appears distinct from food allergic disease (*see* Chapter 4) found in atopic patients in whom enteropathy is rarely found, though both require withdrawal of the offending proteins and foods from the diet. Primary milk protein enteropathy, especially in infants, must be distinguished from coeliac disease by serial biopsies (Walker-Smith *et al.* 1978) in conjunction with dietary withdrawal and challenge.

Lactose intolerance in coeliac patients
Lactase activity may be temporarily depressed in the brush border area of the enterocyte cells of the villi in coeliac patients. Treatment with a gluten-free diet alone is all that is required in the majority. A gluten-free diet with temporary exclusion of milk and lactose is however indicated in about 5% of patients with symptomatic secondary intolerance to milk or lactose (Walker-Smith 1979). Secondary sucrase deficiency is virtually never of clinical importance in coeliac patients. A gluten-free, milk protein-free minimal lactose diet is described in Tables 3.8 and 3.9.

Conditions associated with coeliac disease
Liver abnormalities with raised aminotransferase levels can be associated with a severely damaged mucosa, which may be permeable to toxic substances that are absorbed. Hepatic dysfunction improves with a gluten-free diet. Other conditions associated with coeliac disease such as diabetes mellitus, IgA deficiency, cystic fibrosis, require specific treatment in addition to treatment with a gluten-free diet.

REFERENCES

ANDERSON C. M. (1960) Histological changes in the duodenal mucosa in coeliac disease. *Arch. Dis. Childh.* **35**, 419.

ANDERSON C. M., GRACEY M. & BURKE V. (1972) Coeliac disease; some still controversial aspects. *Arch. Dis. Childh.* **47**, 292–8.

CICLITIRA P. J., ELLIS H. J., EVANS D. J. & LENNOX E. S. (1985) A radioimmunoassay for wheat gliadin to assess the suitability of gluten-free foods for patients with coeliac disease. *Clin. exp. Immunol.* **59**, 703–8.

COOK D. M., EVANS N., LLOYD A. & STEWART J.S. (1970) Normal serum and red-cell folate levels in a child with coeliac disease. *Lancet* **1**, 571–2.

DICKE W. K. (1950) Coeliakie: een onderzoek naar de nadelige invloed van sommige graansoorte op de lijder aan coeliakie. MD thesis, Utrecht, and *Transactions of the 6th International Congress of Paediatrics*, p. 117. Zurich.

DISSANAYAKE A. S., TRUELOVE S. C. & WHITEHEAD R. (1974) Lack of harmful effect of oats on small intestinal mucosa in coeliac disease. *Brit. med. J.* **4**, 189–91.

DHSS (1980) *Present Day Practice in Infant Feeding*, No. 18. London: HMSO.

EDITORIAL (1977) Third International Coeliac Symposium. *Lancet* **2**, 1215.

EGAN-MITCHELL B. & McNICHOLL B. (1972) Constipation in childhood coeliac disease. *Arch. Dis. Childh.* **47**, 238–40.

GROLL A., CANDY, D. C. A., PREECE M. A., TANNER J. M. & HARRIES J. T. (1980) Short stature as the primary manifestation of coeliac disease. *Lancet* **2**, 1097–9.

HOLMES G. K. T., STOKES, P. L., SORAHAN T. M. *et al.* (1976) Coeliac disease, gluten free diet and malignancy. *Gut* **17**, 612.

KASARDA D. D., QUALSEL C. O. & MECHAM D. K. *et al.* (1978) A test of toxicity of bread made from wheat lacking alpha gliadins coded by 6A chromosome. In *Perspectives in Coeliac Disease* (eds. McNicholl B., McCarthy C. F. & Fottrell, P. E.), p. 55. Lancaster: MTP Press.

KUITUNEN, P., VISAKORPI J. K., SAVILAHTI E. & PELKONEN P. (1975) Malabsorption syndrome with cow's milk intolerance. Clinical findings and course in 54 cases. *Arch. Dis. Child.* **50**, 351–6.

LLOYD-STILL J. D., GRAND R. J., KON-TAIK K. & SHWACHMAN H. (1972) The use of cortiscosteroids in coeliac crisis. *J. Pediat.* **81**, 1074.

McNEISH A. S., ROLLES C. J., NELSON R., *et al.* (1974) Factors affecting the differing racial incidence of coeliac disease. In *Coeliac Disease* (eds. Hekkens W., Th. J. M. & Peña A. S.), pp. 350. Leyden: Stenfert Kroese.

MEEUWISEE G. W. (1970) Diagnostic criteria for coeliac disease. *Acta paediat. scand.* **59**, 461–3.

MYLOTTE M., EGAN-MITCHELL B., FOTTRELL P. F. *et al.* (1973) Incidence of coeliac disease in the west of Ireland. *Brit. med. J.* **1**, 703–5.

PACKER S. M., CHARLTON V., KEELING J. W. *et. al.* (1978) Gluten challenge in treated coeliac disease. *Arch. Dis. Childh.* **53**, No. 6, 449.

RUBIN C. E., BRANDBORG L. L., FLICK A. L., *et al.* (1962) Biopsy studies on the pathogenisis of coeliac sprue. In *Intestinal Biopsy* (eds. Wolstenholme G. E. W. & Cameron M. P.), p. 67. Edinburgh: Churchill Livingstone.

SAKULA J. & SHINER M. (1957). Coeliac disease with atrophy of the small intestine mucosa. *Lancet* **2**, 876.

SHELDON SIR WILFRED (1969) Prognosis in early adult life of coeliac children treated with a gluten free diet. *Brit. med. J.* **2**, 401–4.

STOKES P. L. & HOLMES G. K. J. (1974) Coeliac disease; malignancy. *Clinics in Gastroenterology* **3**, 159.

VERKASOLO M., KUITUNEN P., LEISTI S. & PERHEENTUPA J. (1978) Growth failure from symptomless coeliac disease. *Helv. paediat. Acta* **33**, 489–95.

VISAKORPI J. K. & IMMONEN P. (1967) Intolerance to cow's milk and wheat gluten in the primary malabsorption syndrome in infancy. *Acta paediat. scand.* **56**, 49–56.

WALKER-SMITH J. A. (1979) Coeliac disease. In *Diseases of the Small Intestine in Childhood*, 2nd Edition (ed. Walker-Smith J.A.). London: Pitman Medical.

WALKER-SMITH J. A., HARRISON M., KILBY A. *et al.* (1978) Cow's milk sensitive enteropathy. *Arch. Dis. Childh.* **53**, 375–80.

WALKER-SMITH J. A. & KILBY A. (1977) Small intestinal enteropathies. In *Essentials of Paediatric Gastroenterology* (ed. Harries J. T.). Edinburgh: Churchill Livingstone.

WATT J., PINCOTT J. R. & HARRIS J. T. (1983) Combined cow's milk protein and gluten-induced enteropathy: common or rare? *Gut* **24**, 165–170.

WHO (1979) Proposed draft standard for gluten-free products. *Codex Alimentarius* Commission ALINORM 79/26 Appendix 2 Step 8. pp. 19–20.

Recipes

GLUTEN-FREE COOKING HINTS

Gluten-free flours have different cooking properties to ordinary flour due to the lack of gluten, which has specific elasticity properties which play an important role, especially in bread-making. Gluten-free flour therefore requires different cooking techniques, e.g. bread is made as a batter consistency, and biscuits and pastry are less crumbly if kneaded, and left in the refrigerator or a cool place for half an hour before rolling and cutting.

Many household recipes can be adapted for use in gluten-free diets, provided that care is taken to omit or replace unsuitable ingredients with the gluten-free equivalent. Gluten-free flours are mostly plain flours, so a gluten-free baking powder must be added separately. Most recipes can be cooked with any of the gluten-free flours so long as baking powder is added appropriately, but trial and error is needed to get successful baking. The *Coeliac Society Handbook* contains a number of gluten-free recipes.

GLUTEN-FREE BAKING POWDER

This can be made from either of the following recipes or a gluten-free commercial baking powder can be purchased. A basic guide is to use two level 5 ml teaspoons of baking powder to 250 g (8 oz) gluten-free flour for cakes, puddings or sponges and one level 5 ml teaspoon of baking powder to 250 g (8 oz) gluten-free flour for biscuits, pastry and batters.

Gluten-free baking powder

(a) 100 g (4 oz) cornflour (gluten-free)
    75 g (3 oz) bicarbonate of soda
    50 g (2 oz) cream of tartar
    50 g (2 oz) tartaric acid

(b) 100 g (4 oz) cream of tartar
    50 g (2 oz) bicarbonate of soda
   100 g (4 oz) ground rice or cornflour (gluten-free)

Using dry utensils, measure the ingredients and sieve together several times to mix thoroughly. Always use a dry spoon for measuring. Store in an air-tight tin.

VARIATIONS TO BASIC RECIPES

The following flavourings are suitable for all recipes:

1 Vanilla essence or other essence flavouring, ground ginger, cinnamon, mixed spice (gluten-free), instant coffee, chocolate (gluten-free) or cocoa.
2 Dried fruit and nuts, e.g. sultanas, raisins, currants, mixed peel, walnuts, almonds or glacé cherries, may be added to recipes, although the fruit tends to sink to the bottom of cakes.
3 Icing may be used on cakes. Butter icing, water icing, jam or fresh cream may be used as decoration or filling. Marzipan can be used, provided it is a gluten-free brand. Royal icing made from egg-white and icing sugar is suitable, and sugar flowers or decorations made from this will be gluten-free. Commercial equivalents may not be gluten-free.

Basic gluten-free milk-free bread

340 g (12 oz) gluten-free milk-free flour
  (select from Table 3.3)
  1 tsp salt
30 g (1 oz) lard, or Tomor margarine, or
  30 ml (1 oz) vegetable oil
  1 egg
30 g (1 oz) fresh yeast or 15 g ($\frac{1}{2}$ oz) dried
  yeast
  1 tsp sugar
340 ml (12 oz) warm water

Add salt to gluten-free flour and rub in the fat. Cream together the sugar and yeast and add the warm water. If dried yeast is used stand until frothy. Mix all ingredients into a batter including the egg and pour into a well-greased tin. Allow to stand in a warm place for about 20 minutes, until doubled in-size. Cook at 200°C (400°F), regulo 5, for 20 minutes. Remove loaf from the tin and place it on the oven shelf for a further 15 minutes.

Basic sponge or sponge cakes (gluten-free milk-free)

100 g (4 oz) gluten-free milk-free flour
  (Table 3.3) or cornflour (check brand)
  $\frac{1}{2}$ tsp gluten-free baking powder
90 g (3 oz) glucose/sugar
  2 eggs
  1 tbsp hot water

Beat eggs and sugar to a stiff foam, then fold in the gluten-free flour and baking powder. Fold in hot water. Place into two greased sponge tins and bake for 15 to 20 minutes in a hot oven, 220°C (425°F), regulo 6. Alternatively, place mixture in small cup cases and cook for 8 to 10 minutes.

Basic biscuit recipe

55 g (2 oz) gluten-free milk-free flour (Table
  3.3) or cornflour (check brand)
45 g (1$\frac{1}{2}$ oz) Tomor margarine or permitted
  fat
  1 egg yolk
30 g (1 oz) glucose/sugar
1 to 2 drops vanilla essence

Cream margarine and sugar together. Add gluten-free flour, egg-yolk and essence. Knead into a dough. Roll out and cut into shapes. Place on a greased tray. Cook in oven at 190°C (375°F), regulo 4, for 15 minutes.

Flapjack biscuits*

110 g (4 oz) Tomor margarine or permitted fat
  85 g (3 oz) sugar or 100 g golden syrup
110 g (4 oz) gluten-milk-free flour (Table 3.3)
  55 g (2 oz) rolled oats*
  $\frac{1}{2}$ teaspoon gluten-free baking powder
1 to 2 drops vanilla essence
  2 tsp water
*Only if oats permitted.

Cream fat and sugar then work in gluten-free flour, oats and baking powder. Spread on well-greased flat baking tin. Bake in oven 190°C (375°F), regulo 4 for 20 minutes. Cut into 20 fingers while still warm.

CHAPTER 4

Food intolerance and allergy

Food intolerance occurs when food contains components which are either toxic, or toxic to certain individuals, or when the nature of the reaction is as yet unknown. Food allergy may be the cause of symptoms but should be distinguished from other clinical conditions which are related to food. This subject has recently been reviewed by the joint committees of the Royal College of Physicians and the British Nutrition Foundation, chaired by Professor Lessof (1984), entitled 'Food Intolerance and Food Aversion'. The First and Second Fison's Food Allergy Workshops, chaired by Professor Coombs (1980 & 1983), have also sought to define food allergic disease, current diagnostic criteria and management.

Food intolerance is the term used to describe an abnormal but reproducible, unpleasant or adverse reaction to a specific food or food ingredient and is not psychologically based. This occurs even when the affected person cannot identify the food given, for example when it is disguised in a flavoured test meal.

Food allergy is a form of food intolerance where there is evidence of an abnormal immunological reaction to food due to sensitization by food antigens which do not provoke abnormal reactions in the majority.

Food aversion incorporates psychological avoidance, e.g. food refusal in toddlers or anorexia nervosa in adolescents, whereas psychological food intolerance is avoidance of food for psychological reasons because of unpleasant bodily reactions caused by emotions associated with food which do not occur if the food is given in a disguised form (Lessof 1984). A number of vague and fluctuating symptoms are reported by such patients, who are often unduly suggestible. An unsupported diagnosis of allergy may initially have been suggested by the medical advisor which may be reinforced by contact with organizations purporting to be able to diagnose food allergy by dubious techniques. Sometimes the intolerance lies not with the patient, but with his family. This is known as 'intolerance of food by proxy', Munchausen syndrome by proxy or Meadow's syndrome (Editorial

1983a, Warner & Hathaway 1984, Meadow 1985). Severe dietary restrictions are imposed on these children by their parents, in the mistaken belief that food allergy is the cause of a variety of symptoms, usually related to the child's behaviour. Such families cannot accept that the child's behaviour is related to family problems and not physical illness.

Clinical conditions which cause reproducible adverse reactions to food are collectively called by some workers 'food idiosyncracy' in order to differentiate them from food allergy (Soothill *et al.* 1976), and are summarized in Fig. 4.1. A number of mechanisms may be responsible. Further details are given in the review by Lessof (1984).

1   Enzyme deficiencies.

(a)   Lactase deficiency in people who do not tolerate milk because they cannot digest lactose (*see* Chapter 1).

(b)   Inherited disorders of protein digestion and degradation (*see* Chapters 9 and 10) such as the various hyperammonaemias and organicacidaemias. The patient with only partial enzyme deficiency or intermittent forms of these conditions may unconsciously select an appropriate low-protein diet to control symptoms by disliking and avoiding foods such as milk, eggs, meat or fish, which the parents assume is because the child is allergic to them.

2   Pharmacological reactions associated with food.

(a)   Caffeine from coffee beans, tea leaves and kola nuts used to flavour cola drinks is a stimulant drug, and clinical effects including insomnia, migraine, palpitations and bouts of rapid heart beat can occur in some people by taking only moderate quantities of caffeine-containing drinks. Caffeine is addictive and sudden withdrawal can also cause headache, irritability and lassitude, and may account for 'weekend migraine' in those who take a large quantity of caffeine during the week but not at weekends.

Fig. 4.1

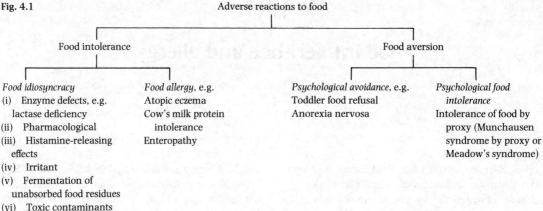

(b) Vasoactive amines include histamine, tyramine, tryptamine, phenylethylamine, octapamine, syrephrine and serotonin, which are present in many foods, including chocolate, cheese, yeast extracts, bananas, avocado pears, and pickled fish. Abnormal clinical effects include facial flushing, headache, urticaria, oedema and abdominal symptoms, including pain, flatulence, constipation and diarrhoea. Histamine-induced symptoms can mimic allergy, but this usually requires larger quantities of the offending substance compared to the often minute quantity of antigen needed for an abnormal immune response.

(c) Monosodium glutamate is a flavouring added to food which in some people causes 'Chinese restaurant syndrome' (Kwok's syndrome) and can mimic myocardial infarction; asthma, headache, thirst and a feeling of bloatedness have also been reported. The latter are probably related to the high sodium content of Chinese food rather than to the glutamate.

3 Histamine-releasing effect in unsensitized individuals, e.g. reactions to strawberries, shellfish and paw paw.

4 Irritant effect on the mucous membranes of the mouth and bowel by highly spiced foods or very hot coffee.

5 Fermentation of unabsorbed food residues (fibre) causing an indirect effect in the lower bowel.

6 Toxic effect of constituents.

(a) Natural toxins, such as the lectins in raw beans and soya known as haemagglutinins. These lectins are heat-labile and so are destroyed by boiling, thus removing the toxic property.

(b) Microbial and insect infestation which occurs during food storage and processing, e.g. storage mites which infest cereals, dried milks, cheese, sugar and dried fruit can cause allergic asthma and dermatitis; storage fungi such as *Aspergillus* spp., *Erwinia herbicola* and other bacteria and their spores are known to be allergic and can cause respiratory symptoms in grain workers.

(c) Additives are widely used to inhibit microbial and chemical changes in food on storage, e.g. nitrite to inhibit *Clostridium* and antioxidants to prevent fat rancidity. A steadily increasing number of reports associate intolerance to food additives with clinical disorders usually considered to be allergic in origin, e.g. urticaria, angioedema and asthma. Substances reported to provoke such reactions include tartrazine (Juhlin 1981), benzoates (Michaëlsson & Juhlin 1973), sulphur dioxide (Freedman 1977) and antioxidants such as butylated hydroxyanisole and butylated hydroxytoluene (Juhlin 1980).

(d) Unidentified mechanisms.

FOOD ALLERGY

Although there is widespread interest in food allergy, there are no accurate figures on its prevalence. Different diagnostic criteria, screening tests and the variety of symptoms connected with food allergic disease together with author bias are responsible for different studies quoting incidences varying from 0·3 to 20% (Ogle & Bullock 1977) of children who suffer from, or have suffered from, symptoms caused by some form of dietary intolerance. Cow's milk protein intolerance is the most common form of food allergy in young children and was reported to have a prevalence of 0·2 to 7·5% by Bahna and Heiner (1980).

The incidence of food intolerance is greatest in infancy and decreases with age. Small intestinal mucosal damage demonstrated by serial small intestinal biopsies (Walker-Smith 1985) occurs as a result of food intolerance almost exclusively in young children, apart from coeliac disease resulting from gluten intolerance which affects all age groups (*see* Chapter 3). Once established, hypersensitivity reactions do not always persist indefinitely, e.g. cow's milk protein intolerance and other types of food allergy in many infants and some children are transient (Dannaeus & Inganas 1981). More than 40% of infants with intolerance to food grow out of the problem in two to two and a half years (Ford & Taylor 1982).

Genetic and environmental factors

Individuals are predisposed to a number of diseases by genetic factors and this is true of some types of food intolerance, particularly those caused by enzyme defects. Allergic disorders are more common in the children of atopic parents (Buisseret 1982). The links between gluten sensitivity and HLA-B8 and DW3 genotypes (Dansset & Svejgaard 1977) and the atopic eczema and HLA haplotype A1-B8 are well documented (Soothill *et al.* 1976).

Atopic people have a family history of allergy, react to skin-prick tests to antigens such as pollen, dust mite and cat dander, tend to have symptoms of eczema, hay fever and asthma, are immune-deficient, and frequently react to foods from a number of different categories and therefore are more prone to multiple food allergy.

Approximately one in three of all people are potentially atopic (Hagy & Settipane 1969), but the number who actually experience the characteristic disorders of eczema, asthma and hay fever is less than this. Many potential atopics apparently never suffer any ill effects as a consequence of their immunological abnormalities (Atherton 1982). Genetic predisposition must be accompanied by environmental factors in order to acquire the disorder. For example, monozygotic twins are not necessarily both affected by coeliac disease or atopic eczema; breast-feeding

may reduce the risk of atopic eczema in the genetically vulnerable infant (Soothill *et al.* 1976, Matthew *et al.* 1977, Saarinen *et al.* 1979).

Various types of inherited immune deficiency can also predispose to atopic disease, including deficiency of immunoglobulin A, or of complement (C2), and defects of the mechanisms that stimulate the phagocytic function of leucocytes or defects of T-cells (Lessof 1984).

Antibody IgA controls the absorption of antigens. Food antigens induce the formation of secretory IgA antibody, which complexes with these antigens within the intestinal lumen, thereby reducing their absorption (immune exclusion) (Swarbrick *et al.* 1979). The production of secretory IgA is immature in infants, who are therefore less able to limit antigen absorption. Breast-feeding contributes IgA to the infant during this vulnerable period. Exposure to antigens in the vulnerable period of immune immaturity may predispose the infant to allergy. Taylor and his colleagues (1973) found that infants who developed atopy in the first months of life had low IgA levels. The differences in gut flora found in breast- and bottle-fed babies also influence antibody response to absorbed antigens.

Gastroenteritis and similar conditions cause vascular changes and inflammation of the gut mucosa, which may allow abnormal entry of food antigens (Harrison *et al.* 1976). Small intestinal damage can result (Walker-Smith 1979, 1985). In particular viral disorders in infants with a family history of atopy provoke food allergic disorders (Frick *et al.* 1979, Manuel & Walker-Smith 1981, Walker-Smith 1985).

Increased permeability of the gut can also occur due to a local effect of histamine and may occur in such patients as those with urticaria who are sensitive to histamine. Certain foods are either rich in histamine themselves or trigger histamine release from mast cells and so theoretically provoke the disorder.

Immune responses to food

The gut is probably the major port of entry of antigens which provoke a reaction in a susceptible organ; however, antigens may reach the target organ by other routes, such as inhalation or skin contact. The role of inhaled antigens, such as dust mite faeces, cat dander and grass pollens, in precipitating allergic response in patients with eczema, asthma and hayfever is well recognized. Airborne particulate antigens are largely deposited in the oropharynx, but rapidly pass to the gastrointestinal tract, and only a very small proportion enter the lower airways (Wilson *et al.* 1973).

The gut wall is protected by a mucous coating, by a tight junction between the mucosal cells, and by the immunological tissues beneath them (Lessof 1984). Virtually all foods, many partially digested food constituents, food additives, drugs and other swallowed substances (micro-organisms and contaminants) may act as antigens within the gut and elicit a specific immune response involving antibody and cells. Before immune responses can occur, or immunological tolerance can be induced, it is necessary for the antigen to gain access to the tissues of the body. Small amounts of food antigen penetrate the normal gastrointestinal surface epithelium at various sites including the cells overlying the Peyer's patches.

Once an allergic response has been stimulated by an antigen (and this may be minimal or maximal), it is only the particular circumstances (such as the degree, the location and other factors) which determine whether the subsequent encounter with the same antigen results in immunity and protection (prophylactic) or hypersensitivity which is harmful (antiphylactic). A subsequent encounter with the antigen in a sensitized individual may give an undesirable reaction. Certain foods and additives (Table 4.1) more commonly cause food intolerance as a result of hypersensitivity, though no food is totally exempt.

The diagnosis of food allergy as a cause of food intolerance implies the presence of an abnormal immune response to one or more foods. It is, however, important to note that immune responses to food can often be found in normal individuals who do not exhibit food intolerance.

Four different types of allergic reactions which have been identified help to explain the different type, severity and time intervals encountered in reactions to food. Coombs and Gell (1975) have classified these reactions which produce tissue damage:

Type I anaphylactic or immediate hypersensitivity, occurring within minutes (usually 10 to 15) of exposure to the antigen. This type of reaction is responsible for general anaphylaxis, hay fever, allergic asthma, urticaria and some other clinical situations.
Type II cytotoxic reactions are seen in blood transfusion reactions, some allergic drug reactions and in some autoallergic diseases.
Type III reactions induced by antigen/antibody complexes causing inflammation several hours after exposure to the antigen. Extensive tissue

Table 4.1 Foods and additives most commonly implicated in food intolerance.

(a) Foods.

Milk	Wheat
cow	Rye
goat	Other cereals
Egg	Yeast
Fish	Potato
Soya	Chocolate
Cheese	Citrus fruit and tomato
Pork	Berry and pip fruit
Ham and bacon	Nuts
Chicken	Spices
Beef	Sugar(s)
Lamb	

(b) Additives.

	E Number
Azo dyes	
tartrazine	E102
sunset yellow	E110
new coccine/ponceau 4R (red)	E124
Amaranth	E123
Erythrosine BS (red dye No. 3)	E127
Benzoate derivatives	E210 to 219
Monosodium glutamate	621
BHT (butylated hydroxytoluene)	E321
BHA (butylated hydroxyanisole)	E320
Salicylate	
Sulphur dioxide	E220
Sodium nitrite	E249
Sodium nitrate	E251
Sodium metabisulphite	E223

damage and lesions may be produced, but the reactions are not usually life-threatening. There are many situations under which these reactions may occur.
Type IV delayed hypersensitivity or cell-mediated immunity with a delay of 1 to 2 days after antigen exposure, so that the relationship between a specific food and the reaction is not usually obvious.

In any individual more than one type of reaction can occur in concert, and the type of reaction involved in a particular disease may not be clear, as illustrated by coeliac disease where there is controversy as to whether the disease is primarily a toxic or an allergic phenomenon, and the type of reaction is open to question; some consider it to be mainly type IV, but types III, II and even I may also be involved.

The tendency to develop hypersensitivity reactions depends on the amount of antigen absorbed and the nature and quantity of circulating antibody or the number of sensitized lymphocytes and their distribution. Protective factors include (a) normal digestion of the antigens; (b) an intact gastrointestinal epithelium; (c) presence of secretory IgA antibodies which are able to bind antigen without causing inflammatory reactions; and (d) the 'cleansing' function of liver phagocytic cells on immune complexes and particular antigen, which are removed from the portal blood before they reach the systemic circulation (Lessof 1984).

To cure food allergy, it may be necessary to recreate the conditions which allow spontaneous recovery in children or to find ways of recreating immunological suppression or oral tolerance. For example, desensitization by injections has been established with respiratory antigens, but results of oral desensitization regimes are disappointing, and there is, as yet, no control trial evidence that it works.

Clinical manifestations of food intolerance and allergy

Food intolerance is an appropriate term when no immunological basis can be established for an adverse but reproducible reaction to food. However, there are enormous variations in the normal child's reactions to food which can be misinterpreted as an adverse

Table 4.2 Clinical conditions related to food intolerance. Adapted from information in Coombs (1980) and Lessof (1984).

System	(i) Considered proven that the condition is at least in some cases caused by food allergic reaction	(ii) A food allergic cause is considered possible but other possibilities are equally or more probable on present evidence
Systemic	Anaphylaxis	Cot death
Upper respiratory tract	Rhinitis Nasal polyps	Sinusitis
Eye	Conjunctivitis	
Lung	Asthma Allergic alveolitis	
Alimentary tract	Oral ulceration and geographic tongue Oesophagitis Coeliac disease Cow's milk protein enteropathy Multiple food intolerance without enteropathy Colitis	Erosive gastritis Infantile colic Bowel mobility disorders Irritable bowel syndrome Vomiting/diarrhoea Failure to thrive in infants Crohn's disease Pruritis ani
Skin	Urticaria and angiodema Atopic eczema Dematitis herpetiformis	
Joints		Arthritis
CNS	Migraine	Behavioural disorders Epilepsy
Genitourinary or renal		Enuresis
Cardiovascular system	Cardiac arrhythmias	

reaction due to disease (David 1985). It is therefore essential that clinicians have a clear knowledge of normal child physiology and development and the variations in normality at different ages (Illingworth 1983). However, food intolerance and allergy are associated with a wide range of symptoms (Table 4.2) (Coombes 1980, 1983, Lessof 1984):

1   The symptoms are known to result from hypersensitivity reaction to antigens, e.g. anaphylaxis, angioedema and urticaria.

2   The symptoms are non-specific, and occur frequently or predominantly for other reasons, but may be due to intolerance, e.g. diarrhoea, vomiting, failure to thrive, infantile colic and migraine. The latter require the confirmation of food intolerance by dietary withdrawal and challenge, and to make a diagnosis of food allergy an 'allergic' reaction to the food in question must be established. There may be delay between food ingestion and onset of symptoms making it difficult to identify the food(s) implicated.

1   Anaphylaxis, angioedema

These conditions are classically and obviously associated with food allergy due to a type I immune reaction causing an immediate reaction. The offending food is usually easily identified by the patient or his parents or from the dietary history. Skin-prick tests and IgE antibody tests are usually positive. Intradermal skin tests and open food challenge are potentially dangerous and unnecessary for diagnostic purposes. Double-blind challenges are contraindicated. Often a reaction to a food is more severe following a period of exclusion (David 1984). In the event of a severe reaction occurring, adrenaline should be administered immediately. Previous anaphylaxis in a patient, i.e. collapse, hypotension, loss of consciousness or respiratory obstruction, requires admission to hospital for any proposed challenge with the specific food that provoked such a reaction. It is recommended that at least a year should elapse before reintroduction is attempted, and adrenaline, resuscitation equipment and an anaesthetist should be available during the initial part of the oral challenge. It is suggested that a skin-prick test should be done first; a very severe reaction may indicate special caution and, perhaps, the deferment of reintroduction. If there is no skin reaction or only a mild (skin-prick test) reaction 1 ml of 1:20 diluted milk or 1 mm³ of the food under test can be administered. If a reaction occurs, including swelling, itching, redness or pain,

no further milk or test food is given. If no reaction occurs within 20 minutes, a second test dose of 1 ml of full-strength milk or 1 cm³ of food can be given, and the patient is kept under observation for 24 hours. Provided there is no reaction to the test doses, frequent, gradually increasing doses are given at intervals of at least 20 minutes, reaching a normal-size serve for the child's age by the fourth day, e.g. after the initial test doses $\frac{1}{4}$, $\frac{1}{2}$, $\frac{3}{4}$ then full-strength milk or formula is given in daily increments, whilst milk substitute feeds are decreased proportionally. After successful reintroduction the patient should take milk or the reintroduced food as a regular part of the diet. Some patients may develop symptoms (e.g. diarrhoea or skin rash) hours or several days after reintroduction of the food; withdrawal may then be necessary. David (1984) has recently reported four children who had delayed anaphylaxis up to 24 hours after an ingested food following a period of dietary elimination treatment for atopic eczema.

2   Gastrointestinal symptoms

Symptoms include diarrhoea, vomiting, abdominal pain, malabsorption, failure to thrive, enteropathy with small intestinal damage, gastrointestinal blood loss or colitis, and multiple food intolerance. Cow's milk protein is the commonest antigen concerned and intolerance to it may occur singly or in conjunction with multiple food allergy. Only a small number of children who have food intolerance have gastrointestinal symptoms (Lessof 1984). Many have or develop later other more obvious allergic disorders. Acute milk intolerance in infants has a sudden onset, with vomiting and occasionally pallor and a shock-like state. Anaphylaxis is rare, but the risk of it must not be overlooked (De Peyer & Walker-Smith 1977). Diarrhoea usually follows the onset of vomiting, and the clinical syndrome is very similar to acute gastroenteritis and may be secondary to it. Secondary lactose intolerance with or without sucrose intolerance (*see* Chapter 1) may coexist. Treatment is by complete withdrawal of milk proteins, lactose and, if necessary, sucrose.

Gastroenteritis predisposes to cow's milk enteropathy, especially in infants (Harrison *et al.* 1976), and serial small intestinal biopsies can provide objective diagnostic evidence (Walker-Smith 1985). Small intestinal damage is best documented in coeliac disease (*see* Chapter 3) and cow's milk intolerance (Walker-Smith 1979), but also occurs with soya (Ament & Rubin 1972), chicken, rice, fish and egg (Vitoria *et al.* 1982). The use of a hypoallergic milk formula during the recovery phase following gastroenteritis may reduce the incidence of this syndrome (Manuel & Walker-Smith 1981). Not all patients show mucosal damage or enteropathy in conjunction with gastrointestinal food intolerance.

Skin tests in these patients are of little value in diagnosis, as are total antibody and IgE antibody measurements. Dietary manipulation, withdrawal and challenge can be misleading because of the variation in onset and duration of symptoms. Response to a milk-free diet does not confirm food intolerance and challenge is essential before long-term treatment is considered. However, the appropriate time for challenge will vary according to the initial diagnosis and symptoms. For example, infants who have had acute milk intolerance, or intolerance following gastroenteritis, enteropathy or colitis may benefit from a period of several months on an appropriate elimination diet before challenge and reintroduction of a normal diet, by which time the patient may have outgrown the temporary intolerance, and diagnosis can only be made in retrospect.

3 Atopic eczema

Eczema is a distinct cutaneous response to various stimuli. Atopic eczema is largely a disease of children and affects at least 5% of all children at some time. It typically starts in infants, but rarely in the first four weeks of life. A highly irritating rash appears on the face then spreads to the limbs. Subsequently the rash disappears from the face and settles in the limb flexures. The severity of the disease fluctuates with a general trend to eventual spontaneous resolution in about 95% of cases (Atherton 1982). This distinctive pattern of eczema occurs almost exclusively in atopic individuals who frequently have or subsequently develop asthma and/or hay fever. Elevated serum IgE levels precede and tend to predict the appearance of atopic eczema in infants (Matthew *et al.* 1977). Skin moisturizers and weak topical corticosteroid treatment are needed in all patients with eczema, and, if properly administered, suffice in the majority (75%) of cases (Atherton 1985). Only when this approach fails is food allergy diagnosis and antigen avoidance warranted.

Allergic disease clearly plays an important role in infants and children with eczema (Atherton, 1982 & 1985). House dust mite, pollens, dander from pets and other contact allergens are implicated (Mitchell *et al.* 1982), and nutritional deficiencies of zinc (Aggett & Harries 1979) and essential fatty acids may be important (Wright & Burton 1981). Food intolerance is a common factor and diet can be useful. A

double-blind crossover trial of diet in eczema by Atherton *et al.* (1978) showed that 14 out of 20 children aged 2 to 8 years improved on a diet eliminating milk, egg, beef and chicken; the diet also excluded fish and other foods to which the child was known to react. Even in those whose eczema improved on such a diet there was not always complete clearance of the disease, suggesting all antigens had not been excluded, and/or factors other than food antigens were contributing to the symptoms. Hill and Lynch (1982) reported 5 out of 10 children with eczema who improved on an elemental diet used for an extended period of time. Patients with eczema who have not improved on an empirical diet may benefit from a trial of an oligoantigenic diet, and such a trial is currently being undertaken in a group of patients at the Hospital for Sick Children, Great Ormond Street, London. Preliminary results in 19 children who have completed the trial to date show five who have failed to respond to two different oligoantigenic diets and 14 who have responded and have completed the reintroduction phase. In nine children double-blind challenges have been undertaken and eight patients reported provocation of their eczema with the challenge food and not the placebo (Atherton 1985). Further results are awaited.

Skin-prick tests are not reliable in identifying which foods are implicated (Atherton *et al.* 1978). Reaction from antigen ingestion may be delayed for several days; anaphylactic and immediate reactions are rare but occasionally can occur (David 1984). This makes it particularly difficult to identify the foods implicated without careful dietetic manipulation and objective assessment of symptoms. Milk and egg remain the commonest antigens associated with atopic eczema of childhood (*see* later, Table 4.9, milk- and egg-free diet). However, artificial colourings and preservatives, particularly the azo dyes and benzoate derivatives, frequently exacerbate eczema, warranting their exclusion, alone (*see* later, Table 4.14) or in conjunction with the exclusion of milk, egg, chicken and perhaps fish (Atherton 1985). Subsequent food challenges following remission of symptoms are needed to identify which items are implicated in the individual. In the author's experience, beef seems less commonly implicated than chicken or fish, and hence an initial empirical diet excluding milk, egg, chicken, the azo colours and preservatives, and perhaps also fish (*see* later, Table 4.10), is now considered more appropriate than the diet used in the trial by Atherton *et al.* (1978). Other allergens can be implicated, especially soya, goat's milk, various fruits, wheat and rye, in which case a trial of an oligoantigenic diet may be warranted to determine which antigens are involved. This is discussed later under management. Adults with atopic eczema have less success with dietary treatment (Barnetson & Merrett 1980) than children, though a number have a history of food intolerance, suggesting a dietary trial is probably warranted in this group of patients.

4 Urticaria

Acute contact urticaria is most common in children and is usually of short duration and self-limiting. Food proteins are frequently the provoking agent and lips may be swollen within minutes of contact with the food. Another common cause is contact with animals (Atherton 1985). Chronic symptoms persisting more than three months usually have identifiable causes in the majority of children, but not always in adults (Lessof 1984).

'Ordinary' urticaria due to food allergy is well documented in all age groups (August 1980, Atherton 1985). In Halpern's (1965) study, 44% of children with urticaria had food sensitivities. Because reactions mostly occur only 1 to 2 hours after ingestion of the offending food the association between antigen and symptoms is easily identified. Sensitivity tends to be severe, even anaphylactic, especially after a period of allergen elimination for a few weeks, whereas repeated exposure may lead to a state of unreactivity or masking (Ros *et al.* 1976). Stress and intercurrent infections exacerbate reactions.

Many foods and other antigens have been identified in patients with urticaria, including milk, egg, nuts, fish, shellfish, cheese, wheat, yeast, strawberries, tyramines, azo dyes, benzoate derivatives, other preservatives and antioxidants, salicylates, and various fruits, especially citrus and berry fruits. Table 4.1 gives a comprehensive range of foods and additives implicated in food allergic disease, almost all of which have been implicated in at least some patients with urticaria (Lockey 1971, Michaëlsson & Juhlin 1973, James & Warin 1971). The most appropriate diet approach is either omission of the foods implicated by the history, an empirical diet free from azo dyes and non-nutritive additives (colouring and preservative) (Table 4.14) or an oligoantigenic diet trial to identify the foods implicated.

5 Asthma and rhinitis

Adverse reactions to inhaled allergens (pollens) are well established, and reactions to ingested foods have been documented. The importance of food in causing respiratory disease has been poorly evaluated and a precise diagnosis is difficult (Wilson & Silverman 1985). Response to exclusion of the offending food may take days or weeks (Coombs 1980). Challenge tests with foods may not produce a change in lung function but bronchial reactivity may be altered (Wilson *et al.* 1982).

Pharmacological approaches to therapy are relatively simple and efficacious, regardless of allergic status. Desensitization to respiratory inhaled antigens by injections has been successful.

Aspirin, and many foods have been implicated, especially milk, egg, the azo dyes, metabisulphite, and wheat and other cereals, the latter probably because of a cross-reaction between pollens and cereals. When warranted dietary manipulation can be used to try and identify the offending foods concerned with the symptoms in an individual. A careful history may identify the foods concerned in precipitating or exacerbating symptoms (Wilson & Silverman 1985). Dietary elimination and challenge is more difficult in identifying causative allergens because of the variability of asthma from time to time, because of the delayed reaction to foods when they do occur and because other factors may need to co-exist with the food allergen for an adverse reaction to occur, e.g. exercise and provoking food, temperature of food, etc. (Wilson & Silverman 1985).

6 Migraine

It is well recognized that foods can provoke migraine. Until recently the foods implicated have been thought to be those containing tyramine and other vasoactive amines. A recent study of children with severe migraine by Egger and colleagues (1983) showed that 93% of 88 children recovered on an oligoantigenic diet, and causative foods were identified by sequential reintroduction and confirmed by double-blind controlled trial in 40 of the children. Seventeen children had symptoms with only one food, but most patients responded to several foods and one child reacted to 24 foods but was well on a nutritionally adequate diet excluding these. In all, 55 different foods were involved, suggesting an allergic rather than an idiosyncratic pathogenesis. Associated symptoms, asthma, eczema, abdominal pain, fits and behaviour disorders, also improved on the diet and the successfully treated children no longer developed migraine when challenged with non-specific stimuli, such as blows on the head, exercise and flashing lights, while they were on their diet. The dietary items to which more than five of the children reacted were cow's milk, egg, chocolate, orange, wheat, rye, cheese, tomato, benzoic acid, tartrazine, fish, pork, beef, maize, oats, soya, tea, coffee and goat's milk. Because so many dietary items are implicated an empirical diet approach is unlikely to identify the causative food in the majority, and therefore an oligoantigenic diet or modification of this approach is necessary (Carter *et al.* 1985). This is only warranted in severe and frequent migraine and therefore careful clinical assessment of patients before embarking on dietary manipulation is essential.

7 Behavioural disorders and hyperactivity

The terms hyperactivity, hyperkinesis or the hyperactive child syndrome are used loosely and many clinical features have been described, but the result is disruptive behaviour and under-achievement at school. The cause is unknown. The distinction between hyperactivity and other forms of behaviour disturbance is vague, and evidence linking it to food intolerance has been poor (Lessof 1984).

Behaviour disorders are seen in some children with atopic symptoms such as eczema and asthma, and in patients with migraine. Improvement in behaviour was reported by the parents of the children when an elimination diet aimed at treating the atopic symptoms was instigated (Egger *et al.* 1983). Whether this improvement is due to the diet, secondary to the improvement of the clinical disease, or is a placebo effect, which such a diet inevitably causes, is not clear. Recently, a double-blind trial in 76 children with severe behavioural disorders and hyperkinetic syndrome has been undertaken by Egger *et al.* (1985), in a similar way to the migraine trial reported above, in order to investigate the role of food intolerance in these children. Results are encouraging, and in those who responded (62 of the original 76 patients) to the oligoantigenic diet, provoking foods were identified during a reintroduction phase and confirmed by double-blind trials using randomized placebo and challenge food which had previously provoked symptoms. The proportion of patients with atopic diseases was identical in those who responded and non-responders. All of the children reacted to at least one food, 34 of the 50 children for whom full data were available reacted to fewer than seven foods, but two patients reacted to 30 foods. The commonest foods causing reactions were benzoic acid and tartrazine, which were usually involved together, but no child reacted to these alone and 46 other foods were implicated, including milk, soya, chocolate, wheat, egg, cheese, grapes, oranges, maize, oats and fish. This trial establishes that the contribution of diet to behaviour disorders must be taken seriously but further research is required to establish the optimal regimen for treatment in the majority.

Earlier Feingold posed the hypothesis that ingested low molecular weight chemicals (salicylates, natural and medicinal; artificial food colours; artificial flavours) were important in the development and maintenance of hyperactivity in children (Feingold *et al.* 1973, Feingold 1974). More recently the diet recommendations have been revised to exclude preservatives, e.g. sodium benzoate, nitrates, nitrites and antioxidants, especially butylated hydroxytoluene (BHT), and butylated hydroxyanisole (BHA), but the role of natural salicylates now receives less attention (Feingold & Feingold 1979). Until the recent work of Swain *et al.* (1984) there had been no accurate data on the salicylate content of foods. The same food varies in salicylate depending on where it is grown, and current analysis methods are difficult and often unreliable, and hence different dietary lists vary considerably. The author has thus relied on not theoretical lists of salicylate- and benzoate-containing foods but individual response to foods which provoke symptoms on elimination and challenge.

Several crossover control diet studies, with various minor diet modifications, have been carried out to try and establish whether the improvement claimed is related to the additive-free 'Feingold' diet (Connors *et al.* 1976, Harley *et al.* 1978a, Williams *et al.* 1978, Levy *et al.* 1978). Challenge experiments have also been carried out giving a test dose of additive or placebo in a cookie or candy to children who have responded to the additive-free diet (Goyette *et al.* 1978, Harley *et al.* 1978b, Augustine *et al.* 1980, Swanson & Kinsbourne 1980). Reviews of these studies are reported by Stare *et al.* (1980), the Editorials in the *Lancet* (1979, 1982) and by the Concensus Development Conference on Hyperactivity (1982). The latter concluded that 'the diet should not be universally applied', but that it may be effective in a few cases. Though a small sub-group may be vulnerable to additives, the observed improvement may be due to other factors such as the placebo effect of the regimen itself, change in family dynamics, increased attention devoted to the child that such a regimen demands, or nutritional status.

It is difficult to identify which children will respond to dietary manipulation. The potential benefits of the diet, which is harmless in itself, must be balanced with the harmful long-term educational impact of communicating to a child that his behaviour is controlled by what he eats, particularly when this is not true for the majority. The use of a placebo treatment carries other risks, such as making a scapegoat of the child, neglect of other beneficial treatments, or loss of self-esteem, and the diet can become a punishment, as it 'deprives' the child of many foods enjoyed by peer groups and family.

Other dietary modification hypotheses have been put forward, such as a link with essential fatty acid metabolism or abnormal carbohydrate metabolism in patients with hyperactivity and behavioural disorders. A pilot study to investigate essential fatty acid supplements in these children is being conducted. Essential reactive hypoglycaemia has become a popular diagnosis by the lay public and press. Johnson *et al.* (1980) found that hypoglycaemia with normal meals and lifestyles only occurs in a tiny minority; symptoms are related to low blood glucose concentrations and are relieved by carbohydrate. Claims that hypoglycaemia is responsible for ill-health in adults have not been substantiated by objective evidence (Johnson *et al.* 1980) and there have been no systematic studies in children to indicate that hypoglycaemia *per se* is responsible for ill-health (Lessof 1984).

A positive correlation between consumption of sugar and behaviour was found by Prinz *et al.* (1980), who suggests that sugar intake may be a contributing factor to behavioural disorders in some sensitive children. There is a need for further controlled studies with varying sugar intakes and the investigation of the possible mechanisms involved. Others have suggested a relationship between diet and behaviour (Wurtman 1983, Schauss 1983) which requires further investigation. Egger *et al.* (1985) also found that some patients reacted adversely to the addition of sugar to the basic oligoantigenic diet in their study in children with the hyperkinetic syndrome; five reacted to both beet and cane sugar, three to cane sugar and one only to beet sugar out of a total of 55 children tested, though numerous other foods and additives were also implicated, as discussed above.

8   *Infantile colic*

Many children with cow's milk protein intolerance are found in retrospect to have had infantile colic (Minford *et al.* 1982). However, this is a relatively common problem, affecting 16% of infants, and it occurs in breast-fed infants and those on both cow's milk and soya formulae. Jakobsson and Lindberg (1978) found that withdrawal of milk from the diet of breast-feeding mothers gave improvement, but this was an uncontrolled study. A subsequent controlled trial by Evans *et al.* (1981) did not confirm this finding. Correlation between colic and food intolerance therefore remains to be proven, but may be more important in those who subsequently develop atopic symptoms.

DIAGNOSIS

The clinician and dietitian have complementary roles in the diagnosis and management of food intolerance (Lessof 1984).

Clinical diagnosis should first exclude other causes of the presenting symptoms including a thorough review of differential diagnoses (McCarty & Frick 1983), e.g. enzyme deficiencies, inborn errors of metabolism, cystic fibrosis.

When a severe reaction occurs immediately after ingesting food the precipitating cause is obvious. A careful history including diet, appetite, other symptoms and family history is essential. No patient should be put on an inappropriate and unnecessary diet because of inadequate investigation.

Self-diagnosis and treatment of food allergic disease is often attempted by the public when dietetic and medical advice is not forthcoming, as illustrated by the number of self-help groups, private clinics and media which provide well-meaning, though sometimes inaccurate and inappropriate advice (David 1985). Elimination diets are difficult, expensive and potentially dangerous, can lead to deficiency diseases and growth retardation (Tripp *et al.* 1978, Goldsborough & Francis 1983, David 1985) and may prevent appropriate treatment of the underlying cause (Editorial 1982, Warner & Hathaway 1984, David 1985).

The index of suspicion for food allergy is increased when there is a family history of food allergic disease, diseases associated with other allergic symptoms, e.g. asthma, eczema, and when atopy is detected by positive skin-prick tests and/or RAST tests to antigens such as dust mite and pollen.

At present, there are no laboratory tests which alone will diagnose food intolerance and identify the foods requiring elimination for treatment. A number of tests are available to identify individuals in whom immune responses are qualitatively and/or quantitatively different from normal (Lessof 1984).

Tests used to verify an allergic (immune) response in a patient with an adverse reaction to food include skin-prick tests, radio-allergosorbent test (RAST), tests for IgE antibody, and measurement of other antibodies and complexes. At present simple skin-prick tests are as informative as more elaborate tests (May 1979), but are limited due to the quality of antigen test materials available. Both false-positive and false-negative tests occur. Such tests are therefore only a guide to the foods involved and need verification by dietary manipulation. Preliminary studies on immunological tests largely used in research, such as Clq binding and LIF, which provide information on immune complex- and cell-mediated food sensitivity, may prove useful diagnostic tools in the future (McCarty & Frick 1983).

Sequential jejunal biopsy showing enteropathy is useful in some patients with symptoms of gastro-intestinal allergy, e.g. cow's milk protein intolerance (Manuel *et al.* 1979), and intolerance of other food proteins (Vitoria *et al.* 1982), soya (Ament & Rubin 1972) and gluten (Walker-Smith 1970). Unlike un-treated gluten-sensitive enteropathy, cow's milk en-teropathy is variable in severity and is patchy in dis-tribution; although a flat mucosa may occur, more often lesser degrees of mucosal abnormality are found (Walker-Smith 1979, 1985). Some patients with ali-mentary food intolerance, however, have a normal small intestine mucosa.

Serial respiratory function tests can be used in res-piratory diseases to show an association between an ingested food and a drop in peak flow values, thus identifying the food concerned (Wraith 1980).

There are a number of other tests which have not been shown to be of value (Cant 1985, David 1985). These include the pulse test, sublingual food test, Rin-kel's intradermal skin test, cytotoxic food test and hair tests. Radionics, radiaesthesia, psionic medicine and dowsing are all forms of extrasensory perception for which there is no scientific basis.

Diagnosis, at least in part, depends on dietary eli-mination of the food antigens and the disappearance of symptoms, and return of the same symptoms on challenge with the suspected food. Improvement on an elimination diet may take up to three or four weeks, and initially symptoms may temporarily wor-sen, possibly due to a withdrawal effect (Egger *et al.* 1985). Only if symptoms improve on an appropriate elimination diet should the possibility of food intoler-ance be pursued.

DIAGNOSTIC ELIMINATION DIETS

These are summarized in Fig. 4.2 and fall into four categories:

I Single incriminated food exclusion
This is appropriate when it is obvious from the his-tory and symptoms that the patient will require ex-clusion of one (or two) foods, often of relatively little nutritional importance. Shellfish or strawberries, for example, are easily avoided, and with a little care regarding savoury foods, tomato or onion, elimina-tion is no hardship.

II Empirical diet
An appropriate empirical diet, according to symptoms and the history of the patient, can be selected when type I reactions are involved, or when only a few foods are implicated or specific foods are commonly associated with the symptoms. For example, cow's milk protein is frequently implicated in post-gastro-enteritis enteropathy; milk and egg are commonly implicated in children with atopic eczema and/or asthma; the azo dyes, colourings and preservatives are often associated with urticaria. Examples of vari-ous empirical diets are given later in Tables 4.8 to 4.14, and a milk-free diet can be devised by modifi-

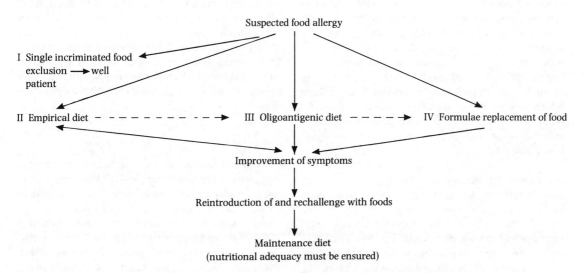

Fig. 4.2 Dietary diagnosis of food intolerance. From Goldsborough and Francis (1983) with permission.

cation of Table 1.8. These diets are socially inconvenient and unless appropriately supplemented by the use of a nutritionally adequate milk substitute in young children, and substitutes for bread, they can be inadequate for growth, and without adequate instruction dietary compliance may fail (*see* Table 4.6) (Goldborough & Francis 1983, Hathaway & Warner 1983).

III   Diets containing few foods (oligoantigenic diet)
This approach is used:

(i)   In patients who have a slow response to foods when several days may elapse after ingestion before symptoms occur.

(ii)   When multiple foods are suspected or involved; for example, 55 different foods were implicated in the migraine study in children by Egger *et al.* (1983).

(iii)   Where withdrawal of individual foods fails and the suspicion of food intolerance remains, and it is therefore necessary to use a diet containing only a few foods which are not common antigens in an oligoantigenic diet.

Such a diet classically permits only one meat, one cereal, one fruit, one vegetable, and a milk substitute or calcium and vitamin supplement, depending on the child's age, together with an oil, salt and water (Table 4.3). The choice of foods is somewhat arbitrary, but will vary according to the clinical syndrome and the patient's preferences. Imaginative cooking is necessary to produce attractive meals from such a limited range of foods. Even so, such a diet requires home preparation of all food, and dedication and motivation of patient and parents. It is socially unacceptable to many families and is expensive. A modified oligoantigenic diet (Table 4.4) permits a wider range of selected foods and is more practical, though still very restricted (Carter *et al.* 1985). Even so, such a diet should only be used for 5 to 20 days before review and introduction of additional foods. Infants and young children should be given a suitable milk substitute with such diets to ensure its nutritional adequacy.

IV   Formulae replacement diets
Only in extreme circumstances should conventional foods be temporarily withdrawn from the diet of children and replaced with a formula diet appropriately selected for age and suitability. In infants formulae replacement of milk-based feeds is better tolerated, but the introduction of solids at an appropriate age is important to social and developmental progress

subsequently. When a formula diet is used, the nutritional adequacy of the diet depends on the product used, its formulation and the quantity consumed. A milk substitute can be selected from Table 1.4, 1.7 or 2.9. A number of new peptide- and amino acid-based products have recently become available which could prove useful in these situations once they are evaluated. The merits of each product must be considered carefully. Those based on amino acids are potentially less likely to cause sensitization than those based on peptides, which should be of low molecular weight. However, they are very unpalatable. The origin of each ingredient must be scrutinized for suitability for the patient, e.g. glucose polymers are usually of maize origin, and will be unsuitable in patients who are intolerant of maize, products containing soya oil will be contraindicated in those intolerant to soya, and non-nutritive additives such as flavourings, emulsifiers and antioxidants must be considered carefully, together with the nutritional adequacy of the product for different age groups.

Formulae diets are monotonous, often unpalatable, and expensive, and patient compliance of such regimens is poor. Such diets should be used only for a very limited time, e.g. 5 to 20 days, as the sole source of nutrition except in young infants.

If no improvement has occurred within three weeks on the selected diagnostic diet, either it still contains food(s) to which the patient is intolerant, or factors other than food antigens are contributing to symptoms. If food allergy or intolerance is still suspected and symptoms are known to be delayed, as in asthma, the diagnostic diet may need to be continued for a further period, up to six or eight weeks in total, otherwise an alternative diet can be selected. If an oligoantigenic diet fails the alternative diet should ideally contain no food in common with the first diet. The alternative diet should only be used for a three-week trial period. If no improvement occurs the diet should be abandoned and the clinical situation reassessed.

REINTRODUCTION OF FOODS

Open food challenges are an essential part of the diagnosis of delayed and multiple food intolerance, and are necessary in order to devise the long-term maintenance diet, except in those patients who have type I immune reactions to a single food. Reintroduction of foods is particularly important for those patients on elimination diets from groups III and IV above, which are extremely limited and of dubious nutritional adequacy for growth. After a limited period of

Table 4.3 Examples of two oligoantigenic diets. From Carter *et al.* (1985) with permission.
   To be used for only three weeks.
   Use only the foods listed or selected according to the individual requirements.

Diet A	Diet B
Turkey *or* chicken	Lamb *or* rabbit
Cabbage, sprouts, broccoli, cauliflower	Carrots, lettuce, celery, cucumber
Potato and potato flour, plain potato crisps	Rice and rice flour
Banana *or* peaches and apricots	Apples and apple juice *or* pears
Tomor margarine, soya oil	Sunflower oil
Water	Water

NB Calcium and vitamin supplements are essential with both diets, unless a milk substitute is used:

Calcium gluconate, three 1 g tablets daily
or Calcium lactate, six 300 mg tablets daily $\Big\}$ Each is approximately 300 mg elemental calcium

   Abidec, 0·6 ml daily, or three Ketovite Tablets plus 5 ml Ketovite Liquid* daily.

Possible additions to either of above	*Comment*
Selected milk substitute for age, e.g.	Essential in infants and very young children.
Infants: Pregestimil, Pepdite 0–2, Neocate (SHS).	
Children: Unflavoured 028 Elemental Diet (SHS), Pepdite 2 +, Nutranel, Flexical.	
Spring water, home-made soda water.	
Sugar	Could select cane or beet. Use sparingly or not at all.
Arrowroot, sago, tapioca.	
Salt and pepper in cooking.	
Gravy browning, e.g. Crosse & Blackwell.	Contains caramel E150.
Sodium bicarbonate, cream of tartar.	
Baking powder made with rice flour (e.g. Sainsbury's).	
Ener-G egg replacer (GF Dietary Supplies).	Contains potato flour.
For B above, Puffed Rice Cakes (Living Foods).	
For B above, Country Basket Rice Cakes (Newform Foods).	Contain sesame seeds.
Avoid: Coloured toothpastes, medicines containing artificial colour and/or preservatives.	

*Contains benzoate in present formulation

5 to 20 days and clinical improvement on one of the diets suggested, single foods previously eliminated are introduced openly in a planned sequence one after another, and withdrawn again if symptoms recur. An appropriate final dose is a normal-size serving for age on a daily basis, but the first administration may have to be a much lower dose given under observation or even hospitalization in those who have had a type I immune reaction such as anaphylaxis, angioedema or other severe reactions. Often a reaction to a food is more severe following a period of exclusion (David 1984). Two small test doses of the food with two adults present are recommended in the first in-

stance. A suggested protocol for milk or food introduction for patients at risk of severe reactions is given on p. 82. In patients with less severe and delayed food reactions a full-size serve could be given immediately after the two test doses. Before assuming a particular food will not provoke symptoms, a full serve should be given for 3 to 7, or in patients with very delayed symptoms 14, consecutive days, depending on the anticipated delay of symptoms in the individual. The order in which foods are introduced is largely a matter of patient preference and previous history, but the nutritional aspects and practicalities of the diet should also be considered. It is ideal to

Table 4.4   Modified oligoantigenic diet. From Carter *et al.* (1985) with permission.
To be used for 3 to 4 weeks only.
This diet may need to be altered to suit the individual child.
Use only the foods listed.

Meat	Lamb, chicken, turkey Offal from these meats if liked
Cereal	Rice flour, potato flour, arrowroot Rice Krispies, Ricicles (contain malt) Rice crackers available from health food shops, e.g. Country Basket Rice Cakes (Newform Foods), Puffed Rice Cakes (Living Foods) Rice grain, brown or white
Vegetables	Cabbage, sprouts, broccoli, cauliflower, leeks, courgettes, marrow, carrots, turnips, parsnips, swede, onion, garlic, celery, lettuce, cucumber, cress, chicory Potatoes, roast or chips in permitted oil, boiled, baked or mashed without added milk.
Fruit	Apple, pear, banana, peaches, apricots, plums, nectarines, pineapple, melon, grapes, cherries Fresh, stewed, or tinned in natural juice.
Fats	Milk-free margarine, e.g. Tomor. Low-fat spread, e.g. Safeway's or Sainsbury's, Granose or Vita- quell margarine Vegetable oil, preferably sunflower
Milk	None in older children Selected milk substitute for age is essential in infants and very young children e.g. Pepdite 0–2, Pregestimil, Neocate, *or* Flexical, Nutranel, Pepdite 2 +, or Unflavoured 028 Elemental Diet
Beverages	Pure unsweetened juices from above fruits, tap water, soda water, spring water

Miscellaneous	Salt, pepper, pure herbs, e.g. bouquet garni
	Plain or ready-salted plain potato crisps (preferably only 1 packet per day)
	Bicarbonate of soda, cream of tartar for baking, baking powder which is grain-free (except rice),
	    e.g. Sainsbury's
	Special jams which are free from added sugar, colour and preservatives and contain only permitted
	    fruits
	Sugar used sparingly or not at all. Select either cane or beet sugar

Avoid	Coloured toothpaste, medicines containing artificial colour and/or preservative

NB   A calcium and vitamin supplement is recommended with this diet if no milk substitute is used:

  Calcium gluconate, three 1 g tablets daily ⎫
or Calcium lactate, six 300 mg tablets daily ⎬ Each is approximately 300 mg elemental calcium.
   Abidec, 0·6 ml daily ⎭

Biscuits, fruit crumbles, etc. can be made with rice and potato flour, permitted margarine and sugar, provided a small
    quantity of sugar is not contraindicated.

introduce items singly, e.g. wheat is given as whole-meal flour or cereal before bread which contains many ingredients and yeast; milk is given before cheese, etc. Table 4.5 gives a suggested list for reintroducing foods. Once a food has been reintroduced, it should be given regularly in the diet.

Patient support and supervision of the diet during food reintroductions are essential by both clinician and dietitian. Close liaison between members of the team is essential, in order to provide adequate support to the patient and a proper diagnosis ultimately.

A diet diary which objectively records symptoms is essential, and should also record intercurrent infections, pilfering and other facts, so that medical and dietetic staff can determine when and how to test any reactions to food by double-blind challenge. Confusion frequently occurs during diagnostic dietary manipulations unless careful supervision is maintained, because many patients do not realize that reactions may take some days to occur and outside influences such as stress and intercurrent infections can precipitate symptoms, making it difficult to interpret results. Response to a food may be different on different occasions.

The criteria of Goldman *et al.* (1963) suggested that three challenges with similar adverse reactions should be performed on patients with food intolerance before diagnosis of food allergy could be established. However, this is more appropriate as a research tool, is unacceptable to many parents and is not ethical if an antigen provokes a severe reaction and/or anaphylaxis.

Double-blind challenge

Foods which provoke symptoms on open reintroduction can be confirmed at a later date using carefully matched and disguised antigen and placebo given in random sequence under double-blind conditions (Carter *et al.* 1985). This is important to help exclude food fads, food aversion disorders and the placebo effect of dietary treatment, and verifies that symptoms are associated with the particular food. A history of a food causing a severe reaction, anaphylaxis or immediate reaction is a contraindication for this form of provocation.

Poorly defined symptoms require assessment by an outside objective observer who, together with the patient (and parents), should be unaware of the sequence of the double-blind food challenges.

Capsules have been used to disguise test doses of food which provoke symptoms in tiny quantity, or food dyes, colours, preservatives and similar additives (August 1980, Egger *et al.* 1983). Coded tins of food challenge materials, soups, cookies and candies of test material and placebo, have been prepared by manufacturers (Swanson & Kinsbourne 1980, Egger *et al.* 1983, Atherton 1985) and are useful for home testing. Soups, drinks, puddings, cakes and cookies can be prepared (in the diet kitchen and frozen) in which test doses of a food reported to cause a reaction are disguised in one batch and not in a similar batch. Both batches should appear and taste identical, apart from coding known only to the person preparing the items and not to the worker instructing the patient in their use. The difficulty is to disguise an average-size serve of the test food, e.g. one egg, in a reasonable quantity which can be given on 3 to 7, and

occasionally 14, consecutive days (Carter *et al.* 1985). Also, the food preparation and processing may alter the sensitizing capacity of the test food and must be remembered in assessing results.

Sodium cromoglycate improves or prevents symptoms in some patients with food allergic disease. It has been used by some workers to confirm the diagnosis of suspected food allergy, when symptoms improve with sodium cromoglycate and not when a placebo is administered. However, even large doses of sodium cromoglycate are ineffective when the patient is exposed to large quantities of antigen and dose–response is variable (Syme 1979).

MAINTENANCE DIET

Once it is established that a child is intolerant to a particular food(s), it should be avoided completely, and a suitable diet should be devised. The diet must be nutritionally adequate for growth in children, should be as near normal as possible, and have as few exclusions as possible. The diet should be supervised by a dietitian who has three main responsibilities: first to ensure that the prescribed diet is nutritionally adequate, secondly to ensure the diet excludes the foods to which the patient is intolerant, and thirdly that the diet can be applied practically in the home by supplying a list of suitable foods including accurate and up-to-date lists of manufactured products and recipes. A varied diet encourages compliance. The following foods should be omitted, at least initially, when a child has to avoid soya: bread to which soya flour is added, soya oils and foods fried in soy oils, Tomor margarine containing soya oils, and soya 'milks'. To avoid beef, not only the meat, but also beef fat, gelatine and probably all sources of cow's milk, need to be omitted. Specific additives, not only in food, but in medicines, sweets and toothpaste, must be omitted, once identified as causing a reaction.

Dietary manipulation is difficult, and many practical problems can arise. The symptoms concerned must warrant the diet, and safe alternatives should be used when available, e.g. topical treatment alone is sufficient in the majority of children with atopic eczema.

Food processing may alter the likelihood of antigen response in certain patients, for example cooking and some heat treatments used for canning denature protein structure; hydrolysis of proteins produces smaller molecular weight peptides and amino acids. For example, evaporated milk may be tolerated whereas pasteurized milk causes an allergic reaction,

Table 4.5 Open sequential reintroduction of foods. From Carter *et al.* (1985) with permission.
Each new food should be introduced separately and tested for 3 to 14 days before being allowed freely in the diet. This list is not comprehensive and is only meant as a guide.

The following foods may or may not have been allowed in the initial oligoantigenic diet:

Lamb, chicken, rice, potatoes, banana, apple, peaches and apricots, etc.
They can be introduced one by one at some stage.

Oats	Porridge oats for breakfast and for making flapjacks (if sugar is already allowed), Scottish oatcakes.
Sugar	Introduce either cane or beet sugar.
Beef	Use fresh or frozen beef, any cut cooked by roasting, grilling or boiling. Stews should contain only permitted foods already tolerated.
Wheat	Wholemeal flour or unbleached white flour for cooking, spaghetti, pasta (egg-free), Shredded Wheat, Puffed Wheat, or Shredded Wheat Cubs are tried before giving bread which contains a number of ingredients (*see* Table 4.6) in addition to wheat.
Yeast	Give home-made wholemeal bread, or buy wholemeal bread from a health food shop or local baker after checking there are no additives.
Cow's milk	Fresh pasteurized cow's milk. If milk is tolerated, permit cream, pure plain yoghurt, pale uncoloured butter.
Cheese	If milk is tolerated, test separately. Plain unprocessed cheese, e.g. pale-coloured Cheddar, Lancashire. If cheese is not tolerated, goat's or ewe's cheeses may be tried at a later date.
Cow's milk substitute	If cow's milk is not tolerated, substitutes can be tried one by one (*see* Tables 1.4, 1.7 and 2.9). Soya milk, e.g. Cow & Gate S Formula. Goat's milk, ewe's milk (boiled or pasteurized) may be suitable in older children. Non-dairy or imitation cream. (Dilute 10 ml to 100 ml water. This is not a nutritional substitute for milk but a good vehicle for breakfast cereals, etc.). Some patients will tolerate evaporated milks but not fresh pasteurized milks.
Eggs	Use whole fresh eggs (approximately one per day). If not tolerated, try ducks' eggs later. (Some patients tolerate egg-yolk but not white; others only tolerate well-cooked egg, e.g. hard-boiled or in cakes.)
Fish	Use fresh or frozen fish (not smoked), e.g. cod, plaice, haddock. Try shellfish separately later.
Orange	Pure orange juice, fresh oranges, tinned mandarins if sugar is in the diet, satsumas. If oranges are tolerated all citrus fruit will probably be tolerated.
Chocolate	Ordinary plain or milk chocolate. If diet is milk-free use chocolate which is milk- and butter-free, e.g. Terry's Bitter Chocolate, Sainsbury's Plain Chocolate, Marks & Spencer's Swiss Plain Chocolate, Cote d'Or Plain Chocolate, etc., cocoa.
Tomatoes	Fresh, tinned, puréed. Tomato ketchup which is additive-free, e.g. Heinz, can then be introduced if tomato is tolerated.
Pork	Fresh or frozen, any cuts cooked appropriately.
Baked beans	If tomatoes are tolerated many children like baked beans in tomato sauce. Select a suitable brand, e.g. Heinz.
Rye	This is particularly worth trying if wheat is not tolerated, e.g. Ryvita (original rye crispbread), Ryking (blue pack).

Table 4.5 *continued*

Malt	Rice Krispies, Ricicles, if rice is tolerated. Weetabix, Shreddies if wheat is tolerated. Ready Brek (plain) if oats are tolerated.
Corn	Sweetcorn, popcorn, corn oil, corn flour, maize flour, Cornflakes if malt is tolerated.
Peas and beans	These are likely to cause no reaction if baked beans and/or soya have been introduced satisfactorily. These include peas, runner beans, kidney beans, lentils.
Ordinary white flour	Use white flour in cooking and home-made or additive-free white bread once wheat is tolerated. (Bread contains natural benzoates.)
Soya/propionate preservative	Supermarket white bread contains both these and should be introduced as a separate item.
Artificial colours, some preservatives	Orange squash if orange is tolerated. Choose one containing tartrazine and benzoate preservative. Colours are present in jelly, fruit gums, boiled fruit sweets, jelly beans, etc. (These can only be tried if the diet contains added sugar and each colour should be tested separately.) Tartrazine and benzoic acid can also be tested using capsules containing either tartrazine or benzoic acid.
Nitrites	These are present in cooked or cured meats. This includes ham and bacon if pork is tolerated, beefburgers and corned beef if beef is tolerated. Some water supplies also contain nitrates.
Tea and coffee	As drinks, but only add milk and sugar if tolerated.
Sodium glutamate	Most people ask to use stock cubes or gravy mixes, many of which contain this. Allow the one of their choice after checking other ingredients.

Other foods and manufactured products such as ice-cream, biscuits, can be introduced weekly taking into account avoidance of foods to which the patient is sensitive.

and boiled milk is less sensitizing to guinea-pigs than raw or pasteurized (McLaughlin *et al.* 1981). The newer, modified whey-based infant feeds are less likely to cause sensitization compared to the older type of milks (Manuel & Walker-Smith 1981). Studies using guinea-pigs who react to milk with anaphylactic sensitizing (McLaughlan *et al.* 1981) have done much to clarify this previously confused area.

The initial diet should exclude all traces of the suspect allergen, though subsequent reintroduction may indicate that specific foods are tolerated in individual patients; for example, butter is sometimes tolerated even though milk causes symptoms. A dose-related and/or cooking effect is found in some individuals (Atherton 1985); for example, the amount of egg in a cake is tolerated where egg on its own is not. Such phenomena are unlikely in infants and patients with gastrointestinal symptoms of milk intolerance, where even small traces of antigen can provoke a reaction.

While it is generally known that some patients can tolerate modest amounts of particular foods if they are taken at spaced intervals, but symptoms occur if large quantities are taken on consecutive days, there is little evidence to justify obsessional adherence to rotational diets. There is also a danger that such diets are nutritionally inadequate, particularly for children, and therefore they are not recommended unless the patient is intolerant to a number of different foods whose total exclusion would make an impractical regimen, and the symptoms are sufficiently severe to warrant such an approach (Carter *et al.* 1985).

Nutritional adequacy of the diet

Inadequate diets abound, either self-selected or devised by those without expert knowledge of nutrition, and they can be harmful (Tripp *et al.* 1979, Goldsborough & Francis 1983, David 1985).

The nutritional adequacy of an elimination diet depends largely on the food or foods being excluded. Some patients only need to exclude a single food, for example nuts, shellfish, tomatoes or strawberries. None of these is difficult to remove from the diet and its exclusion is not likely to cause nutritional deficiencies. Other patients, however, need to exclude foods which have much greater nutritional and social implications, e.g. milk, egg, wheat. Cow's milk is a common food allergen, especially in young children. Of the recommended intake for age, a two-year-old obtains 100% calcium, 50% protein, 24% energy and 100% riboflavin from 500 ml (1 pint) of cow's milk. It is convenient and versatile and is used to incorporate other foods into the diet, such as cereals. In addition, cheese, yoghurt and many other foods are made from or contain milk, and therefore must be excluded from a diet free of cow's milk protein. Such a diet is likely to be nutritionally inadequate, particularly in infants and children under school age, unless a suitable replacement of milk is given. Examples of milk substitutes free of cow's milk protein are given in Tables 1.4 and 2.9. The most suitable products for infants are Pregestimil and Pepdite(s), which are made from protein hydrolysates, or soya protein isolate modified formulae, such as Formula S (soya), Prosobee or Wysoy. Goat's milk should not be used for infants under six months of age and ewe's milk should not be used before one year old, as they are too high in protein and solute and cannot be easily modified to meet the nutritional requirements for infant feeding (Francis 1986). Goat's and ewe's milk are commonly sold unpasteurized and therefore the author recommends that they be boiled for two minutes to reduce microbial contamination. Ewe's milk should be diluted with an equal amount of water. When goat's or ewe's milk provides a major part of the diet, vitamins A, D and C and a source of vitamin B_{12} and folic acid should be given. Soya drinks that are only made from soya beans and sugar are not nutritional replacements for cow's milk. They are generally lower in energy, calcium, zinc availability and vitamins, and therefore are only a social replacement of milk (*see* Table 1.7) and should never be given as a sole source of nutrition, or for infants and young children as milk substitutes.

Despite the increasing number of cows' milk substitutes available, problems still arise. The appropriate milk substitute is not always recommended or prescribed, many products are unpalatable or expensive, and cheap alternatives are often used in error. Some patients react to soya and/or goat's milk as well as cow's milk, making these unsuitable substitutes. There is still a need for manufacturers to develop more acceptable low-allergen products which meet the nutritional needs of young children and infants.

It can take many weeks or even months to reintroduce foods singly to an oligoantigenic diet. It is therefore essential that the basic diet is nutritionally adequate for the individual patient for whom it is devised. Diets place great demands on the mother and family to provide interesting and nutritious meals. The more foods excluded, the more difficult and demanding this becomes. Very few manufactured foods can be used, and most meals have to be prepared in the home from basic ingredients; this is difficult for the mother who has come to rely on 'convenience foods'.

Diets should be continually assessed in the light of clinical findings; updated information on product changes is essential. The diet should be abandoned if of no benefit, if it is worse than the symptoms of the disease, or when the need for it is outgrown.

Compliance

The dietitian and parents should ensure that the prescribed diet excludes all sources of the suspected food allergens. New legislation on food labelling enables easier identification of ingredients (MAFF 1982), but the terminology used by manufacturers is often confusing to the lay public.

Patients fail to comply with exclusion diets for a number of reasons. Sometimes the decision is deliberate: the patient finds the diet too limiting, too expensive or too much trouble. Children on very strict diets may pilfer foods due to boredom or hunger, or just the desire to be the same as their contemporaries. The mother may be unable to adhere to the diet prescription because of guilt about the diagnosis, her emotional relationship with the child, inability to deprive the child of what she feels are basic needs, or to exert appropriate discipline. At other times noncompliance may be due to a genuine mistake, for example due to insufficient instruction or misinterpretation of food labels (Table 4.6).

Modern technology allows the development of multi-ingredient products containing a wide range of non-nutritive additives. Manufacturers only have to list some of these by category, e.g. antioxidant, others by name or their EEC code number (e.g. tartrazine = E102). This makes compliance more difficult than ever in a convenience food-oriented society. The Ministry of Agriculture, Fisheries and Food has published details on food labelling entitled: *Look at the Label* (MAFF 1982).

REVIEW

Children on complex exclusion diets should be seen regularly by the clinician and dietitian, and growth should be monitored.

Food allergy is frequently temporary, and children have a habit of getting better, irrespective of treatment. Infants with cow's milk and/or lactose intoler-

Table 4.6 Non-compliance with diet—some causes and misconceptions.

Baby cereals, savouries and desserts, particularly the instant powder varieties, frequently contain milk powder, soya and wheat; certain brands are colouring- and preservative-free.

Bread contains not only wheat, but yeast, soya, flour whiteners and shelf-life extenders, propionate preservative and natural benzoates.

Butter and table margarines may contain yellow dyes or carotene.

Casein(ate) and whey are the names of milk proteins added to many manufactured foods. EM40 and lactein contain milk proteins and lactose; EM40 is mostly used in meat products including cured meats such as ham, lactein is used in bakery products.

Chocolate (plain dark) contains milk and/or butter in most brands.

Coffee creamers, e.g. Coffee-mate and Compliment, contain casein(ate); Pareve-mate (kosher) although milk-free contains tartrazine.

Crisps contain antioxidants, the oil used is rarely identified and flavoured crisps contain a number of artificial flavours, colouring and preservatives, and may contain milk protein and/or lactose, even in the 'salt & vinegar' type.

Farina is frequently of wheat origin.

Food labels mostly state 'permitted preservatives or colour' or 'E' numbers without detailing the chemicals used.

Fruit juices, drinks and cordials frequently contain azo dyes and benzoate derivatives, as do sweets, candy, carbonated beverages.

Hydrolysed vegetable proteins can be of either soya or wheat origin or mycoprotein.

Hydrolysed whey sugar contains up to 10% milk protein. It can be used in confectionery.

Medicines and toothpaste frequently contain flavourings, colouring and preservatives. They may also contain sugar or sorbitol.

'Non-milk fat' milks and ice-cream are often misinterpreted as milk-free.

Products and packaged foods, such as meat, sausages, paté, bread, frozen foods, contain preservatives to extend shelf-life.

Peppermints, even white ones, contain either oil of wintergreen or peppermint essence and may contain other additives.

Skimmed milk powder and/or whey is added in the manufacture of all table margarines, rendering them unsuitable for use in milk-free diets; vegetable and polyunsaturated margarines are not exempt though some brands of low-fat spreads and all kosher and vegan margarines are milk-free.

Textured vegetable proteins are usually of soya origin.

Wheat starch is unsuitable on a wheat and/or cereal-free diet but may be classified as gluten-free if its purity is within the *Codex Alimentarius* gluten-free definition (p. 66).

ance(s), particularly post-gastroenteritis whether accompanied by enteropathy or not, frequently are symptom-free on a normal diet by one year old (Walker-Smith 1979). The optimal time of rechallenge or reintroduction of a normal diet in patients on maintenance diets for food allergic disease is a matter of opinion and debate. Often a genuine mistake with or without a reaction gives a clue, and therefore patients should be encouraged to keep a diary of such events. If a mistake does not provoke a reaction, a formal open challenge should be arranged, as sometimes a reaction is dose-related or is only obvious when a food is given on repeated occasions. At least a yearly review of both the need for the diet and its nutritional adequacy, together with practical aspects of the maintenance diet, such as new or revised product information, school meal, social eating and holiday catering hints, is essential.

PREVENTION

There has been much debate about the suggestion that allergy may be prevented by either the maternal diet in pregnancy or infant feeding. Sensitization can occur *in utero*, especially when the diet includes some foods in excess (Michel *et al.* 1980). However, as yet there is no evidence that dietary manipulation in pregnancy will prevent the child getting allergy, but it would seem sensible for women with a history of allergy to avoid *excess* intakes of the common food antigens during the last two months of pregnancy. At present there is no justification for recommending complete avoidance diets (Lessof 1984).

Recently attention has been focused on the role of inhaled allergens and early intercurrent infections in facilitating antigen sensitization in the infant. Dietary manipulation may be less important than avoidance of inhaled antigens by manipulating the birth month away from the pollen season and the house dust mite season, and avoiding household pets (Lessof 1984).

It has been suggested that atopic infants may have a temporary defect of immune function in the first months of life when sensitization may occur (Taylor *et al.* 1973). Exclusive breast-feeding in the first months of life may offer some protection against atopic disease (Matthew *et al.* 1977, Saarinen *et al.* 1979), but others have not confirmed this (Kramer & Moroz 1981). Food intolerance can occur in fully breast-fed infants. Even if breast-feeding offers only some protection against allergy it should be encouraged for as long as possible, with avoidance of all supplements (milk formulae, solids and fruit juices) in early infancy (*see* Chapter 1, Francis 1986), provided growth is satisfactory. Practical help and advice regarding demand breast-feeding is of paramount importance in achieving long-term success. Demand feeding at the breast can meet the nutritional needs of most infants for at least four months and exclusive breast-feeding is often adequate until eight months of age and occasionally even into the second year of life (Ahn & MacLean 1980). Human milk provides optimal nutrition and a relatively low-antigen feed, as well as positive immunological protection from microbes. It contains small amounts of protein derived from the maternal diet. Supplementary formulae and solids, however, introduce large amounts of additional antigens. Sensitization can occur later in life, but the infant is most vulnerable. Food antigens from the mother's diet may possibly, though rarely, sensitize some infants, and may trigger disease in an infant previously sensitized by complementary or supplementary feeds. The mother during lactation may need to avoid milk, eggs and other foods to which she has allergic reactions (Cant 1984, Cant & Bailes 1984).

The nutritional adequacy of the maternal diet is essential, and particular attention should be paid to the intake of calcium, folic acid, riboflavin and iron.

The desirable length of time to continue breast-feeding is uncertain, especially for those whose parents have atopic disease and who are therefore at greater risk. Extended partial breast-feeding (even into the second year) in conjunction with suitable weaning solids has been reported by Saarinen *et al.* (1979) to reduce the risk of allergy, particularly eczema.

Should breast-feeding not be possible, Glaser & Johnstone's (1953) work suggested that a degree of allergy prevention could be achieved by the use of a soya formula rather than a cow's milk formula, but this has not been confirmed (Taitz 1982) and there may be disadvantages in the use of soya (Editorial 1983b, Zoppi *et al.* 1983).

There is some evidence that modern modified milks cause less sensitization than older formulae and cow's milk because of heat treatment (McLaughlin *et al.* 1981, Manuel & Walker-Smith 1981). A liquid concentrate evaporated formula, or hydrolysed protein formula, such as Pregestimil or Pepdite 0–2, may be preferable in the child at high risk of atopy who is unable to be breast-fed.

Weaning should be discouraged until at least 4 to 6 months. The late introduction of solids may decrease the risk of eczema but not asthma (Lessof 1984). Provided growth and nutrition are adequate, a delay in introducing solids until six months may be preferable. From six months of age solids should be gradually introduced, including a dietary source of iron such as purée meat, liver or cereals. Fruit and vegetables should also be introduced. Highly sensitizing foods like milk, egg, wheat and nuts, and probably fish, citrus and berry fruits, are best avoided for an arbitrary period, until at least six months and possibly until one year in those whose parents are atopic or allergic to these foods. The order in which foods are introduced is a matter of debate as no data are available to indicate the optimal regimen. Single and sequential introduction of new foods may be advisable in the child at high risk of atopy, as reported by Cant (1984) and Cant and Bailes (1984).

COMMONLY USED EMPIRICAL AND MAINTENANCE DIETS

The dietitian will be able to adapt and modify the appropriate regimen from the diets given or devise a suitable regimen for the individual patient.

Cow's milk-free diet

Cow's milk is one of the commonest food antigens and intolerance to it may occur singly or in conjuction with multiple food allergy. Lactase deficiency, both secondary and, less commonly, primary, is a relatively common enzyme deficiency and also requires omission of milk from the diet (*see* Chapter 1). Differentiation between milk protein and lactose intolerance should ideally be made, although some patients have symptoms of both, and by excluding milk or using a milk substitute of appropriate type either or both may be simultaneously eliminated. The protein constituents of milk are the cause of milk allergy and human milk or boiled goat's milk (which contain lactose) may be satisfactory substitutes. Cross-reaction can occur between cow's milk and beef, in which case both need to be omitted, and similarly between egg and chicken (Atherton 1985).

Lippard (1936) showed that, whatever age cow's milk is introduced into a child's diet, milk antibody can be detected in the blood. Despite this, only a relatively small number go on to have milk protein intolerance, and in the majority it is a transient phenomenon of childhood. Cow's milk contains β-lactoglobulin, which is absent from human milk, and together with the casein and whey proteins from cow's milk is responsible for cow's milk protein intolerance (Visakorpi & Immonen 1967, Frier *et al.* 1969). Whey-based modified milks have a higher β-lactoglobulin content than those based on diluted cow's milk. The extra whey is added to improve the casein:whey ratio and amino acid profile compared to human milk, and hence the whey-based modified milks have a higher biological value of the protein than cow's milk or casein. β-lactoglobulin sensitivity is possibly commoner in infants fed whey-based milks, and casein sensitivity commoner in those fed the diluted modified cow's milk formulae. The modern infant formulae are, however, less sensitizing than earlier formulae (Manuel & Walker-Smith 1981).

McLaughlin *et al.* (1981) have shown that different types of milk cause differing degrees of sensitization in guinea-pigs. The degree of sensitization is in reverse proportion to the heat treatment (time and temperature exposure) used in processing and hence the degree of protein denaturation. Hydrolysis of the protein also reduces its sensitizing capacity; clinical experience supports this theory, at least in paediatric gastroenterology (Manuel & Walker-Smith 1981). Pregestimil and Nutramigen, which are hydrolysed casein formulae, are less sensitizing than soya formulae. Ten per cent of infants fed soya formulae because of cow's milk intolerance subsequently become intolerant to soya (Editorial 1983b). Liquid evaporated milks are less sensitizing than powder or fresh milk. By inference: liquid concentrate Gold Cap SMA (Wyeth) is less sensitizing than Gold Cap SMA powder; the ready-to-feed type of formulae, including Aptamil, Milumil, Osterfeed, Ostermilk, Premium and SMA, are less sensitizing than the reconstituted powder format of the same formulae. Boiled goat's milk was less sensitizing than fresh goat's milk in guinea-pigs (McLaughlin *et al.* 1981).

In the treatment of milk protein and/or lactose intolerance all sources of milk, casein, whey, butter, cheese, cream, yoghurt, foods containing non-milk fat solids, and, unless the degree of hydrolysis is known, hydrolysed whey, casein(ate) and lactalbumin, should be excluded. Table 1.8 gives details of a milk- and lactose-free diet. The young child, and particularly the infant, requires a nutritionally adequate milk substitute. Tables 1.4 and 2.9 list suitable products for different age groups, and give details of the source of protein each contains.

For the infant, of the formulae currently available, Pregestimil, Pepdite 0–2, or the module feed based on Comminuted Chicken (Table 1.18) is the most appropriate; Nutramigen is suitable for those over three months of age. The new Neocate amino acid- and peptide-based formulae such as the Pepdite range may prove useful for the young child, and Elemental 028 (unflavoured) amino acid formula may be useful for the older child, as an alternative to Flexical. The soya formulae have proved useful milk substitutes, at least in some patients with atopic eczema, asthma and other conditions related or caused by cow's milk sensitivity, and in those with lactase deficiency.

Goat's milk is the least suitable alternative, because it can induce allergy, has a high solute content, contains lactose, and because of the risk of microbial contamination of raw milk. It should not be used for infants under six months. Microbial contamination can be reduced by boiling for two minutes, which possibly decreases the risk of inducing sensitization and allergy. In addition to vitamins A, D and C, a source of B_{12} and folic acid supplement (e.g. three Ketovite Tablets plus 5 ml Ketovite Liquid) should be given if goat's milk is used as a major source of nutrients, as goat's milk anaemia related to folic acid deficiency has been documented. Ewe's milk is now available, and has similar disadvantages to goat's milk, but its role as an alternative milk in children with allergy is still being evaluated. It is unsuitable for infants under one year old and should be boiled and diluted with an equal quantity of water, i.e. half-strength, for children, and vitamin supplements are advised. Goat's milk powders are available and mostly reconstitute to whole milk. When *no* other alternative is available a simple modification of goat's milk to reduce the high solute content is possible (Table 4.7). This recipe does not meet the recommendations for an artificial feed for infants (DHSS 1980), as it still contains more protein and solute than recommended, but if goat's milk is diluted further the vitamin, essential fatty acid and trace mineral content will be inadequate.

For the school-age child requiring a milk-free diet a calcium supplement (400 mg elemental calcium per

Table 4.7 Goat's milk modification.

	Protein (g)	Fat (g)	Carbohydrate (g)	Energy kJ	kcal
75 ml boiled goat's milk 25 ml boiled water } 100 ml 5 g sugar	2·5	3·4	8·5	302	75

Vitamins A, D, C, B₁₂ and folic acid, e.g. three Ketovite Tablets and 5 ml Ketovite Liquid, are recommended.

Goat's milk is not recommended for infants under six months unless no other suitable milk substitute is available, in which case the above dilution is suggested. Goat's milk powders mostly reconstitute to whole goat's milk. This recipe does not meet the recommendations of the DHSS (1980) for artificial feeds for young infants but has a reduced protein and solute compared to whole goat's milk.

day) may suffice, rather than a milk substitute, provided adequate protein, energy and riboflavin are taken from natural foods. A social replacement of milk can be useful, for example Granose Soya-Milk Liquid, Plamil (Plantmilk), Pareve-mate (Carnation kosher coffee creamer) or a milk-free non-dairy imitation cream (Table 1.7).

Although there are no generally agreed criteria for milk challenge, whole cow's milk is usually used as the initial test dose(s), and the child is graded onto an appropriate formula for age if no reaction occurs. A scheme for lactose and milk challenge and their reintroduction in different clinical situations is described in Chapter 1, p. 40. In patients with cow's milk enteropathy sequential jejunal biopsies before and after milk challenge are indicated (Walker-Smith 1979 & 1985). Follow-up of patients with milk intolerance, both while on a diet and subsequently after milk challenge, is essential to ensure adequate growth and to rule out relapse, which may only show as chronic symptoms such as failure to thrive.

Frequently, atopic patients react to more than one category of food. Various combinations of diets, excluding other foods and milk, will be required by different patients. Egg is another common antigen which often has to be excluded. The following diets are therefore provided:

Table 4.8 Egg-free diet.
Table 4.9 Milk- and egg-free diet.
Table 4.10 Milk-, egg-, chicken-, azo dye- and preservative-free diet with or without fish.

Reactions to wheat, often in combination with rye intolerance, as in coeliac disease, occur in patients with allergy symptoms unrelated to the gastrointestinal tract, such as asthma, and such patients need a wheat-free diet with or without rye exclusion. The gluten-free diet given in Table 3.1 can be adapted for use by these patients. A milk-, egg- and wheat-free diet is given in Table 4.11 and a milk-, egg-, wheat-, azo dye- and preservative-free diet is given in Table 4.12. Patients with food allergy rarely tolerate wheat starch-based products (Francis 1980, Lessof 1984) and therefore gluten-free wheat starch-based breads and flours should be omitted, at least initially, from a wheat-free diet for food allergy. Suitable products are listed in Table 4.13.

Non-nutritive additives, preservative, flavourings and colourings

Chemical substances were added to food to enhance its flavour and act as preservatives long before modern food technology was developed, e.g. salt was used as a preservative; sodium nitrite is traditionally added to the liquid in which bacon is pickled; hops act as a preservative in beer. However, a large number of additional substances have been introduced relatively recently, e.g. food colours; flavours and sweeteners; flour improvers; bleaches; 'shelf' extenders, emulsifiers, stabilizers; antioxidants; preservatives, antibiotics, insecticides; nutritional supplements, vitamins, minerals; and possibly unintentional additives from wrappings, machinery and processing. Many additives are necessary to prevent food spoilage, particularly for urban populations. To imitate the taste and smell of natural food frequently requires an intricate and complex range of chemicals, e.g. to produce imitation pineapple flavour necessitates a mixture of up to 10 pure chemicals and seven natural oils. Additives are carefully scrutinized before new products are permitted by law, and regulations control their use. In processed foods labels must indicate their addition by either category and in some cases by name or EEC (E) number. Many additives are natural colours or nature identical (MAFF 1982).

For the majority, such additives cause no adverse reaction. However, a minority of patients are intoler-

Table 4.8 Egg-free diet.
A normal diet can be modified to exclude egg provided the following precautions are taken.

The following foods must be excluded:

Egg in all forms: boiled, scrambled, poached, fried.
Cakes, biscuits, meringues, containing egg.
Manufactured foods containing egg and egg albumen (scrutinize the ingredients list on all packet labels before use).

Manufactured items likely to contain egg or albumen:
Mayonnaise and salad cream
Fish in batter and fish fingers
Lemon curd
Rice pudding
Meringue and meringue mix
Marshmallow
Soft-centred sweets and chocolate
Egg noodles
Fresh spaghetti
Fried rice.

Egg replacers:
These have no food value but are useful in cooking.

(a) Edifas A (methylethylcellulose) available from ICI Ltd, or Bow Products Ltd. It must be made into a solution before use; it replaces the binding property of egg in recipes.

Soak 3·5 g ($\frac{1}{8}$ oz) in 30 ml (1 oz) hot water, stir. When cold add a further 30 ml (1 oz) cold water to make 60 ml (2 oz) of Edifas solution. Use 60 ml (2 oz) of solution to replace one egg in a recipe.

(b) Ener-G egg replacer (potato starch, tapioca and cellulose) by Ener-G Foods Inc., available from GF Dietary Supplies (U.K.).

For each egg in a recipe substitute:
1 tsp Ener-G egg replacer ⎫
2 tbsp water   ⎬ = 1 whole egg
Mix thoroughly   ⎭

If the recipe calls for unbeaten eggs, stir egg replacer into water (do not beat). If recipe calls for beaten egg-whites use an electric whisk and beat the egg replacer with water until stiff.

If the recipe calls for egg-yolks only, use half the amount of water for each egg.

Other liquids may be substituted for water if preferred.

---

ant of them. A diet excluding non-nutritive additives is given in Table 4.14. Because of their widespread use in processed food, a diet excluding non-nutritive additives must be based on primary foods such as meats, fruits, cereals, vegetables and milk. The azo dyes, benzoate derivatives and salicylates which are closely related chemically have been particularly implicated in urticaria (Lockey *et al.* 1971). Adverse reactions to the azo dyes, which are derivatives of coal tar, have been recorded for over 30 years. Naturally occurring salicylates and benzoates in some fruits and vegetables and benzoates in bread may also cause a reaction in some patients sensitized to these chemicals, but there are no accurate lists of such foods and

therefore it is preferable to identify foods which provoke symptoms by elimination and challenge. The labels of all processed and manufactured foods must be scrutinized, and only those products free from added artificial colours, preservatives or the relevant 'E' numbers (MAFF 1982, Hanssen 1984), as appropriate for the diet concerned, should be used.

August (1980) has pointed out that many patients who are prescribed azo-free, or colouring- and preservative-free, diets will be given antihistamine and other medicines, many of which contain preservatives, and a number of which are coloured, e.g. many tablets contain azo dyes, especially those coloured orange, red, green or yellow. White tablets and gelatine capsules may be satisfactory. Toothpaste, lozenges, and vitamin preparations containing synthetic flavourings, colourings and preservatives should be avoided.

The success of an additive-free diet depends on the enthusiasm of the doctor and dietitian and the skill and determination of the patient and his parents, firstly in eliminating non-nutritive additives from the diet, then in identifying the specific additives which are responsible for symptoms, and, not least, the long-term maintenance diet preparation which requires continual vigilance in scrutinizing foods and products. The patients and their parents must be committed largely to home-prepared foods from primary ingredients. Social eating must be planned very carefully, particularly when there is risk of severe reactions, such as anaphylaxis, angioedema or hypotension and, to a lesser extent, urticaria.

CONCLUSION

The dietary approach to the management of food intolerance is particularly complex and can lead to nutritional difficulties and social disruption. The complementary roles of clinician and dietitian in diagnosis and treatment are essential, in order to avoid unnecessary dietary restrictions and yet provide a varied and nutritionally adequate practical regime when required. Such diets should be continually reviewed, updated and discontinued as soon as no longer necessary for treatment.

Table 4.9 Milk- and egg-free diet.
Eggs, milk and all manufactured products containing milk, egg, casein, whey, butter, and albumen must be excluded from the diet. This diet needs modification for infants. The diet should be continually reviewed, appropriately adjusted, new foods introduced or eliminated and updated with information of product changes.

(a)   Allowed and forbidden foods.

Foods allowed	Foods forbidden
Milk substitute—*see* Tables 1.4 and 1.7.	Milk, cream, cheese, butter, ordinary margarine, eggs, egg albumen.
	Casilan, Coffee-mate, Fast Pints, Five Pints, Compliment.
	Galactomins and products containing casein, whey, milk solids, caseinate, etc.

Meat
  Beef, lamb, pork, veal, rabbit
Offal
  Liver, kidney
Poultry
  Chicken, turkey
Fresh fish, if permitted
	Sausages, unless milk-free.
	Fish fingers and fish in batter unless milk- and egg-free.
	Tinned meat, ham, fish, etc. unless brand and ingredients are checked.

Milk-free margarine: Tomor, Telma Soft Margarine. Safeway's and Sainsbury's low-fat spread. Vegetable oils, pure fats, lard, Trex, Spry.	

Cereals
  Wheat, rye, barley, oats, rice, flour, semolina, sago (cooked without milk or with milk substitute).
Macaroni, spaghetti.
Breakfast cereals
  Weetabix, Cornflakes, Rice Krispies, Shreddies, bran, All-bran.
Baby cereals
  Robinson's Baby Rice, Farex Weaning Food, Milupa Rice Cereal, Farley's Original Rusk.
	Milk puddings, e.g. custard, creamed rice.
	Non-milk fat products, instant custard.
	Egg noodles, macaroni cheese, tinned spaghetti with or without cheese, e.g. spaghetti hoops, Italian spaghetti, fresh spaghetti.
	Baby cereals fortified with egg and/or milk solids, e.g. Farley's Breakfast Cereal.
	Swiss-type cereals and muesli, Special K.
	Farley's Low-Sugar Rusks.

Sugar, jam, honey, jelly, syrup. Marmite, Bovril, Oxo, Bisto. Salt and pepper, herbs, spices, essences.	Hydrolysed milk sugar Lemon curd Salad cream, mayonnaise.

Table 4.9 (a) *continued*

Foods allowed	Foods forbidden
Bread, e.g. wholemeal, Hovis, plain white milk-free, Vit-Be, granary breads.	Milk bread, Procea.
Cakes and biscuits known to be free of milk and egg.	Cakes and biscuits containing egg and/or milk.
Egg substitutes (Table 4.8)	Eggs, egg-white, meringues, etc.
Tea, coffee, cocoa, drinking chocolate.	Horlicks, Ovaltine, Bournvita.
Boiled sweets, lollies, pastilles, gums, Terry's Bitter Chocolate.	Fudge, toffee.
	All types ice-cream (including non-milk fat types).
	Milk chocolate, some plain dark chocolate, diabetic chocolate.
	Opal Fruits, plain chocolate, e.g. Suchard, Bournville Chocolate, Chocolate Shapes, etc.
Fruit—all varieties.	Fruit pies and crumbles.
Vegetables without butter, milk or egg.	Instant potato containing milk and/or butter.
Potatoes, plain crisps.	Mashed potato containing milk and/or butter.
	Potato salad, flavoured crisps, vegetable salad.
Fruit juices and squash, fizzy pop, Coke, Pepsi, Lucozade, Pareve-mate (kosher)	
	Cream, tinned and packet soups.
Tinned or processed foods known to be free of milk and egg, etc. Check every label before use.	Manufactured and processed food unless checked to be free of milk, eggs, whey, milk solids, egg powder.

(b)   Milk- and egg-free diet—sample menu.

Breakfast	Weetabix, Cornflakes or porridge
	Sugar
	Milk substitute
	Bacon and tomato
	Milk-free bread or toast
	Milk-free margarine, etc.
	Marmalade, jam, honey, Marmite, Bovril
	Milk substitute, flavoured with tea or coffee or cocoa
Mid-morning	Fruit juice or milk substitute
Lunch	Meat, chicken, fish, etc. ⎫
	Potato—roast, boiled, chips ⎪ Cook without milk, butter or egg.
	Vegetables, pulses ⎬
	Gravy ⎭
	Fruit, jelly
	Special custard made with milk substitute and suitable custard powder
	Suitable fruit pie, tart (made without milk, butter or eggs)
Tea	Suitable milk- and egg-free biscuit or cake
	Milk substitute

Table 4.9 (b)   *continued*

Supper	Meat, chicken, fish, etc. ⎫
	Salad or vegetables or pulses ⎬ Cook without milk, butter or egg.
	Chips or plain crisps; rice; macaroni ⎭
	Milk-free bread
	Milk-free margarine, etc.
	Marmite, jam, honey, peanut butter
	Milk-free/egg-free biscuit or cake
	Fruit or jelly
	Milk substitute flavoured with tea or coffee
Bedtime	Milk substitute
	Fruit

Vitamin supplement as appropriate

(c)   Milk- and egg-free weaning diet—sample menu (to use in conjunction with milk substitute feeds as appropriate for age, e.g. Cow & Gate S Formula or Pregestimil).

Breakfast	Robinson's Baby Rice, Farley's Rusk, Milupa Plain Rice Cereal
	Mix with milk substitute feed as prescribed
Lunch	Sieved or minced meat
	Boiled potato, may be mashed but without milk, butter or egg
	Sieved vegetables
	Special custard made with milk substitute and plain custard powder
	or Baby food known to be free of milk and egg
Tea	Fruit purée and suitable custard as lunch
	or Baby food free of milk and egg

Table 4.10   Milk-, egg-, chicken-, azo colouring- and preservative-free diet, with or without fish. Empirical diet for use in atopic eczema and/or urticaria.

The diet is used for some forms of food allergic disease. It is used for a trial period (normally 6 to 8 weeks) to see if the symptoms improve. It is essential that the diet has appropriate adjustments such as food reintroduction and updating of information about manufactured products. Mostly natural fresh foods and home-cooked foods should be used whenever possible.

This diet needs modification for infants.

Milk, eggs and chicken and all manufactured products containing these items must be excluded from the diet. This includes foods containing milk, cream, cheese, skimmed milk powder, non-fat milk solids, casein, sodium caseinate, whey, butter, hydrolysed milk sugar, egg and egg powder, albumen, chicken and chicken fat. For example, even Chipsticks or salt and vinegar crisps can contain milk, so only use manufactured foods with a comprehensive list of ingredients which should be continually checked.

Colourings and preservatives
A number of non-nutritive additives—colours, flavourings, preservatives and antioxidants—are permitted in food manufacture. It is best to avoid, if possible, foods to which they are added. The following have been found a particular problem in patients with atopic eczema and/or urticaria:

Azo dyes which are derivatives of coal tar, including tartrazine (orange–yellow) E102, sunset yellow E110, and new coccine E124 (Ponceau 4R) red.

Benzoic acid and its derivatives, which are preservatives, E210 to E219 inclusive.

Salicylate or aspirin sensitivity can occur in some patients sensitive to azo dyes.

Table 4.10 *continued*

It is necessary to check every food package and container very carefully: in many cases specific colourings and preservatives are not listed by name. When in doubt the food should not be given. Food with labels which state 'permitted preservative or colouring' should not be given.

All syrup medicines, including some vitamins, coloured tablets (especially orange, red, green or yellow ones), coloured toothpaste and sweets should also be omitted.

(a) Allowed and forbidden foods.

Allowed foods	Forbidden foods
Milk substitute—*see* Tables 1.4 and 1.7	Milk, cream, cheese, all ordinary and vegetable margarines, yoghurt, evaporated milk, ice-cream.
	Instant Whip, Casilan, Coffee-mate, Fast Pints, Five Pints, Compliment, Pareve-mate.
	Galactomins and products containing casein, whey, milk solids, etc.
Meat: Lamb, pork, beef, veal, rabbit, turkey, duck, goose.	Chicken, chicken liver, chicken stock cubes.
Buy fresh meats from butchers rather than pre-packed meats from supermarkets.	Supermarket packaged meats, frozen meats.
	Sausages, beefburgers, frankfurters, salami.
	Canned meats, e.g. corned beef.
	Some hams and bacons, especially smoked products.
	Stuffing and forcemeat.
	Processed meats.
	Ham and other cured meats may contain whey protein or EM40.
Fish (only if permitted and no known reactions in the past). Fresh fish including shellfish.	Fish in batter, fish fingers, ready-cooked fish. Fish canned in tomato sauce may contain colouring. Smoked fish, e.g. smoked haddock, smoked salmon, kippers.
Tinned and frozen fish provided no milk and/or egg and/or colouring and/or preservative have been added.	
Egg substitutes—*see* Table 4.8.	Eggs, meringues, etc.
	Albumen
	Foods containing egg, e.g. cake.
Fats: Milk-free margarine containing natural carotene and known to be free of artificial colouring, e.g. Tomor margarine	Butter
	Margarines containing artificial yellow colouring and/or milk solids.
Vegetable oils, lard, dripping.	Chicken fat
Cereals: 100% wholemeal flour, cornflour, baking powders (check ingredients), rice, oats, semolina, sago, tapioca, barley (cooked without milk).	White flour
	Coloured custard powders
	Milk puddings, e.g. creamed rice.
Home-made wholemeal bread, Allinson's Windmill, Prewett's, Goswell's wholewheat bread, Ryvita.	White and brown breads, milk breads.
Breakfast cereals free of milk and/or colourings and/or preservatives, e.g. Weetabix, Shredded Wheat, Puffed Wheat, porridge oats, Kellogg's Cornflakes, Rice Krispies, Jordan's Muesli, etc.	Cereals containing milk, e.g. Kellogg's Special K, Swiss-type cereals.
	Cereals containing artificial colourings and/or preservatives, e.g. Sugar Puffs, Kellogg's Puffa Puffa Rice.
Baby cereals: Robinson's Baby Rice, Milupa Plain Rice Cereal, Farley's Original Rusk, Farex Weaning Food.	Baby cereals fortified with milk and/or egg, e.g. Farley's Low-Sugar Rusk, Liga Rusk, Farley's Breakfast Cereal.
Macaroni, spaghetti.	Egg noodles, fresh spaghetti containing egg, macaroni cheese, tinned spaghetti and baked beans containing colouring and preservatives and/or cheese.
	Green lasagne.

Table 4.10 (a)   *continued*

Foods allowed	Foods forbidden
Home-made cakes and biscuits using the permitted ingredients.	Commercial cakes, pastries, pies, biscuits, and mixes. Cakes and foods containing lactein.
Vegetables: It is safer to use fresh vegetables—wash well. Frozen and canned vegetables should be checked for milk products and/or colouring and/or preservative.	Canned and frozen vegetables containing milk and/or colouring and/or preservatives, e.g. instant potato containing milk and/or butter. Ready-prepared salads, e.g. potato salad. Tomato-flavoured savoury foods, e.g. tomato paste and tomato ketchup may contain artificial colouring.
Home-made soups using permitted ingredients.	Cream, some tinned and packet soups.
Plain crisps.	Chipsticks and flavoured crisps.
Fruit: Fresh fruit is suitable, but should be washed to remove any sprays used in growing or to enhance keeping. Canned fruit mostly contains fruit and added sugar only, but check label.	Tinned rhubarb frequently has added colouring.
Miscellaneous: Sugar, golden syrup, treacle, honey. Home-made jams without colouring and preservatives. Salt, pepper, fresh herbs and spices. Bisto gravy powder, Marmite, Heinz Tomato Ketchup and processed foods which have been scrutinized for suitability of their ingredients.	Commercially made jams containing colouring and/or preservatives, lemon curd. Ketchup, sauces, pickles, chutneys containing colourings and/or preservatives. Gravy mixes, salad cream, mayonnaise containing egg flavouring and essences.
Drinks: Milk substitute, water, mineral water, soda water. Natural permitted fruit juices, Baby Ribena. Cocoa, e.g. Bournville, Cadbury's Drinking Chocolate, tea and pure coffee. Colourless fizzy drinks free of preservative.	Milk, milk-shake powders and syrups. Horlicks. Ovaltine, Bournvita. Build-Up Instant teas Fruit squashes Fizzy coloured drinks, e.g. Coke, Pepsi, shandy, Lucozade. Alcoholic beverages
Sweets: home-made sweets and milk-free toffee. Home-made ice-lollies made from permitted ingredients. Pascall's Murray Mints, Marks & Spencer's Soft Mints. Terry's Bitter Chocolate, Sainsbury's Plain Chocolate (ingredients should be checked).	Chocolate, milk toffee, fudge. All coloured sweets and ice-lollies. Jellies, pastilles, lozenges.
Nuts (only if permitted), e.g. shelled or salted peanuts, cashew nuts, fresh coconut.	Dessicated coconut, dry roasted peanuts.

(b)   Milk-, egg-, azo colouring- and preservative-free diet with or without fish—sample menu.

Breakfast	Natural permitted fruit juice
	Suitable cereal, e.g. Weetabix, Shredded Wheat, Jordan's Muesli
	Sugar
	Milk substitute
	Wholemeal bread
	Milk-free margarine, honey, home-made marmalade, jam
	Milk substitute—tea or coffee if permitted

Table 4.10 (b)   *continued*

Lunch/supper (Can be adapted to a packed meal for school)	Fresh lamb, pork, beef, turkey ⎫ Potato, rice, pasta ⎬ Cooked without milk or egg Wholemeal bread and milk-free margarine ⎭ Fresh vegetables Fresh fruit, home-made cake or dessert using permitted ingredients
Snacks	Milk substitute Natural permitted fruit juice Fresh fruit or permitted dried fruit or nuts* Home-made cakes or biscuits using permitted ingredients
Vitamins	Only use Children's Clinic Vitamin A, D, C, Drops, or Abidec 0·6 ml and/or white ascorbic acid tablets.
Medicines	Use only white tablets or those specifically prescribed. *Do not give* syrup medicines, cough mixtures, and medicines containing flavouring, colouring, preservatives.
Toothpaste	Use only white toothpaste or use a little salt instead.
Soap	Plain white, unscented soap is preferable. If eczema or urticaria is a symptom soap should be avoided.

*Do not give whole nuts to children under ≃ four years old.

Table 4.11   Milk-, wheat-, egg-free diet.

This diet must be modified for the individual needs of the patient, especially in the case of infants. The diet should be continually reviewed, appropriately adjusted, new foods introduced or eliminated and updated with information on product changes.

Wheat.   Wheat, and all foods containing wheat, must be excluded from the diet, e.g. ordinary bread, biscuits, cakes, wheat-based breakfast cereals. Rye, barley and oats intolerance can be associated with wheat intolerance, but these foods are not necessarily excluded and gluten-free products are not necessarily suitable.

Milk protein.   Cow's milk and all foods containing cow's milk should be omitted. This includes casein, non-fat milk solids, whey, cheese, butter. A number of substitutes for cow's milk are available.

Egg.   Eggs and all foods containing eggs must be excluded. This includes egg albumen.

(a)   Allowed and forbidden foods.

Foods allowed	Foods forbidden
Milk substitute appropriate for age (*see* Tables 1.4 and 1.7).	Cow's milk, baby milks, dried and evaporated milks, yoghurt, cream, ice-cream, coffee creamers, milk-shake powders, filled milks. Galactomin and products containing casein or caseinate, whey, milk solids, etc.
Milk-free margarines, Tomor kosher margarine, Granose margarine, Telma soft margarine, Vitaquell margarine, and milk-free low-fat spreads. Vegetable oils, lard and cooking fats.	Butter, cheese, all table margarines containing whey solids.
All meats, fish, poultry, ham, bacon, offal.	Manufactured meat products, e.g. meat paste, sausages, fish fingers, beefburgers and made-up dishes, etc. unless checked as milk-, egg-, wheat-free.

Table 4.11 (a) *continued*

Allowed foods	Forbidden foods
Egg replacer (*see* Table 4.8)	Eggs, albumen, egg-whites, meringues.
All fruit, natural fruit juice.	
Pulses; Beans, peas, lentils, gram, dahl, etc.	Made-up vegetable dishes (e.g. potato salad) unless checked as milk-, egg- and wheat-free.
Vegetables, fresh, tinned, frozen or dried (without butter, milk, egg, flour, etc.).	
Plain crisps	Flavoured crisps, Chipsticks, 'MacDonald's' chips.
All cereals (except wheat), rice, corn, maize flour, cornflour, soya, arrowroot, rice flour, ground rice, sago, tapioca, potato flour, buckwheat, rice bran, soya.	Wheat, wheat starch, semolina, macaroni, spaghetti, pasta, farina, wheat crispbreads.
Rye, oats, barley if permitted	Gluten-free products based on wheat starch.
Rye crispbread, Ryvita, Ryking, oatcakes (*see* Table 4.13)	
Use special recipes for making biscuits, cakes and bread from permitted flour, e.g. rice flour or potato flour.	Ordinary bread, cakes, meringues.
Porridge, Ready Brek (plain), Farex Weaning Cereal, Rice Krispies, Ricicles, Cornflakes, Puffa Puffa Rice, Frosties, Robinson's Baby Rice, Milupa Plain Rice Cereal.	Special K, Weetabix, Farley's Rusks, Wheat Flakes, Puffed Wheat, Shredded Wheat, Farley's Breakfast Cereal, Milupa Rice Dessert containing milk, muesli.
Maize-based custard and blancmange powders if free of cow's milk.	Instant Whip, Angel Delight, tinned and packet custard mixes, jelly creams, made-up desserts.
Jelly, gelatine.	
Cream of tartar, bicarbonate of soda, wheat-free baking powder, yeast (bakers' and brewers').	Baking powder containing flour filler.
Bovril, Marmite, Osem Instant Bouillon Cubes, Telma Kosher Beef Stock Cubes.	Oxo, Bisto, stock cubes.
	Soups, sauces, gravy mixes containing forbidden ingredients.
	Mayonnaise, salad cream.
Salt, pepper, pure herbs and pure spices, vinegar.	Ready-mixed mustard and spices sometimes contain flour.
Tea, coffee, cocoa, instant coffee.	Bengers, Ovaltine, Horlicks, drinking chocolate unless brand is checked.
Carbonated beverages, squash, cordial.	
Glucose, sugar, jam, honey, marmalade, syrup.	Lemon curd, mincemeat (sweet), hydrolysed milk sugar.
Milk-free chocolate, boiled sweets and fruit gums.	Filled chocolate, milk chocolate, Smarties, Kit Kat, Mars Bars, Opal Fruits, dark chocolate containing butter, Chocolate Shapes, liquorice, fudge, toffee.
Salted peanuts.	Dry roasted peanuts.
Tinned or processed foods known to be free of wheat, milk and eggs.	Manufactured and processed food unless checked to be free of wheat, milk and egg.
Scrutinize labels before using manufactured products.	

(b)   Milk-, wheat-, egg-free diet—sample menu.

Breakfast	Porridge, Cornflakes, Rice Krispies, Ricicles, Frosties, Ready Brek (plain)
	Sugar
	Milk substitute
	Bacon or ham
	Permitted crispbread or oatcakes or wheat-free bread (*see* Table 4.13)
	Milk-free margarine
	Jam, marmalade, Bovril, honey, Marmite
	Tea, coffee, fruit juice
Lunch and/or supper	Meat or poultry (fresh or frozen)
or	Ham or bacon or fish
	Gravy made with meat juices and maize cornflour
	Potatoes—roast, jacket, boiled, chips Cooked without milk, egg, wheat flour
	Rice, pasta, pulses
	Vegetable/salad
	Permitted crispbread or oatcakes
	Milk-free margarine
	Fruit, fresh or tinned
	Pudding with milk substitute or using special recipes
	Natural fruit juice etc.
Snacks	Fresh fruit, dried fruit, nuts
	Plain crisps
	Permitted crispbread or oatcakes (*see* Table 4.13)
	Milk-free margarine, etc.
	Honey, jam, Bovril, Marmite
	Cake, biscuits, etc. from recipes provided
	Tea or coffee or fruit juice

Table 4.12   Milk-, egg-, wheat-, azo dye- and preservative-free diet.
   This diet demands home-prepared meals from basic natural ingredients. If manufactured foods are included, the ingredients list must be continually scrutinized and products avoided if a detailed list of ingredients is not included. This diet should be continually reviewed, appropriately adjusted, new foods introduced or eliminated and updated with information on product changes.

(a)   Use only the following foods.

Milk substitute	Milk substitute as appropriate for age (*see* Table 1.4 or 1.7), e.g. Nutramigen, Pregestimil, Pepdite, Soya S Formula, Prosobee, Wysoy.
	If permitted boiled goat's milk plus vitamins A, D, C, folic acid and vitamin B_{12}.
Meat, poultry, fish	Buy fresh meat from a butcher whenever possible, rather than pre-packed meats from supermarkets, or use frozen meat.
	Avoid prepared dishes, beefburgers, fish fingers, meat extenders, gravy mixes.
	Smoked fish and meat, e.g. smoked, smoked bacon, Breakfast Slices.
	Ham and bacon may be suitable.

Table 4.12 (a) *continued*

Fruit, vegetables and pulses, potato, plain crisps	Fresh, frozen or canned in syrup or brine only (check that no colouring or preservatives are added). Dried fruit and nuts—shelled or salted only. *Avoid* made-up dishes such as baked beans, potato and vegetable salads, pies, 'MacDonald' type chips, flavoured crisps, dry roast peanuts, etc. Bananas and peas contain natural benzoic acid.
Beverages	Fresh squeezed fruit juices, natural fruit juices without colour and preservatives, e.g. Baby Ribena, colourless lemonade, e.g. 7-Up (provided citrus and berry fruits are permitted). Tea, coffee, instant coffee, cocoa, drinking chocolate. *Avoid* milk-shake syrups and powders, squashes and cordials, instant teas, coke, etc.
Cereals and flours	Maize, rice (white and brown), soya, pulses, buckwheat, ground rice, rice flour, corn (maize) flour, soya flour, potato flour. Kellogg's Cornflakes and Rice Krispies. Rice bran, soya bran. Sago, tapioca, arrowroot, wheat-free baking powder, e.g. Rite-Diet Gluten-Free Baking Powder. Bicarbonate of soda, cream of tartar, yeast (brewers' and bakers'). *Avoid* wheat, flour, bread, biscuits, semolina, macaroni, pasta, custard powder, instant puddings and desserts. Rye, oats, barley if permitted (wheat intolerance can be associated with intolerance to these cereals and occasionally all cereals need to be avoided).
Suitable bread and biscuits replacements	Rye crispbread, Ryvita, Ryking, Scanda Crisp, oatcakes, pumpernickel, rye and barley bread free of wheat. } If permitted *See also* Table 4.13 for wheat-, milk-, egg-free special products (those marked * are free of azo dyes and preservatives).
Sugars	Glucose, jam (without colouring, preservative), honey, golden syrup, treacle, toffee, white peppermints, barley sugar, peanuts (shelled or plain salted), peanut butter. Sugar (cane and beet). *Avoid* boiled sweets, chocolate, dry roast peanuts and flavoured crisps. All branded sweets unless they have a comprehensive list of ingredients to check suitability: e.g. Opal Fruits contain hydrolysed milk and tartrazine; Chocolate Shapes contain egg albumen; Bournville Chocolate contains butter.
Flavourings	Salt, pepper, Bovril, fresh herbs and vinegar, Marmite. *Avoid* essences, spices, curry powder, stock cubes, gravy mixes, prepared mustard. Food colourings, preservatives (*see* Table 4.15).
Vegetable oils, lard	Milk-free margarines, e.g. Tomor margarine, Telma margarine, Granose margarine, Vitaquell margarine or milk-free low-fat spread. E101, E160 and E161 are permitted. *Avoid* butter and ordinary margarines which contain whey/milk and/or colouring.
Miscellaneous	Egg substitutes (*see* Table 4.8) have no food value but are useful as a binder in recipes. Rice bran, soya bran.

(b) Milk-, egg-, wheat-, azo dye- and preservative-free diet—sample menu.

Breakfast	Porridge, Kellogg's Rice Krispies or Cornflakes Sugar Milk substitute Optional bacon, ham or fish (unsmoked and no milk, egg, flour) Wheat-free bread or rye crispbread (*see* Table 4.13) Milk-free margarine Marmite, honey or permitted ham/marmalade, peanut butter Tea, coffee with milk substitute or fresh fruit juice
Snack	Fruit, salted peanuts, plain crisps, permitted rye crispbread or permitted biscuits Milk substitute or fresh fruit juice
Lunch and supper	Meat, fish, poultry, ham Gravy made from meat juices and cornflour } Unsmoked and no milk, egg, flour Potato, rice, pulses Vegetables and/or salad Fruit Wheat-free bread and/or rye crispbread or GF Brand Gluten-Free Crackers Milk-free margarine Marmite, honey or permitted jam/marmalade, peanut butter Fresh fruit juice or milk substitute with tea, coffee
Vitamin and mineral supplements	Abidec drops (0·6 ml) are recommended with this diet, at least in children under two years. Some patients will require a more comprehensive vitamin supplement, e.g. Cow & Gate Supplementary Vitamin Tablets, 6 to 12 daily, plus 5 ml Ketovite Liquid. If no milk substitute is given a calcium supplement is required as either: calcium gluconate, three 1 g tablets *or* } Each supplies approximately 300 mg elemental calcium. calcium lactate, six 300 mg tablets

Table 4.13 Wheat-, milk-, egg-free products which are commercially available (also free of azo dyes, benzoate and salicylate).

Biscuits

*†Puffed Rice Cakes with or without salt	La Source de Vie Living Foods
*†Country Basket Rice Cakes with or without salt	Country Basket Newform Foods
*†Brown Rice Snaps	Edward & Sons
*GF Brand Thin Wafer Bread	GF Dietary Supplies
GF Brand Gluten-Free Crackers	GF Dietary Supplies
*GF Brand Fruit Bran Biscuits	GF Dietary Supplies
*Rite-Diet Gluten-Free Sweet Biscuits (also Lincoln, Shortcake, Sultana and Savoury)	Welfare Foods Ltd
Rite-Diet Gluten-Free Custard Creams	Welfare Foods Ltd
†Rite-Diet Low-Protein Sweet Biscuits	Welfare Foods Ltd
†Rite-Diet Low-Protein Vanilla Cream-Filled Wafers	Welfare Foods Ltd
*Rite-Diet Gluten-Free Digestive Biscuits	Welfare Foods Ltd
*Rite-Diet Gluten-Free Chocolate Chip Cookies	Welfare Foods Ltd
*Aglutella Azeta Cream-Filled Low-Protein Gluten-Free Wafers	GF Dietary Supplies
†Rite-Diet Low-Protein Cream-Filled Biscuits (chocolate flavour)	Welfare Foods Ltd

Table 4.13 *continued*

If permitted, rye and oats
   *†Ryvita Original Rye Crispbread
   *†Ryvita Dark Rye Crispbread
   *†Ryking Light, blue packet
   *†Ryking Dark, brown packet
   *†Scanda Crisp
   *†Sliced rye bread   Springhill Packed
   *†Sliced pumpernickel   Springhill Packed
   *†Girdle oatcakes   Patersons
   *†Wholefood oatcakes without bran   Vesson Ltd
   *†Scottish oatcakes   Nairns

Pasta
   †Aproten: anellini, tagliatelle, rigatini   Ultrapharm (Carlo Erba) Ltd
   †Aglutella Pasta and Semolina   GF Dietary Supplies
   †Rite-Diet Low-Protein Pasta, macaroni, short-cut spaghetti,   Welfare Foods Ltd
     rings

Miscellaneous
   *†Rite-Diet Gluten-Free Baking Powder   Welfare Foods Ltd
   *†Baking Powder   Sainsbury

Bread mixes
   *†Ener-G Brown Rice Baking Mix   GF Dietary Supplies
   *Trufree Special Dietary Flours 1 to 7   Larkhall Laboratories/Cantassium Co.
   *Rite-Diet Soya Bran   Welfare Foods Ltd
   *†Ener-G Rice Bran   GF Dietary Supplies

Egg replacers for use in baking
   Ener-G egg replacer   GF Dietary Supplies
   Edifas A (methylethylcellulose)   ICI and Bow Products Ltd

*Free of non-nutritive additives.
†Soya-free.
Labels should be scrutinized for ingredients as changes occur frequently.

Table 4.14   Diet free of food additives.
   This diet is used for some forms of suspected food allergic disease or food intolerance. It is used for a trial period (about four weeks) to see if symptoms improve.

   This diet needs modification for infants.

   The diet should exclude the additives found in manufactured foods. These are food colours, preservatives, emulsifiers, stabilizers, flavours, and others such as the bleaching agent in ordinary white flour. Most of these additives have been designated 'E' numbers. Non-food sources of these additives should also be avoided, such as the colour and preservative in most medicines, some vitamin preparations, and coloured toothpaste. Some people are sensitive to salicylates, i.e. aspirin, Dispirin. Some additives are 'natural' or nature-identical and are not forbidden. A number of E numbers are mentioned below and in Tables 4.1(b) and 4.15.

   Some children have cravings for certain foods, e.g. sugar. However, it is important that the diet should be as varied as possible and no one food should be taken in especially large amounts, particularly:
      Milk—not more than 500 ml (one pint) per day.
      Bread—. . . slices per day appropriate for age.
      Sugar—use added sugar sparingly.

   This diet involves using home-cooked food wherever possible.

(a) Allowed and forbidden foods.

Foods allowed	Foods forbidden
Meat	
Buy fresh meat from the butcher rather than pre-packed meats from the supermarket. Beef, lamb, veal, turkey, chicken, rabbit, liver, kidney. Fresh frozen meats.	Meats containing colour and/or preservative, e.g. canned meat, sausages, beefburgers, salami, luncheon meat, corned beef, ham, bacon, meat dishes with colour and preservative, stuffing and forcemeat.
Fish	
Fresh fish and shellfish. Tinned and frozen fish provided no preservatives are added, e.g. canned tuna, sardines, salmon, etc.	Fish in batter, fish fingers, ready-cooked fish, smoked fish, e.g. smoked haddock, kippers.
Eggs	
All types allowed.	Egg substitutes
Milk	
Whole and skimmed milk, cream, evaporated and condensed milk, plain yoghurt. Home-made milk puddings (and some canned ones, e.g. rice pudding, but check labels). Home-made ice-cream (or suitable additive-free brand).	Flavoured milks and yoghurts. Custard powder, instant whips, ice-cream, Dream Topping, etc. Coffee-mate, Compliment, Five Pints, Fast Pints, etc.
Cheese	
Plain cheeses, e.g. Cheddar, Cheshire, Wensleydale, etc. If these are coloured it is usually with a natural colour (carotene, E160). Cottage cheese, curd cheese.	Processed cheese, highly coloured cheese. Flavoured cheeses and cheese dips.
Fats	
Butter and margarine containing natural colour (carotene, E160). Many margarines contain 'natural' flavour and emulsifiers, e.g. Sainsbury's blue and green label and sunflower margarines, Flora, Blue Band, Stork, Summer County, Echo, Tomor. Vegetable oils, lard, dripping.	Margarines containing the following antioxidants: BHA (E320), BHT (E321), gallates (E310, E311, E312). Krona margarines.
Flour	
Wholemeal or wholewheat flour. Unbleached white flour from wholefood shops. Other wholegrain flours, e.g. rye, etc.	Ordinary white flour.
Bread	
Home-made wholemeal bread, or wholemeal bread without preservative from some supermarkets, your local baker who bakes his own bread, or health food shops.	White bread, supermarket brown bread with preservatives which are called propionates (E280–E283).
Cereals	
Rice (brown and white), flaked and ground rice, semolina, sago, tapioca, cornflour, arrowroot, spaghetti (wholemeal and white), macaroni, pasta, barley, rye, oats.	Green lasagne
Breakfast cereals	
Weetabix, Shredded Wheat, Puffed Wheat, Sugar Puffs, porridge oats, muesli, Rice Krispies, Ricicles, Cornflakes, Frosties, plain Ready Brek, etc.	Breakfast cereal with preservative or colour.

Table 4.14 (a)   *continued*

Foods allowed	Foods forbidden
Cakes, biscuits, puddings Home-made with permitted ingredients, e.g. egg custard, rice pudding, flapjacks, wholemeal shortbread, jelly made with natural fruit juice and gelatine. Additive-free cookies from health food shops, but these are expensive and not essential. Some shop-bought crispbreads, e.g. Ryvita, Ryking, oat-cakes and others, but check labels.	Shop-bought cakes and biscuits, pies, puddings, mixes, jelly, all food colours and essences, custard and blancmange powders.
Fruit Fresh fruit should be washed well to remove sprays used in growing or to enhance keeping. Canned fruit usually contains fruit and sugar only and some fruit is now canned in natural juice, however check labels as some fruits, e.g. rhubarb, blackcurrants, may have added colour. Sunmaid raisins.	Dried fruit, e.g. raisins, sultanas, usually are coated with mineral oil. Dried apricots, etc. usually have a preservative (sulphur dioxide, E220).
Vegetables Wash fresh vegetables well. Frozen and canned vegetables may be suitable, but check for colouring in some canned vegetables, mint in frozen peas, etc. Potatoes—boiled, roast, jacket and chips. Dried pulses, e.g. lentils, chick-peas, kidney beans. Canned baked beans and spaghetti in tomato sauce without added colour, e.g. Heinz. Plain ready-salted potato crisps. Pickles, sauces and ketchup without additives, e.g. Heinz tomato ketchup.	Ready-prepared salads, canned vegetables with colour e.g. tinned peas, bottled beetroot, mint flavour in peas. Ready-peeled potatoes containing 'whitener' used in commercial catering. All flavoured crisps and those containing BHA (E320) and BHT (E321). Most commercial sauces and pickles contain food additives; these include salad cream, mayonnaise, soy sauce, chilli sauce.
Soup Home-made using permitted ingredients.	Packet and tinned soups
Gravy Use meat juices or home-made stock and thicken with cornflour to make gravy. You may find in health food shops additive-free stock cubes, e.g. Hügli, and a savoury soya product called Miso. Marmite and Bovril.	All stock cubes and gravy mixes contain additives, usually monosodium glutamate.
Drinks Milk, water, soda water, bottled water, e.g. Perrier, tea, coffee, cocoa, drinking chocolate, natural fruit juice without additives (these sometimes contain an antioxidant, E300, which is a nature-identical ascorbic acid or vitamin C). Fizzy drinks free of additives, e.g. Appletise, Kiri, 7-Up. Baby Ribena.	Fruit squash, Coke, Pepsi, Lucozade, most fizzy drinks including diet drinks and diet 7-Up. Wine, cider, alcoholic drinks. Milk-shake, milk-shake syrups and powders, e.g. Nesquick, Build-Up, etc.
Miscellaneous Sugar (white, icing and brown), golden syrup, honey.	Coloured sugar crystals and jelly.

Table 4.14 (a) *continued*

Foods allowed	Foods forbidden
Home-made jam and lemon curd. Shop-bought jam free of preservative and colour.	The cheaper commercial jams containing preservative and colour. Shop lemon curd
Salt, pepper, pure herbs and spices. Marmite, Bovril. Malt vinegar, spirit vinegar.	Ready-prepared mustard. Cider and wine vinegar.
Gelatine, rennet.	
Sweets Home-made sweets and toffee. Barley sugar Plain and milk chocolate. Home-made ice-lollies from natural fruit juices.	All sweets and candies, filled chocolates, Smarties, etc. Commercial ice-lollies, cough syrups and lozenges.
Nuts Both shelled and in shells. Salted peanuts, ground almonds, fresh coconut. Peanut butter.	Dry roasted peanuts Dessicated coconut
Baby foods Most are labelled 'no added colour and preservatives' but ingredients lists should still be scrutinized.	Baby foods with additives, especially the dried savoury varieties and juices.

(b)   Additive-free diet—sample menu.

Breakfast	Natural fruit juice Cornflakes, porridge, Weetabix, etc. A little sugar Milk Wholemeal bread or Ryvita, etc. Butter or suitable margarine Honey or home-made or additive-free marmalade or jam or peanut butter Egg—optional Tea, coffee
Main meals	Fresh meat, fish or egg Home-made casseroles or grilled, roast, fried meat or fish Fresh vegetables, cooked or raw Potatoes (roast, chipped, baked, mashed, etc.) Rice or pasta Fruit, pure plain yoghurt, egg custard, home-made puddings, e.g. fruit crumble
Snacks: packed lunch	Milk or natural fruit juice or Appletise Fruit, plain potato crisps, nuts, Sunmaid raisins Home-made cake or biscuits Wholemeal bread sandwiches with meat, peanut butter, Marmite, egg, tinned tuna, etc.
Vitamins	Use only Children's Clinic Vitamin A. D. C Drops, pure cod-liver oil, Abidec 0·6 ml daily or ascorbic acid tablets.

114   *Chapter 4*

Table 4.14 (a)   *continued*

Medicines	Use only white tablets or those specifically prescribed.
	It may be wise to avoid salicylates, e.g. aspirin, Disprin.
	Also avoid syrup medicines, cough mixtures, all medicines containing colour and preservatives. The doctor should be consulted before changing any prescribed medicines but remind him or her that the child is avoiding colours and preservatives each time a prescription is required.
Toothpaste	Use white toothpaste.

Table 4.15   Additives in foods.

These are found in many manufactured foods, e.g. soft drinks and squashes, sweets and jellies, packet mixes, cakes, preserves, etc. They are also present in most medicine preparations.

Colours

Many of the colours used are coal tar and azo dyes. These are the food additives most frequently implicated in intolerances. The most commonly used one is tartrazine (E102). Not all of them have an E prefix. They are:

E102, E104, E107, E110, E122, E123, E124, E127, E128, E131, E132, 133, E142, E151, 154, 155, E180.

Other colours are from natural sources or are synthetic but 'nature-identical'. These are least often implicated in intolerances. They are:

E100, curcumin (turmeric root).
E101, riboflavin (vitamin B_2, usually produced synthetically).
E150, caramel.
E153, carbon black (banned in the U.S.A.)
E160, E161, naturally occurring yellow colours, e.g. carotene, annatto.
E162, beetroot red.
E163, anthocyanins (plant pigments).
E170, calcium carbonate.
E171–5, metals.

Preservatives

E280–3 propionates are preservatives in both white and brown supermarket bread. They are also found in pre-packed cakes and pastry.

E210–E219 inclusive are benzoic acid and benzoates. These are preservatives in soft drinks and other manufactured foods and medicines. Like the azo dyes they seem to be some of the commonest implicated in intolerances. Benzoates also occur naturally.

E249–E252 inclusive are nitrates and nitrites. These are preservatives in cooked meats such as corned beef, ham, bacon, beefburgers, hamburgers, sausages, paté. Nitrates also occur in some water supplies.

E220, sulphur dioxide, and E221–E227 inclusive, sulphites, are very commonly used preservatives.

E230–E232 inclusive, biphenyl and related compounds. Used for treatment of skins of citrus fruit to inhibit mould growth.

E260, acetic acid, is present in many pickles and chutneys. There are no known toxicological problems. E261–E263 are related compounds (acetates). Occurs naturally in vinegar.

E200–E203 inclusive are sorbic acid and sorbates. These are found in a wide variety of manufactured foods, e.g. yoghurt, processed cheese, frozen pizza, pre-packed cake.

E239, hexamine, is a fungicide not commonly used.

234, nisin, is a preservative in cheese, clotted cream, some canned foods.

E270, lactic acid, is a naturally occurring substance with no known problems. Present in confectionery, infant milks, salad dressing.

E290, carbon dioxide, is a natural gas in fizzy drinks.

Antioxidants

These additives prevent food from spoiling when in contact with the oxygen in the air. An example of this is rancidity in oils and fats. Antioxidants have numbers E300–320. Many of them are natural or nature-identical, e.g. E300 (vitamin C). Others may be implicated in intolerances, e.g. E320 (BHA) and E321 (BHT) and possibly E310–E312 (gallates).

Emulsifiers and stabilizers

E322–E494 (not totally inclusive) These are many and varied and are present in a large number of manufactured foods. Many of them are safe and natural.

Flavour enhancer

621, monosodium glutamate.
622, 623, 627, 631, 635, other flavour enhancers.
This is present in packet snacks, e.g. crisps, pork pies and sausages, packet soup, stock cubes and gravy mixes.

Bleaching agents

Ordinary white flour has been treated with bleaching agents, e.g. chlorine dioxide, potassium bromate. They do not have E numbers.

REFERENCES

AGGETT P.J. & HARRIES J.T. (1979) Current status of zinc in health and disease states. *Arch. Dis. Childh.* **54**, 909–17.

AMENT M.E. & RUBIN C.E. (1972) Soy protein—another cause of the flat intestinal lesion. *Gastroenterology* **62**, 227.

AHN C. & MACLEAN W.C. (1980) Growth of the exclusively breast-fed infant. *Amer. J. clin. Nutr.* **33**, 183–92.

ATHERTON D.J. (1982) Atopic eczema. *Clinics in Immunology and Allergy* 2(1) 77–100.

ATHERTON D.J. (1985) Skin disorders and food allergy. *J. roy. Soc. Med.* Suppl. No. 5, Vol. **78**, 7–10.

ATHERTON D.J., SEWELL M., SOOTHILL J.F., WELLS R.S. & CHILVERS C.E.D. (1978) A double-blind controlled crossover trial of an antigen-avoidance diet in atopic eczema. *Lancet* 1, 401.

AUGUST P.J. (1980) Urticaria. In *Proceedings of The First Food Allergy Workshop* chaired by Professor R.R.A. Coombs, pp. 76–81. Medical Education Services Ltd.

AUGUSTINE G.J. & LEVITAN H. (1980) Neurotransmitter release from a vertebrate neuromuscular synapse affected by a food dye. *Science* **207**, 1489–90.

BAHNA S.L. & HEINER D.C. (1980) *Allergies to milk.* New York: Grune & Stratton.

BARNETSON R. ST C. & MERRETT T.G. (1980) Atopic eczema. In *Proceedings of the First Food Allergy Workshop* chaired by Professor R.R.A. Coombs, pp. 69–75. Medical Education Services Ltd.

BIDDER R.T., GRAY O.P. & NEWCOMBE R. (1978) Feingold diet. *Arch. Dis. Childh.* **53**, 574–9.

BOOTH I.W. & HARRIES J.T. (1984) Inflammatory bowel disease in childhood. *Gut* **25**, 188–202.

BUISSERET P.D. (1982) Allergy. *Sci. Amer.* **247**, 82–91.

CANT A.J. (1984) Diet and the prevention of childhood allergic disease. *Hum. Nutr.; Appl. Nutr.* **38A** (6), 455–68.

CANT A.J. (1985) Food allergy in childhood. *Hum. Nutr.; Appl. Nutr.* **39A**, 277–93.

CANT A.J. & BAILES J.A. (1984) How should we feed the potentially allergic infant? *Hum. Nutr.: Appl. Nutr.* **38A** (6), 455–68.

CARTER C.M., EGGER J. & SOOTHILL J. (1985) A dietary management of severe childhood migraine. *Hum. Nutr.: Appl. Nutr.* **39A**, 294–303.

CONNERS C.K., GOYETTE C.H., SOUTHWICK D.A., LEES J.M. & ANDRUTONIS P.A. (1976) Food additives and hyperkineses: a controlled double-blind experiment. *Pediatrics* **58**, 154–66.

CONSENSUS DEVELOPMENT CONFERENCE (1982) Refined diets and childhood hyperactivity. Held at The Office for Medical Applications of Research, National Institute of Health, Bethesda, Maryland. *J. Amer. med. Ass.* **248**(3), 290–2.

COOMBS R.R.A. Chairman (1980) *Proceedings of The First Food Allergy Workshop.* Medical Education Services Ltd.

COOMBS R.R.A. Chairman (1983) *Proceedings of the Second Food Allergy Workshop.* Medical Education Services Ltd.

COOMBS R.R.A. & GELL P.G.H. (1975) Classification of allergic reactions responsible for clinical hypersensitivity and disease. In *Clinical Aspects of Immunology*, 3rd Edition (eds. Gell P.G.H. & Coombs R.R.A.), p. 761. Oxford: Blackwell Scientific Publications.

DANNAEUS A. & INGANAS M. (1981) A follow up study of children with food allergy. Clinical care in relation to serum IgE and IgG antibody levels to milk, egg and fish. *Clinical Allergy* **11**, 533–9.

DANSSET J. & SVEJGAARD (1977) *HLA and disease.* Copenhagen: Munksgaard.

DAVID T.J. (1984) Anaphylactic shock during elimination diets for severe atopic eczema. *Arch. Dis. Childh.* **59**, 983–6.

DAVID T.J. (1985) The overworked or fraudulent diagnosis of food allergy and food intolerance in children. *J. roy. Soc. Med.* Suppl. 5, Vol. **78**, 21–31.

DE PEYER E. & WALKER-SMITH J.A. (1977) Cow's milk intolerance presenting as necrotizing enterocolitis. *Helv. paediat. Acta* **32**, 509.

DHSS (1980) *Artificial Feeds for the young Infant* Report No. 18. London: HMSO.

EDITORIAL (1979) Feingold regime for hyperkinesis. *Lancet*, 617–18.

EDITORIAL (1980) Pathogenesis and mechanisms. In *Proceedings of the First Food Allergy Workshop*, chaired by Professor R.R.A. Coombs, pp. 21–2. Medical Education Services Ltd.

EDITORIAL (1982) Food additives and hyperactivity. *Lancet*, 662–3.

EDITORIAL (1983a) Meadow's and Munchausen syndrome. *Lancet* 1, 456.

EDITORIAL (1983b) Milk substitutes. *Drug Therapeutic Bulletin.*

EGGER J., CARTER C.M., WILSON J., TURNER M.W. & SOOTHILL J.F. (1983) Is migraine food allergy? A double-blind controlled trial of oligoantigenic diet treatment. *Lancet* **2**, 865–9.

EGGER J., CARTER C.M., GRAHAM P.J., GUMLEY D & SOOTHILL J.F. (1985) Controlled trial of olioantigenic treatment in the hyperkinetic syndrome. *Lancet*, 540–5.

EVANS R.W., FERGUSSON D.M., ALLARDYCE R.A. & TAYLOR B. (1981) Maternal diet and infantile colic in breast fed infants. *Lancet* 1, 1340–2.

FEINGOLD B.F. (1974) *Why Your Child is Hyperactive.* New York: Randum House.

FEINGOLD B.F. & FEINGOLD H.S. (1979) *The Feingold Cookbook for Hyperactive Children.* New York: Randum House.

FEINGOLD B., GERMAN D.P., BRAHAM R.M. & SIMMERS E. (1973) *Adverse Reactions to Food Additives.* Read before the annual convention of the American Medical Association, New York.

FORD R.P.K. & TAYLOR B. (1982) Natural history of egg hypersensitivity. *Arch. Dis. Childh.* **57**, 649–52.

FRANCIS D.E.M. (1980) Dietary management. In *Proceedings of the First Food Allergy Workshop*, chaired by Professor R.R.A. Coombs, pp. 85–94. Medical Education Services Ltd.

FRANCIS D.E.M. (1986) *Nutrition for Children.* Oxford: Blackwell Scientific Publications.

FREEDMAN B.J. (1977) Asthma induced by sulphur dioxide, benzoate and tartrazine contained in orange drinks. *Clinical Allergy* 7, 407–15.

FRICK O.L., GERMAN D.F. & MILLS J. (1979) Development of allergy in children 1. Associated with virus infections. *Journal of Allergy Clinical and Immunology* 63, 228.

FRIER S., KLETTER B., GERY I., LEBENTHAL E. & GEIFMAN M. (1969) Intolerance of milk protein. *J. Pediat.* 75, 623.

GLASER J. & JOHNSTONE D.F. (1953) Prophylaxis of allergic disease in the newborn. *J. Amer. med. Ass.* 153, 620.

GOLDMAN A.S., ANDERSON D.W. JR, SELLERS W.A., SAPERSTEIN S., KNIKER W.T. & HALPERN S.R. (1963) Milk allergy 1. Oral challenge with milk and isolated milk proteins in allergic children. *Pediatrics* 32, 425.

GOLDSBOROUGH J. & FRANCIS D.E.M. (1983) Dietary management. In *Proceedings of the Second Food Allergy Workshop*, chaired by Professor R.R.A. Coombs, pp. 89–94. Medical Education Services Ltd.

GOYETTE C.H., CONNERS C.K., PETTI T.A. & CURTIS L.E. (1978) Effects of artificial colours on hyperkinetic children. A double-blind challenge study. *Psychopharmacol. Bull.* 14, 39–40.

HAGY G.W. & SETTIPANE G.A. (1969) Bronchial asthma, allergic rhinitis and allergy skin tests amongst college students. *J. Allergy* 44, 323–32.

HALPERN S.R. (1965) Chronic hives in children. An analysis of 75 cases. *Amer. Allergy* 23, 589.

HANSSEN M. & MARSDEN J. (1984) *E for Additives*. Wellingborough: Thorson Publishers Ltd.

HARLEY J.P., RAY R.S., TOMASI L., EICHMAN P.L., MATHEWS C.G., CHUN R., CLEELAND C.S. & TRAISMAN E. (1978a) Hyperkinesis and food additives testing the Feingold hypothesis. *Pediatrics* 61, 818–28.

HARLEY J.P., MATTHEWS C.G. & EICHMAN P. (1978b) Synthetic food colours and hyperactivity in children. A double-blind challenge experiment. *Pediatrics* 62, 975.

HARRISON M., KILBY A., WALKER-SMITH J.A., FRANCE N.F. & WOOD C.B.S. (1976) Cow's milk protein intolerance—a possible association with gastroenteritis, lactose intolerance and IgA deficiency. *Brit. med. J.* 1, 150.

HATHAWAY M.J. & WARNER J.O. (1983) Compliance problems in the dietary management of eczema. *Arch. Dis. Childh.* 58, 463–4.

HILL D.J. & LYNCH B.C. (1982) Elemental diet in the management of severe eczema in childhood. *Clinical Allergy* 12, 313–5.

ILLINGWORTH R.J. (1983) *The Normal Child—Some Problems of the Early Years*, 8th Edition. Edinburgh: Churchill Livingstone.

JAKOBSSON I. & LINDBERG T. (1978) Cow's milk as a cause of infantile colic in breast fed infants. *Lancet* 2, 437–9.

JAMES J. & WARIN R.P. (1971) An assessment of the role of *Candida albicans* and food yeasts in chronic urticaria. *Brit. J. Dermatol.* 84, 327.

JOHNSON D.D., DORR K.E., SWENSON W.M. & SERVICE J. (1980) Reactive hypoglycaemia. *J. Amer. med. Ass.* 243, 1151–5.

JUHLIN L. (1980) Incidence of intolerance to food additives. *Int. J. Dermatol.* 19, 548–51.

JUHLIN L. (1981) Recurrent urticaria: clinical investigation of 330 patients. *Brit. J. Dermatol.* 104, 369–81.

KRAMER M.S. & MOROZ B. (1981) Do breast-feeding and delayed introduction of solid foods protect against subsequent atopic eczema. *J. Pediat.* 98, 546–50.

LESSOF M.H. (1984) Food intolerance and food aversion. A joint report of the Royal College of Physicians and the British Nutrition Foundation chaired by Professor M.H. Lessof *J. roy. Coll. Phys. Lon.* Vol. 18, No. 2.

LEVY F., DUMBRELL S., HOBBES G., RYAN M., WILTON N. & WOODHILL J.M. (1981) Hyperkinesis and diet. A double-blind crossover trial with a tartrazine challenge. *Med. J. Aust.* 1, 61–4.

LIPPARD V.W., SCHLOSS O.M. & JOHNSON P.A. (1936) Immune reactions induced in infants by intestinal absorption of incompletely digested cow's milk proteins. *Amer. J. Dis. Child.* 51, 562.

LOCKEY S.D. (1971) Reactions to hidden agents in foods, beverages and drugs. *Ann. Allergy* 29, 461.

MCCARTY E.P. & FRICK O.L. (1983) Food sensitivity: keys to diagnosis. *J. Pediat.* 102, 5, 645–52.

MCLAUGHLIN P., ANDERSON K.J., WIDDOWSON E.M. & COOMBS R.R.A. (1981) Effect of heat on the anaphylactic-sensitising capacity of cow's milk, goat's milk and various infant formulae fed to guinea pigs. *Arch. Dis. Childh.* 56, 165–71.

MAFF (1982) *Look at the Label* London: HMSO.

MANUEL P.D. & WALKER-SMITH J.A. (1981) A comparison of three infant feeding formulae for the prevention of delayed recovery after infantile gastroenteritis. *Acta paediat. belg.* 34, 13–20.

MATTHEW D.J., TAYLOR B., NORMAN A.P., TURNER M.W. & SOOTHILL J.F. (1977) Prevention of eczema. *Lancet* 321–4.

MAY C.D. (1979) Food hypersensitivity. In *Comprehensive Immunology* (series eds. Good R.A. & Day S.B.), Vol 6 *Cellular, Molecular and Clinical Aspects of Allergic Disorders* (eds. Gupta S, & Good R.A.), p. 321. New York: Plenum Press.

MEADOW R. (1985) Management of Munchausen syndrome by proxy. Personal practice. *Arch. Dis. Childh.* 60, 385–393.

MICHAELSSON G. & JUHLIN L. (1973) Urticaria induced by preservative and dye additives in food and drugs. *Brit. J. Dermatol.* 88, 525.

MICHEL F.B., BOUSQUET J., GREILLIER P., ROBINET-LEVY M. & COULOMB Y. (1980) Comparison of cord blood immunoglobin E concentrations and maternal allergy for the prediction of atopic diseases in infancy. *J. Allergy clin. Immunol.* 65, 422–30.

MINFORD A.M.B., MACDONALD A. & LITTLEWOOD J.M. (1982) Food intolerance and food allergy in children: a review of 68 cases. *Arch. Dis. Childh.* 57, 742–7.

MITCHELL E.B., CROW J., CHAPMAN M.D., JOUHAL S.S., POPE F.M. & PLATTS-MILLS T.A.E. (1982) Basophils in allergen induced patch test sites in atopic dermatitis. *Lancet* 1, 127–30.

OGLE K.A. & BULLOCK J.D. (1977) Children with allergic

rhinitis and/or bronchial asthma treated with elimination diet. *Ann. Allergy* **39**, 8.

PRINZ R.J., ROBERTS W.A. & HANTMAN E. (1980) Dietary correlates of hyperactive behaviour in children. *J. cons. clin. Psychol.* **48**, No. 6, 760–9.

ROS A.M., JUHLIN L. & MICHAELSSON G. (1976) A follow up study of patients with recurrent urticaria and hypersensitivity to aspirin, benzoates and azo dyes. *Brit. J. Dermatol.* **95**, 19.

SAARINEN U., KAJOSAARI M., BACKMAN A. & SIIMES M. (1979) Prolonged breast-feeding as prophylaxis for atopic disease. *Lancet* **2**, 163.

SCHAUSS A.G. (1983) Nutrition and behaviour. *J. appl. Nutr.* **35**, 1, 30.

SOOTHILL J.F. (1983) The atopic child. In *Paediatric Immunology* (eds. Soothill J.F. Hayward A.R. & Wood C.B.S)., pp. 248–71. Oxford: Blackwell Scientific Publications.

SOOTHILL J.F., STOKES C.R., TURNER M.W., NORMAN A.P. & TAYLOR B. (1976) Predisposing factors and the development of reaginic allergy in infancy. *Clin. Allergy* **6**, 305.

STARE F.J., WHELAN E.M. & SHERIDAN M. (1980) Diet and hyperactivity: is there a relationship? *Pediatrics* **66**(4), 521–5.

SWAIN A.R., DUTTON S.P. & TRUSWELL A.S. (1985) Salicylates in food. *J. Amer. diet. Ass.* **85**, 950–9.

SWANSON J.M. & KINSBOURNE M. (1980) Food dyes impair performance of hyperactive children on a laboratory learning test. *Science* **207**, 1485–7.

SWARBRICK E.T., STOKES C.R. & SOOTHILL J.F. (1979) Absorption of antigens after oral immunization and the simultaneous induction of specific systemic tolerance. *Gut* **20**, 121.

SYME J. (1979) Investigation and treatment of multiple intestinal food allergy in childhood. In *The Mast Cell: Its Role in Health and Disease* (eds. Pepys J. & Edwards A.M.), p. 438. London: Pitman Medical.

TAITZ L.S. (1982) Soy feeding in infancy. *Arch. Dis. Childh.* **57**, 814–15.

TAYLOR B., NORMAN A.P., ORGEL H.A., STOKES C.R., TURNER M.W. & SOOTHILL J.F. (1973) Transient IgA deficiency and pathogenesis of infantile atopy. *Lancet* **2**, 111.

TRIPP J.H., FRANCIS D.E.M., KNIGHT J.A. & HARRIES J.T. (1979) Infant feeding practice: a cause for concern. *Brit. med. J.* **2**, 707–9.

VISAKORPI J.K. & IMMONEN P. (1967) Intolerance to cow's milk and wheat gluten in the primary malabsorption syndrome in infancy. *Acta paediat. scand.* **56**, 49.

VITORIA J.C., CAMERERO C., SOJO A., RUIZ A. & RODRIGUEZ-SORIANO J. (1982) Enteropathy related to fish, rice, and chicken. *Arch. Dis. Childh.* **57**, 44–8.

WALKER-SMITH J.A. (1979) *Diseases of the Small Intestine in Childhood*, 2nd Edition. London: 'Pitman Medical.

WALKER-SMITH J.A. (1985) Food allergies and bowel disease. *J. roy. Soc. Med.*, **78**, Suppl. No. 5, 3–6.

WARNER J.O. & HATHAWAY M.A. (1984) Allergic form of Meadow's syndrome (Munchausen by proxy). *Arch. Dis. Childh.* **59**, 151–6.

WILLIAMS J.I., CRAN D.I., TAUSIG F.T. & WEBSTER E. (1978) Relative effects of drugs and diet and hyperactive behaviours. An experimental study. *Pediatrics* **61**, 811–17.

WILSON A.F., NOVEY H.S., BERKE R.A. & SURPRENANT E.L. (1973) Deposition of inhaled pollen and pollen extract in human airways. *New Engl. J. Med.* **288**, 1056–8.

WILSON N. & SILVERMAN M. (1985) Diagnosis of food sensitivity in childhood asthma. *J. roy. Soc. Med.* **78**, Suppl. No. 5, 11–16.

WILSON N., VICKERS H., TAYLOR G. & SILVERMAN M. (1982) Objective test for food sensitivity in asthmatic children: increased bronchial activity after cola drinks. *Brit. med. J.* **284**, 1226–8.

WRAITH D. (1980) Respiratory diseases. In *Proceedings of the First Food Allergy Workshop*, chaired by Professor R.R.R. Coombs, pp. 64–8. Medical Education Services Ltd.

WRIGHT S. & BURTON J.L. (1982) Oral evening-primrose-seed-oil improves atopic eczema. *Lancet* **2**, 1120–2.

WURTMAN R. (1983) Behavioural effect of nutrients. *Lancet*, 1145–7.

ZOPPI G., GASPARINI R., MANTOVANELLI F., GOBIO-CASALI L., ASTOLFI R. & CROVARI R. (1983) Diet and antibody response to vaccination in healthy infants. *Lancet* **2**, 11–14.

Recipes

*Recipes for use in various allergy diets. The ingredients must be scrutinized for suitability before use in any particular diet.

Wheat substitutes
There are several types of flour which can be used for baking when wheat is not allowed. Some of the possibilities are soya flour, cornflour, rice flour, sago flour, potato flour, rye flour, maize flour and buckwheat flour. Many of the following recipes use rice flour, which is convenient and fairly readily available. Most health food shops sell wholemeal rice flour, and Indian food shops and some supermarkets sell a white rice flour which is good for cooking. The most common brand is 'Encona'. Gluten-free flours are not necessarily wheat-free (*see* Table 4.13).

Egg substitutes
Some of the following recipes use Ener-G egg replacer which contains methylcellulose. It can be obtained from health food shops or by mail order from GF Dietary Supplies.

Milk substitutes
A variety are available; most can be used in cooking but the hydrolysates may give the recipe an unusual taste.

Baking powder   (wheat-free, milk-, egg-, colour-, preservative-free)

  60 g (2 oz) tartaric acid
  60 g (2 oz) cream of tartar
100 g ($3\frac{1}{2}$ oz) bicarbonate of soda
  90 g (3 oz) ground rice or potato flour

Mix ingredients thoroughly and store in an airtight jar.

Cooking with potato flour
Where grain flours are very restricted, potato flour, e.g. Encona, Cantassium, can be useful. It is not very easy to work with, but biscuits and shortbread can be made adequately.

*The majority of these recipes have been devised by C. Carter, Research Dietitian.

Potato shortbread   (milk-, egg- wheat-, cereal-, colour-, preservative-free)

90 g (3 oz) potato flour
60 g (2 oz) milk-free margarine
30 g (1 g) castor sugar

Make as for ordinary shortbread, i.e. work the ingredients together and press into a 6-inch mould or flan ring. Bake at 180°C for about 30 minutes. Sprinkle with castor sugar and cut through into segments while still hot. Leave to cool before removing from baking sheet. This shortbread will not go golden brown like ordinary shortbread, so do not overcook it.

Melting moments   (milk-, egg-, wheat-, cereal-, colour-, preservative-free)

120 g (4 oz) milk-free margarine
  30 g (1 oz) icing sugar
120 g (4 oz) potato flour

Cream together the ingredients. Force through a large star nozzle into fancy shapes on a greased baking sheet or pipe into paper cases. Bake at 190°C for about 15 to 20 minutes. Do not overcook as they do not go brown. Remove when cool.

Fruit cake   (milk- and egg-free, wheat-free if rice flour is used, cereal-free if potato flour is used)

120 g (4 oz) permitted flour
100 g ($3\frac{1}{2}$ oz) milk-free margarine
2 tsp mixed spice
  75 g ($2\frac{1}{2}$ oz) brown sugar
  75 g ($2\frac{1}{2}$ oz) sultanas, raisins, peel
  15 g ($\frac{1}{2}$ oz) chopped nuts
2 tsp Ener-G egg replacer powder
4 tbsp water
2 tsp baking powder (wheat-free)

Cream margarine and sugar. Mix Ener-G egg replacer with the water; add to margarine and sugar. Add other ingredients. Mix well.

Cook for approximately ½ hour at 200°C. Ice with 'butter icing', using milk-free margarine and icing sugar, or water icing.

Rice Krispies or Cornflake cakes
(milk-, egg-, wheat-, colour-, preservative-free)

45 g (1½ oz) cocoa
120 g (4 oz) golden syrup
60 g (2 oz) milk-free margarine
60 g (2 oz) sugar
90 g (3 oz) Rice Krispies or Cornflakes

Melt syrup, sugar, margarine and cocoa in a saucepan. Fold in the cereal. Spoon into paper cases and leave to set.

Banana cake   (milk-, egg-, wheat-, colour-, preservative-free)

120 g (4 oz) rice flour or permitted flour
1 rounded tsp baking powder
60 g (2 oz) milk-free margarine
120 g (4 oz) castor sugar
60 ml (2 tbsp) water
1 large banana, mashed
2 tsp egg replacer and 4 tbsp water

Mix flour and baking powder. Put fat, sugar and water in a saucepan and heat to dissolve sugar and melt margarine. Put this mixture in a mixing bowl and beat in the egg replacer, banana, and then the flour. Pour into two 6-inch diameter cake tins lined with greased foil or greaseproof paper. Alternatively, pour the mixture into individual paper baking cases, half filling each with mixture. Bake the cake at 180°C for at least 30 minutes until well browned. Bake small cakes at 190°C for about 20 minutes.

Rice shortbread   (milk-, egg-, wheat-, colour-, preservative-free)

90 g (3 oz) rice flour
60 g (2 oz) milk-free margarine
30 g (1 oz) castor sugar

Mix flour and sugar, and work in the margarine by hand. Shape and roll into a round, 6 inches in diameter, or press into a 6-inch diameter flan ring. Bake on a greased baking sheet at 180°C until lightly browned. Cut into segments while still hot and sprinkle with castor sugar.

Fruit crumble   (milk-, egg-, wheat-, colour-, preservative-free)

180 g (6 oz) sugar
180 g (6 oz) rice flour
90 g (3 oz) milk-free margarine
500 to 750 g (1 to 1½ lb) permitted fruit, e.g. apple, rhubarb

Preheat oven to 180°C. Rub margarine into the flour until the mixture resembles breadcrumbs. Stir in half the sugar. Put the remaining sugar and the fruit into a pie dish. Cover with the crumble mixture and bake for about 30 minutes.

Scotch pancakes   (milk-, egg-, wheat-, colour-, preservative-free)

120 g (4 oz) rice flour or other permitted flour
¼ tsp bicarbonate of soda
½ tsp cream of tartar
30 g (1 tbsp) sugar
1 tsp egg replacer in 2 tbsp water
180 ml (6 fl oz) water or milk substitute to mix

Have ready a hot griddle, or non-stick or heavy frying pan, which has been lightly oiled. Mix dry ingredients and add egg replacer, and stir in enough milk or water to give a thick batter which is the consistency of thick cream. Pour the mixture in spoonfuls on the hot pan. When bubbles begin to rise to the surface of the pancakes, turn them over and cook until golden brown on both sides. It takes 4 to 6 minutes.

Flapjacks (milk-, egg-, wheat-, colour-, preservative-free)

120 g (4 oz) rolled oats
90 g (3 oz) milk-free margarine
60 g (2 oz) golden syrup
60 g (2 oz) moist brown sugar
$\frac{1}{4}$ tsp ground ginger if allowed

Melt margarine. Add sugar and syrup. Work in oats and ginger. Press into a greased 7-inch diameter sponge tin. Bake at 160°C for about 30 minutes. Cut into wedges while still hot and then allow to cool in tin.

Crunchies (milk-, egg-, wheat-, colour-, preservative-free

120 g (4 oz) milk-free margarine
90 g (3 oz) castor sugar
1 tsp golden syrup
3 tsp boiling water
120 g (4 oz) rice flour or permitted flour
1 tsp baking powder
60 g (2 oz) rolled oats

Cream together the fat and sugar. Beat in the syrup and water. Stir in flour, raising agent and oats. Divide into approximately 28 balls and place apart on a greased baking sheet. Flatten slightly and bake for about 15 minutes at 180°C until golden brown.

Bread (milk-, egg-, wheat-, colour-, preservative-free)

1 tsp salt
360 g (12 oz) rice flour
or, preferably,
360 g (12 oz) mixed flours,
e.g.
{ 180 g (6 oz) cornflour + 60 g (2 oz) soya
   flour + 120 g (4 oz) rice flour
30 g (1 oz) milk-free margarine
{ 120 ml (4 fl oz) boiling water plus 240 ml
   (8 fluid oz) milk substitute (cold)
or
360 ml (12 fl oz) warm water
1 tsp sugar

30 g (1 oz) fresh yeast or 7 g ($\frac{1}{4}$ oz) (1 tsp) dried yeast

Mix yeast, sugar, milk substitute and water together, and allow to just start frothing. Add salt to flour and rub in fat. Make a well in the centre and pour in the yeast mixture. Mix well to a smooth batter. Pour batter into a greased loaf tin and allow to stand in a warm place for 20 minutes or until loaf has doubled in size. Keep covered with a damp cloth. Bake for 20 minutes in an oven at 200°C. Remove loaf from tin and continue baking on the oven shelf for a further 15 minutes. Cool on a wire tray.

Basic shortcrust pastry (milk-, egg-, wheat-, colour-, preservative-free)

240 g (8 oz) rice flour
120 g (4 oz) milk-free margarine or solid
   vegetable fat
Pinch salt
50 to 60 ml (about 2 tbsp) water

Make like ordinary pastry. It is much more brittle than ordinary pastry.

Apple or carrrot cake (milk-, egg-, wheat-, colour-, preservative-free)

120 g (4 oz) rice flour
1 rounded tsp baking powder
1 level tsp bicarbonate of soda
Pinch salt
60 g (2 oz) castor sugar (or soft brown
   sugar)
90 g (3 oz) golden syrup
90 ml (3 fl oz) sunflower oil
2 tsp Ener-G egg replacer and 2 tbsp water
120 g (4 oz) grated carrot or grated apple.

Sieve flour, raising agents and salt. Mix in the sugar and carrot or apple. Beat together the oil, egg replacer and syrup, and add to the flour mixture. Pour into an 8-inch diameter sponge tin lined, preferably, with greased foil. Bake at 180°C for 45 minutes.

Syrup cookies (milk-, egg-, wheat-, colour-, preservative-free)

120 g (4 oz) rice flour
Pinch salt
½ tsp bicarbonate of soda
½ tsp baking powder
60 g (2 oz) castor sugar
60 g (2 oz) golden syrup
70 g (2½ oz) milk-free margarine

Sift together the flour, salt, raising agent, and add sugar. Weigh the syrup and margarine into a pan and heat to melt and dissolve. Stir into dry ingredients and form into small balls. Place well apart on greased foil on a baking sheet. Flatten slightly and bake at 180°C for about 10 minutes until golden. The cookies will spread out during cooking, and will still be soft when cooked. They harden on cooling.

*Sponge (wheat- and milk-free)

100 g (4 oz) milk-free margarine
100 g (4 oz) castor sugar
2 eggs
100 g (4 oz) cornflour or permitted flour(s)
1 to 2 tsp wheat-free baking powder
1 to 2 drops vanilla essence

Cream margarine and sugar, beat in eggs. Fold in sifted flour and baking powder. Add essence and a little water to mix to a soft dropping consistency. Place in a greased tin and bake 20 to 25 minutes in a moderate oven, 180°C.
Or steam in a greased pudding basin for 1½ hours with a little jam, fruit or syrup in the bottom of the basin.
Or place 1 to 2 teaspoons into paper cup cases and bake 10 to 12 minutes in hot oven, 190°C. Decorate with water glacé icing.

Scones (milk-, egg-, wheat-, colour-, and preservative-free)

150 g (5 oz) cornflour or permitted flour (s)
1 tsp wheat-free baking powder

* NB Contains egg.

45 g (1½ oz) milk-free margarine
15 g (½ oz) sugar or 1 pinch salt for savoury scones
Water (or milk) to mix

Rub margarine into flour. Add sugar or salt. Mix to a soft dough with water. Shape into a ½-inch thick round with a little extra cornflour. Place onto a greased baking sheet. Cut into small scones. Bake for 8 to 10 minutes at 200°C. Serve cut in half and 'buttered' with jam.

Apple cake (milk-, egg-, wheat-, colour-, preservative-free)

90 g (3 oz) sugar
60 g (2 oz) milk-free margarine
180 g (6 oz) rice flour
90 ml (½ cup) cold tea
500 g (2 large) cooking apples
1½ tsp baking powder (wheat-free)
½ tsp bicarbonate of soda

Put sugar, tea and margarine into pan and heat until boiling. Cool. Stir in sifted dry ingredients, and add the peeled chopped apples (chopped not grated). Put into 6½-inch cake tin. Cook in 140°C oven for 1 to 1½ hours.

Meringues (egg-free; also milk-, wheat-, cereal-, colour-, and preservative-free)

5 g Edifas A powder, soaked in 45 ml hot water
135 ml (4½ oz) cold water
180 g (6 oz) castor sugar
Pinch of salt

Allow Edifas A to soak in hot water, whisking occasionally. When cool, add cold water. Mix together salt and Edifas A solution. Whisk to a stiff foam with an electric mixer on maximum for approximately 15 to 20 minutes. Add half the sugar and whisk to a peak. Fold in rest of sugar. Pipe onto greaseproof paper, dust with a little castor sugar. Dry in a slow oven 140°C for 1½ hours. Store in an airtight tin.

Banana bread   (wheat-free, milk-, egg-,
  colour-, preservative-free)

240 g (8 oz) rice flour
3 rounded tsp wheat-free baking powder
240 g (8 oz) mashed bananas
1 tsp egg replacer and 2 tbsp water
60 g (2 oz) milk-free margarine
60 g (2 oz) sugar
Milk substitute or water

Mix flour and baking powder and rub in the
margarine. Add sugar, egg replacer and
banana and enough 'milk' or water to give a
very sticky consistency. Bake in a loaf tin
lined with greased paper or foil for 45
minutes at 180°C.

Date and rice bubble balls   (milk-, egg-,
  and wheat-free)

60 g (2 oz) milk-free margarine
240 g (8 oz) dates
120 g (4 oz) sugar
4 cups of Rice Krispies
½ tsp vanilla essence (optional)
60 g (2 oz) coconut (optional)

Place dates, margarine and sugar in a
saucepan and gently cook until the dates are
soft. Add vanilla. Pour the mixture into the
Rice Krispies (and coconut) in a large bowl.
Cool slightly and stir well to mix. Gently
shape into balls (size of a golf ball) with
your hands while still warm so the Rice
Krispies adhere to the date mixture. Cool.
Keep in an airtight tin.

Honeycomb toffee   (milk-, egg-, wheat-,
  colour-, preservative-free)
60 g (2 oz) 4 level tbsp golden syrup
60 g (2 oz) 4 level tbsp sugar
1 tsp bicarbonate of soda

Weigh or measure the syrup and sugar into
a saucepan and bring to the boil over a low
heat. Boil gently for 10 minutes. Stir in the
bicarbonate of soda, pour into a greased tin,
or preferably a tin lined with greased foil.
Leave to set.

Ice-cream using milk substitute
  (milk-, egg-, wheat-, colour-,
  preservative-free)

500 ml (1 pint) milk substitute
150 g (5 oz) sugar
2 tsp Ener-G egg replacer and 4 tbsp water
30 g (1 oz) milk-free margarine
30 g (1 oz) arrowroot or cornflour

Place egg replacer, water, sugar, margarine
and arrowroot in a bowl and beat on speed
1 of an electric mixer, increasing to speed 3,
until creamy (2 min). Heat milk to
simmering point and pour over the mixture
while continuing to beat for 30 seconds.
Pour all back into a saucepan and cook over
a low heat, beating until the mixture boils
and thickens. Remove from the heat and
allow to cool. Freeze until solid film forms
around sides and bottom of tray. Turn into a
bowl and beat for one minute at speed 3.
Pour back into tray and freeze.

Milk pudding using milk substitute
  (milk-, egg-, wheat-, colour-,
  preservative-free)

45 g (1½ oz) ground rice, flaked rice,
  cornflour, tapioca, etc.
5 g (1 knob) milk-free margarine
30 g (2 tbsp) sugar
500 ml (1 pint) milk substitute

Place all ingredients in a saucepan and bring
to the boil, stirring well. Simmer gently,
stirring frequently, until cooked. A double
saucepan is good for this.

Baked rice pudding   (milk-, egg-,
  wheat-, colour-, preservative-free)

45 g (1½ oz) Carolina or pudding rice
5 g (1 knob) milk-free margarine
30 g (2 tbsp) sugar
500 ml (1 pint) milk substitute

Put all ingredients into a 1½-pint pie dish
and bake in the oven for about 3 hours at
150°C. Stir occasionally; sprinkle with
nutmeg if permitted.

Fruit fool (milk-, egg-, wheat-, colour-, preservative-free)

Cook and purée 500 g (1 lb) of fruit, e.g. cooking apples (or use a tin of apple purée). Combine with 300 ml ($\frac{1}{2}$ pint) of milk pudding made with milk substitute. Chill.

Fondant (milk-, egg-, wheat-, colour-, preservative-free)

150 ml ($\frac{1}{4}$ pint) water (generous measure)
500 g (1 lb) granulated sugar
Pinch of cream of tartar

Put the water in a pan, add sugar and allow it to dissolve slowly. Then bring it to the boil; add cream of tartar and boil to 120°C (you will need a sugar thermometer for this). Pour the boiled fondant on to a slab and allow it to cool for a few minutes until a skin starts to form. Using a spatula, collect up the mixture, then continue to work it with a forward and back movement. When it becomes opaque and firm, scrape it up and knead well until it is an even texture throughout. If no marble slab is available let the syrup cool in a bowl for about 15 minutes and work it until it is thick. The fondant may be stored in a jar or used immediately. Roll out and cut into shapes.

RECIPES USING POTATOES

Shepherd's pie (serves 4 to 6) (milk-, egg-, wheat-, colour-, preservative-free)

750 g (1 lb) potatoes
500 g (1 lb) cooked mince lamb (or beef)
2 chopped onions
90 g (3 oz) milk-free margarine
A little milk substitute, or water
Salt and pepper
Stock or water

Peel potatoes, boil and mash with salt and pepper, 60 g (2 oz) of the margarine and milk substitute or water. Fry onions in the remaining margarine until soft. Mix with meat, moisten with stock or water and place in a greased pie dish. Cover with mashed potato, forking the top. Bake in a hot oven for 20 to 30 minutes, 230°C, until heated through and brown on the top.

Potato and celery soup (milk-, egg-, wheat-, cereal-, colour-, preservative-free)

500 g (1 lb) potatoes
Half a head of celery
2 onions
30 g (1 oz) milk-free margarine
500 ml (1 pint) stock or water
150 ml ($\frac{1}{4}$ pint) milk substitute or water
Salt and pepper
Chopped parsley

Separate the sticks of celery, wash and cut into pieces. Peel the potatoes and cut into quarters. Peel and slice the onions. Melt the margarine in a saucepan, add celery and onion and cook gently for a few minutes. Add potatoes, stock and seasoning. Bring to the boil and simmer gently until the vegetables are cooked. Rub through a sieve or put in a liquidizer. Add milk substitute if allowed. Reheat, adjust seasoning and sprinkle with freshly chopped parsley to serve.

Potato cakes or **'bubble and squeak'** (milk-, egg-, wheat-, cereal-, colour-, preservative-free)

Any left over mashed potato can be formed by hand into 'patties' or cakes and coated with any type of permitted flour and then fried (in permitted oil) on both sides until crispy and well browned. 'Bubble and squeak' can be made by adding any leftover permitted vegetables, e.g. carrots or cabbage, to the mashed potato.

Potato and carrot soup (milk-, egg-, wheat-, cereal-, colour-, preservative-free)

750 g (1$\frac{1}{2}$ lb) potatoes
500 g (1 lb) sliced carrots

1 small sliced onion
90 g (3 oz) milk-free margarine
1 tsp sugar (optional)
1200 ml (2 pints) stock or water
Salt and pepper
Chopped parsley

Peel potatoes and dice roughly. Melt half
the margarine in a saucepan, add onion and
cook until soft but not brown. Add potatoes
and carrots, stir, add sugar and a little salt.
When the vegetables have absorbed the
margarine, add stock or water and cook until
vegetables are tender. Rub through a sieve
or put in a liquidizer. Reheat, adjust
seasoning and add more stock or water if
necessary. Add remaining margarine and stir
in fresh parsley.

Lamb rissoles (milk-, egg-, wheat-, cereal-, colour-, preservative-free)

60 g (2 oz) cooked minced lamb
120 g (4 oz) mashed potato (mashed with
    milk-free margarine)
Potato flour or other flour to coat
Sunflower oil
Salt and pepper

Combine the lamb with mashed potato.
Mould the mixture into rissoles or croquette
shapes, coat with 'flour' and deep fry in oil
until golden brown.

Potato scones (milk-, egg-, wheat-, cereal-, colour-, preservative-free)

500 g (1 lb) boiled potatoes
120 g (4 oz) rice flour or other permitted
    flour
Salt to taste

Mash the potatoes well. Add the flour and
salt and knead well. Roll out thinly on a
floured board. Prick with a fork, cut into 12
to 15 rounds or triangles, and cook quickly
on a lightly greased heavy frying pan or
griddle. Alternatively, they may be baked in
a very hot oven, 260°C, for about 10

minutes. Turn them over half-way through
cooking. Serve the scones hot with milk-free
margarine and golden syrup. Any leftovers
are tasty fried for breakfast.

Potato pan mash (milk-, egg-, wheat-, cereal-, colour-, preservative-free)

500 g (1 lb) mashed potatoes
A little milk-free margarine or sunflower oil
Salt and pepper

Heat the fat in the frying pan. Add the
mashed potato, smooth over and cook
gently until crispy brown underneath. Fold
over with a fish slice or palette knife and
slide on to a warm plate. They can be filled
with a suitable filling, e.g. fried onions or
mushroom if permitted.

Duchesse potatoes (milk-, egg-, wheat-, cereal-, colour-, preservative-free)

Mash some cooked potatoes with salt,
pepper, margarine, milk substitute or water
until soft enough to pipe. Put the mixture in
a large forcing bag with a large star nozzle
and pipe potato in pyramids on to a greased
baking sheet. Bake in a hot oven or under
the grill until browned. This mixture may
also be made into potato 'nests'.

Sauté potatoes (milk-, egg-, wheat-, cereal-, colour-, preservative-free)

Peel potatoes and partly cook in salt water
for about 10 minutes. Drain well and dry off
in a pan over low heat. Cut the potatoes
into chunky pieces. Heat some sunflower oil
in a frying pan, add the potatoes and fry on
all sides until crisp and brown. They are
delicious mixed with sliced cooked onions,
or chicken livers if permitted.

Lancashire hot pot (serves 4–6)
(milk-, egg-, wheat-, cereal-, colour-, preservative-free)

500 to 750 g (1 to 1½ lb) potatoes
750 g (1½ lb) middle neck of mutton or lamb
2 large onions
2 sheep kidneys
Salt and pepper
300 ml (½ pint) stock (from bones or water using permitted meat and vegetables)

Cut meat into neat pieces. Peel potatoes and slice about ¼-inch thick. Slice onion thinly. Put layers of meat, potato, and onions into a greased casserole. Season well and finish with a layer of potatoes. Add about ½ pint of stock or water and cover with a lid. Bake in a slow oven, 160°C, for 2½ to 3 hours, removing the lid for the last half hour to brown the potatoes. Add small dabs of milk-free margarine on the potatoes if they go dry during cooking.

CEREAL-FREE RECIPES

Treacle tarts (cereal-free)

240 g (8 oz) basic potato shortbread dough
4 dessertspoons syrup
30 g (1 oz) potato flour
30 g (1 oz) sugar

Make up dough and mould pieces into cake tray moulds. Cook in 180°C oven for approximately 8 minutes. Meanwhile, combine syrup, flour and sugar, and heat in a thick-based saucepan. Cook till this resembles a thick paste (adding more flour if necessary). Remove tart cases from the oven and fill the centres with this mixture. Return to oven for approximately 10 to 15 minutes. Serve hot or cold.

Goat's milk custard (wheat-, cereal-, egg-, colour-, preservative-free)

50 g (2 oz) arrowroot
500 ml (1 pint) goat's milk
Sugar to taste

Mix arrowroot with a little cooled goat's milk to a smooth paste. Warm the rest of the goat's milk, add to the arrowroot mixture and return to the pan. Stir well and bring to a gentle boil. Cook for 2 minutes.

Goat's milk fudge (wheat-, cereal-, egg-, colour-, preservative-free)

300 ml (10 oz) goat's milk
800 g (27 oz) granulated sugar
100 g (3½ oz) milk-free margarine

Pour milk into a saucepan and bring slowly to the boil. Add sugar and margarine, and heat slowly till they dissolve, stirring well. Bring to the boil, cover and leave to boil for 2 minutes. Uncover, then boil steadily for 10 to 15 minutes. Remove from the heat and cool for 5 minutes. Beat until thick and creamy. Place in a greased tin, mark into squares, and leave to cool.

Syrup toffee (wheat-, cereal-, egg-, milk-, colour-, preservative-free)

75 ml (2½ oz) water
100 g (3½ oz) golden syrup
450 g (15 oz) granulated sugar
50 g (1¾ oz) milk-free margarine

Pour water and syrup into a saucepan. Bring to the boil. Add sugar and margarine. Heat slowly, stirring well, until the sugar dissolves and the margarine melts. Bring to the boil, cover the pan and boil gently for 2 minutes. Uncover, continue to boil, stirring occasionally for 12 to 15 minutes (till it forms a round ball when dropped into cold water if rolled with the fingers). Pour into a greased tin and leave until hard.

MILK- AND EGG-FREE RECIPES

Yeast-free Irish soda bread*(milk-, egg-free)

750 g (1½ lb) wholemeal flour
300 ml (½ pint) goat's milk or permitted milk
  substitute
1 tsp cream of tartar
1 tsp bicarbonate of soda
1 tsp salt

Mix dry ingredients in a basin and make a
well in the centre. Add enough milk to make
a thick dough. Stir with a wooden spoon;
the mixing should be done lightly and
quickly. Add more milk if too stiff. Flatten
into a circle about 1½ inches thick. Put on a
baking sheet and cut a large cross over it.
Bake at 190°C for about 40 minutes.

Wholemeal scones* (milk-, egg-free)

Raising agent
30 g (1 oz) bicarbonate of soda } Mix thoroughly and keep in airtight jar
60 g (2 oz) cream tartar

Scone
240 g (8 oz) wholemeal flour
Pinch salt
2 tsp raising agent
60 g (2 oz) milk-free margarine
Up to 15 g (2 oz) of sugar (optional)
120 ml (4 fl oz) goat's milk (approximately)

Mix the flour and raising agent and add salt.
Cut and rub in the fat. Stir in sugar if used.
Mix in the milk to give a soft dough. Turn
on to a floured board and either:
  (a) Divide mixture into two and shape
  into two rounds about ½ inch thick.
  Place well apart on a greased sheet and
  cut each through into eight segments,
  but do not separate.
  (b) Shape into one round, roll out ½
  inch thick and cut into rounds with a
  2½-inch cutter and place on a greased
  sheet. Bake at 240°C for 7 to 10
  minutes.

* NB Contains wheat.

Melting moments   (milk-, egg-, colour-, preservative-free)

120 g (4 oz) milk-free margarine
30 g (1 oz) icing sugar
90 g (3 oz) flour (permitted)
30 g (1 oz) cornflour

Cream margarine and sugar. Sift in the flours
and work into the creamed mixture. Force
through a star pipe into fancy shapes on a
greased baking sheet. Bake at 140°C for
about 10 minutes until cooked through but
only very lightly browned.

Viennese fingers   (milk-, egg-, colour-, preservative-free)

Make mixture for melting moments. Using a
large star nozzle, pipe lengths of mixture on
a greased baking sheet. When cooked,
sandwich together with 'butter-cream' made
with icing sugar and milk-free margarine or
with non-dairy imitation cream.

Corn oil cake   (milk-, egg-, colour-, preservative-free)

120 g (4 oz) flour (permitted)
1 rounded tsp baking powder
1 level tsp bicarbonate of soda
Pinch of salt
60 g (2 oz) castor sugar
90 g (3 oz) golden syrup
90 ml (3 fl oz) corn oil
2 tsp Ener-G egg replacer and 4 tbsp water
120 g (4 oz) grated carrot or grated apple

Sieve flour, raising agent and salt. Mix in the
sugar and carrot. Beat together the oil, egg
replacer, and syrup and add to the flour
mixture. Pour into an 8-inch diameter
sponge tin lined with greased foil and bake
at 180°C for 45 minutes.

Apple scones   (milk-, egg-, colour-, preservative-free)

240 g (8 oz) flour (permitted)
1 to 2 level tsp baking powder

60 g (2 oz) milk-free margarine
60 g (2 oz) sugar
1 medium cooking apple grated
150 ml ($\frac{1}{4}$ pint) water or milk substitute

Mix the flour and raising agent. Rub in the fat. Stir in the sugar and apple, and finally the milk or water. Roll out thickly and cut into rounds. Place on a greased baking sheet brush with water or milk substitute and sprinkle with brown sugar. Bake at 200°C for about 20 minutes.

Eggless fruit cake   (milk-, egg-free)

240 g (8 oz) self-raising flour
$\frac{1}{2}$ tsp mixed spice
60 g (2 oz) milk-free margarine
120 g (4 oz) sugar
180 g (6 oz) dried fruits
$\frac{1}{2}$ tsp bicarbonate of soda
150 ml ($\frac{1}{4}$ pint) milk substitute or water
15 ml (1 tbsp) vinegar

Sieve dry ingredients and rub in fat. Add sugar, and fruit. Put bicarbonate in a basin, mix smoothly with milk substitute and add vinegar, then pour at once into dry ingredients. Mix quickly and put into prepared shallow square tin. Bake at 180°C for about 30 minutes until well risen and firm to touch.

Ginger parkin   (milk-, egg-, colour-, preservative-free)

240 g ($\frac{1}{2}$ lb) golden syrup
90 g (3 oz) milk-free margarine
120 g (4 oz) soft brown sugar
120 g (4 oz) self-raising flour
$\frac{1}{2}$ tsp baking powder
1 rounded tsp ground ginger
240 g ($\frac{1}{2}$ lb) medium oatmeal
90 ml ($\frac{1}{2}$ teacup) milk substitute or water

Melt syrup, margarine, and sugar in a large pan. Add milk and stir in all dry ingredients.

Pour into a greased 7- or 8-inch square baking tin and cook for 1 to 1$\frac{1}{2}$ hours at 150°C. It is best kept a week before eating.

Oat macaroons*   (milk-, wheat-, colour-, preservative-free)

60 g (2 oz) cornflour or potato flour or permitted flour
120 g (4 oz) castor sugar
60 g (2 oz) rolled oats or ground rice
1 egg-white if permitted
Jam
1 egg-white stiffly beaten ⎫
Juice of $\frac{1}{2}$ lemon   ⎬ For icing
60 g (2 oz) icing sugar   ⎭

Mix cornflour, oats, and sugar together. Work in egg-white. Place a little cornflour onto a pastry board and rolling pin. Roll out and cut into rounds, about 1 cm ($\frac{1}{4}$ inch) thick. Spread with jam. Place on greased baking sheet. Mix icing ingredients together and spread over pastry. Bake in a cool oven, 150°C, for about 10 to 15 minutes. Cool before removing from sheet.

Arrowroot biscuits   (milk-, egg-, wheat-, cereal-, colour-, preservative-free)

90 g (3 oz) potato flour
60 g (2 oz) arrowroot
60 g (2 oz) castor sugar
90 g (3 oz) milk-free margarine

Cream sugar and margarine. Fold in the flours. Although this mixture is fairly sticky it can be rolled out with a rolling pin using plenty of arrowroot to stop it sticking. Cut into rounds with a biscuit cutter and place the rounds on a greased baking sheet. Bake at 190°C for about 20 minutes. Sprinkle with sugar and remove when cool. They will be a pale golden colour when cooked.

* NB Contains egg.

CHAPTER 5

Juvenile diabetes mellitus

Introduction

Diabetes mellitus is defined as a state of chronic hyperglycaemia. The aetiology has recently been reviewed by Farquhar (1979) and Gamble (1980). The classical symptoms of juvenile diabetes mellitus are an acute onset, with polyuria, polydipsia, recent weight loss, raised blood sugar, glucosuria and frequently acetonuria. Growth of the child is subsequently impaired (Starkey 1967). The β-cells of the islets of Langerhans in the pancreas fail to produce adequate insulin necessary for the normal metabolism of carbohydrate (Oakley *et al.* 1975). Insulin is also needed to inhibit the breakdown of protein to amino acids, gluconeogenesis and lipolysis as well as being necessary for the entry of glucose into the cells and its conversion to glycogen (Starkey 1967).

Juvenile diabetes mellitus is insulin-sensitive and requires injections of insulin for control. The aim of treatment is to normalize blood glucose levels and obtain a fully active child who leads a normal life within the limits of the diabetic regimen, grows adequately, and gains weight within the normal range, avoiding secondary obesity which can frequently occur, or growth failure which results from poor control (Oakley *et al.* 1975, Craig 1977). The degenerative long-term complications of diabetes are multifactorial, but, at least in part, are thought to be related to the degree of diabetic control achieved (Tchobroutsky 1978, Belton & Farquhar 1984).

Insulin

The juvenile diabetic requires insulin therapy, as the hypoglycaemic drugs alone are ineffective. A normal pancreas releases insulin in response to blood glucose levels. Multiple subcutaneous injections of soluble insulin, or mixed insulins, is, at present, the best means of achieving normoglycaemia throughout the 24 hours in the patient with diabetes, but in practice insulin is injected usually only once daily in the young child and twice daily during adolescence. As yet, continuous infusion of insulin is impractical for the majority and is reserved for the minority of patients who are difficult to control. There are a number of different insulins available, Fig. 5.1 gives a summary of the mode of action of the commonly used types. All insulin supplied in the U.K. is now 100 strength (100 units in each 1 ml). Although the delayed-action insulins have made the regimen more tolerable for children, their use is now being questioned, as there is a suspicion that the advantages may have been gained at the expense of optimal control and at increased risk of complications ultimately. The monocomponent and purified insulins are not interchangeable with each other, or with conventional insulin. Porcine insulin differs from human insulin in only one amino acid and has a slightly shorter onset and duration than equivalent insulin of bovine origin, which differs in three amino acids. Human insulin is now available but its advantages compared with cost are still being evaluated.

Treatment of diabetic ketoacidosis and insulin requirements and dose adjustment for children are given in detail by Craig (1977) and Belton and Farquhar (1984). The response to stress, variation in absorption from patient to patient and between different sites in the same patient and the Somogyi effect (Somogyi 1959) mean that each child must be treated on an individual basis.

Insulin should be given not more than 30 minutes before a meal. Mealtimes should be as regular as possible, though practical advice can be given to the family regarding the 'Sunday lie-in', holidays and special occasions. For example, if insulin and breakfast are given 1 to $1\frac{1}{2}$ hours later than usual then the mid-morning snack and lunch should be delayed for an hour compared to usual; the day's remaining meals can be delayed by an hour or given at the usual time. If mass or communion is taken 'fasting', 1 to 2 exchanges of fruit juice should be given half an hour before or at the usual breakfast time, insulin will be delayed until after mass and then followed by the usual quantity of carbohydrate normally given at breakfast.

Fig. 5.1 Insulin: onset, peak and duration of action of different insulins.

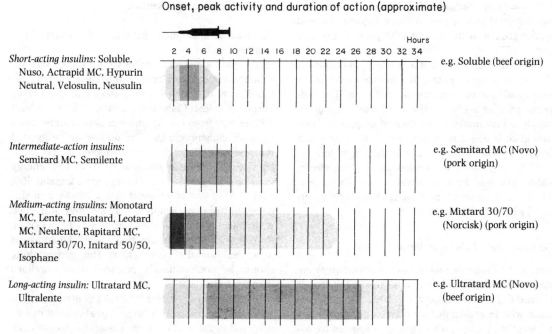

Onset, peak activity and duration of action (approximate)

Short-acting insulins: Soluble, Nuso, Actrapid MC, Hypurin Neutral, Velosulin, Neusulin — e.g. Soluble (beef origin)

Intermediate-action insulins: Semitard MC, Semilente — e.g. Semitard MC (Novo) (pork origin)

Medium-acting insulins: Monotard MC, Lente, Insulatard, Leotard MC, Neulente, Rapitard MC, Mixtard 30/70, Initard 50/50, Isophane — e.g. Mixtard 30/70 (Norcisk) (pork origin)

Long-acting insulin: Ultratard MC, Ultralente — e.g. Ultratard MC (Novo) (beef origin)

All insulins supplied in the UK are now 100 strength (100 units/1 ml)

When mixing insulins in the syringe the shorter acting insulin should be drawn into the syringe first and the mixed insulin should be given immediately after it is drawn up. Monocomponent and purified insulins are not interchangeable with each other or with conventional insulins.

The dose of insulin is adjusted according to blood glucose levels, aiming to keep them ideally in the normal range of between 3 and 10 mmol/l* throughout the 24 hours. During periods of illness a sudden increase in the insulin dose may be required with return to the previous dose on recovery. The dose can be expected to increase gradually with age. As a result of extra exercise during the summer months and holiday periods the insulin dose may need to be temporarily decreased. Frequently this also occurs following the diagnosis and initial control of diabetes, as the pancreas may partially recover during the so-called 'honeymoon period'. The parents and child should be informed that this is a temporary phenomenon. The occasional child has late-onset diabetes and does not require insulin, but this is very uncommon (Craig 1977, Belton & Farquhar 1984).

Need for dietary control

The maintenance of normoglycaemia is considered the best protection against long-term complications. Fluctuations in blood glucose levels are inevitable with the present insulins, injection techniques and the unpredictable appetite and activity of children (Belton & Farquhar 1984). A controlled dietary intake has short-term benefits in avoiding large swings in blood glucose levels, allows easier stabilization and minimizes episodes of hypoglycaemia and ketoacidosis. However, it remains to be seen what contribution the new dietary recommendations, modern insulins, various treatment regimens and methods of monitoring control will have on long-term prognosis (Kinmonth & Baum 1982). Although there are difficulties in maintaining children on a diet, problems also occur with a 'free diet' which can become overrestricted in carbohydrate, especially where parents think that sugar and carbohydrate foods are harmful and subsequently eliminate many foods from the diet.

---

*Plasma glucose measured in mmol/l × 18·02 = mg/100 ml.

A measured carbohydrate diet in these circumstances is often welcome. Variety is possible if the diet is well understood and adequate information is available. An over-restricted diet or poor diabetic control can lead to poor growth in the patient with juvenile diabetes (Craig 1977).

The psychological effect of a 'free diet' in childhood followed by dietary control in adolescence or adulthood should not be forgotten, as well as the psycholoptical effect of a diet on the child. Any change in lifestyle is best made at the time of diagnosis when motivation is at a maximum. The best control and compliance will be achieved by imposing as few restrictions as possible, by families sharing together a healthy diet, and by approaching as closely as possible the achievement of normoglycaemia throughout each 24 hours.

Diet for juvenile diabetes mellitus

There is no evidence that a low total carbohydrate intake is beneficial, and quite a bit to suggest that it is harmful. The need is for a regulated carbohydrate intake with increased dietary fibre in order to lower and lengthen post-prandial glucose curves, so avoiding hyperglycaemic peaks and urinary loss (Belton & Farquhar 1984).

Nutrients are not metabolized in isolation, but within complex interrelated pathways. Carbohydrate consumption directly affects post-prandial blood glucose levels. However, to some extent protein and fat as well as carbohydrate ultimately affect diabetic control. Dietary energy intake is therefore an important consideration in diabetics and in the child must be adequate for growth but not so excessive as to cause obesity or refusal of food.

Energy intake
The dietary energy intake for the well-controlled diabetic is similar to that for a normal child. The overweight child with diabetes requires some restriction of the energy intake, whereas at the time of diagnosis some patients require a higher energy intake temporarily to allow for catch-up growth or correction of the weight loss that has occurred before diagnosis. Considerable energy loss occurs in the untreated or poorly controlled diabetic who has glycosuria. The 24-hour urine glucose loss (Foman et al. 1974) will give an indication, and may exceed 200 g, accounting for a large energy loss (3200 kJ; 800 kcal) with subsequent poor growth and/or weight loss (Craig 1977). The situation is worsened if thirst is satisfied with sweetened drinks and if periodic hunger leads to

pilfering, frequently of high-carbohydrate and energy foods. Improved control with diet and adjustment of the insulin dosage is essential.

Carbohydrate intake in the diet of juvenile diabetes mellitus
In the past a reduced carbohydrate intake was recommended, e.g. 40% energy from carbohydrate, but this is now considered unnecessary and is probably harmful (*British Diabetic Association 1980). At least 45% energy from carbohydrate is now recommended by most diabetic clinics. The author has suggested that the normal diet for young children in this country should provide approximately 10 to 15% energy from protein, 35 to 40% of energy from fat, and 50% energy from carbohydrate (Francis 1984), and this energy distribution is appropriate for the young child with diabetes mellitus. However, it may be beneficial if an even higher carbohydrate, lower fat intake is prescribed for the older child. The carbohydrate should be predominantly provided from unrefined carbohydrate.

In Asian countries and Japan 70 to 80% energy is provided from carbohydrate and good control can be achieved in diabetes on such a regimen (Hirata et al. 1970). Experimental studies (Simpson et al. 1979) using diets containing 60 to 85% energy from carbohydrate have confirmed that such diets are well tolerated by insulin-dependent adults with diabetes. When treatment is adequate carbohydrate handling is restored to a state similar to that of normal subjects (Brunzell et al. 1974). *Dietary Recommendations for Diabetics in the 1980s* (*British Diabetic Association, 1980, Nutrition Sub-committee) gives evidence supporting the need for the increased carbohydrate, reduced fat, lowered salt intakes that are now recommended.

Carbohydrate prescription
The carbohydrate intake should be controlled and measured. The quantity prescribed will depend on age, activity, meal pattern and energy requirement of the individual. Table 5.1 gives suggested carbohydrate intakes according to the recommended energy intakes for age.

Many pre-school aged children find the bulk of a high-fibre–high-carbohydrate–low-fat diet unacceptable, in which case a temporary compromise of a lower carbohydrate higher fat intake is recommended in order to avoid, as far as possible, the inevitable

---

* British Diabetic Association, 10 Queen Anne Street, London, W1M 0BD. Telephone 01–323–1531.

Table 5.1 Guide to the intake of carbohydrate (g) per day for children of different ages with diabetes mellitus.

Age in years	Boys			Girls		
	Carbohydrate (g/day)			Carbohydrate (g/day)		
	(I)	(II)	(III)	(I)	(II)	(III)
1	135	180	165	125	140	150
2	155	175	195	145	160	180
3–4	175	195	215	170	190	205
5–6	195	215	240	190	210	230
7–8	220	245	270	215	235	260
9–11	255	285	315	230	255	280
12–14	300	330	365	240	270	295
15–17	345	360	400	240	270	295

Based on recommended amounts of energy for different age groups.

   (I)   Carbohydrate supplying $\simeq$45% energy intake (energy kcal $\times$ 0·113, kJ $\times$ 0·027).

   (II) Carbohydrate supplying $\simeq$50% energy intake (energy kcal $\times$ 0·125, kJ $\times$ 0·03).

   (III) Carbohydrate supplying $\simeq$55% energy intake (energy kcal $\times$ 0·138, kJ $\times$ 0·033).

toddler food refusals. A gradual change of diet to a higher carbohydrate intake of unrefined carbohydrates should be made once the child becomes accustomed to the diabetic regime.

Some adolescent boys will need 13 000 kJ (3000 kcal) per day and therefore a diet containing 400 g carbohydrate per day may be appropriate during the rapid growth period of adolescence. However, adolescent girls mature at an earlier age and rarely need more than 250 to 300 g of carbohydrate prescribed daily.

The normal appetite regulation with self-selected intake of protein-containing foods (lean meat, fish), moderate restriction of fat intake and encouragement of a generous intake of fruit and vegetables, together with the carbohydrate prescription, mainly from bread, cereals and potatoes, ensures an adequate energy intake for growth, provided good diabetic control is achieved with insulin.

Carbohydrate distribution

The carbohydrate prescription is distributed between three meals and three snacks, according to the mode of action and duration of the insulin selected (Fig. 5.1), the time of meals, family meal pattern and the child's activity.

Adequate carbohydrate should be given to cover overnight needs by the inclusion of a late night or bedtime snack made up of unrefined carbohydrate, ideally with a high fibre content, and some protein,

e.g. a wholemeal bread sandwich and glass of milk.

Patients treated with one injection of an intermediate or long-acting insulin, with or without a short-acting insulin, require an approximately evenly distributed carbohydrate with individual modification for different mealtimes and activity, e.g. 200 g carbohydrate daily would theoretically be divided:

   40 g carbohydrate for breakfast at 8 a.m.
   20 g carbohydrate mid-morning at 10.30 a.m.
   50 g carbohydrate for lunch at 12.30 p.m.
   20 g carbohydrate for snack at 3.30 p.m.
   50 g carbohydrate for evening meal at 6 p.m.
   20 g carbohydrate for bedtime snack at 8 p.m.

When soluble or short-acting insulin alone is used twice-daily, the carbohydrate given at breakfast and the evening meal following the injected insulin should be slightly greater than the carbohydrate given at lunchtime, e.g. 200 g carbohydrate daily would theoretically be divided:

   40 g carbohydrate for breakfast at 8 a.m.
   30 g carbohydrate mid-morning at 10.30 a.m.
   40 g carbohydrate for lunch at 12.30 p.m.
   20 g carbohydrate for snack at 3.30 p.m.
   40 g carbohydrate for evening meal at 6 p.m.
   30 g carbohydrate for bedtime snack at 8 p.m.

Individual adjustment of the carbohydrate distribution should be made according to blood glucose profiles and from time to time as indicated by changes in activities and school schedules.

Type of carbohydrate

Traditionally, simple sugars have been eliminated from the diet of diabetic patients in order to reduce the carbohydrate intake, and because they cause a rapid rise in blood glucose. Steel *et al.* (1983) showed no glycaemic difference between 20 g carbohydrate mid-morning snacks in insulin-dependent diabetics whether the food was predominantly fructose, sucrose or starch. They concluded that the exclusion of sweet food may not be necessary or even desirable, and that fructose-containing foods have no advantage over starch-containing foods. Other workers have demonstrated that refined starches have a similar effect to glucose (Wahlquist *et al.* 1978) and that sucrose can be less acutely hyperglycaemic than glucose or starch, possibly due to the fructose component of sucrose (Thompson *et al.* 1978).

A mixture of carbohydrate and fibre reduces the magnitude of the glycaemic curve more than the same amount of carbohydrate alone (Haber *et al.* 1977). Pectin, guar gum and pulses (beans) appear to be especially effective (Jenkins *et al.* 1979, Belton & Farquhar 1984), but all dietary fibre is probably beneficial, and is thought to slow down the rate of carbohydrate absorption and appears to have a therapeutic value in the diet of diabetics (Jenkins *et al.* 1980). Refined carbohydrates, with the exception of treatment for hypoglycaemia, during intercurrent illness, or as 'treats', are best replaced by wholegrain cereals, wholemeal bread, pulses and fruit. Fig. 5.2 divides the foods containing carbohydrate into three groups with different physiological effects related to their content of fibre. Vegetables are also a useful source of dietary fibre and should be encouraged.

Accompanying nutrients may also affect post-prandial glycaemia as the presence of fat or protein will delay the rate of carbohydrate absorption (Estrich *et al.* 1967). In order to avoid hyperglycaemic peaks it is recommended that meals and snacks should normally contain some high-fibre carbohydrate foods (Table 5.2a), together with some protein and small amounts of fat.

Fructose and sorbitol are not recommended, and refined carbohydrates should be used sparingly. Further work on guar gum and pectin supplements is needed before these can be recommended routinely

for children with diabetes, and palatable and acceptable means of including them in the diet must be found. Guar has been used as a powder, granules, or as a crispbread.

Measurement of carbohydrate (exchanges)

The same amount of carbohydrate should be given at the same time each day, but this does not necessarily have to be from the same food. Table 5.2 lists foods that provide 10 g carbohydrate exchanges when eaten in the amount stated, based on information from the British Diabetic Association (1982). The table is divided into three sections, according to the type of carbohydrate and fibre content, corresponding to Fig. 5.2. The amounts of food are described in two ways; a measure using standard measuring spoons (1 teaspoon = 5 ml, 1 tablespoon = 15 ml) and the weight of the food in grams and approximate ounce equivalent. Standard measuring spoons are available from the British Diabetic Association. Scales should weigh in 5 g ($\frac{1}{4}$ oz) increments. During the learning phase patients are encouraged to weigh foods in order to familiarize themselves with the size of exchanges. Each meal's prescription of carbohydrate can be made up by combinations of these foods, but

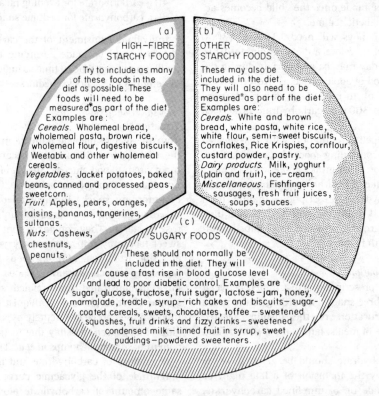

Fig. 5.2   Carbohydrate-containing foods. A list of carbohydrate exchange foods is given in Table 5.2.

at least some carbohydrate should be high in fibre selected from Table 5.2a.

Many manufactured foods can be included in the diet provided their carbohydrate content is known. *Carbohydrate Countdown* published regularly by the British Diabetic Association provides a list of products, including manufactured foods, and their carbohydrate and energy content.

Protein

Protein is necessary for growth in children, and 10 to 15% dietary energy from protein is recommended. The protein and energy intake of the diet is not specifically controlled except for moderate restriction of total dietary energy in the overweight patient. Table 5.3 lists a number of foods which contain negligible carbohydrate including the first-class protein sources such as meat, egg and fish. Protein is also provided from some foods which contain carbohydrate (Table 5.2, 10 g carbohydrate exchange foods) such as milk, pulses (beans and peas), bread and cereals. The inclusion of 1 to 2 serves of the first-class protein foods and 2 to 3 carbohydrate exchanges from milk or skimmed milk, together with the protein contribution from cereals and bread, will supply an adequate intake of protein. Vegetarians should include pulses and nuts as part of their carbohydrate prescription to replace the first-class protein sources in order to provide adequate protein for growth needs.

Fat

Total dietary fat intake should be limited in patients with diabetes. An increased carbohydrate prescription necessitates the reduction of the dietary fat intake, otherwise the total energy intake will be excessive. In order to reduce the fat intake of the diet, any meat used should be lean, cheese should be used in moderation, poultry and fish used more frequently than meat, and fats should be used sparingly.

Patients with diabetes have an increased long-term risk of atherosclerosis and disability or death from cardiovascular disease (Keen & Thomas 1978). Dietary measures are therefore desirable to lower serum cholesterol levels and the hyperlipidaemia associated with diabetes. Although a reduced fat intake is recommended, as yet such a diet has not been proved to reduce vascular mortality, and other factors such as dietary sodium intake, obesity and smoking are also relevant.

An association of hyperlipidaemia with atherosclerosis in juvenile diabetes has been established (Court *et al.* 1978). The control of hyperlipidaemia in diabetes is achieved primarily by careful control of the diabetes (Court *et al.* 1978) and a measure of satisfactory control is by the measurement of blood lipid levels at intervals. Kaufman *et al.* (1975) have demonstrated that serum cholesterol levels can be strikingly reduced in children with diabetes by adjusting the dietary polyunsaturated to saturated fatty acid ratio. Prophylactic use of predominantly polyunsaturated fats has been recommended for diabetics by some workers (British Diabetic Association 1980). The diet can be adapted by using the polyunsaturated natural vegetable oils for cooking (e.g. safflower, sunflower, soya or corn oil) in place of the saturated and hard fats (*see* Chapter 7). However, recent work on long-chain *trans* fatty acids produced during the manufacture particularly of margarine, including some claiming to be high in polyunsaturated fatty acids (PUFA), makes their use of debatable value. *Trans* fats are lower in traditional fat sources. Further work to evaluate the role of *trans* fats is urgently needed, but they appear to act similarly to saturated fatty acids in the body (DHSS 1984). In the meanwhile only margarines solely of vegetable origin and labelled high in PUFA can be recommended without reservation. Emphasis on a reduction in total fat intake rather than the type of fat is now considered of greater importance, together with good diabetic control, in hopefully reducing the incidence of cardiovascular disease associated with diabetes.

Vegetables and fruit

Many vegetables and some fruits have a beneficial high fibre content. A selected range of vegetables and limited list of fruit contain negligible quantities of carbohydrate (Table 5.3) and should be encouraged. A number of miscellaneous items and suitable carbohydrate-free drinks are also suitable for inclusion in the diet.

Sodium

Because there may be a relationship between dietary sodium, hypertension and cardiovascular disease (British Diabetic Association 1980, DHSS 1984) extra added salt at the table and highly salted foods should be discouraged. A small quantity of salt in cooking, and that naturally occurring in foods, milk, bread, cereals, is in order.

Proprietary 'diabetic' products

These products are not necessary, though a number are available (Table 5.4). They are expensive and some contain sorbitol and/or fructose which have no advantage over other carbohydrates in the diet for the child with diabetes. Sorbitol is slowly absorbed

Table 5.2 Lists of foods that provide 10 g carbohydrate (exchanges) when eaten in the amount stated.

(a) *Exchanges of carbohydrate* high in dietary fibre.
   Approximate amounts are listed using the standard measures provided by the British Diabetic Association.
   tsp: level 5 ml teaspoon.
   tbsp: level 15 ml tablespoon.

Food	Approximate measure	Weight g	≃oz
Cereals			
Wholemeal flour	2 tbsp	15	½
Wholemeal bread		25	1
Wholemeal spaghetti, uncooked, or other uncooked wholemeal pasta	20 short (10″) strands	15	½
Brown rice, uncooked	1 tbsp	10	⅓
Digestive or wholemeal biscuits	1	15	½
Oats, uncooked	3 tbsp	15	½
All Bran	5 tbsp	20	¾
Branbuds	4 tbsp	20	¾
Muesli (unsweetened)	2 tbsp	15	½
Puffed Wheat	15 tbsp	15	½
Shredded Wheat	⅔ of 1 biscuit	15	½
Spoon-size Cubs	12 to 14	15	½
Weetabix	1 biscuit	15	½
Weetflakes	4 tbsp	15	½
Vegetables			
Jacket potato	1 egg-sized	50	2
Baked beans	4 tbsp	100	3½
Broad beans—cooked	10 tbsp	150	5
Red kidney beans—raw	2 tbsp		
Chick-peas—raw	2 tbsp	20	¾
Lentils—raw	2 tbsp		
Mung beans—raw	2 tbsp	30	1
Cooked dhal	—	90	3
Beetroot	2 small	100	4
Parsnip—cooked	1 small	75	3
Peas—processed or marrowfat	7 tbsp	75	3
Plantain, green, raw, peeled	Small slice	30	1
Sweetcorn—canned or frozen	5 tbsp	60	2
Sweetcorn on the cob	½ medium cob	45	1½
Sweet potato, boiled	1 small slice	50	2
Yams	—	30	1
Nuts			
Chestnuts (weight with skin)		30	1
Peanuts—fresh shelled or roasted and salted		120	4

Table 5.2 (a) *continued*

Food	Approximate measure	Weight g	≃oz
Fruit—fresh fruit or fruit tinned in water or stewed without sugar			
Apples			
Eating, whole	1 medium	110	4
Cooking, whole	1 medium	125	4
Stewed without sugar	6 tbsp	125	4
Apricots			
Fresh, whole	3 medium	160	6
Dried, raw	4 small	25	1
Bananas			
With skin	5½″ in length	90	3
Peeled	3½″ in length	50	2
Bilberries, raw	5 tbsp	75	3
Blackberries, raw	10 tbsp	150	5
Blackcurrants, raw	10 tbsp	150	5
Cherries, fresh, whole	12	100	4
Currants, dried	2 tbsp	15	½
Damsons, raw, whole	7	120	4
Dates			
Fresh, whole	3 medium	50	2
Dried without stones	3 small	15	½
Figs			
Fresh, whole	1	100	4
Dried	1	20	¾
Grapes, whole	10 large	75	3
Greengages, fresh whole	5	90	3
Guavas, fresh, flesh only	1	70	2½
Mango, fresh, whole	⅓ of a large one	100	4
Melon, all types, weighed with skin	large slice	300	11
Nectarine, fresh, whole	1	90	3
Orange, fresh, whole	1 large	150	5
Paw paw, fresh, whole	⅙ of a large one	80	3
Peach, fresh, whole	1 large	125	4
Pears, fresh, whole	1 large	130	5
Pineapple, fresh, no skin or core	1 thick slice	90	3
Plums			
Cooking, fresh, whole	4 medium	180	6
Dessert, fresh, whole	2 large	110	4

(b) *Exchanges of carbohydrate* high in starch but low in fibre.

Food	Approximate measure	Weight g	≃oz
White or brown bread	½ large thick slice	20	¾
	⅔ large thin slice	20	¾
	1 small slice	20	¾
Pitta bread	⅓	20	¾

Table 5.2 (b) *continued*

Food	Approximate measure	Weight g	≏oz
White spaghetti, uncooked	⎫	10	⅓
Other white pasta, uncooked	⎬ 6 long (19") strands	10	⅓
White pasta, cooked		40	1½
Spaghetti tinned in tomato sauce	⎭	80	3
Potatoes			
Boiled	1 egg-sized	50	2
Mashed	1 small scoop	50	2
Roast	½ medium	40	1½
Chips	4 to 5 average	30	1
Crisps	1 small packet	20	¾
White rice			
Raw	1 tbsp	10	⅓
Boiled		30	1
White flour	1½ tbsp	10	⅓
Arrowroot/custard powder	1 tbsp	10	⅓
Cornflour	1 tbsp	10	⅓
Sago/tapioca/semolina	2 tsp	10	⅓
Pastry	—	20	¾
Semi-sweet biscuits	2	15	½
Cream crackers	2	15	½
Crispbread	2	15	½
Kelloggs Waffles	1	—	—
Cornflakes	5 tbsp	10	⅓
Rice Krispies	6 tbsp	10	⅓
Special K	8 tbsp	15	½
Milk—whole or skimmed	—	200	7
Dried skimmed milk powder	10 tsp	20	¾
Evaporated milk	6 tbsp	90	3
Plain yoghurt	1 carton	160	6
Fruit yoghurt	½ carton	60	2
Unsweetened fruit juices			
Apple/pineapple	6 tbsp	90	3
Blackcurrant/orange	7 tbsp	100	4
Grapefruit juice	8 tbsp	120	4
Fish fingers	2	60	2
Sausages, English-type	2 large/ 3 chipolatas	90	3
Snackpot—Beef Risotto	¼ pot	15	½
Birds Eye Minced Beef Pancake	1	50	1½
Findus Lasagne	⅙ of 16 oz packet	70	2½
Findus Moussaka	¼ of 14 oz packet	100	3½
Birds Eye Chicken Pie	⅓	50	1½
Birds Eye Sausage Rolls	1	35	1¼
Bowyers Pork Pie	⅓ of individual (5 oz) pie	50	1½
Findus French Bread Pizza	¼	30	1
Sainsbury's Individual Cheese and Tomato Pizza	⅓	—	—

Table 5.2 (b) *continued*

Food	Approximate measure	Weight g	≏oz
Heinz Ready to Serve Soups			
Cream of Chicken		180	6
Cream of Mushroom		220	8
Cream of Tomato		90	3
Oxtail		150	5
Pea & Ham		100	4

(c) *Exchanges of refined carbohydrate* foods.

The foods on this list are *high in sugar* and should *not normally* be included in the diet. They may be used in the case of hypoglycaemia, in illness or possibly before strenuous exercise. They are not recommended for use in the regular daily diet.

Food	Approximate measure	Weight g	≏oz
Lucozade	4 tbsp	60 ml	2
Sugar	2 tsp	10	⅓
Glucose tablets	3	10	⅓
Glucose	2 tsp	10	⅓
Honey/jam*/marmalade*	2 tsp	15	½
Mincemeat/lemon curd	1 tbsp	15	½
Golden syrup/black treacle	1 tbsp	15	½
Nesquik	2 tsp	10	⅓
Drinking chocolate	—	15	½
Lemonade (fizzy)*	—	180 ml	6
CocaCola*, Pepsi Cola*	—	100 ml	3½
Ribena (undiluted)*	1 tbsp	15 ml	½
Squashes (undiluted)*	2 tbsp	35 ml	1¼
Jelly cubes*	—	15	½
Jelly made with water*	—	70	2½
Ice-cream plain types dairy and non-dairy		40	1½

*Sweetened variety.

and therefore only slowly affects the blood sugar, has a laxative effect, and has the same energy value as other carbohydrates.

Fructose is an intensely sweet sugar and its effect on blood glucose is controversial. Steel *et al.* (1983) found no practical difference in glycaemic effect between fructose and other 20 g carbohydrate snacks in insulin-dependent diabetics. It is therefore not recommended for children with diabetes, unless calculated as part of their carbohydrate prescription. Many of the proprietary diabetic products are less desirable in the diet and in palatability than the traditional equivalents, though some of the latter should only be used in moderation or for treats in the diet.

Table 5.3 Non-carbohydrate foods (those containing little or no carbohydrate).

These may be taken in normal amounts without measurement. They have very little effect on blood glucose.

Protein foods
  Meat (do not fry)
    Lean poultry, beef, lamb, pork, veal, ham, meat paste, bacon, liver, kidney, continental sausages, salami, paté, frankfurters.
  Fish
    All fresh, frozen, smoked or tinned fish, fish paste.
  Eggs
  Cheese (in moderation)
    Cottage, Edam, Cheddar, etc.

Fruits (do not add sugar)
  Blackcurrants, gooseberries, loganberries, lemons, rhubarb, olives, blackberries, avocado pear, $\frac{1}{2}$ grapefruit per day is permitted.

Vegetables
  Broccoli, cabbage, and all greens, carrots, celery, cauliflower, courgettes, cucumber, French and runner beans, leeks, lettuce, marrow, mushrooms, onions, frozen peas, peppers, swede, turnip, tomato.

Drinks
  Water, clear soup, Marmite, Oxo, Bovril, soda water, unsweetened tomato juice, coffee, tea, sugar-free drinks.

Miscellaneous
  Salt, pepper, mustard, vinegar, herbs, spices, essences and food colours, yeast, gelatine, Worcester sauce, pickles.
  Tomato ketchup, salad cream, brown sauce—up to 2 teaspoons daily of each.
  Gravy—not too thick.
  Bran.
  Almonds, brazils, walnuts.
  Peanut butter—up to 2 teaspoons daily.
  Saccharin tablets and liquid. Aspartame, Acesulfame K.

Fats
  Should be used sparingly.
  Low-fat spreads may be used.
  Polyunsaturated margarines, vegetable oils, butter, margarine, ghee.
  Grilling is preferable to frying.
  Fried foods and cream should be given only as treats.

Table 5.4 Proprietary products for diabetics.

These are *not* essential. Most are very expensive, but some may be useful. Others are not recommended.

The following are useful
Sweetening agents
  Saccharin tablets, e.g. Sweetex, Hermesetas, Saxin, can be used to sweeten drinks or foods. Sweetex Liquid or a liquid sweetener can be made by dissolving saccharin tablets in a little hot water; this is useful for sweetening puddings, cereals, or fruit. To sweeten milk-pudding or stewed fruit it is better to add saccharin after cooking to avoid a bitter taste.

  Aspartame (Canderel, Nutrasweet) and Acesulfame K are new artificial sweeteners which can be used similarly to saccharin.

  Sorbitol, a powdered sweetener, e.g. Sionin, may be useful in cakes and biscuits. However, in large quantities it may give abdominal pain and/or diarrhoea and should be restricted to a maximum of 15 g ($\frac{1}{2}$ oz) daily).

Diabetic squashes and sugar-free drinks are particularly useful, but it is essential to check that no glucose, fructose, or sugar has been added. Low-calorie and dietetic squashes are not necessarily suitable and therefore ingredients must be checked.

Suitable brands include:
  Boots Diabetic Squash
  Roses Dietetic Squash
  Diet Pepsi, OneCal
  Slimline drinks, Tab

Fruit canned without sugar, i.e. unsweetened or sweetened with sorbitol. These all contain carbohydrate from the fruit and must be counted as exchanges in the diet. Check the label carefully for details of carbohydrate content.

Diabetic pastilles and sweets and sugar-free chewing gum containing saccharin and a small amount of sorbitol e.g. Boots sugarless pastilles, Skels, Orbit sugar-free gum. A few may be included in the diet each day.

Diabetic sugar-free jelly crystals.

The following are *not* recommended
Diabetic sugar-free jam and marmalade usually contain sorbitol and are expensive—use those free from added sugar, but only in moderation. It is preferable to use savoury spreads such as Marmite, Bovril, meat paste, or fish paste or peanut butter.

Diabetic chocolate—all brands contain some carbohydrate as well as sorbitol. It is very high in energy and expensive. Use only brands free from added sugar or specially prepared for diabetics, e.g. Wander, Boots, Cadbury. Eaten in small amounts (up to 15 g [$\frac{1}{2}$ oz] in any one day), it does not need to be counted as part of the diet. Larger amounts are not recommended, as this may cause diarrhoea, and would need to be counted as carbohydrate exchanges.

Table 5.4 *continued*

Diabetic cakes and biscuits—all contain carbohydrate, and are very expensive. They must be counted as carbohydrate exchanges in the diet. Check the label for details of carbohydrate content. They have no advantage over ordinary biscuits and cakes of known carbohydrate content. Those made for slimming, are *not* suitable.

Do not use other sugars as sweetening agents such as fructose, fruit sugar, glucose, lactose, glucose polymers, Caloreen, Calonutrin, Maxijul, Hycal, powdered sweeteners containing carbohydrate such as Sweet'n'Low, etc.

Slimming products such as biscuits and meal replacement drinks are not suitable for diabetics.

RECIPES FOR DIABETIC DIETS

A number of cookery books are now available and recipes can also be selected from traditional sources, provided the principles of the diet are understood.

> *The Diabetics' Cook Book* (1982) by J. Mann, published by Martin Dunitz.
> *Better Cookery for Diabetics* (1982) by J. Metcalfe is available from the British Diabetic Association.
> *Cooking the New Diabetic Way* (1983) by J. Metcalfe is available from the British Diabetic Association.

These books have a number of recipes, which are high in fibre and suitable for all the family. The carbohydrate and energy content of each recipe is given.

CHILDREN

Table 5.5 provides an example of a 270 g carbohydrate diet for a diabetic child of 8 to 9 years receiving one injection of an intermediate-action insulin before breakfast.

INFANTS

(a) *Transient neonatal diabetes* is very rare and is temporary, even though insulin in minute doses may be required for a period of a few months. Ketosis is not a feature. Normal infant feeds should be given, with several small doses of insulin per day to normalize the blood glucose (Oakley *et al.* 1975, Craig 1977).
(b) *Infants of diabetic mothers* are not diabetic themselves, but in the neonatal period are at risk

of hypoglycaemia and should therefore be given oral or intravenous glucose soon after birth and frequent feeds in the first few days of life.
(c) *Infantile diabetes mellitus*. This is also very rare, especially in the first few months of life, and can be misdiagnosed. Normal infant feeds and vitamins, together with appropriate weaning solids as applicable for age, should be given with multiple doses of soluble or short-acting insulin to normalize blood glucose. Frequent blood glucose monitoring is recommended, especially as urine tests are both relatively impractical and unreliable. The mother should be given reassurance and a guide to carbohydrate intake, but a strict system of timing and measuring meals is inappropriate and likely to lead to food refusal, which can be dangerous. Carbohydrate replacement with fluids is appropriate if meals are refused, but care is necessary to avoid a diet of inadequate nutritional intake. The total dietary intake must be adequate for growth and should be increased with appetite. Infant feeds and weaning solids should be gradually changed to three meals and two snacks per day by the end of the first year; however, a late evening (10 p.m.) milk feed is continued until the child is around two years of age and able to go to bed a little later, when a bedtime snack may replace the late evening feed.

Hypoglycaemia should be avoided, but it can be difficult to notice signs in a sleeping child who may be pale anyway (Craig 1977). Blood glucose home monitoring is extremely helpful in determining whether the child is or is not hypoglycaemic, should there be any doubt.

After the first two years of age a yearly increment in the carbohydrate prescription is usually appropriate during childhood and should be used as an appropriate occasion to review the dietary regimen and gradually introduce a higher carbohydrate–lower fat dietary regimen based on the principles outlined above.

Food refusal

The diet must be adequate in all nutrients and excess emphasis on one dietary nutrient can lead to an imbalance of others, e.g. concern with carbohydrate intake can lead to exclusion of meat and vegetables. Inadequate intake of protein, trace nutrients and fibre can result when natural carbohydrates (milk, bread, cereals and fruit) are replaced with refined carbohydrate and sugars. This is a particular concern in pre-school age children who are difficult eaters and

Table 5.5 Example of 270 g carbohydrate diet for a diabetic child of 8 to 9 years receiving one injection of intermediate-action insulin before breakfast.

The carbohydrate would be divided through the day as follows

Time	Meal	Exchanges	Carbohydrate (g)
7.30 to 8.00 a.m.	Breakfast	6	60
10.30 a.m.	Mid-morning	3	30
12.30 p.m.	School dinner	6	60
4.00 p.m.	Snack/tea	3	30
6.00 p.m.	Evening meal	6	60
8.00 to 9.00 p.m.	Bedtime	3	30

Give insulin before breakfast

			Carbohydrate (g)	
Breakfast	Milk 200 ml		10	
	Wholegrain cereal and/or fruit, two exchanges		20	
	Grilled bacon or ham or fish or egg (optional)		Nil	60
	Wholemeal bread, four exchanges		40	
	Margarine*/butter (use sparingly)		—	
Mid-morning	Milk 200 ml, e.g. school milk		10	30
	Fresh fruit and/or biscuits, two exchanges		20	
School dinner	Meat/cheese/fish/chicken		Nil	
	Wholemeal bread, four exchanges	As sandwiches or as a picnic tuck-box	40	
	Butter/margarine (use sparingly)		—	60
	'Free' vegetables or salad		Trace	
	Fresh fruit and/or natural yoghurt, two exchanges		20	
Snack/tea	Wholemeal bread or biscuits, two exchanges		20	
	Fruit, one exchange		10	30
	Margarine*/butter (use sparingly)		—	
Evening meal	Lean meat, chicken, fish		Nil	
	'Free' vegetables		Trace	
	Potatoes, three exchanges		30	60
	Baked beans, two exchanges		20	
	Fruit or dessert, one exchange		10	
Bedtime	Peanut butter/meat/cheese			
	Wholemeal bread, three exchanges	As sandwiches	30	30
	Butter/margarine* (use sparingly)			

* Use margarines high in PUFA.
To make this example suitable for twice-daily insulin, e.g. soluble insulin before breakfast and evening meal, extra carbohydrate could be given at breakfast and bedtime and the lunch and afternoon tea snack proportionally decreased.

in whom toddler 'food strikes' are relatively common, even in normal children, especially when the level of parental anxiety is great. As in normal children who refuse to eat, these episodes are best ignored, but guidance and practical advice are essential, and parents require a great deal of support at such time. Milk and savoury snack foods are particularly useful, rather than traditional meals. A lower intake of carbohydrate and higher intake of protein and fat may be desirable at such times. It is essential that uneaten carbohydrate be replaced with another food or drink of equal carbohydrate value, thus avoiding food battles and yet preventing hypoglycaemia. The type of carbohydrate intake is unimportant at such times.

In prolonged food refusal, or if the child is at risk of malnutrition, psychiatric advice with praise and reward behaviour modification techniques may be needed. Temporarily a period of 'free diet' may be applicable (Craig 1977) in order to reduce tension related to food.

School meals and social eating

The child should be taught to become as independent as possible by school age. Some supervision is essential, especially in junior and primary school. The diabetic is required to eat a set amount of carbohydrate at regular intervals, which will include mid-morning and lunch and possibly mid-afternoon snacks at school. The type of school dinner service provided varies from area to area. A suitable packed meal of sandwiches and fruit is the most appropriate unless the child can return home for lunch. The latter at first appears most appropriate but deprives the child of the 'social eating' which a meal at school provides, and is impractical if the school is some distance from the child's home or the mother goes out to work. Junior and primary schools rarely provide a choice of menu, therefore if the child is to have the meal provided the school meals organizer needs to be informed of the diet requirements. A positive attitude is essential, as the idea of 'no sugar and no sweets' is often already ingrained into adult personnel. The hardest thing to achieve is provision of enough of the right type of carbohydrate and ensuring that the carbohydrate is actually consumed. The child should have some idea of the amount of potato, baked beans, rolls, fruit, milk and even sausages and chips he is permitted, so that the first course of the meal can be incorporated into the diet plan. School puddings are usually not only high in refined carbohydrates but fluctuate enormously in their carbohydrate content, e.g. from fruit to treacle tart, the former too low in carbohydrate on its own, and the latter too high. A set number of carbohydrate exchanges as fruit and biscuits or yoghurt sent from home is recommended (with the chance of exchanging one or other for ice-cream or fruit when these are on the menu). Snack food for the mid-morning break and after school should also be provided by the parents in convenient items such as peanuts, fruit or digestive-type biscuits. Unsweetened school milk can be incorporated into the menu when provided. Snack time should be planned if possible to coincide with between-lesson breaks, but in the case of delay the child should eat his snack in an as 'matter of fact' way as possible in class.

The schoolteacher and school meal organizer should be informed of the diabetic's need for punctual snacks and meals, the risk and symptoms of hypoglycaemia and their prevention (*see* p. 140) so that the child is not delayed when a meal or snack is due. The teacher should be informed that apparent lack of co-operation on the part of a child with diabetes is most likely due to hypoglycaemia. The school should have an emergency supply of suitable foods for snacks, pre-games and treatment of hypoglycaemia.

Children who have diabetes should be encouraged to go out for meals and to parties, as eating out is an important part of social life and helps teach the child independence. Explanation to the adult responsible for the young child regarding meal arrangements is necessary. With co-operation and forethought suitable arrangements can be made. Egg on toast, cheese sandwiches, crisps or peanuts in small bags, semi-sweet biscuits and fruit are easily measured and are popular carbohydrate-containing foods. Sugar-free drinks can be supplied, and at parties small quantities of jelly and ice-cream 'treats' can be included. At parties the child should have adequate carbohydrate, as the extra excitement and exercise can precipitate hypoglycaemia. The psychological boost of a meal 'off diet' may occasionally be appropriate.

In restaurants and cafes simple foods can be selected, e.g. sandwiches, rolls, crisps or egg and chips, and the portions assessed, any excess being left. Made-up dishes with sauces should be avoided. Omelettes, grills, roasts and salads are all suitable; starters may include melon, tomato juice or avocado vinaigrette or prawn cocktail (no sauce); a small glass of pineapple or orange juice contains approximately 10 g carbohydrate, or the child may follow the American tradition and order iced water. Holidays when there is a choice menu pose little problem. Where there is a set menu a word to the waiter or glance at the menu in advance can be helpful without drawing undue attention to the diabetic.

Travel for diabetics requires some forethought. An insulin kit and some easily carried foods, cheese and biscuits and a can or two of sugar-free drinks, together with sugar cubes and sweetened drink in case of hypoglycaemia, should be kept in the hand-luggage in case of delays at airports, fog, traffic jams, closed motorway restaurants and breakdowns. Adjustment for international time-zone change may be necessary if travelling overseas, and a few extras should be carried to substitute for 'foreign foods' of unknown content. Extra carbohydrate intake or a reduction in the insulin dosage may be necessary to compensate for the extra activity undertaken on holidays, which includes sightseeing, sports, etc.

Picnics and outings require similar precautions with plenty of food and drinks for the whole day, including adequate to cover the additional needs of exercise (*see below*) as well as emergencies. An emergency food supply (e.g. kept in the car glove-box and replenished as soon as used) could contain packets of suitable biscuits, cans of sweetened drink with a small plastic measuring cup and packets of sugar cubes. Even 'key' self-opening small tins of meat or fish could be included in case of delayed meals.

EXERCISE

Regular exercise taken by diabetics appears to improve, and correlate with, the degree of metabolic control and will reduce the insulin requirements (Belton & Farquhar 1984). Some exercise should be included daily, except during periods of ketoacidosis, which should be corrected before particularly acute exercise is encouraged or taken (Sherwin & Koivisto 1981). Although exercise reduces blood glucose its effect is unpredictable, especially in children. Extra carbohydrate is recommended before exercising if more than the usual amount is anticipated.

Strenuous exercise is best avoided just before a meal is due. Games like football, tennis, squash or swimming lower the blood glucose quickly, and therefore sugar or refined carbohydrates (Table 5.2c) are needed beforehand, and possibly during and afterwards.

In prolonged exercise, such as long walks, a day at the seaside, a game of cricket or golf, the extra carbohydrate is better to be in the form of starch and high-fibre foods (Table 5.2a and b), as these foods slowly release glucose into the bloodstream.

The amount of extra carbohydrate for different activities will vary from child to child; an extra 20 g is recommended initially, but more may be required, for example hourly on a long hike or during a day at the seaside. As much as 40 to 60 g carbohydrate in addition to the daily prescription may be needed.

A blood glucose level taken after and/or during prolonged exercise will give a guide as to whether adequate extra carbohydrate has been taken, and the regimen can be adjusted subsequently.

HYPOGLYCAEMIA

Hypoglycaemia causes more anxiety to parents than it deserves. It usually results from a temporary excess of insulin, due to the dose given, delayed food intake, increased exercise or unusual exposure to cold such as wet, wind or inadequate clothing (Belton & Farquhar 1984).

Symptoms and signs of hypoglycaemia occur when the blood glucose level falls below 3 mmol/l. A blood glucose level will confirm if the signs are because of hypoglycaemia. It can be prevented in many but not all cases if additional carbohydrate is given appropriately before exercise and the dietary carbohydrate intake is arranged to cover the peak of insulin activity or time of recurrent hypoglycaemia attacks. Late meals and inadequate carbohydrate intake can also be causes of hypoglycaemia and can be prevented by carrying suitable carbohydrate snack foods to use if delays occur, e.g. in traffic hold-ups.

Parents and child need to know the features of hypoglycaemia, which include sweating, pallor, dizziness, restlessness at night or waking as if in a dream or a change of behaviour, e.g. tantrum or sudden quietness. Each patient with diabetes usually has the same symptoms of hypoglycaemia on repeated occasions.

Parents are frequently frightened by hypoglycaemia, especially if it occurs during the night when there may be a delay in recognition of the signs. However, measurable lasting damage is rare. It often helps if they can witness hypoglycaemia (mild) in their child during the initial stabilization in hospital. Schoolteachers, club leaders, etc. should be made aware of the possibility of hypoglycaemia, and its prevention and treatment. A child may not always recognize the symptoms, or may be incapable of co-operation and co-ordination in order to be able to help himself. A diabetic identity disc or bracelet should be worn at all times.

Hypoglycaemia is treated by giving carbohydrate in an easily absorbable, usually concentrated, form such as sugar, glucose or Lucozade, although any carbohydrate-containing food can be used in an emergency. A carbohydrate source, such as sugar cubes, should always be carried for the treatment of hypoglycaemia. 'If in doubt treat as hypoglycaemia' is a practical rule for inexperienced personnel who suspect the child of being hypoglycaemic. At least 10 g carbohydrate should be given immediately and repeated in 5 to 10 minutes if symptoms continue, e.g. 10 carbohydrate is contained in three sugar lumps or two teaspoons of glucose or sugar which can be given in a small drink or 60 ml Lucozade or 100 ml (sweetened) Coke, or 180 ml other fizzy drinks; glucose tablets, although easy to carry, are less practical as they crumble, are difficult to chew and one tablet usually contains only 3 g carbohydrate.

Severe hypoglycaemia (particularly if the child is unable to swallow) can be treated with an injection of glucagon which has the reverse action of insulin and is a secretion of the alpha-cells of the pancreas.

It is injected in the same way as insulin and parents can be taught how and when to use it. It liberates glucose from liver glycogen, resulting in a rise in blood sugar which brings the child around. As soon as the child has recovered sufficiently to swallow, oral glucose must be given, followed by a snack containing carbohydrate. Urgent medical help must be obtained if the child remains unconscious or does not immediately respond to treatment.

Spontaneous recovery from hypoglycaemia can occur and the blood glucose becomes normal; this should be remembered when evaluating the blood glucose and urinary glucose record charts and reported hypoglycaemia.

However, children may fake hypoglycaemia in order to gain attention or to get 'sweets', and this possibility should not be overlooked if the blood glucose taken at the time by parent or responsible adult does not suggest hypoglycaemia. Cheating with test results is also possible.

ILLNESS AND HYPERGLYCAEMIA

Hyperglycaemia in treated diabetics (blood glucose levels in excess of 12 mmol/l and may be in excess of 20 mmol/l) is usually associated with illness and may be accompanied by ketoacidosis. Urine tests will repeatedly indicate 2% or more sugar, often with positive acetone tests. Vomiting, nausea and abdominal pain may be present as a result of the ketoacidosis. Insulin must continue to be given, although the dose will probably need to be increased or supplemented with short-action insulin. Dietary carbohydrate should be continued or replaced with fluids of an equivalent carbohydrate content, as suggested in

Table 5.6 Replacement of carbohydrate in illness.

For example, if the meal to be replaced = 40 g carbohydrate, substitute one of the following;
  (a) 240 ml (8 oz) Lucozade. (Give as sips over an hour or two.)
or (b) 8 heaped tsp (40 g, 1⅓ oz) sugar dissolved in water and flavoured with lemon juice or diabetic squash.
or (c) 200 ml (8 oz) milk
  + 15 g (½ oz) drinking chocolate
  + 2 tsp (10 g, ⅓ oz) sugar
  + 1 digestive biscuit (15 g, ½ oz.)
or (d) 180 ml (6 oz) cream of tomato soup (ready to serve)
  + 40 g (1½ oz) white bread, may be toasted
  Butter/margarine.

Insulin should be continued or the dose temporarily increased, as indicated by blood glucose estimations.

Table 5.6. The foods listed in Table 5.2c are particularly useful at such times. Protein and fat intake can be ignored during short-term illness, and the diet is then reintroduced as tolerated when the appetite indicates. In cases of nausea or vomiting, Lucozade (60 ml [2 oz] = 10 g carbohydrate) or 'de-fizzed' sweetened Coke, dry ginger or Pepsi (100 ml [3½ oz] = 10 g carbohydrate) is most valuable, particularly if given as sips slowly over an hour or two. If persistent vomiting of carbohydrate replacements occurs, hospitalization is necessary.

Monitoring of diabetic control

The belief is growing that a steady state of normoglycaemia protects the diabetic from long-term complications. Control can be monitored by a number of parameters. The usual tests are blood and urinary sugars which indicate the fluctuation in day-to-day blood glucose levels and so indicate the need for daily adjustment to the treatment regimen. However it has become obvious that urine tests are not only messy and unsociable, especially for the teenager, but are incapable of adequately indicating to what extent a steady state of normoglycaemia has been achieved (Belton & Farquhar 1984). Blood glucose estimates give the best indication of the value at a particular time. Blood glucose profiles are essential during stabilization and home monitoring indicator sticks are now available with or without reflectance meters, e.g. BM-Test Glycemic*, Dextristix*. Some children will accept a daily blood glucose profile regimen, but blood testing can be traumatic for the young child. From about 10 years of age many children prefer blood to urine testing, or will accept a compromise of, say, three days per week of each. If the latter is the case one day of each routine should be at the weekend, on one weekday the tests could be taken before the three main meals, and the other weekday the tests taken about 1½ hours after meals, at bedtime and occasionally at 3 a.m. The blood collection can be made easier with the Mini-lancet*, Hypoguard*,

---

* BM-Test Glycemic. The Boehringer Corporation (London) Ltd, Southern Industrial Estate, Bracknell, Berks, RG12 4YS, *or* Bell Lanes, Lewes, East Sussex, BN7 1LG.
Dextristix. Ames and Miles Pharmaceuticals, Strawberry Hill, Newbury, Berks, RG13 1JA.
Autolet, Owen Mumford Ltd, Medical Division, Brook Hill, Woodstock, Oxon.
Hypoguard Ltd, Dock Lane, Melton, Woodbridge, Suffolk, IP12 1PE.
Mini-lancet. Clean Chemical Sweden, AB, S-781, 93 Borlänge, Sweden. UK agent, Hypoguard Ltd.

Autolet* or similar pricking device. It is essential that hands are warm to get an adequate drop of blood and should be washed before collecting the blood not only in the interests of hygiene, but in order to obtain a correct reading, as fingers contaminated with glucose from glucose tablets or glucose-loaded urine can interfere with the result.

Spontaneous monitoring of blood glucose is now possible with an in-dwelling sensor and spontaneous insulin administration from a reservoir. This is known as the closed-loop system or 'artificial pancreas'. However, this is very expensive and at present impractical for routine use in the majority.

Blood lipids and growth are used to give an idea of overall control on a long-term basis. Blood lipids are elevated at diagnosis but slowly return to normal once control is satisfactory. Continued hyperlipidaemia or poor growth indicates poor control (Starkey 1967, Court et al. 1978).

Haemoglobin A_1C is used as an index of diabetic control over the preceding few weeks, but care must be taken in comparing different results because of the difference in methodology and the reference range from different laboratories (Belton & Farquhar 1984).

Twenty-four hour fractional urine tests to measure total glucose and urea output in four-hourly periods by day and 12 hours overnight (Foman et al. 1974) give an indication of the total glucose loss and can be used occasionally as another parameter.

Control is not just a matter of blood glucose and insulin balance, as the body's response is dependent on a number of hormones which are interrelated. The effect of adrenaline release as a result of stress is well known, and this, as well as the hormonal response to hypoglycaemia seen in the Somogyi effect (Somogyi 1959), is related to blood glucose control. The diabetic child's behaviour can be either the result or the cause of poor control. Lack of co-operation is frequently due to hypoglycaemia, but diabetes can be used as a weapon against parents. Careful assessment of the facts is therefore essential. The seeming paradox of a normal blood glucose being found after a reported symptomatic hypoglycaemic attack may be the result of hormone activity normalizing blood glucose so that both facts are true.

Teaching of the diabetic regimen
Parents, and the child when he is old enough, need to be taught about diabetes in an initial and an ongoing programme. A team approach is a useful means of covering all aspects of the diabetic regimen (Paxinos & Ferguson 1978). Instruction should include the following details:

The diet
Insulin and how to give the injection,
Hypoglycaemia,
Exercise and the precautions necessary,
Blood glucose, urine sugar and acetone testing,
Hyperglycaemia and ketoacidosis implications,
When to contact the doctor for advice regarding insulin adjustment,
The need for diabetic identification to be worn at all times and the need to carry sugar for the treatment of hypoglycaemia.

It is ideal if the parents can 'live in' during any periods of hospitalization; this gives the opportunity of observing the regimen at first hand, while learning the details and theory. A specialist community nurse or health visitor can give valuable back-up support to the family at home. Some units have adequate community facilities so that even juvenile diabetics can be stabilized at home.

It should be remembered that the child will need to learn about his diabetes to become an independent adult, and should be encouraged to take responsibility for his regimen as soon as he is able, initially with parental supervision. At first this may be limited to the colour of the tests and counting diet exchanges, then coping with his own school dinner and later giving his own insulin injections.

Camps organized by the British Diabetic Association have proved a valuable training time for many young diabetics. The Association also produces various booklets for parents and children on diabetes and its treatment, and a regular magazine entitled *Balance*.

Complications

Short-term complications of hypoglycaemia, p. 140, and ketoacidosis with hyperglycaemia in association with infections, p. 141, are by far the commonest problems experienced by the child with juvenile diabetes mellitus and require alteration of diet and insulin regime albeit temporarily. Review of the regimen in order to prevent recurrence, and instruction regarding management, should be given as appropriate. The possibility of impotent insulin and over- or under-dosage of insulin must also be considered. Poor control over a period of time may deplete the number of insulin receptors available, but these can be made available again by effecting good control and by exercise. Psychological factors also play a part in causing recurrent ketoacidosis, especially in young adolescents (Belton & Farquhar 1984).

Temporary loss of visual acuity in ketoacidosis is due to osmotic pressure changes within the vitreous humour of the eye as a result of dehydration and may continue for some weeks.

The Somogyi (1959) effect of fluctuating blood glucose levels is well described, though the mechanism causing it has been disputed (Faber *et al.* 1980, Gale *et al.* 1980, Lyen *et al* 1980).

Long-term complications of retinopathy, nephropathy, peripheral and autonomic neuropathy and atherosclerosis and their aetiology have been the cause of endless debate and research (Belton & Farquhar 1984). There is increasing evidence that good control and maintenance of normoglycaemia is the best protection against the development of these complications. In those initially diagnosed in childhood or adolescence complications may occur as early as at 30 to 40 years of age. This has led to increasing pressure on children and their parents to achieve perfect control as represented by consistent normoglycaemia. Adverse emotional reactions in diabetic children can result. The professional team's role is to exert the long-term pressure required to obtain compliance with the minimum of disturbance, and thus achieve the goal of consistent normoglycaemia in their patients.

REFERENCES

BELTON N.R. & FARQUHAR J.W. (1984) Diabetes mellitus. In *Chemical Pathology and The Sick Child* (eds. Clayton B.E. & Round J.M.), pp. 265–95. Oxford: Blackwell Scientific Publications.

BRITISH DIABETIC ASSOCIATION (1980) The Nutrition Sub-committee of the Medical Advisory Committee. *Dietary Recommendations for Diabetics for the 1980s*. London: British Diabetic Association.

BRITISH DIABETIC ASSOCIATION (latest edition) *Carbohydrate Countdown*. London: British Diabetic Association.

BRUNZELL J.D., LERNER R.L., PORTE D. & BIERMAN E.I. (1974) Effects of a fat free high carbohydrate diet on diabetic subjects with fasting hyperglycaemia. *Diabetes* 23, 138.

COURT J.M., DUNLOP M. & HILL M. (1978) A study of plasma-lipid concentration in diabetic children. *J. hum. Nutr.* 32, No. 4, 285–8.

CRAIG O. (1977) *Childhood Diabetes and its Management. Postgraduate Paediatrics Series* (ed. Apley J.). London: Butterworths.

EDITORIAL (1976) Control of diabetes and insulin antibodies. *Brit. med. J.* 1, 484.

ESTRICH D., RAVNICK A., SCHLERF G., FUKAYAMA C. & KINSELL L. (1967) Effects of co-ingestion of fat and protein upon carbohydrate induced hyperglycaemia. *Diabetes* 16, 232.

FABER O.K., BINDER C. & LAURITZEN T. (1980) In search of the Somogyi effect. *Lancet* 2, 701.

FARQUHAR J.W. (1979) Juvenile diabetes mellitus: possibility of prevention. *Arch. Dis. Childh.* 54, 569–80.

FOMAN B.H., GOLDSTEIN P.S. & GENERAL M. (1974) Management of juvenile diabetes mellitus: usefulness of 24 hour fractional quantitative urine glucose. *Pediatrics* 53, 257.

FRANCIS D.E.M. (1984) Should we be advising low fat diets in UK? *Health Visitor* 57, 145–6.

GALE E.A.M., KURTZ A.B. & TATTERSALL R.B. (1980) In search of the Somogyi effect. *Lancet* 2, 279–82.

GAMBLE D.R. (1980) The epidemiology of insulin-dependent diabetes with particular reference to the relationship of virus infection to its etiology. *Epidemiol. Rev.* 2, 49–70.

HABER G.B., HEATON K.W., MURPHY D. & BURROUGHS L.F. (1977) Depletion and disruption of dietary fibre. *Lancet* 2, 679.

HIRATA Y., NAKAMURA Y. & KUKU M. (1970) Characteristics of the treatment of diabetes in Japan. In *Diabetes Mellitus in Asia 1970* (eds. Tsuji S. & Wada M.), pp. 216–20. Amsterdam: Excerpta Medica.

JENKINS D.J.A., TAYLOR R.H., NINEHAM R., GOFF D.V., BLOOM S.R., SARSON D. & ALBERTI K.G.M.M. (1979) Combined use of guar and acarbose in reduction of postprandial glycaemia. *Lancet* 2, 924–7.

JENKINS D.J.A., WOLEVER T.M.S., TAYLOR R.H., BARKER H.M., FIELDEN H. & JENKINS A.L. (1980) Effect of guar crispbread with cereal products and leguminous seeds on blood glucose concentrations of diabetics. *Brit med. J.* 281, 1248–50.

KAUFMAN R.P., ASSAL J.P., SOELDNER J.S., WILMSHURST E.G., LEMAIRE J.R., GLEASON R.E. & WHITE P. (1975) Plasma lipid levels in diabetic children. Effect of diet restricted in cholesterol and saturated fat. *Diabetes* 24, 672–9.

KEEN H. & THOMAS B. (1978) Diabetes mellitus. In *Nutrition in the Clinical Management of Disease* (eds. Dickerson J.W.T. & Lee H.A.), pp. 118–43. London: Edward Arnold.

KINMONTH A.L. & BAUM J.D. (1982) Disorders of carbohydrate metabolism. In *Textbook of Paediatric Nutrition*, 2nd Edition (eds. McLaren D.S. & Burman D.), pp. 266–84. Edinburgh: Churchill Livingstone.

KOCHHAR S.P. & MATSUI T. (1984) Essential fatty acids and *trans* content of some oils, margarine and other food fats. *Food Chemistry* 13, 84–101.

LYEN K.R., FINEGOLD D. & BAKER L. (1980) In search of the Somogyi effect *Lancet* 2, 700–1.

MÄKI M., HÄLLSTRÖM O., HUUPONEN T., VISIKARI T. & VISAKORP J.K. (1984) Increased prevalence of coeliac disease in diabetes. *Arch. Dis. Childh.* 59 (8), 739.

MANN J.I. (1984) What carbohydrate foods should diabetics eat? *Brit. med. J.* 288, 1025–26.

OAKLEY W.G., PYKE M. & TAYLOR K.W. (1975) *Diabetes and its Management*, 2nd Edition. Oxford: Blackwell Scientific Publications.

PAXINOS R. & FERGUSON R. (1978) Juvenile diabetes—a team approach. *J. hum. Nutr.* 32, 4, 294–6.

POND H. (1973) Diabetes mellitus. In *Recent Advances in Paediatrics* (eds. Gairdner D. & Hull D.), p. 317. Edinburgh: Churchill Livingstone.

SHERWIN R.S. & KOIVESTO V. (1981) Keep in step: does exercise benefit the diabetic? *Diabetologia* **20**, 84–6.

SIMPSON R.W., MANN J.I., EATON J., CARTER R. & HOCKADAY T.D.R. (1979) High carbohydrate diets and insulin dependent diabetes. *Brit. med. J.* **2**, 523.

SOMOGYI M. (1959) Exacerbation of diabetes by excess insulin action. *Amer. J. Med.* **265**, 169.

STEEL J.M., MITCHELL D. & PRESCOTT R.L. (1983) Comparison of the glycaemic effect of fructose, sucrose and starch containing mid-morning snacks in insulin dependent diabetics. *Human Nutrition: Applied Nutrition* 37 A, No. 1, 3–8.

STARKEY G. (1967) Growth pattern in juvenile diabetes. *Acta Paediat. Suppl.* **177**, 80.

TCHOBROUTSKY G. (1978) Relation of diabetic control to development of microvascular complications. *Diabetologia* **15**, 143.

THOMAS L.H., JONES P.R., WINTER J.A. & SMITH H. (1981) Hydrogenated oils and fats: the presence of chemically modified fatty acids in human adipose tissue. *Amer. J. clin. Nutr.* **34**, 872–86.

THOMPSON R.G., HAYFORD J.T. & DANWEY M.M. (1978) Glucose and insulin response to diet. Effect of variations in sources and amount of carbohydrate. *Diabetes* **27** (10), 1020–6.

WAHLQUIST M.L., WILMSHURST E.G., RICHARDSON E.N. (1978) The effect of chain length on glucose absorption and the related metabolic response. *Amer. J. clin. Nutr.* **31**, (11) 1998–2001.

CHAPTER 6

Nutrition for children with cystic fibrosis

Cystic fibrosis is a multiorgan disorder characterized by chronic pulmonary disease, pancreatic insufficiency, liver dysfunction and abnormally elevated sweat electrolytes (Kopel 1972, McCollum & Harries 1977, Wilckens *et al.* 1983). The basic defect remains unknown, but the manifestations of the disease can be accounted for by a generalized disorder of the exocrine and mucus-secreting glands. The clinical and pathological features of cystic fibrosis (CF) are a direct consequence of obstruction of the small ducts by mucus.

It is primarily a Caucasian disease with an incidence of approximately one in 2000 births in England with a carrier frequency of 5% and is transmitted as an autosomal recessive trait (Danks *et al.* 1965). It is the commonest inborn error of metabolism, other than familial hypercholesterolaemia, requiring dietary modification, and is the commonest cause of pancreatic insufficiency and possibly malabsorption in children (Robinson & Norman 1975).

Compared with other organic substances the fucose content of glycoproteins obtained from the excretions of the secretory glands is increased compared to normal subjects. The sodium, chloride and sometimes potassium concentrations in sweat are increased due to defective ductular reabsorption. It has been suggested that essential fatty acid deficiency commonly seen in CF may represent a primary abnormality (Chase 1976).

Chronic pulmonary disease with secondary respiratory infections usually dominates the clinical picture and determines the ultimate prognosis. Management of the respiratory disease is therefore of prime importance and is dealt with by others (Mearns 1974, Anderson & Goodchild 1976, Hodson *et al.* 1983, Wilckens *et al.* 1983, Lawson 1984). It is not considered further in this text.

The nutritional state of the child, however, does affect the course of the disease; the child needs to be well-nourished before control of infection can be really effective and, conversely, chest infection must be reduced before good nutrition can be achieved.

The nutritional disturbances may arise as a consequence of malabsorption and/or result from inadequate intake in the presence of increased metabolic demands that occur as a consequence of the respiratory disease (Silk 1984).

Over the years, there has been improvement in the morbidity and mortality of CF (Robinson & Norman 1975, Anderson & Goodchild 1976, Phelan & Landau 1979, Wilckens *et al.* 1983). Various assessments of survival suggest that 80% of patients reach their 19th year (Shwachman & Holsclaw 1969) and other workers suggest that 70% reach their 17th year (Robinson & Norman 1975). The quality of life of survivors is also important. Early diagnosis and treatment are very important factors in the prevention of lung damage and in the ultimate prognosis (Wilchens *et al.* 1983) so that intensive birth-screening programmes should be seriously considered now that reliable techniques (Heeley *et al.* 1982) are available. General improvement in living standards may be partially responsible for the improved prognosis (Brimblecombe & Chamberlain 1973).

Clinical features

A wide spectrum of symptoms occurs in patients with CF and the child's appearance may vary from severely malnourished to a healthy one (McCollum & Harries 1977). Chronic recurrent respiratory infections may be the presenting feature in some patients, and in 15 to 20% there may be no initial evidence of pancreatic dysfunction. In others gastrointestinal symptoms may precede respiratory disease, but by two years of age approximately 75% of patients have developed pulmonary symptoms.

Meconium ileus in the newborn period is the presenting factor in about 5% of patients (Chazalette *et al.* 1977). This is a serious condition of neonatal intestinal obstruction requiring either prompt surgery or treatment with gastrograffin enema under X-ray control (Anderson & Goodchild 1976). The problems of infants following surgery are similar to those of any infant with gut resection or multiple malabsorption (*see* Chapter 1).

If sodium intake is inadequate, sodium depletion, with hypovolaemia, dehydration and shock, can occur in hot weather, with pyrexia, or due to electrolyte losses in sweat. The routine use of low-solute milks in infants and discouragement of highly salted foods for the general population heightens the necessity for awareness of this problem in patients with CF.

Gastrointestinal manifestations
Weight gain and growth are frequently retarded in untreated patients, despite a good appetite; there is abdominal protuberance, lack of subcutaneous fat, poor muscle tone and pronounced steatorrhoea, with the passage of a number of oily, large, bulky, foul-smelling stools (Kopel 1972). Rectal prolapse or intestinal obstruction in the older child due to faecal impaction and meconium ileus in the newborn are also seen in some patients (Anderson & Goodchild 1976, Hodson *et al.* 1983).

Pancreatic dysfunction
Patients with CF show a major and progressive loss of pancreatic function in approximately 80% of cases; 10% show partial loss, while the remaining 10% show little evidence of malfunction (Anderson & Goodchild 1976), although impairment of water and bicarbonate secretion by the pancreas may still exist (Kopel 1972). The low level of trypsin is the most striking finding in the analysis of the pancreatic juice from patients with CF, as well as the reduced volume and low bicarbonate ion content. Faecal losses of fat and nitrogen are considerable in untreated patients due to the lack of pancreatic enzyme lipase required for the hydrolysis of fat, trypsin for the digestion of protein to small peptides and amino acids and amylase for the hydrolysis of starch (Table 1.1).

Hypoalbuminaemia can occur as a result of the losses due to malabsorption of protein and the increased requirements of nitrogen and energy due to catabolism. It is sometimes seen with associated oedema and anaemia in infants or in association with haemodilution due to liver or heart failure. Hypoalbuminaemia has been particularly noted when infants with CF are fed soya milk formulae (Torstenson *et al.* 1970) but also occurs with cow's milk feeds (Harries & Muller 1971).

Degradation of unabsorbed protein by endogenous bacteria in the large intestine may result in the formation of undesirable products such as phenolic acids which may then be absorbed (Seakins *et al.* 1970,

Dolan *et al.* 1970). Analysis of the faeces shows a heavy pattern of amino acids and related compounds which can be directly related to the type and amount of protein in the diet.

Fat and nitrogen balances indicate that pancreatic replacement therapy decreases fat and nitrogen excretion; stool bulk and number are decreased and the child's weight gain is improved (Gibbons R. S. 1969).

Loss of fat-soluble vitamins due to steatorrhoea gives rise to deficiencies. Vitamin E blood levels in children with CF are frequently reduced (Harries & Muller 1969) and deficiency has been reported (Bye *et al.* 1985). Vitamin A deficiency with xerophthalmia and raised intracranial pressure has been reported. Demineralization of bone has been noted even though serum calcium and phosphorus levels are normal, probably caused by malabsorption, although calcium balance studies were not conclusive. Vitamin K deficiency is occasionally observed and may lead to hypoprothrombinaemia and bleeding (Muller & Harries 1969). The effectiveness of water-miscible fat-soluble vitamin supplements has been demonstrated by Harries & Muller (1971) and supplements are now routinely advised.

Recurrent abdominal pain of varying severity and location is not uncommon. Constipation can occur, and may be accompanied by colicky pain and vomiting (Kopel 1972), and is known as meconium ileus equivalent (Anderson & Goodchild 1976, Dodge 1983). The faeces tend to become solid at a point in the gut where they should be liquid. These firm and sticky (adherent) faecal masses will usually be passed normally, but often they can be helped by either temporarily decreasing pancreatin supplements or increasing the fat content of the diet whilst continuing pancreatin. N-acetylcysteine and Tween 80 orally or Tween 80 as a gastrograffin enema has been used to relieve symptoms (Kopel 1972). Flatulence can be troublesome in some patients. The possibility of pancreatitis (and appendicitis) as a cause of pain in these patients should not be overlooked (Anderson & Goodchild 1976).

Small intestinal mucosal function
There is good evidence that the small intestinal structure is abnormal. Mucosal dysfunction may contribute to the malabsorption (McCollum & Harries 1977). The normal microvilli from small intestinal biopsies have been reported to be covered with a coarse fibrillar substance, probably mucus (Freye *et al.* 1964).

Disacchariduria and reduced mucosal lactase in patients have been documented and implicate an intestinal factor (Gibbons I. S. E. 1969). Lactose intolerance of clinical significance is rare but occasionally occurs, and is more common than sucrose intolerance. Infants who have needed intestinal surgery for meconium ileus may acquire a temporary disaccharide intolerance to lactose and sucrose (*see* Chapter 1).

Reduced L-anyl-L-phenylalanine hydrolase activity has been reported in patients with CF (Morin *et al.* 1976).

The coexistence of coeliac disease with CF is rare and is probably a chance association, but has been documented (Hide & Burman 1969), and has been seen in a small number of patients in the author's clinic.

Disturbance of bile salt metabolism
There is defective ileal absorption of bile salts and consequently increased faecal losses of bile salts (Weber *et al.* 1973, Goodchild *et al.* 1975). These abnormalities are reduced by pancreatic supplements or treatment with a low-fat diet (McCollum & Harries 1977). The concentration of bile salts in duodenal fluid is reduced, with a marked increase in the ratio of glycine:taurine conjugated bile salts (McCollum *et al.* 1976). These abnormalities can be anticipated to interfere with the formation of bile salt micelles, impair solubilization of dietary fat and fat-soluble vitamins, and interfere with vitamin E metabolism (Harries & Muller 1971, McCollum & Harries 1977). Free bile salts enhance the colonic absorption of dietary oxalate which may explain the hyperoxaluria which also occurs in patients with cystic fibrosis who may therefore have a risk of renal oxalate stones in later life (Ogilvie *et al.* 1976).

Liver involvement
The incidence of hepatic cirrhosis increases with age (Kopel 1972, Anderson & Goodchild 1976, Hodson, *et al.* 1983) and may result in liver failure with portal hypertension and ascites. Jaundice is unusual. The factors responsible for liver involvement remain obscure. A low-fat diet, usually in the range of 20 to 30% dietary energy, i.e. 25 to 50 g daily for children, is indicated with a high energy and high protein intake. If portasystemic encephalopathy and/or hyperammonaemia due to liver failure is present, protein intake must be reduced temporarily and monitored subsequently (*see* Chapters 8 and 10). A very high carbohydrate intake with some MCT supplements is indicated to achieve an adequate energy intake. Moderate salt restriction may be recommended if ascites are present, but careful clinical observation and monitoring of electrolytes is essential to ensure sodium depletion does not occur from sweat losses.

Glycosuria and diabetes
Diabetes is a well-recognized associated disorder which is assumed to be secondary to pancreatic islet cell destruction. It appears to be similar to the late-onset adult type rather than the classical juvenile diabetes (Anderson & Goodchild 1976). Many patients have glucose intolerance for several years prior to the development of clinical diabetes. They may show glycosuria but ketosis is rare. The number of patients who require treatment is increasing. Oral hypoglycaemic agents are useful, though insulin may be required in the older patient (*see* Chapter 5 regarding diabetes mellitus). A nutritionally adequate diet is essential, as is adequate pancreatin supplementation for optimal absorption. The diet should include 50 to 70% energy from carbohydrates with adequate total protein (15 to 20% energy) and 30 to 35% energy from fat sources selectively high in polyunsaturated fatty acids (PUFA), with sufficient total dietary energy to permit growth and maintain weight in the normal range for age. High-fibre foods are not tolerated well by patients with CF and therefore mixed meals incorporating protein foods with refined carbohydrates (starches and sucrose) should be used as an acceptable means of avoiding post-prandial blood glucose peaks in these patients (Steel *et al.* 1983).

Diagnosis

To make the diagnosis of CF there should be evidence of pancreatic insufficiency and/or pulmonary involvement, together with a sweat sodium in excess of 70 mmol/l in an adequate volume of sweat (more than 100 mg) on at least two separate collections, performed by a laboratory which has experience in the technique (McCollum & Harries 1977, Anderson & Goodchild 1976). A blood-spot immunotrypsin test has proved a reliable additional test in confirming the diagnosis (Heeley *et al.* 1982).

Various screening programmes to detect CF in the newborn are now available (Prosser *et al.* 1974, Heeley *et al.* 1982, Wilckens *et al.* 1983). As yet there is no routine test to distinguish carriers of the abnormal gene nor antenatal detection of the affected fetus.

The profound effect on both family and child of a diagnosis of CF, which is a life-threatening disease, necessitates care in establishing the correct diagnosis, and subsequently appropriate genetic counselling.

Treatment

Since the basic abnormality has not been defined, and since clinical manifestations vary, management will differ from patient to patient according to their symptoms. The aim of treatement is to prevent pulmonary obstruction and infections and to maintain satisfactory growth and nutrition. The major cause of morbidity and mortality in patients with CF is due to the pulmonary manifestations. The state of nutrition depends on both the control of the pulmonary disease and the malabsorption. Specific nutritional deficiencies can occur and growth failure is common (Chase *et al.* 1979, Shepherd *et al.* 1983, Silk 1984). Lapey *et al.* (1974) found that growth failure and the state of nutrition correlated more closely with the degree of pulmonary disease than with the degree of pancreatic insufficiency. The effect of infection, with subsequent periods of catabolism, often at frequent intervals, and the progressive pulmonary insufficiency resulting in oxygen lack, alter the metabolism and utilization of essential nutrients (Anderson & Goodchild 1976). During infections a poor appetite, and nutrient losses due to faecal, sputum and sweat losses, together with the increased demands of catabolism, result in weight loss and growth failure (Kraemer *et al.* 1978). In general, the younger the child and the better the state of the lungs, the better the nutritional status and growth. After the age of eight years, a progressive decline in growth rate compared to normal was reported by Berry *et al.* (1975), whereas the children under eight years maintained weight one standard deviation below the mean. The poor growth was associated with low concentrations of serum albumin and urea nitrogen. Similar findings were reported by Yassa *et al.* (1978), but in their patients both height and weight progressively declined with age in the older children. Puberty is delayed and thereafter growth tends to deviate more dramatically from normal, which is partly because of the delayed puberty but also because clinical deterioration often occurs at this age (Silk 1984).

ENZYME REPLACEMENT THERAPY

Except for the 10 to 15% of patients who have normal pancreatic function enzyme replacement therapy is indicated. Pancreatin preparations are normally extracts of hog pancreas containing lipase, amylase and trypsin (protease). Some also contain proteolytic enzymes from plant origin and bile salts. A variety of products are available in different forms and strengths to suit individual needs (Table 6.1). The basic form is a powder, either loose or in premeasured capsules, which should normally be opened and the contents only consumed.

The degree of steatorrhoea and azotorrhoea and the response to replacement therapy varies widely from patient to patient, but generally speaking fat and nitrogen excretion are improved, but are not completely normal, with pancreatin supplementation. This may be related to the instability of the administered enzymes in the acidic environment of the stomach and duodenum, as well as to impaired micellar solubilization of the products of lipolysis (Anderson & Goodchild 1976, McCollum *et al.* 1976). Enteric-coated granules and tablets theoretically overcome the disadvantage of the enzyme instability compared to powdered pancreatin preparations. Enteric coating on tablets and granules should be light to ensure optimal release of the enzymes (Anderson & Goodchild 1976). The duodenal juice of the patient with CF is usually in the range of pH 6·5 to 7·5 and such pH may inhibit enzyme activity. It is for these reasons that some patients benefit from sodium bicarbonate supplements. It is also recommended that pancreatin should not be given on an empty stomach, but rather during a meal or between the courses of a meal when the food acts as a buffer to the stomach acidity. Some workers have used cimetidine to improve digestion (Cox *et al.* 1979).

Few clinical trials comparing different pancreatin preparations are reported in the literature. One trial comparing Pancrex and Nutrizym showed little difference between these preparations regarding their ability to control steatorrhoea (Goodchild *et al.* 1975). Newer pancreatin preparations (Pancrease and Creon) are becoming available which improve absorption and allow a higher fat and energy intake, thus improving growth (Parsons *et al.* 1980).

To achieve optimal absorption of nutrients it is important that pancreatin actively mixes with the food and must, therefore, be taken with all meals and snacks. The enteric-coated preparations should be swallowed whole. The powder or content of capsules can be mixed with a little water or feed, and given by spoon. In the case of babies, it is given immediately before or halfway through the feed. In older children it is mixed with a little fluid or with items such as jam or honey (Francis 1979) and taken during the meal. Once mixed, it should be taken within one hour as the mixture is an excellent bacterial medium. As pancreatin curdles milk and gives an unpleasant taste and appearance to food, it is not recommended that it be mixed in feeds or sprinkled on food (Anderson & Goodchild 1976). For convenience sometimes the use of two different pancreatin preparations has practical advantages, e.g. tablets for use with school lunch, powder or capsules for a more flexible dose being used at home. Pancreatin preparations have an unusual taste and smell, not unlike protein hydrolysates, and many children take them with difficulty. In these patients the enteric-coated tablets and granules are particularly useful, provided that they can be swallowed. They are taken with the meals and snacks.

The dose of pancreatin prescribed for the child should be adequate to achieve optimal absorption of nutrients and should not be regarded as fixed; parents can be taught to adjust the dose with the type of meal or snack, and in particular its fat content. Dietary treats, birthdays and special occasions should be permitted, but will probably need a larger dose of pancreatin to cover the extra fat and starch content. A small ($\frac{1}{2}$) dose of pancreatin is required with snacks of low fat or starch content; none is required when sweets, candy, sugary drinks and/or fruit are taken alone.

Normal stools, even with large doses of pancreatin, may not be achieved, and provided growth is adequate, and stool bulk, consistency and odour are at an acceptable level, the dose need not be increased further. However, a change to a different pancreatin preparation should be considered, particularly if growth retardation is a feature.

There is no contraindication to large doses of pancreatin except for the rare occurrence of hyperuricosuria after extremely high doses. Particularly in infants, pancreatin may cause localized perioral and perianal irritation and soreness. The use of a local barrier cream is helpful.

In rare cases, pancreatin powder can cause wheezing in sensitive persons, including members of the patient's family, in which case tablets or granules should be used rather than the powder.

NUTRITION IN CYSTIC FIBROSIS

Adequate nutrition is important for both health and normal growth. Many children with CF are in a chronic state of catabolic stress and/or starvation (Chase *et al.* 1979, Shepherd *et al.* 1983) and growth failure is common (Silk 1984).

There is now strong evidence to show that protein–energy malnutrition decreases immune function and predisposes to the risk of infection (Dowd & Heatley 1984). In patients with CF decreased immunocompetence and infection coexist. Specific nutritional de-

ficiencies occur not only prior to diagnosis, but subsequently in treated patients (Chase *et al.* 1979, Bye *et al.* 1985), and a number of these deficiencies are related to poor growth and impaired immunity. This is true for zinc (Dowd & Heatley 1984), and impaired immunity has been related to deficiency of pyridoxine (Axelrod & Trakatellis 1964), vitamin A (Bhaskaram & Reddy 1975) and vitamin C (Neumann *et al.* 1975). Since immunity is impaired in CF (Raeburn 1977) and there are severe and repeated respiratory infections which together with resultant lung damage are directly related to ultimate prognosis, an aggressive approach to nutrition, in order to maintain or improve nutritional status and growth, is rational. There have been a number of reports of nutritional repletion in order to improve immunity in CF (Mullin & Kirkpatrick 1981, Shepherd *et al.* 1980). The aim of dietetic management should be to provide optimal nutrition at all times, both as a prevention of impaired immunity and growth failure (Farrell *et al.* 1984), and, by nutritional support, as repletion nutrition in those in whom poor nutritional status occurs.

Protein

The child with CF should have adequate protein (and energy) intake for growth. Table 6.2 gives suggested intakes, but these must be adjusted individually. Children with CF have an increased need for protein due to malabsorption, and extra protein intake is needed during episodes of catabolism. To overcome malabsorption a higher intake is necessary to increase net protein absorption.

Protein is not utilized for growth unless adequate energy intake is achieved; thus the protein becomes an expensive form of energy. The protein intake may be higher than some children from low-income groups receive, but can usually easily be met by including foods high in protein (e.g. meat) at two to three meals daily, and 500 to 1000 ml (approximately 1 to 2 pints) of milk, full-fat, reduced-fat or skimmed, or occasionally an appropriate milk substitute (e.g. MCT 'filled' milk, MCT Pepdite, Portagen, Pregestimil, Flexical or Triosorbin [Table 7.9]), is indicated. Homogenized and goat's milks are usually suitable, if the child is on Creon or Pancrease.

'Filled' milks such as 'Five Pints', Coffee-mate, and Compliment are unsuitable as they contain fat; as it is not butterfat they are labelled 'non-milk fat'. Ice-creams all contain fat and are best reserved for treats two or three times per week.

Low-fat yoghurt (natural and fruit-flavoured) and

Table 6.1   Pancreatin supplements for use in cystic fibrosis.

Product	Dose as recommended by manufacturer	Theoretical dose equal to 1 × 5 ml teaspoon Pancrex V Forte Powder	Enzyme activity
Pancreatin BNF 1978		—	Protease, 1400 units Lipase, 20 000 units Amylase, 24 000 units } per g
Pancrex V Powder (Paines & Byrne Ltd) 1 g, i.e. 1 level 5 ml teaspoon	For neonates—100 mg/kg/feed initially. For young children—0·5 to 2 g per meal	—	Free protease, 1400 BP units Lipase, 25 000 BP units Amylase, 30 000 BP units } per g
Pancrex V Forte Tablets (delayed-release coating), three tablets equivalent to 1 g Pancrex V Powder	For older children and adults 2 to 6 tablets per meal. Tablets should not be chewed.	3	Free protease, 330 BP units Lipase, 5600 BP units Amylase, 5000 BP units } per tablet
Pancrex V Capsules '340 mg'	For young children—content of 2 to 5 capsules per meal. (*Do not* sprinkle on food or allow whole capsules to be taken.)	3	Free protease, 430 BP units Lipase, 8000 BP units Amylase, 9000 BP units } per capsule
Pancrex V Capsules '125 mg'	For infants—content of 2 to 4 capsules per feed. (*Do not* sprinkle on food or allow whole capsules to be taken.)	8	Free protease, 160 BP units Lipase, 2950 BP units Amylase, 3300 BP units } per capsule
Pancrex V Capsules '62·5 mg'	Use as appropriate when infant on small frequent feeds, e.g. two-hourly.	16	Free protease, 87·5 BP units Lipase, 1562·5 BP units Amylase, 1875 BP units } per capsule
Nutrizym (Merck) Sugar-coated tablets (Each tablet has an enteric-coated pancreatin core and a shell of bromelains. The bromelains—proteolytic enzymes—are active within the pH range 3 to 8.)	1 to 2 tablets or more with meals.	3	Protease, 400 BP units Lipase, 9000 BP units Amylase, 9000 BP units Bromelain, 50 mg Ox bile, 30 mg } per tablet
Cotazym Capsules* (Organon Labs Ltd)	Content of up to 6 capsules/day. (*Do not* sprinkle on food or allow whole capsules to be taken.)	3	Protease, 500 BP units Lipase, 14 000 BP units Amylase, 10 000 BP units } per capsule
Pancrease (Ortho-Cilag) Enteric-coated microspheres in hard gelatin capsules	1 to 2 during each meal, 1 with snacks. The capsules can be opened and the microspheres taken with a drink or in a spoonful of soft foods not requiring chewing.	4 to 6	Protease, 330 BP units Lipase, 5000 BP units Amylase, 2900 BP units } per capsule

Table 6.1 *continued*

Product	Dose as recommended by manufacturer	Theoretical dose equal to 1 × 5 ml teaspoon Pancrex V Forte Powder	Enzyme activity	
Creon (Duphar) Small pancreatic pellets in enteric coating as a gelatin capsule.	1 to 3 capsules per meal. Capsules taken whole or the contents taken similarly to Pancrease.	2 to 3	Protease, 210 BP units Lipase, 8000 BP units Amylase, 9000 BP units	per capsule

* Cotazym B is rarely suitable for children with cystic fibrosis due to the low enzyme content (5400 units lipase).

Pancreatin powder, if mixed with liquid or feeds, should be used within one hour.

It is optimal *not* to give pancreatin on an empty stomach, so the dose given during a meal/feed is preferable, e.g. between the first and second course, mixed with a spoonful of jam or honey or taken with a drink during the meal.

Pancreatin should be given with *all* meals and snacks other than fruit, juices or boiled sweets.

Table 6.2 Protein and energy suggested intakes for children with cystic fibrosis (per kg per day).

Age In years	Protein (g)	Energy* Minimum		High	
		kJ	kcal	kJ	kcal
0 to 1	3 to 4 (max. 6)	540 to 420	130 to 100	840	200
1 to 3	4 to 3	420 to 375	100 to 90	630	150
3 to 10	3 to 2·5	335 to 300	80 to 70	420	100
Teenage	2·5 to 1·5	300 to 200	70 to 45	335	80

* At least normal recommended intakes for age rather than weight should be encouraged in children who are underweight.

cottage cheese are excellent low-fat sources of protein.

Meat, chicken, turkey, white fish and shellfish, eggs and cheese are high in protein. The author suggests two serves per day for toddlers and thereafter try and include three serves daily. Visible fat should be removed, and normally frying should be avoided, unless PUFA oil is used. It is recommended that casseroles, mince and stews are cooked in advance and chilled to remove the fat before reheating. Chicken and turkey are particularly low in fat. Pork, duck, goose, paté and oxtail are high-fat meats and are not advisable, though some hams and lean pork are suitable. Egg-yolk, cheeses and fatty fish like sardines and kippers are all higher in fat than lean meat and should be used with an increased dose of pancreatin. Several low-fat cheeses (Tendale and Shape) are now available.

Textured vegetable protein, Protoveg and pulses (peas and beans) are low in fat and useful cheaper proteins which can be used instead of meat occasion-ally or mixed with meat in mince, casseroles and stews. They should be soaked and cooked well till tender, but should not entirely replace fresh meat. They contain fibre and starch and can cause flatulence, so large quantities are not recommended. This makes it difficult to achieve adequate nutrition and growth for cystic fibrosis children on a vegetarian diet.

Energy

The need for dietary energy is greater in children with CF than in normal children, and may be 50 or even 90% above the theoretical requirement for age and actual weight. Energy requirement should always be calculated on expected weight for age, rather than actual weight, in patients with CF.

Provided protein and energy requirements are met, and malabsorption is controlled with pancreatin, adequate weight gain should result. When well, the child's appetite is usually good. The provision of adequate energy intake can be a problem, especially when the child is unwell, and appetite poor (see p. 157).

Fat

Dietary restriction of fat is an area of controversy, and opinion varies from strict low-fat diet to no restriction at all. The amount of steatorrhoea is individual and depends on the degree to which steatorrhoea and bile salt losses are controlled by pancreatin (Harries & Muller 1969, Cox *et al.* 1979). Fat provides dietary energy, fat-soluble vitamins and essential fatty acids, concentrates energy density and permits a certain degree of variety. The degree of steatorrhoea is dependent not on dietary intake of fat but on residual lipase and colipase activity. The proportion of fat absorbed remains constant irrespective of intake, and therefore losses can be compensated for by either an increase intake with resultant large, oily stools, or reduced intake with subsequent risk of low energy intake. Fat tolerance may deteriorate during infections. The pancreatin dose should be adjusted to minimize faecal losses.

A normal diet usually contains 10 to 15% energy from protein, 45 to 55% from carbohydrate and 30 to 50% from fat, the latter in infants. In the child on the older type of pancreatin preparation, fat intake usually needs to be restricted to about 30% energy intake, but should be as generous as possible. Those on Creon or Pancrease usually tolerate a normal to high fat intake. The occasional patient needs no restriction, as pancreatic enzyme activity is normal. Over-restriction of fat decreases energy intake which may be detrimental and is unnecessary (Macdonald 1984). The energy deficit must be replaced with an increased carbohydrate, and to some extent protein, intake.

If a reduced fat intake is necessary, a diet permitting lean meat, fish, egg, cheese, cereals, bread, fruit and vegetables and milk (reduced 2% fat) with the omission of visible fats and fried foods is advised. Either a low-fat spread or sparing use of, preferably, a margarine high in polyunsaturated fatty acids (PUFA) is permitted.

Essential fatty acids may be important in CF (Chase 1976, Hubbard 1980, Crawford *et al.* 1984), as a low plasma level of linoleic acid is commonly found. The diet should not be so low in fat as to be deficient in essential fatty acids. As fat is poorly absorbed it is important to bear this in mind by providing in the diet a generous proportion of fat as PUFA, especially linoleic acid. Dodge *et al.* (1976) reported essential fatty acid deficiency in an infant with CF on an artificial diet. Elliott (1976), in an uncontrolled study,

reported some improvement in patients following essential fatty acid supplementation. Further controlled studies are required to confirm these observations. Meanwhile, the dietary fats high in PUFA should be selected; fish and poultry should be encouraged and margarines or low-fat spreads selected for their PUFA content (*see* Table 7.11), and cooking fat should be replaced with either a vegetable oil rich in PUFA (Table 7.11) or MCT oil.

The criteria used in determining the individual's intake are the number and bulk of stools, child's weight gain, presence of abdominal discomfort, rectal prolapse and liver dysfunction. Pancreatin should be increased with meals containing a higher fat content, e.g. school dinner, fish and chips cooked in ordinary fat, or treats of cream cake or ice-cream, and during infection when protein and energy needs are greatest. Fat tolerance and, therefore, energy intake and weight gain can often be improved by either adjustment of the pancreatin dose or a change to an alternative preparation, e.g. Creon or Pancrease.

Rectal prolapse or liver disease requires a definite low-fat diet, in children usually 25 to 50 g fat per day, or approximately 20% energy from fat, (*see* Chapter 7, p. 165). It is especially important that the energy deficit in such diets is replaced in a tolerated form, usually as carbohydrate and/or MCT. MCT is less dependent on pancreatic lipase for absorption, but there is added benefit if MCT is given with pancreatin supplements (Forstner *et al.* 1980). These are of no medicinal value (McCollum & Harries 1977), however they can add variety and energy to an otherwise low-fat diet.

MCT can be useful in children with a large appetite resulting from malabsorption, because they can replace some dietary fat and increase dietary energy density (Gracey *et al.* 1970). These children are more likely to suffer abdominal distension and even pain, which improves when the appetite becomes more normal. A number of MCT-containing products are available (*see* Tables 7.8 and 7.9).

Carbohydrate

Carbohydrate energy intake must be increased to provide the increased energy needs and to compensate for the decreased intake of fat, and may need to supply 60 to 70% energy in the diet. Disaccharides, and particularly sugars, are usually tolerated well, do not require pancreatic enzymes for digestion, and are practical, palatable and acceptable (Francis 1979) including fruit, fruit juice, sugar, Coke and candy. Glucose polymers can be a useful supplement to the energy intake, but should not be used to such an extent as to suppress appetite for other foods which provide other nutrients.

Glucose polymers are 5 to 8 glucose molecules linked by α-1–4 bonds. Maltase in the intestinal mucosa is of more importance than pancreatic amylase in their digestion. They have a lower osmolality than mono- and disaccharides for the same per cent solution and provide a source of energy without the risk of a high osmolar load.

Starch is largely dependent on pancreatic amylase for digestion and is often less well absorbed than the sugars. However, it is a useful source of energy, and an adequate to generous intake should be provided in the diet. Pancreatin supplements should be given with starch-containing foods, including cereals, bread, biscuits, potato, and pulses, which coincidentally also provide some protein and a little fat.

Undigested starch passes into the large intestine where it is acted on by bacteria, forming gas, which results in abdominal distension and flatulence. This can be largely overcome by adequate pancreatin supplements. High-fibre foods, pulses, wholegrain cereals, wholemeal bread and bran, are not encouraged, as they increase faecal output and frequently cause flatulence, which is less well controlled by pancreatin supplements.

Fruit and vegetables add carbohydrate, energy, vitamins and minerals to the diet, as well as provide variety, and are usually well-tolerated by patients with CF. Onions, pips, skin, nuts and dried fruit may need to be avoided if they cause flatulence.

A reduced carbohydrate intake is not appropriate in patients in whom there is evidence of glucose intolerance, but hypoglycaemic drugs or insulin should be used to increase carbohydrate utilization as necessary. A guide to carbohydrate distribution throughout the day should be provided in order to normalize hyperglycaemic peaks where possible (*see* Steel *et al.* 1983). Adequate total energy and protein intakes are still essential (*see* p. 151).

Vitamins

Patients with CF even with treatment may have depleted stores of some vitamins (Silk 1984). Vitamin C stores have been considered low in some patients even on 50 mg vitamin C supplements. Vitamin B_{12} levels are low due to impaired absorption, but this is improved with pancreatic supplementation. Vitamin A levels are low on conventional supplements, as are serum 25-OH cholecalciferol levels in some patients. Vitamin E levels are invariably low unless supplements are given (Harries & Muller 1971). Vitamin K deficiency with bleeding secondary to hypothrombin-

aemia may also occur, and supplements may well be required (Silk 1984). Vitamin deficiencies, particularly of fat-soluble vitamins, are a feature of untreated patients. A water-miscible form of fat-soluble vitamins A, D, E and possibly K is recommended for all patients with CF. A supplement of Abidec 0·6 ml (Parke Davis) is usually adequate, together with vitamin E, 1 mg/kg of water-miscible α-tocopherol acetate *or* 10 mg/kg per day of fat-soluble vitamin E (Harries & Muller 1971, Taylor *et al.* 1973). Vitamins K and B_{12} may also be required in some instances. Alternatively, a comprehensive vitamin supplement such as three Ketovite Tablets plus 5 ml Ketovite Liquid (Paines & Byrne), or 6 to 12 Cow & Gate Supplementary Vitamin Tablets plus 5 ml Ketovite Liquid, is indicated in patients with growth failure or poor nutritional status.

Trace minerals

Preliminary studies on trace minerals suggest these are poorly absorbed in patients with CF, and deficiency states have been described for zinc, iron, selenium, iodine, cobalt, copper, chromium, molybdenum, manganese and vanadium (Silk 1983). Malabsorption, steatorrhoea, poor nutrition, and synthetic diets all predispose to trace mineral deficiency. Supplements may be appropriate for individuals. Further work is necessary to determine optimal intakes or possible supplements for use in the future (*see* Francis 1986), particularly in the light of at least one fatality in a young child with CF who was receiving selenium supplements (Hubbard *et al.* 1980). Zinc supplements have been used to improve growth in patients with growth retardation and low plasma zinc levels (Dodge & Yassa 1978).

Salt

Increased sodium excretion occurs through sweat in CF. Salt supplements may be required routinely in tropical countries, or during summer holidays in hot climates and with pyrexia. In this country salt supplements are rarely needed for the older child, but adequate salt intake should be encouraged by adding salt in cooking and to meals at the table. Salt tablets (300 mg sodium chloride = 5 mmol sodium) or sodium bicarbonate supplements can be prescribed if necessary.

Infants may require higher intakes of sodium to that provided by modified milks and some milk substitutes, but the intake must be carefully monitored to prevent both sodium depletion and hypernatraemia. This is particularly important if faecal losses are high, such as in patients with an ileostomy as a result of surgery for meconium ileus, and during infections.

Diet in infants with cystic fibrosis

Infants who are diagnosed in the neonatal period from screening programmes, sibship or meconium ileus should ideally be breast-fed; small doses of pancreatin are given at each feed (Dinwiddie 1983).

Human milk, especially from the infant's own mother, is ideal both for nutrition and because it gives the baby a number of protective factors (Francis 1986). The protein and particularly the type of fat are in an easily digestible form. Lipase, the enzyme needed to digest fat, is also present in human milk. Lipase is heat-labile and therefore is lost on pasteurization of expressed breast milk. Unprocessed expressed breast milk, ideally from mother to her own child, is recommended for those infants too ill to breast-feed. 'Drip' breast milk, because of its lower energy content, is not recommended. Expressed breast milk can be fortified, if necessary, with 5 g

Pregestimil powder to each 100 ml to increase the nutrient value (Table 6.3).

Women who themselves have CF (but not heterozygotes) may not be able to breast-feed their infant, as their milk may be too high in electrolytes for the infant, and the mother's own nutritional status may deteriorate due to the increased nutritional demands of lactation (Welch et al. 1981). The milk should be analysed for electrolytes and the infant weighed regularly to ensure adequate nutrition (Welch et al. 1981).

If adequate breast milk is not available for the infant with CF, or the mother chooses not to breast-feed, a modified feed with a reduced fat but containing essential fatty acids and a slightly higher protein should be selected. Pancreatin is required at each feed time. Adequate energy intake is essential and electrolyte intake should compensate for sweat and faecal losses; at least 2 to 3 mmol/kg per day of both sodium and potassium are recommended.

Skimmed milk alone and MCT 1 (Cow & Gate) are unsuitable for infants because of their protein and

Table 6.3 Feeds for infants with cystic fibrosis.

100 ml	Protein (g)	Carbo-hydrate (g)	Fat (g)	Energy kJ	kcal	Sodium (mmol)	Potassium (mmol)	Calcium (mmol)	Phosphorus (mmol)	Iron (μmol)	Zinc (μmol)	Copper (μmol)
Human milk (mature)	1·3	7·2	4·1	289	69	0·6	1·5	0·9	0·5	1·3	4·3	0·6
Fortified human milk												
100 ml human milk (EBM)	1·3	7·2	4·1	289	69	0·6	1·5	0·9	0·5	1·3	4·3	0·6
+ 5 g Pregestimil powder	0·6	3·1	0·9	97	23	0·5	0·6	0·5	0·5	7·7	2·2	3·4
Total	1·9	10·3	5·0	386	92	1·1	2·1	1·4	1·0	9·0	6·5	4·0
*Cystic mixtures**												
(a) 6·5 g Gold Cap SMA	0·8	3·6	1·8	138	33	0·3	0·7	0·6	0·5	6·0	2·9	0·4
4·3 g Marvel	1·6	2·2	0·1	65	16	1·0	1·8	1·3	1·3	0·4	2·8	0·2
6·5 g Caloreen	Nil	6·5	Nil	104	26	0·1	Trace	—	—	—	—	—
Water to 100 ml												
Total	2·4	12·3	1·9	307	75	1·4	2·5	1·9	1·8	6·4	5·7	0·6
(b) 6·2 g Premium	0·8	3·7	1·8	138	33	0·4	0·9	0·7	0·5	4·5	3·1	0·3
4·6 g Marvel	1·7	2·4	0·1	69	16·5	1·1	1·9	1·4	1·4	0·4	3·1	0·2
6·5 g Polycal	Nil	6·5	Nil	104	26	0·1	Trace	—	—	—	—	—
Water to 100 ml												
Total	2·5	12·6	1·9	311	75·5	1·6	2·8	2·1	1·9	4·9	6·2	0·5

* Recipes (a) and (b) can be made using the scoop in the SMA or Premium packet for each ingredient as follows:

2 level scoops Gold Cap SMA or Premium powder ⎫
2 level scoops Marvel granules   ⎬   Total volume approximately 130 ml
2 level scoops Caloreen or Polycal   ⎪
4 measured ounces boiled water   ⎭

Vitamin supplements including A, D, E and K are essential.
Alternative brands of modified milk and glucose polymers can be calibrated to provide a suitable formula or formula selected from Table 1.4.

solute content, and they do not provide essential fatty acids or adequate energy. The regular modified milks are usually too high in fat and others contain butter-fat, which is poorly absorbed even in normal infants and is low in essential fatty acids. However, whey-based modified formulae can be adapted (Table 8.3) to obtain a feed containing approximately 2 g protein, 2 g fat high in essential fatty acids, 10 g carbohydrate and 275 to 315 kJ (65 to 75 kcal) per 100 ml. MCT is not necessary, but can be used as an energy supplement in addition to or as part replacement of the carbohydrate.

An appropriate feed is made by diluting a modified whey-based milk containing a vegetable–animal fat combination; protein is increased with skimmed milk powder and the energy with added carbohydrate (e.g. glucose polymer). A feed which is easily converted into practical scoop measures for home use is given in Table 6.3. Alternatively, one of the newer pre-term infant formula feeds can be selected, e.g. Low Birth Weight SMA which contains some MCT would be appropriate, but it is only available to hospitals as a ready-to-feed formula.

Adequate volume of feed should normally be offered on demand at least five times daily. Initially 200 ml/kg per day is recommended, and the volume of feeds should not be reduced too soon in order to prevent a decrease in nutritional intake before an adequate intake of weaning solids can compensate the protein, energy and essential fatty acid deficits. Growth is the best guide and is usually adequate, as chest involvement is minimal in these patients, at least in early infancy. As solids are introduced from about four months, the offered feed volume is reduced to 150 ml/kg per day and later to 100 ml/kg per day and a change to a 2% fat follow-on milk such as Progress would be appropriate. From about 10 months the modified milk can be omitted and replaced with full-strength skimmed or reduced-fat milk, plus added carbohydrate. At one year of age, solids should provide the major nutritional intake, and 500 ml (1 pint) of follow-on milk, or skimmed or reduced-fat milk with added carbohydrate is appropriate, essential fatty acids being provided from solids. Vitamin supplements such as Abidec and vitamin E, or three Ketovite Tablets plus 5 ml Ketovite Liquid, and fluoride drops to protect teeth if the water supply is low in fluoride, are recommended.

Meconium ileus

Infants treated for meconium ileus with gastrograffin enema have similar nutritional needs to other infants with CF. Those in whom surgery has been necessary,

especially when an ileostomy has been performed, have special nutritional problems in the post-surgery phase. Malabsorption is a major problem and parenteral nutrition is usually necessary (Dinwiddie 1983). Treatment should be appropriate to symptoms in addition to conventional therapy for cystic fibrosis, including pancreatin with oral feeds. A feeding programme as described in Chapter 1 for multiple malabsorption syndrome and protracted diarrhoea may be necessary. There is a high incidence of temporary disaccharide intolerance, large losses of protein and electrolytes in stools, and fat absorption is poor. Great care is necessary to ensure these infants do not become dehydrated, or hyponatraemic, with the risk of hypovolaemia and collapse, especially as fluid and electrolyte losses are increased with an ileostomy, pyrexia, and in those nursed in an incubator. Electrolyte and fluid balance is critical; at least 3 mmol/kg per day of both sodium and potassium are commonly needed, and an oral fluid requirement of 200 to 300 ml/kg per day may be necessary. Initially a small frequent feeding regimen is recommended, e.g. hourly feeds initially, or a continuous nasogastric or naso-jejunal feeding regimen administered by syringe pump may be required. Adequate protein (4 g/kg per day) and energy (540 to 840 kJ, 130 to 200 kcal/kg per day) are necessary to promote healing and growth. Pregestimil and MCT Pepdite 0–2, which are 'predigested' and disaccharide-free (Table 1.4), or Low Birth Weight SMA, are the most appropriate feeds if human milk is either not tolerated or unobtainable. Alternatively a module feed based on Comminuted Chicken (Tables 1.6 and 1.18) or peptides may be indicated (Chapter 1, p. 38). The regimen is tailored to the child's clinical needs and as improvement occurs a more normal feeding regimen is gradually introduced.

The disaccharide intolerance is usually temporary, and after clinical improvement or closure of the ileostomy a change can be made to a feed used in the regular treatment of CF (Table 8.3). Sucrase activity is rarely depleted so as to cause clinical sucrose intolerance and recovers more readily than lactase activity when it is affected. By the time weaning solids are introduced conventional foods containing sugar are usually permitted, though added sugar may be replaced with glucose or glucose polymers.

Weaning solids for infants with CF

Solids are normally introduced between three and six months in the usual manner; some infants with CF may even benefit from their introduction at an earlier age than average if weight gain is poor, in order to increase nutrient intake. However, the occasional patient will be overweight, though far less often than in the normal population.

Initially solids with a low fat content are advised until fat tolerance is assessed. Starch-containing foods, cereals and puddings are permitted, but require a slightly increased dose of pancreatin. Cereals, fruit-flavoured cereals and fruit purées are usually the first solids introduced. Savouries are then introduced, e.g. puréed lean meat, potato, fat-free gravy, and vegetables or commercially available low-fat strained foods, e.g. Heinz Turkey Dinner. Because chicken and turkey breast are low in fat but contain essential fatty acids, and because the availability of minerals such as iron and zinc from meat is better than from cereals, these foods should be included in the diet from about four to six months and well before a change from the milk substitute or infant cystic formula to reduced-fat milk.

From six months of age a *little* salt can be added to savoury foods. Between eight and nine months, egg-yolk, which is quite high in fat but an excellent source of protein, B vitamins and iron, is cautiously introduced, at first 2 to 3 times per week and later one egg can be given 3 to 4 times per week. The range and quantity of solids are quickly expanded (Table 6.4) using the guidelines for the older child's diet (*see later*, Table 6.5). At this stage feeds can be decreased to four per day and some offered from a cup. The consistency of foods offered should be changed from purées to mashed foods and finger foods should be offered to encourage chewing by 8 to 10 months to avoid later food refusal of lumps. A crust with a little honey or Marmite is a useful finger food. Self-feeding should be encouraged by about one year of age.

The quantity of special infant formula should not be reduced too quickly, as it is an important source of energy and essential fatty acids as well as protein, minerals and vitamins. Custard and puddings can be made with reduced-fat milk.

Many toddlers are faddy about food. Parental anxiety is understandable but only encourages the child to seek attention through food. Self-feeding with frequent opportunities to eat, e.g. 5 to 6 times per day, is advisable. Pancreatin can be given after meals, the dose being judged on the quantity eaten. Refused meals can be replaced with drinks of an appropriate special feed. Force-feeding should be avoided. Praise and reward schemes are a positive way of encouraging the child, but parental temptation to 'nag' the child about eating must be resisted. If the diet or indeed other aspects of treatment become a battle-

Table 6.4   Example of a weaning menu for a child with cystic fibrosis.

Breast-feeds or suitable infant feed (*see* Table 6.3) or an alternative such as Pregestimil should provide the major nutritional intake; pancreatin mixed with a little water should be given from a spoon immediately before or halfway through the feed or meal.

a.m.	Cereal, e.g. baby rice, Farex Weaning Food
	Sugar
	Infant feed to mix with cereal
	Optional toast and honey or Marmite (no butter, margarine)
Noon	Homogenized or minced turkey, chicken or lean meat or grilled fish
	Potato, mashed ⎫ No added fat or butter. A
	Puréed vegetables ⎬ little salt may be added.
	Fat-free gravy, e.g. Bisto made with water or vegetable water
	Custard made with infant feed or low-fat yoghurt
	Fruit purée or mashed banana
Snack	Fruit juice
	Crust of bread and honey or Marmite or suitable rusk
p.m.	As noon or a.m.
	or
	Boiled egg
	Bread and Marmite or Bovril
	Puréed fruit and jelly or low-fat yoghurt or low-fat mousse
	or
	Commercial baby weaning food (savoury and/or dessert)

ground between parents and child, early advice and support are necessary from the specialist cystic clinic or paediatrician.

Meals for older children with cystic fibrosis

Meals should be selected from conventional foods which are prepared in such a way as to reduce the fat content, if necessary, and yet provide adequate protein and energy. An example of a suitable diet is given in Table 6.5. The diet should be as near normal as possible. Frequent meals and snacks (six per day) are advised. Supplements to increase protein and energy intakes are advised if nutritional status is poor. Suggestions are given later in Table 8.6 (*see also* Tables 7.6, 7.8 and 7.9). However, synthetic foods are rarely needed, and are monotonous, expensive and often unpalatable; if nutritional status is very poor and/or malabsorption is a feature, then, for example, one of the Peptide range, Pregestimil and/ or Flexical as an enteral feed by nasogastric or naso-jejunal continuous or overnight feeding regimen may be useful to achieve nutritional repletion (Silk 1984).

Liberal amounts of salt in cooking or added at the table should be encouraged to compensate losses from sweat.

Many household recipes are suitable or if necessary can be adapted to reduce or omit fat. For example, two egg-whites can replace one whole egg. A low-fat spread can be used in place of other fats except for frying, but the water content of the recipe will need to be reduced. Half the quantity of butter or PUFA margarine can be used in many recipes without altering the result. Savoury pies can be made with potato instead of pastry, home-made 'ice-cream' can be made from evaporated milk or custard with folded-in beaten egg-white. The Cystic Fibrosis Trust* produces a low-fat cookery book (Wrigley 1983). A variety of lower fat convenience foods are more widely available than previously.

Participation in school lunch, tea with friends or a party can be important to a child on a diet and should be encouraged. Advice to the mother or school meals supervisor can prevent many problems which could arise when unsuitable items such as fried fish and chips or doughnuts are on the menu; grilled fish or fish fingers and boiled potato, or a boiled egg, or beans with toast and low-fat spread, yoghurt or fruit are suitable substitutes. Most children can manage school lunch menus with extra pancreatin to cover the higher fat content. Alternatively, a packed lunch box can be easily prepared.

Teeth care

Teeth care is essential because the diet is relatively high in sugar and sweet foods. Fluoride tablets, drops or the use of fluoride toothpaste reduces the risk of dental caries if there is no fluoride in local water and is recommended, together with regular teeth cleaning routines and dental check-ups.

Infections and illness

Requirements of protein and energy are elevated during catabolism associated with infections but fat tolerance may be temporarily reduced, and appetite poor. It is important to maintain adequate intakes during infections and periods of poor appetite (Parsons *et al.* 1980) to prevent weight loss and muscle wasting (Shepherd *et al.* 1983) if at all possible. Replacement

---

* The Cystic Fibrosis Trust, 5 Blyth Road, Bromley, Kent, BR1 3RS, offers practical support to patients and their families.

supplements such as fluids and easily eaten foods which are palatable, high in protein and energy, but moderate to low in fat are ideal, and should be continued until catch-up growth has been achieved. Suitable items include low-fat yoghurt, milk jelly, low-fat mousse, high-protein milk-shakes or soup, Build-Up, Complan or Kellogg's Two-Shakes (*see* Recipes, Table 6.6). From about two years, half to one of the recipes, according to age, is used as a meal replacement or a supplement to the diet. For the younger child, the suggested adapted infant feed (Table 6.3) is more appropriate, and for those using a 'milk substitute' e.g. Pepdite, Pregestimil, Flexical or MCT 'filled' milk this should form the basis of the replacement, appropriately supplemented if necessary, administered by nasogastric or nasojejunal feeding regimen if necessary.

PROBLEMS DUE TO MALABSORPTION

Apart from malnutrition and growth retardation (*see* pp. 149 & 161) the major problems are abdominal distension, flatulence and abdominal pain. Relief of these symptoms may be given by increasing the dose of pancreatic enzymes. Starchy foods may be responsible for these symptoms or excess fibre from pulses or cereals. A reduction of high-fibre foods may be indicated if extra pancreatin does not suffice. Avoidance of a starchy bedtime snack can help to overcome early morning flatulence, in which case a suitable 'milk' shake is an ideal alternative. Decreased dietary fat may also alleviate these symptoms, but care must be taken not to over-restrict energy intake coincidentally.

Rectal prolapse occurs quite often in young children with CF (Anderson & Goodchild 1976) and as a cause of rectal prolapse CF should always be considered. This is one occasion where a temporary stricter low-fat diet is advisable, so that the number and bulk of stools can be kept to a minimum. The amount of fibre and residue in the diet may also have to be decreased until symptoms are relieved. Replacement of the energy deficit of the reduced dietary fat is essential with glucose polymers and/or MCT as appropriate and adequate pancreatin supplement to reduce stool bulk.

The occasional patient with CF has clinical lactose intolerance, but this is rare except in infants following surgery for meconium ileus. In the infant Pregestimil or MCT Pepdite 0–2 is the milk substitute most suitable, or a low-fat adaptation of the Comminuted Chicken or peptide module regimen (Table 1.4 and Table 1.18).

Table 6.5 Example of a menu for a child with cystic fibrosis requiring a reduced fat intake.

On waking	Fruit juice, or cup of tea with skimmed milk* and sugar or glucose polymer
Breakfast	Cereal, skimmed milk* and honey or glucose or sugar
	Ham, fish, grilled lean bacon or egg
	Toast or bread (high-fibre and wholemeal types are not recommended)
	Low-fat margarine, or scraping of polyunsaturated margarine
	Honey, jam, jelly marmalade, Marmite, Bovril
	Skimmed milk* and sugar
	Pancreatin
Mid-morning	Skimmed milk* and sugar or milk-shake
	Sandwich or biscuits (low-fat semi-sweet or crispbread type)
	Piece of fruit
	Pancreatin
Lunch	Meat or fish (trim off fat and do not fry or add butter)
	Jacket, boiled, mashed potato or reconstituted instant potato, rice, spaghetti
or	Bread and low-fat spread or scraping of polyunsaturated margarine
	Fat-free gravy, e.g. Bisto
	Salt to taste
	Vegetables, salad, peas, beans, lentils in small quantities
	Fruit, fresh, tinned or stewed, or jelly or plain sponge pudding (not suet or pastry) or low-fat yoghurt
	Pancreatin
Tea	Fruit juice, skimmed milk*, tea or coffee with sugar
	Bread and low-fat margarine or scraping of polyunsaturated margarine
	Jam, honey, Marmite, Bovril or cottage cheese
	Semi-sweet biscuits, sponge cake, low-fat cake, meringues or sweets
	Piece of fruit
	Pancreatin
Supper	Lean chicken, meat, fish, egg or cheese, fat-free gravy, salt to taste
	Potatoes, vegetables or bread and low-fat margarine or scraping of polyunsaturated margarine
	Fruit or jelly or low-fat yoghurt or sponge cake
	Skimmed milk*, tea or coffee with sugar
	Pancreatin
Bedtime	Skimmed milk* drink and sugar or milk-shake
	Semi-sweet biscuits, low-fat cake or sandwich
	Piece of fruit
	Pancreatin
Vitamins	0·6 ml Abidec daily plus vitamin E
or	3 Ketovite Tablets plus 5 ml Ketovite Liquid plus vitamin E
Fluoride tablets	Recommended if there is no fluoride in local water supply. Teeth-cleaning to remove plaque is very important with high-carbohydrate diets.
* 'Milk'	500 to 1000 ml (1 to 2 pints) skimmed, reduced-fat or full-fat milk plus 2 to 3 tablespoons honey, glucose polymer or sugar per 500 ml (1 pint) for drinks, cereal and puddings
Treats	(Provided weight and stools are satisfactory, these can be given as treats but a little extra pancreatin should be given with them.)
	1 One or two ice-creams per week (avoid Cornish ice-cream, but remember non-milk fat ice-cream is not actually low in fat).
	2 Four squares chocolate or one chocolate-coated biscuit.
	3 $\frac{1}{2}$–1 packet crisps or a few chips.

Table 6.5 *continued*

School meal suggestions

Provided growth is satisfactory and pancreatin is given to help digest food, no food is actually forbidden, although it is advised that fatty and fried food be avoided.

Mid-morning	Skimmed milk* and sugar or milk-shake (send in a plastic bottle from home)
	Sandwich/biscuit and/or fruit
	Pancreatin
School dinner	Meat or fish (trim off fat and avoid fried items) or well-grilled sausages, beefburger or fish fingers
	Potato, rice, spaghetti (limit roast and chips if possible)
	Vegetables
	Gravy and salt
	Fruit, jelly, sponge-type puddings (avoid suet-type and pastry)
	Low-fat yoghurt
	A little custard or occasional ice-cream
	Drink, fruit juice or water
	Pancreatin (mix at the meal-time and give before or during the meal)
Picnic/home-packed lunch box	Sandwiches or rolls (using low-fat margarine or scraping of polyunsaturated margarine or butter) filled with plenty of sliced meat, cottage cheese, ham, hard-boiled egg
	Salad, pickle, ketchup,
	Baked beans,
	Jam, honey, dates
	Pancreatin
	or
	Salad box with cold meat, hard-boiled egg
	Fish fingers or cooked chicken quarter or drumstick or tub of cottage cheese
	Bread or rolls
	Suitable sponge cake, meringue or low-fat cake
	Low-fat yoghurt
	Sweets
	Soup or drink in flask, canned or bottled fruit juice
	Skimmed milk*
	Fruit
	Pancreatin.

*Reduced-fat or semi-skimmed or full-fat milk or a suitable milk substitute can be selected. 'Filled' milks containing non-milk fat are not suitable, e.g. Five Pints, Coffee-mate.

For the older child a low-lactose milk substitute with reduced fat or MCT is appropriate, e.g. Portagen, or the new complete MCT Cow & Gate milk formula. The minimal lactose diet (Table 1.8) can be adapted to a lower fat regimen if necessary.

SYNTHETIC DIETS AND SUPPLEMENTS IN CF

An artificial diet is usually unnecessary in the routine treatment of CF (McCollum & Harries 1977, Yassa *et al.* 1978, Clayton & Francis 1978) but may be useful to replenish nutritional status (Silk 1984).

The module diet first posed by Allan *et al.* (1973) was based on Albumaid Complete, glucose polymer, MCT oil and Metabolic Mineral Mixture with either an egg-yolk or polyunsaturated margarine for essential fatty acids, and vitamins from Ketovite Tablets plus Liquid. Other food was kept to a minimum. Initial reports on the use of the diet were encouraging, but the regimen was complex, expensive and unpalatable (Allan 1975, Berry *et al.* 1975).

Yassa *et al.* (1978) have published details of a comprehensive trial on a similar module diet in 28 patients compared with 15 controls, all with CF. The artificial diet led to some improvement in height, weight, and subscapular skinfold thickness, and a disproportionate advance of bone age for the group as a whole. Greatest improvement was noted in the young mildly affected patients. Very small patients showed least improvement. Barclay and Shannon

Table 6.6 Replacement meals for use during illness or as nutritional supplements in children with cystic fibrosis.

		Energy kJ	kcal	Carbohydrate (g)	Protein (g)	‡Fat (g)
(a)	200 ml (7 oz) skimmed milk ⎱ Or 45 g skimmed milk powder	284	66	5·0	6·8	0·1
	20 g (¾ oz) skimmed milk powder ⎰ plus water	302	72	10·6	7·2	0·1
	20 g (¾ oz) sugar, glucose polymer or milk-shake powder	320	80	20	—	—
	Total ≃ 200 ml	906	218	35·6	14·0	0·2
(b)	200 ml (7 oz) skimmed milk or 25 g skimmed milk powder plus water	284	66	10·0	6·8	0·1
	plus 1 egg*	306	73	Trace	6·1	5·5
	20 g (¾ oz) glucose polymer or sugar	320	80	20	—	—
	1 to 2 drops vanilla or a little nutmeg					
	Total ≃ 250 ml	910	219	30	12·9	5·6
(c)	300 ml (10 oz) skimmed milk or 38 g skimmed milk powder plus water	426	99	15	10·2	0·3
	38 g (1 sachet) Build-Up (Carnation)†	550	131	26	8·5	0·2†
	Total ≃ 300 ml	976	230	41	18·7	0·5
(d)	100 ml (3½ oz) skimmed milk or 12·5 g skimmed milk powder plus water	142	33	5·0	3·4	0·1
	150 g (1 carton) low-fat fruit yoghurt	560	130	24	7·4	1·5
	Total ≃ 250 ml	702	163	29	10·8	1·6
(e)	200 ml (7 oz) skimmed milk or 25 g skimmed milk powder plus water	284	66	10	6·8	0·1
	1 banana* (100 g)	337	79	19·2	1·1	0·3
	10 g (⅓ oz) skimmed milk powder	151	36	5·3	3·6	0·1
	Total ≃ 250 ml	772	181	34·5	11·5	0·5
(f)	150 ml (5 oz) ready-to-serve tomato soup	345	83	8·9	1·2	5·0
	20 g (¾ oz) skimmed milk powder	302	72	10·6	7·2	0·1
	Water to 200 ml					
	Total ≃ 200 ml	647	155	19·5	8·4	5·1
(g)	150 ml (5 oz) ready-to-serve vegetable soup	239	56	2·3	3·4	0·4
	50 g baked beans	135	32	5·1	2·6	0·3
	Total ≃ 200 ml	374	88	7·4	6·0	0·7
(h)	100 g canned rice pudding	386	91	14·7	3·4	2·5
	100 ml (3½ oz) skimmed milk	142	33	5·0	3·4	0·1
	10 g glucose polymer	160	40	10	—	—
	Total ≃ 200 ml	688	164	29.7	6·8	2·6

Homogenize and serve hot or cold. Those marked:

  * should be used immediately and not more than one raw egg should be given in any one day.

  † Chocolate-flavoured Build-Up slightly higher in fat (≃ 1 g/sachet) and energy content.

  ‡ 15 ml (½ oz) Liquigen MCT emulsion supplying 263 kJ (62 kcal) can be added to each recipe (after heating) if necessary.

Skimmed milk can be replaced with reduced-fat 2% or full-fat milk which will increase the energy content by 74 to 150 kJ (18 to 36 kcal) per 100 ml.

(1975) found similar growth results. Very rapid weight loss occurred on discontinuing the artificial diet (Yassa *et al.* 1978), suggesting fluid retention may have been in part responsible for the weight changes. Some problems with acceptance of the regimen given orally were experienced, but newer predigested formulae, which are nutritionally complete and more palatable, are now available. No significant beneficial effects were observed on lung function, or frequency of chest infection (Yassa *et al.* 1978). However, more recently Shepherd *et al.* (1980) have shown a reduction in infections after a period of parenteral nutrition to improve nutritional status, and pulmonary infections were reduced which cannot be

Table 6.7 Various enteral feeds suitable for use in children with cystic fibrosis as supplements or fluid diets.

		Energy kJ	Energy kcal	Carbo-hydrate (g)	Protein (g)	Fat (g)
(a)	250 ml whole milk ⎱ Or 100 g skimmed milk powder	680	163	11·8	8·3	9·5 LCT
	75 g skimmed milk powder ⎰ plus 20 ml Prosparol/Calogen	1134	266	40·0	27·3	1·0 LCT
	100 g glucose polymer	1600	400	100·0	—	—
	60 ml Liquigen	1050	249	—	—	30·0 MCT
	Water to 1000 ml					
	Total	4464	1078	151·8	35·6	40·5
(b)	152 g Portagen	2960	705	82·4	25	5·3 LCT
						28·8 MCT
	65 g glucose polymer (optional)	1040	260	65	—	—
	Water to 1000 ml					
	Total	4000	965	147·4	25	34·1
(c)	213 g Triosorbin (2½ sachets)	4250	1000	119	40·4	8·1 LCT
	Water to 1000 ml					32·3 MCT
	Total	4250	1000	119	40·4	40·4
(d)	100 g skimmed milk powder	1512	355	52·8	36·4	1·3
	57 g Complan (1 sachet)	1070	253	31	11	9
	65 g glucose polymer	1040	260	65	—	—
	Water to 1000 ml					
	Total	3622	868	148·8	47·4	10·3
(e)	253 g Nutranel (2½ tins)	4200	1000	187·5	40	5 LCT
	Water to 1000 ml					5 MCT
	Total	4200	1000	187·5	40	10
(f)	50 g Albumaid Complete	680	160	Nil	40	Nil
	150 g glucose polymer	2400	600	150	—	—
	20 ml Prosparol/Calogen	370	90	—	—	10 LCT
	60 ml Liquigen	1050	249	—	—	30 MCT
	Water to 1000 ml					
	Total	4500	1099	150	40	40
(g)	227 g Flexical (½ can)	4200	1000	153	22·5	26·4 LCT
	Water to 1000 ml					7·4 MCT
	Total	4200	1000	153	22·5	33·8
(h)	148 g Pregestimil	2871	684	91·2	18·9	15·7 LCT
	Water to 1000 ml					11·4 MCT
	Total	2871	684	91·2	18·9	23·8

An appropriate feed volume should be given to provide nutrient requirement.

Pregestimil and Portagen are the most appropriate for the pre-school age child.

The recommended vitamin supplements for cystic fibrosis should be continued except with (a) and (d) where six Cow & Gate Supplementary Vitamin Tablets plus 5 ml Ketovite Liquid plus vitamin E is required and (f) where three Ketovite Tablets plus 5 ml Ketovite Liquid plus vitamin E is recommended plus 8 g Aminogran or Metabolic Mineral Mixture per day.

ignored. Bradley *et al.* (1979), Shepherd *et al.* (1983) and Silk (1984) have used overnight nasogastric enteral feeding regimens to improve nutrition and growth with different commercial hydrolysate formulae (Nutranel, Vipep [Tuta Labs Australia] or a new formula, Reabilan) in conjunction with *ad libitum* conventional diet. Optimal absorption of protein occurs from peptides of 2 to 3 amino acid residues (Keohane *et al.* 1983, Rees *et al.* 1984). Such formulae should be nutritionally adequate for the patient's individual needs in macro- and micronutrients, including trace elements, vitamins, protein, energy and essential fatty acids. Supplements which require administration by nasoenteral feeding are not recommended unless clinically indicated, but are an important adjunct to conventional nutritional regimes in malnourished patients and/or those with growth failure.

MCT Pepdite 0–2 or Pregestimil is the most appropriate formula for the young infant, many of whom will accept these formulae as a bottle-feed. For the older child, a low-fat MCT 'filled' formula should be selected, e.g. Pepdite 2 +, Portagen, Triosorbin, Nutranel, or Flexical (*see* Tables 6.7 and 7.9), as appropriate for the nutritional needs of the patient. Small doses of pancreatin are required with such feeds. Alternatively, a feed can be devised from appropriate modules, e.g. skimmed milk powder or a hydrolysed protein preparation such as Albumaid Complete, together with glucose polymer, vegetable oil (LCT) to provide essential fatty acids, MCT emulsion, complete vitamins and appropriate mineral or trace element supplements (Table 6.7). Individual calculation of such a regimen is essential in order to prevent the hazards of a nutritionally inadequate regimen, particularly regarding trace nutrients, and the osmolality of the planned feed should be assessed, and should not exceed 500 mmol/kg.

Provided the selected feed has a low osmolality the feed can be introduced as a full-strength enteral feeding regimen (Keohane *et al.* 1984) unless contraindicated, for example post-surgery.

Examples are given in Table 6.7 of various enteral feeds which could be used in appropriate volume to provide a fluid regime or dietary supplement. Artificial and synthetic diets, e.g. Table 6.7 (f), can only be as adequate as current nutritional knowledge and available products permit. For example, the trace elements, chromium, nickel, selenium and zinc, are essential, but little is known about their requirement (*see* Francis 1986), especially in patients with malabsorption such as those with CF.

EMOTIONAL AND SOCIAL IMPLICATIONS OF CF

The implications of an incurable disease on the child and family can be profound, and constant support is needed, and in some families psychiatric help may be beneficial. The quality of life achieved and the demands of the treatment programme including diet, medications, physiotherapy and frequent hospital admissions all contribute to the stress on the family unit. A dietary regimen which is an adaptation of the family meal pattern has considerable benefits for all concerned.

REFERENCES

ALLAN J.D. (1975) Artificial diet in treatment of cystic fibrosis. *Nutrition* 29, 211–6.

ALLAN J.D., MASON A. & MOSS A.D. (1973) Nutritional supplementation in the treatment of CF of the pancreas. *Amer. J. Dis. Child.* 126, 122–6.

ANDERSON C.M. & GOODCHILD M.C. (1976) *Cystic Fibrosis, Manual of Diagnosis and Management.* Oxford: Blackwell Scientific Publications.

AXELROD A.E. & TRAKATELLIS A.C. (1964) Relationship of pyridoxine to immunological phenomena. *Vitamins and Hormones* 22, 591–607.

BARCLAY R.P.C. & SHANNON R.J. (1975) Trial of an artificial diet in the treatment of cystic fibrosis of the pancreas. *Arch. Dis. Childh.* 50, 490–3.

BERRY H.K., KELLOG F.W., HUNT M.M., INGBERG R.C., RICHTERM L. & GUTJAHR C. (1975) Dietary supplement and nutrition in children with cystic fibrosis. *Amer. J. Dis. Child.* 129, 165–71.

BHASKARAM C.R. & REDDY V. (1975) Cell mediated immunity in iron and vitamin deficient children. *Brit. med. J.* 111, 522.

BRADLEY J.A., AXON A.T.R. & HILL G.L. (1979) Nocturnal elemental diet for retarded growth in a patient with cystic fibrosis. *Brit. med. J.* 1, 161.

BRIMBLECOMBE F.S. & CHAMBERLAIN J. (1973) Screening for cystic fibrosis. *Lancet* 2, 1428–31.

BYE A.M.E., MULLER D.P.R., WILSON J., WRIGHT V.M. & MEARNS M.B. (1985) Symptomatic vitamin E deficiency in cystic fibrosis. *Arch. Dis. Childh.* 60, 162.

CHASE H.P. (1976) Fatty acid, prostaglandins and cystic fibrosis. *Pediatrics* 87, 441.

CHASE H.P., LONG M.A. & LAVIN M.H. (1979) Cystic fibrosis and malnutrition. *J. Pediat.* 95, 337–47.

CHAZALETTE J.P., DUTAN G., CHEVALIER G., FILLIAT M. & GALABERT G. (1978) Study of the medium and long term survival of 28 cases of meconium ileus. In *Proceedings of the 7th International Cystic Fibrosis Congress* Paris: L'association Francaise de Lutte contre la Mucosviscidose. Imprimerie Jouvel.

CLAYTON B.E. & FRANCIS D.E.M. (1978) Inborn errors of metabolism in children. *Nutrition in the Clinical Manage-*

ment of Disease (eds. Dickerson J.W.T. & Lee H.A.), pp. 29–48. London: Edward Arnold.

COX K., ISENBERG J., OSHER A. & DOOLEY R. (1979) The effect of cimetidine on maldigestion in cystic fibrosis. *J. Pediat.* **94**, 488–92.

CRAWFORD M., HARE W. & MEARNS M. (1984) Essential fatty acids and nutrition in cystic fibrosis. *Cystic Fibrosis News*, Summer 1984, 4–5.

DANKS D.M., OLAN J. & ANDERSON D.M. (1965) Genetic study of fibrocystic disease of the pancreas. *Ann. hum. Genet.* **28**, 323.

DINWIDDIE R. (1983) The management of the first years of life. In *Cystic Fibrosis* (eds. Hodson M.E., Norman A.P. & Batten J.C.). London: Ballière Tindall.

DODGE J.A. (1983) Nutrition. in *Cystic Fibrosis* (eds. Hodson M.E., Norman A.P. & Batten J.C.), pp. 132–43. London: Ballière Tindall.

DODGE J.A. & YASSA J.G. (1978) Zinc deficiency syndrome in a British youth with cystic fibrosis. *Brit. med. J.* **1**, 411.

DODGE J.A., SALTER D.G. & YASSA J.G. (1976) Essential fatty acid deficiency due to artificial diet in an infant with cystic fibrosis. *Brit. med. J.* **1**, 192–3.

DOLAN T.F., ROWE D.S. & GIBSON L.E. (1970) Edema and hypoprotinaemia in infants with cystic fibrosis. *Clin. Pediat.* **9**, 295–7.

DOWD P.S. & HEATLEY R.V. (1984) The influence of under-nutrition on immunity. *Clin. Sci.* **66**, 241–8.

ELLIOT R.B. (1976) A therapeutic trial of fatty acid supplementation in cystic fibrosis. *Pediat.* **57**, 474.

FARRELL P., SONDEL S., PALTA M. & MISCHLER E. (1984) Prevention of growth retardation in infants with cystic fibrosis. In *Cystic Fibrosis: Horizons, Proceedings of the 9th International Cystic Fibrosis Congress* (ed. Lawson D.), p. 391. Chichester: John Wiley & Sons.

FORSTNER G., GAL G., COREY M., DURIE P., HILL R. & GASKIN K. (1980) Digestion and absorption of nutrients in cystic fibrosis. In *Proceedings of the 8th International Cystic Fibrosis Congress*, pp. 137–48. Toronto: Canadian Cystic Fibrosis Foundation.

FRANCIS D.E.M. (1979) Inborn errors of metabolism—the need for sugar. *J. hum. Nutr.* **33**, 146–54.

FRANCIS D.E.M. (1986) *Nutrition for Children*. Oxford: Blackwell Scientific Publications

FREYE H.B., KURTZ S.M., SPOCK A. & CAPP P. (1964) Light and electron microscopic examination of the small bowel of children with cystic fibrosis. *J. Pediat.* **64**, 575.

GIBBONS I.S.E. (1969) Disaccharides and cystic fibrosis of the pancreas. *Arch. Dis. Childh.* **44**, 63.

GIBBONS R.S. (1969) In *Proceedings of the 5th International Cystic Fibrosis Conference 1969, Paper 26.*

GOODCHILD M.C., MURPHY G.M., HOWELL A.M., NUTTER S. & ANDERSON C. (1975) Aspects of bile acid metabolism in cystic fibrosis. *Arch. Dis. Childh.* **50**, 769–77.

GRACEY M., BURKE V. & ANDERSON C.M. (1970) Medium chain triglycerides in paediatric practice. *Arch. Dis. Childh.* **45**, 445.

HARRIES J.T. & MULLER D.P.R. (1969) Absorption of water miscible and fat soluble preparations of vitamin E in cystic fibrosis. In *Proceedings of the 5th International Cystic Fibrosis Conference 1969, Paper 28* (ed. Lawson D.I.) Cambridge: London Cystic Fibrosis Research Trust.

HARRIES J.T. & MULLER D.P.R. (1971) Absorption of different doses of fat soluble and water miscible preparation of vitamin E in children with CF. *Arch. Dis. Childh.* **46**, 341.

HEELEY A.F., HEELEY M.E., KING D.N., KUZEMKO J.A. & WALSH M.P. (1982) Screening for cystic fibrosis by dried blood spot trypsin assay. *Arch. Dis. Childh.* **57**, 18.

HIDE D.W. & BURMAN D. (1969) An infant with both cystic fibrosis and coeliac disease. *Arch. Dis. Childh.* **44**, 533–5.

HODSON M., NORMAN A.P. & BATTEN J.C. (1983) *Cystic Fibrosis*. London: Ballière Tindall.

HUBBARD V.S. (1980) Nutrient requirements of patients with cystic fibrosis. In *Proceedings of the 8th Congress of Cystic Fibrosis*, p. 149–60.

HUBBARD V.S., BARBERO G. & CHASE H.P. (1980) Selenium and cystic fibrosis. *J. Pediat.* **96**, 421–7.

KEOHANE P.P., GRIMBLE G.K., BROWN B.E. & SILK D.B.A. (1983) Nitrogen absorption from protein hydrolysate in man—significance of peptide chain length composition. *Gastroenterology* **84**, 1206.

KEOHANE P.P., ATTRILL H., LOVE M., FROST P. & SILK D.B.A. (1984) Relation between osmolality of diet and gastrointestinal side effects in enteral nutrition. *Brit. med. J.* **1**, 288, 678–80.

KOPEL F.B. (1972) Gastrointestinal manifestations of CF. *Gastroenterology* **62**, 483.

KRAEMER R., RUDEBERG A., HADORN B. & ROSSI E. (1978) Relative underweight in CF and its prognostic value. *Acta paediat. scand.* **67**, 33–7.

LAPEY A., KATTWINKEL J., DI SANT 'AGNESE & LASTER L. (1974) Steatorrhea and azotorrhea and their relation to growth and nutrition in adolescents and young adults with CF. *J. Pediat.* **34**, 328–34.

LAWSON D. (ed.) (1984) *Cystic Fibrosis: Horizons, Proceedings of the 9th International Cystic Fibrosis Congress*. Chichester: John Wiley & Sons.

MACDONALD A. (1984) High, moderate and low fat diets for cystic fibrosis. In *Cystic Fibrosis: Horizons, Proceedings of the 9th International Cystic Fibrosis Congress*, (ed. Lawson D.), p. 395. Chichester: John Wiley & Sons.

McCOLLUM J.P.K. & HARRIES J.T. (1977) Disorders of the pancreas. In *Essentials of Paediatric Gastroenterology* (ed. Harries J.T.), pp. 335–53. Edinburgh: Churchill Livingstone.

McCOLLUM J.P.K., MATHIAS P.M., SCIBERRAS D. *et al.* (1978) Factors influencing the serum concentration of vitamin E and essential fatty acids in CF. In *Proceedings of the 7th International Cystic Fibrosis Congress*, pp. 316–27. Paris: L'association Francaise de Lutte contre la Mucoviscidose. Imprimerie Jouvel.

MEARNS M. (1974) Cystic fibrosis. *Brit. J. Hosp. Med.* **4**, 497.

MORIN C.L., ROY C.C., BONIN A. & LASALLE R. (1978) Small bowel mucosal dysfunction in patients with CF. In *Proceedings of the 7th International Cystic Fibrosis Congress* (1976). Paris: L'Association Francaise de Lutte contre la Mucoviscidose. Imprimerie Jouvel.

MULLIN T.J. & KIRKPATRICK J.R. (1981) The effect of nutr
tional support on immune competency in patients suffer-
ing from trauma, sepsis and malignant disease. *Surgery*
90, 610–14.

NEUMANN C.G., LAWLOR G.J., STIEHM E.R., SWENDSEID M.E.,
NEWTON C., HERBERT J., ANIMANN A.J. & JACOBS M. (1975)
Immunologic responses in malnourished children. *Amer.
J. clin. Nutr.* **28**, 89–104.

OGILVIE D., MCCOLLUM J.P.K., PACKER S., MANNING J., OYE-
SIKU J., HARRIES J.T. & MULLER D.P.R. (1976) Urinary
output of oxalate, calcium and magnesium in children
with intestinal disorders: a potential cause of renal calculi. *Arch. Dis. Childh.* **51**, 790–5.

PARSONS H., DUMAS A., BEAUDRY P. & PENCHARZ (1980) Dietary counselling and nutritional supplementation in the
treatment of CF and its effect on growth. In *Proceedings of
the 8th International Cystic Fibrosis Congress*, pp. 161–5,
Canada.

PHELAN P. & LANDRAU L. (1979) Improved survival of
patients with CF. *Med. J. Aust.* **1**, 261–70.

PROSSER R., OWEN H., BULL F., PARRY B., SMERKINICH J.,
GOODWIN H.A. & DATHAN J. (1974) Screening for cystic
fibrosis by examination of meconium. *Arch. Dis. Childh.*
49, 597–601.

RAEBURN J.A. (1977) Nutrition and immunity in CF. *Proceedings of the Nutrition Society* **36**, 77–83.

REES R.G., GRIMBLE G.K., KEOHANE P.P., HIGGINS B.E., WEST
M., SPILLER R.C. & SILK D.B.A. (1984) Peptide chain
length of protein hydrolysates influences jejunal nitrogen
absorption. *Gut* **25**, A547.

ROBINSON M.J. & NORMAN A.P. (1975) Life tables for CF.
Arch. Dis. Childh. **50**, 962–5.

SEAKINS J.W.T., ERSSER R.S. & GIBBONS I.S.E. (1970) Studies
on the origin of faecal amino acids in CF. *Gut* **11**, 600.

SHEPHERD R.W., COOKSLEY W.G.E. & COOKE W.D.D. (1980)
Improved growth and clinical nutritional and respiratory
changes in response to nutritional therapy in CF. *J. Pediat.*
7, 351–7.

SHEPHERD R.W., THOMAS B.J., BENNETT D., COOKSLEY W.G.E.
& WARD C. (1983) Changes in body composition and
muscle protein degradation during nutritional supplementation in nutritionally growth-retarded children with
cystic fibrosis. *J. paediat. Gastroenterol. Nutr.* **2**, 439–46.

SHWACHMAN H. & HOLSCLAW D.S. (1969) Complications of
CF. *New Engl. J. Med.* **281**, 500–1.

SILK D.B.A. (1983) *Nutritional Support in Hospital Practice*, p.
51–67. Oxford: Blackwell Scientific Publications.

SILK D.B.A. (1984) Future directions in supplemental nutrition. In *Cystic Fibrosis: Horizons, Proceedings of the 9th
International Cystic Fibrosis Congress* (ed. Lawson D.), pp.
96–114. Chichester: John Wiley & Sons.

STEEL J.M., MITCHELL D. & PRESCOTT R.L. (1983) Comparison
of the glycaemic effect of fructose, sucrose and starch-
containing mid-morning snacks in insulin-dependent diabetes. *Human Nutrition: Applied Nutrition* **37A**, No. 1, 3–8.

TAYLOR B.W., WALL J.L. & FOSBROOKE A.S. (1973) Vitamin
E therapy in CF. *Arch. Dis. Childh.* **48**, 657–8.

TORSTENSON O.L., HUMPHREY G.B., EDSON J.R., WARWICK W.J.
(1970) Cystic fibrosis presenting with severe haemor-
rhage due to vitamin K malabsorption: a report of 3 cases.
Pediatrics **45**, 857–61.

WEBER A.M., ROY C. & MORIN C.L. (1973) Malabsorption of
bile acids in children with CF. *New Engl. J. Med.* **289**,
1001.

WELCH M.J., PHELPS D.L. & OSHER A.B. (1981) Breast feeding
by a mother with CF. *Pediatrics* **67**, 5, 664–6.

WILCKENS B., BROWN A.R., URWIN R. & BROWN D.A. (1983)
Cystic fibrosis screening by dried blood spot trypsin assay:
results in 75000 newborn infants. *J. Pediat.* **102** (3),
383–7.

WRIGLEY M. (1983) *Low Fat Cookery Book for Cystic Fibrosis*,
2nd Edition, CF Research Trust, Brown & Sons, Ring-
wood, Hants.

YASSA J.G., PROSSER R. & DODGE J.A. (1978) Effects of an
artificial diet on growth in patients with CF. *Arch. Dis.
Childh.* **53**, 777–83.

CHAPTER 7

Fat-restricted diets for treatment of disorders of lipid metabolism: low-fat diets with or without medium-chain triglycerides: familial hypercholesterolaemia

Restriction of dietary fat is required in several groups of clinical conditions including disorders of lipid metabolism and absorption, for example cystic fibrosis (*see* Chapter 6) or malabsorption syndromes with steatorrhoea (*see* Chapter 1). This chapter deals with disorders of serum lipoproteins and other conditions requiring low-fat diets.

DIETARY FATS

Thirty to fifty per cent of the dietary energy intake is normally derived from fat. Fat intake in infants is approximately 50% of their energy intake, whilst milk is a major component of diet. Fats play an important role in nutrition as recently reviewed by Gurr (1984). The recommendation for a reduction of fat in the national diet as a whole (James 1983, DHSS 1984) and the implications for children are discussed by Francis (1984, 1986). The recommendation to reduce dietary fat is not intended for children under five years (DHSS 1984).

Fat is largely composed of triglycerides. Only a small proportion is present as free fatty acids, cholesterol esters and phospholipids. Triglycerides are esters of glycerol containing three fatty acids, and the physicochemical properties depend upon the number of carbon atoms present, and the degree of saturation. Polyunsaturated fatty acids (PUFA) contain two or more double bonds. Various nomenclature for fatty acids has been used (Table 7.1). Triglycerides containing fatty acids with 8 to 10 carbon atoms are known as medium-chain triglycerides (MCT) and are absorbed differently to long-chain triglycerides (LCT) which have 12 or more carbon atoms, and comprise most ordinary dietary fat.

The common fats or oils usually contain six or more fatty acids in the product as a whole. There is considerable difference in the fatty acid composition of triglyceride in different groups of food and some of the most important differences are listed below; further information is given in *The Chemical Consti-*

tuents of Natural Fats (Hilditch & Williams 1964). Paul *et al.* (1980) give details of the fatty acid content of foods.

1 The depot fat of most land animals contains considerable proportions of $C_{16:0}$ and $C_{18:0}$, and most of the unsaturated fat is $C_{18:1}$. The milk of ruminants contains significant amounts of $C_{6:0}$ to $C_{12:0}$ fatty acids.
2 The fat of both fresh and sea fish contains high proportions of unsaturated fatty acids.
3 Plant seeds contain fats with a high proportion of $C_{18:1}$, $C_{18:2}$ and $C_{18:3}$. Coconut oil is exceptional in containing about 50% of $C_{12:0}$, and is also particularly rich in the medium-chain fatty acids $C_{8:0}$ and $C_{10:0}$.

The dietary fat currently eaten by the U.K. population on average is composed of dairy products (30·8%), meat (27%), and margarine (13·1%), and other sources account for 29·1% of fat intake (from DHSS [1984] based on household food consumption and expenditure statistics 1981). Saturated and *trans* fatty acids make up approximately 47% fat intake and the P/S ratio of the national diet is currently approximately 0·23. These figures do not take into account foods eaten outside the home, which when taken into consideration increase the non-dairy, non-meat fat intake to 36%. No details regarding the fat content of the diets of children are available.

Trans unsaturated fatty acids are thought to act similarly to saturated fats in the body and these should be taken together when considering P/S ratio of any diet (Thomas *et al.* 1981, DHSS 1984). The use of vegetable oils and polyunsaturated margarines is increasing in at least some sections of the population as a result of dietary recommendations (DHSS 1984). Vegetable oils, although many are rich in polyunsaturated fatty acids (PUFA), vary considerably in their fatty acid composition (*see later*, Table 7.11) and even different batches of an oil will vary (Kochhar & Matsui 1984). Excessive and repeated heating of fats and oils, for example during frying of foods, causes

Table 7.1 Fatty acid nomenclature.

	Shorthand	Systematic	Common name
Saturated fatty acids			
Short-chain	$C_{4:0}$		Butyric
	$C_{6:0}$		Caproic
Medium-chain	$C_{8:0}$		Caprylic
	$C_{10:0}$		Capric
	$C_{12:0}$	Dodecanoic	Lauric
Long-chain	$C_{14:0}$		Myristic
	$C_{16:0}$	Hexadecanoic	Palmitic
	$C_{18:0}$	Octadecanoic	Stearic
	$C_{20:0}$		Arachidic
	$C_{22:0}$		Behenic
	$C_{24:0}$		Lignocenic
Monounsaturated fatty acids			
	$C_{16:1}$	Hexadecenoic	Palmitoleic
	$C_{18:1}$	Octadecenoic	Oleic
	$C_{20:1}$		Eicosenoic
	$C_{22:1}$		Erucic
Polyunsaturated fatty acids			
	$C_{18:2}$	Octadecadienoic	Linoleic*
	$C_{18:3}$		Linolenic*
	$C_{20:4}$		Arachidonic

*Essential fatty acids.

changes in the fat, in general increasing the saturated fatty acids. Hydrogenation of oils in the manufacture of margarines forms saturated and *trans* fatty acids, such that the resultant margarine is quite different in composition, though the choice of component oils is reflected in the final product. For example, higher quantities of *trans* fatty acids are found in margarines containing marine oils, hard margarines are composed largely of saturated fatty acids, and those made solely of vegetable oils such as soya, safflower, sunflower seed oils or corn oils are richest in PUFA and low in *trans* fatty acids (Kochhar & Matsui 1984). Margarines rarely contain more than 50% of their fat as PUFA. Butter although low in PUFA is also low in *trans* fatty acids, as are vegetable oils. The significance of *trans* fatty acids is still not fully understood, but until such time as as they are known to be 'safe' their intake should be limited, at least in children.

FAT ABSORPTION AND TRANSPORT

In healthy individuals, after infancy, approximately 97% dietary fat is absorbed. A diagrammatic representation of fat absorption is given in Fig. 7.1.

Because fats are insoluble in water they are transported in the plasma with proteins, as complex macromolecules, of which there are four main lipoprotein fractions: chylomicron, pre-β-lipoprotein (very low density lipoprotein, VLDL), β-lipoprotein (low density lipoprotein, LDL) and α-lipoprotein (high density lipoprotein, HDL). Each has a specific role and distinct composition.

The proteins found in lipoprotein are referred to as apoproteins. Chylomicrons with a diameter of 400 nm are large enough to be visible; the others are progressively smaller down to HDL which is less than 10 nm diameter. Their different densities reflect differences in their size and make-up. Chlyomicrons and VLDL have only small amounts of protein and carry the bulk of triglycerides, a combination which makes them light and large. In contrast most of the cholesterol (60 to 70%) is carried by LDL which together with HDL has a higher protein content and so is heavier and more dense. The cholesterol in VLDL is largely endogenous, i.e. synthesized by the liver, whereas chylomicrons carry dietary fat absorbed in the intestine. The main protein in HDL is apoprotein A, which facilitates the joining of the ester groups derived from fatty acids onto molecules of free cholesterol. This esterification, which occurs in the

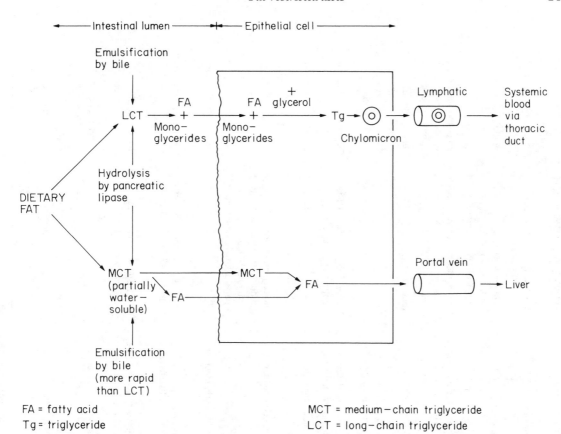

FA = fatty acid   MCT = medium−chain triglyceride
Tg = triglyceride   LCT = long−chain triglyceride

Fig. 7.1 Major factors in the absorption of dietary fat.

serum, is important since about two-thirds of the total body cholesterol is in the ester form. The lipoproteins are in a continual state of flux and are continually being remodelled and changing their composition. Chylomicrons and VLDL acquire apoprotein C from HDL, which also takes unesterified cholesterol from VLDL, adds on an ester group and then passes it back up the line. The focus of research recently has changed from total serum cholesterol to LDL, which carries cholesterol to the tissues, and HDL which appears to carry it away again. Specific tissue receptors on the surface of certain cells bind LDL and take it into the cell where the LDL particle is broken down and cholesterol is released. This then suppresses the cell's own synthesis of cholesterol and the formation of new receptors and also ensures that cells have adequate cholesterol for their needs. This brief summary illustrates the complexity of lipid metabolism, which is discussed by Rifkind and Levy (1977) and Myant (1982). Because of the interest in coronary heart disease lipid research is a fast-growing area.

Although triglycerides constitute the major component of dietary fat, a small amount of dietary cholesterol is also present. The average western adult diet contains approximately 250 to 750 mg cholesterol per day, of which about half is absorbed. However, the adult is able to synthesize 0·5 to 1 g of cholesterol per day, which is at least twice and possibly 3 to 4 times what is taken in the diet. The bulk of the body's cholesterol is found in the cell membranes, where it acts as a stabilizing agent; about one-quarter is in the nervous system where it forms a major component of the myelin sheaths; it is a precursor of bile acids which play a major role in dietary fat and cholesterol absorption and digestion in the intestine; and it is a precursor of oestrogen, testosterone and corticosteroids. The net cholesterol is the result of dietary intake, endogenous synthesis and excretion, e.g. in bile acids and the small amounts which are lost in the faeces. An adult has approximately 145 g cholesterol in his body, of which less than 10% is in the bloodstream, the rest being in the tissues (Myant 1982).

Table 7.2 Summary of lipid disorders (adapted from Lloyd 1982).

Lipoprotein class primarily affected	Primary disorder	Treatment of primary disorder	Secondary disorder*
(a) Hypolipoproteinaemia			
Chylomicrons	Abetalipoproteinaemia	Very low-fat diet (MCT not recommended)	Fat malabsorption
β-lipoprotein	Abetalipoproteinaemia	Vitamins A, D, E, K supplements (vitamin E is particularly important)	Fat malabsorption
	Familial hypobetalipoproteinaemia (physiological in newborn)	Low-fat diet if steatorrhoea is a feature	Hyperthyroidism Hepatic failure Chronic anaemia
α-lipoprotein	Familial α-lipoprotein deficiency (Tangier disease)	None	Hepatic failure
	Familial lecithin cholesterol acyltransferase deficiency (LCAT)	None	Non-specific in acute and chronic illnesses
(b) Hyperlipoproteinaemia			
Chylomicron	Familial lipoprotein lipase deficiency: hyperchylomicronaemia (type I)	Very low-fat diet and MCT to improve palatability	Diabetes mellitus (rarely)
β-lipoprotein	Familial hypercholesterolaemia	Cholestyramine and/or reduced saturated and *trans* fatty acids, plus polyunsaturated fatty acids	Hepatic glycogenosis type III Obstructive jaundice Hyperthyroidism
	Familial hyperbetalipoproteinaemia (type IIa)		
β-lipoprotein	Familial combined hyperlipidaemia (type IIb)		Nephrotic syndrome
Broad β-lipoprotein	Broad beta disease: familial hyperlipidaemia (type III). Rarely seen in children	Reduction of energy to control obesity. Clofibrate effective	Hypothyroidism (rarely)
Pre-β-lipoprotein	Familial hypertriglyceridaemia (type IV). Rarely seen in children	May respond to reduced carbohydrate intake	Diabetes mellitus Nephrotic syndrome Glycogen storage disease types I and IV Hypercalcaemia
Chylomicrons and pre-β-lipoprotein	Familial hyperlipoproteinaemia (type V). Rarely seen in children	Moderate reduction of fat and carbohydrate. Increased protein	Pancreatitis Diabetes mellitus Nephrotic syndrome

*The secondary lipidaemias are normally treated by management regimens aimed to treat the primary condition.

The lipoproteins in plasma can be separated by techniques such as electrophoresis or ultracentrifugation (Lloyd 1982). Both hypolipoproteinaemia and hyperlipoproteinaemia states occur and are reviewed by Lloyd (1982).

Disorders may be due to primary defects that are genetically determined, or a secondary manifestation of other conditions such as diabetes mellitus, nephrotic syndrome, or glycogen storage disease. Five types of lipid pattern can be distinguished and have been classified by WHO (Beaumont *et al.* 1970). Table 7.2 summarizes the lipid disorders based on electrophoresis findings. Lipid patterns are not specific and do not on their own constitute a diagnosis, and they should not be used blindly as an indication for a particular therapy (Lloyd 1982). The conditions in this chapter are largely those related to the primary lipid disorders which respond to dietary modification.

DISORDERS OF LIPID METABOLISM REQUIRING DIETARY FAT RESTRICTION

Abetalipoproteinaemia

This rare inherited condition is due to failure to synthesize chylomicrons and is characterized by complete absence of β-lipoprotein, chylomicrons and pre-β-lipoprotein in the serum, even after a meal of fat (Herbert *et al.* 1983, Lloyd 1982). Malabsorption of fat, fat-soluble vitamin deficiencies including those of vitamins A, E, and K, characteristic red blood cells and progressive neurological manifestations occur, which may be due to vitamin E deficiency. Rickets are not a consistent feature, probably due to vitamin D synthesis from sunlight on skin. The mucosal villi cells are distended with triglyceride. Despite this, approximately 50 to 70% of dietary fat is absorbed, probably via the portal vein route, and MCT which is normally absorbed in the same way may inhibit the absorption of normal dietary fat (LCT) including $C_{18:2}$, the essential fatty acid (Lloyd & Muller 1972). In addition, MCT may exacerbate fatty changes in the liver (Partin *et al.* 1974). Treatment is with a very low-fat diet to control steatorrhoea, without MCT, but with specific supplements of vitamins A, E and K (Lloyd 1982) in addition to supplements required to ensure the nutritional adequacy of the diet. Large doses of vitamin E may prevent or improve the neurological features of the disease (Muller *et al.* 1977). Linoleic acid serum levels are low, but no features attributable to the deficiency are reported. Some linoleic acid (2 to 5 g per day) can be included in the diet, but this reduces the intake of other dietary fat

and there is no evidence of clinical benefit. Lloyd (1982) suggests an intake of only 5 to 20 g dietary fat daily, which needs to be continued throughout life. This necessitates a very high energy intake from carbohydrate (Francis 1979). Such a regimen usually results in excellent catch-up growth and normal physical development (Muller *et al.* 1977).

Familial lipoprotein lipase deficiency. Type I: primary hyperchylomicronaemia or fat-induced hypertriglyceridaemia

This is a rare recessively inherited disorder in which the basic defect is a deficiency in the apoprotein C with resultant inactivation of lipoprotein lipase and hence failure to clear chylomicrons at a normal rate. Clinical features include, especially in infants and young children, failure to thrive, attacks of abdominal pain, eruptive xanthoma and hepatosplenomegaly. Occasionally, the condition is asymptomatic. Serum is milky in the fasting state with gross elevation of triglyceride, 35 to 115 mmol/1* (3000 to 10 000 mg per 100 ml) and lesser elevation of cholesterol (Fredrickson *et al.* 1978).

The condition is treated with a very low-fat diet. Carbohydrate intake is increased to ensure adequate energy (Kwiterovich *et al.* 1973). MCT may be used as a source of energy and to improve the palatability of the diet. Fat-soluble vitamin supplements are required.

During episodes of abdominal pain a 'no-fat' (less than 1 g/day) diet is recommended temporarily. To maintain the fasting serum optically clear as little as 5 g fat/day may be tolerated, however a diet of 5 to 10 g fat/day is used long-term, even though serum lipids remain slightly elevated. This is slightly more practical and as there is as yet no evidence to suggest an increased incidence of atherosclerosis in later life; provided the child remains symptom-free, the higher fat intake is satisfactory (Lloyd 1982). Tolerance of fat does not increase with the age of the child (Lloyd & Wolff 1969) and it is unlikely that most children will manage as much as the 25 to 35 g fat suggested for the treatment of adults (Levy *et al.* 1972). Clinical deficiency of linoleic acid on such low-fat diets has not been observed (Lloyd 1982) and growth rate is usually normal.

Familial hypercholesterolaemia. Type II: familial hyperbetalipoproteinaemia

This is the commonest of the primary hyperlipoproteinaemias, occurring in approximately 1 in 500 of

---

* mmol/1 $\times$ 88·54 = mg/100 ml triglycerides.

the population. The cholesterol-rich β-lipoproteins are present in increased amounts in the serum, due to defective removal of cholesterol, at least in part because the LDL receptors are not produced in adequate numbers. The disorder is inherited as an autosomal dominant; the heterozygotes are the common form with serum cholesterol levels of 7·3 to 13 mmol/l* (280 to 500 mg per 100 ml) compared to normal levels of less than 6·2 mmol/l (240 mg/100 ml). In the heterozygous form xanthomata develop in adult life, and corneal arcus occurs and has also been observed in some children. The condition is associated with a high incidence of premature ischaemic heart disease, especially in males (Slack 1969, Myant & Slack 1973). The object of instituting treatment in children is to attempt to reduce the risk of ischaemic heart disease, although there is as yet no absolute evidence that it will do so in children with familial hypercholesterolaemia (Lloyd 1982).

The homozygous form is rare and much more severe; serum cholesterol may reach up to 25 mmol/l (1000 mg per 100 ml). In the homozygous form tuberous and tendon xanthomata may develop in childhood, and ischaemic heart disease may occur in adolescence. Treatment intervention programmes remain disappointing in this latter group of patients.

Although it has not yet been shown convincingly that lowering the serum cholesterol in familial hypercholesterolaemia can delay the development of atherosclerosis, the results of the Lipid Research Clinic's primary prevention trial (Anonymous 1984) is encouraging. In the trial 3806 asymptomatic men aged 35 to 59 years with primary hypercholesterolaemia ≥ 6·85 mmol/l (≥ 265 mg/100 ml) were treated with diet modification, and in half cholestyramine resin was given (treatment group) and the remainder received a placebo. In this study over seven years, serum cholesterol (total and LDL) was lowered in the treatment group and a 19% reduction in the risk of coronary heart disease (CHD) was observed, angina was decreased by 20%, the development of electrocardiographic signs on exercise testing by 24%, and the rate of treatment by coronary bypass surgery by 21%. No specific advice was given regarding other risk factors such as smoking, exercise or weight to either group. The degree of reduction in plasma lipids was directly related to the dose of cholestyramine taken daily. There was only a 7% reduction in overall mortality due to an increase in deaths from other causes in the treatment group. The reduction in CHD found in this study is consistent with

other trial data and suggests that treatment is justified in those with familial hypercholesterolaemia, and those in the top quintile for plasma cholesterol levels (Oliver 1984). The regimen must be sufficient to lower plasma cholesterol over many years by about 10% and LDL by 15%.

If lowering the serum cholesterol has any effect, such treatment is likely to achieve best results if started early in life, before atheromatous lesions have become too advanced. Screening of children in affected families is therefore recommended. Because of the diagnostic difficulties in infants under one year (Darmady et al. 1972) it is, in general, wise to defer treatment until about one year of age. Studies in human infants relating subsequent serum cholesterol levels to the type of feed used have failed to show any correlation (Friedman & Goldberg 1975).

Treatment of familial hypercholesterolaemia must effectively reduce serum cholesterol long-term, be practical and without side-effects, and any diet used must be nutritionally adequate and acceptable. Many studies have been published showing serum cholesterol levels can be reduced by dietary manipulation (Slack 1969; Fredrickson et al. 1970, Anderson et al. 1973) in both normal and hypercholesterolaemic subjects, although many different regimens have been used to achieve this effect.

DIET IN HYPERCHOLESTEROLAEMIA

The COMA report on diet and cardiovascular disease (DHSS 1984) recommends that those at risk of CHD, such as individuals with hypercholesterolaemia, should decrease saturated and *trans* fatty acid intake to 10% and total fat to not more than 30% of dietary energy. No specific recommendation is given for the consumption of PUFA and monounsaturated fatty acids, but to facilitate the recommendation for saturated fat reduction they recommend a P/S ratio of approximately 0·45 but not more than 1·0. They also recommend a reduction in dietary cholesterol to < 100 mg/4200 kJ (1000 kcal) and an increase of dietary fibre to more than 30 g daily in adults.

These principles can be adapted for children with familial hypercholesterolaemia. Segal et al. (1970) however emphasized the need to reduce dietary fat, and showed the addition of corn oil and its products had no specific hypocholesterolaemia action in children with familial hypercholesterolaemia.

In practice, a dietary prescription of 30% energy from fat requires a diet containing only 8 g total fat for each 1000 kJ, i.e. 33 g total fat for each 1000 kcal. Also, to achieve the desired reduction in

---

* mmol/l × 38·67 = mg/100 ml cholesterol.

saturated fatty acids only half of the fat should be derived from conventional dietary fats such as those in lean meats, cereals, bread (preferably wholegrain varieties), cakes, biscuits, egg, milk and dairy products, in which, on average, 50% of the fat is present as saturated fatty acids. Fat sources rich in PUFA such as safflower, sunflower seed, soya or corn oils should provide 25% of the fat prescription, and the remaining 25% can be provided from polyunsaturated margarines. The latter, however, rarely contain more than 50% PUFA, and so the choice of margarine must be made carefully, the PUFA oils rather than the PUFA margarines being preferred (*see* Table 7.11). The total diet must be nutritionally adequate in protein, and the carbohydrates should preferably be made up of wholegrain cereals, pulses, potato and wholemeal bread, fruit and vegetables.

The need for severe restriction of dietary cholesterol is not convincingly established. Compared with liver synthesis of cholesterol dietary cholesterol is probably insignificant in influencing serum cholesterol in children with familial hypercholesterolaemia. However, many dietary regimens for hypercholesterolaemia recommend restriction of dietary cholesterol (Fredrickson *et al.* 1970, DHSS 1984). Concentrated sources of dietary cholesterol include egg-yolk, chicken-liver, lamb's liver, cod roe, sweetbread and brain; moderately high sources of cholesterol are heart, ox liver, pig's liver, tripe, tongue, shrimps, prawns, cream, Stilton and Cheddar cheese. When considered necessary these high-cholesterol foods can be restricted or avoided. However, as children largely consume cholesterol in conjunction with dietary fat, mostly in the form of eggs and dairy fats, restriction of dietary fat automatically reduces cholesterol intake without the need for undue emphasis on dietary cholesterol (Lloyd 1982), thus simplifying the diet prescription.

Restrictions of ordinary dietary fat to 15 to 20 g/day in children with familial hypercholesterolaemia achieved a reduction of 20 to 24% of the pre-treatment value, which may be insufficient to reduce the serum cholesterol level to acceptable values (Lloyd 1982, Anderson *et al.* 1973).

In practice, the maintenance of a strict diet is difficult over long periods of time, particularly during adolescence. West and Lloyd (1974) and Schlierf *et al.* (1979) both found that only about 20% of patients on follow-up after three years had satisfactory control by diet alone. The patients need to be strongly motivated to continue. As a result, for the majority, drugs, particularly cholestyramine, are more effective, and provided cholesterol levels are satisfactory rigorous

dietary restriction need not be continued (West & Lloyd 1973).

DRUGS IN HYPERCHOLESTEROLAEMIA

Cholesterol-lowering drugs, used in conjunction with dietary manipulation, are necessary in some heterozygous patients, particularly adults (Fredrickson & Levy 1970, Anonymous 1984), to achieve acceptable serum cholesterol levels. In homozygous type II familial hypercholesterolaemia, even with vigorous dietary and drug treatment, results are very disappointing.

Cholestyramine (Questran) is an anion exchange resin that binds bile salts in the gut, preventing reabsorption and thus decreasing the cholesterol pool. In children 0·6 g/kg per day of cholestyramine has been found to be effective, and results in a mean reduction of serum cholesterol of approximately 33% (West & Lloyd 1973). Compliance with treatment is better than with diet, but after five years West and Lloyd (1979) report a compliance rate of only 57%. More recently Wheeler *et al.* (1985) have carried out a trial using bezafibrate in children with familial hypercholesterolaemia with some encouraging preliminary results. Further follow-up is required to assess the safety and effectiveness of this treatment over a longer period before it can be recommended for routine use.

The nutritional status of patients and particularly children given cholestyramine or any drug must be monitored (Lloyd 1982). Cholestyramine induces folate deficiency, and supplements of 5 mg/day of folic acid are recommended. Steatorrhoea occurs in some children and the Lipid Research Trial (Anonymous 1984) found gastrointestinal side-effects in many men in the trial, 68% of those receiving cholestyramine having such complaints after one year and 25% after seven years; heartburn, gas, belching and bloating were common.

Thus 'the risk of correcting risk by drugs may be greater than the uncorrected risk' (Oliver 1982), and the Lipid Research Trial (Anonymous 1984) concludes 'the mode of action, cholesterol lowering potency and possible toxicity of cholesterol lowering drugs must be taken into account before their use is advocated in the prevention of coronary heart disease'.

In any treatment programme aimed at the prevention of coronary heart disease other high risk factors must be corrected or minimized. Exercise should be encouraged to become a life-long habit, overweight should be corrected or avoided, and smoking should be strongly discouraged (DHSS 1974, James 1983, DHSS 1984).

Other conditions requiring low-fat diet treatment

The following conditions also require low-fat dietary treatment. The resultant energy deficit should be replaced by the addition of either carbohydrate and/or MCT, whichever is preferred.

1   DEFECTIVE INTRALUMINAR DIGESTION/ ABSORPTION

(a)   Pancreatic insufficiency
Pancreatic insufficiency, commonly due to cystic fibrosis and more rarely due to Shwachman syndrome, causes a deficiency of lipase needed for the hydrolysis of fat (McCollum & Harries 1977). Pancreatic enzyme replacement therapy with moderate restriction of dietary fat is indicated. Details of the diet required in cystic fibrosis are given in Chapter 6.

(b)   Obstructive jaundice, biliary atresia and disorders of enterohepatic circulation
Obstructive jaundice, such as in infants with neonatal hepatitis or biliary atresia, causes steatorrhoea due to a lack of bile salts necessary for emulsification of fat. A low-fat diet with adequate protein, vitamins, especially A, D, E and K, and minerals and high energy intake is indicated. As a result of treatment and adequate nutrition growth rate may be improved (Burks & Danks 1966, Mowat 1979).

(c)   Malabsorption associated with abnormal intestinal flora
Abnormal intestinal flora occur in the stagnant loop syndrome and interfere with the action of bile salts. Specific treatment is with antibiotics and/or surgery, but a low-fat diet with adequate energy, protein, vitamins and minerals may be helpful in improving the nutritional state prior to the operation (Gracy et al. 1970).

(d)   Loss of absorptive surface
Intestinal resection during the surgical management of gastrointestinal tract abnormalities may cause reduction in absorptive area: short gut syndrome. Fat malabsorption occurs and often in infants multiple malabsorption syndrome results. The management of the latter is dealt with in Chapter 1. Less complex cases may benefit from a slightly reduced fat intake with supplements of the fat-soluble vitamins and vitamin B_{12}, temporarily or long-term.

(e)   Protracted diarrhoea
Protracted diarrhoea, often with multiple malabsorption of uncertain pathogenesis, usually requires withdrawal of disaccharides and cow's milk protein from the diet (see Chapter 1). Reduction of fat is occasionally indicated if steatorrhoea persists (Larcher et al. 1977).

2   DEFECTIVE CHYLOMICRON TRANSPORT: INTESTINAL LYMPHANGIECTASIA: CHYLURIA: CHYLOTHORAX

(a)   Intestinal lymphangiectasia
This is a generalized lymphatic disorder associated with loss of serum protein into the gastrointestinal tract and resultant hypoproteinaemia with oedema (Leyland et al. 1969). The reduction of dietary fat to a minimum, e.g. 5 to 10 g daily, reduces lymph flow, and with additional protein intake usually controls the symptoms; although some protein leak persists, plasma protein returns toward normal. Sodium intake may need to be reduced if oedema is a feature. Carbohydrate and/or MCT is useful, to replace the energy deficit caused by the fat reduction.

(b)   Chyluria and chylothorax
These conditions are caused by disorders of the lymphatic system, and may be the conequence of surgery. In chyluria the patient passes milky urine containing chyle. In chylothorax there is an abnormal communication between the lymphatic system draining the small intestine and the pleural space. A minimal fat intake reduces chyle flow, largely improving clinical problems. In both conditions protein loss occurs, either primarily or as a result of thoracenteses (Tamir et al. 1969), and must be replaced in the diet or by plasma infusions. Treatment is discontinued once clinical improvement occurs.

Minimal and very low-fat diets

It is impossible to design a completely fat-free diet for long-term use. Quantities can be reduced to below 1 g fat daily temporarily and for infants. Skimmed milk alone is unsuitable but this or the high biological whey protein Maxipro can be used with supplements of glucose polymer, vitamins and minerals (Table 7.3) or a MCT 'filled' milk can be selected (Table 7.9). As many of these feeds are high in protein, renal solute load and osmolality, they should be used cautiously in young infants. Appropriate vitamin and mineral supplements should be prescribed

Table 7.3 Minimal fat feeds for infants with lipid disorders.

		Renal solute*	Sodium (mmol)	Potassium (mmol)	Chloride (mmol)	Energy		Carbohydrate (g)	Protein (g)	Fat (g)
						kJ	kcal			
1	*Infants under six months*									
	(a) 5 g skimmed milk powder		1·2	2·1	1·6	76	18	2·2	1·8	Trace
	15 g Maxijul LE¶		Trace	Trace	Trace	240	60	15		
	Water to 100 ml									
	Total‡	12·1	1·2	2·1	1·6	316	78	17·2	1·8	Trace
	(b) 2 g Maxipro HBV		0·2	0·2	N/S	30	7	Trace	1·8	Trace
	15 g Maxijul LE¶		Trace	Trace	Trace	240	60	15		
	0·8 g Metabolic Mineral Mixture		1·4	1·7						
	Water to 100 ml									
	Total§	≃14·2	1·6	1·9	N/S	270	67	15	1·8	Trace
2	*Moderate protein*									
	7 g skimmed milk powder		1·7	3·0	2·2	106	25	3·7	2·5	<0·1
	15 g Maxijul LE¶		Trace	Trace	Trace	240	60	15		
	Water to 100 ml									
	Total‡	16·9	1·7	3·0	2·2	346	85	18·7	2·5	<0·1
3	*High protein*									
	10 g skimmed milk powder		2·4	4·2	3·1	151	36	5·3	3·6	0·1
	10 g Maxijul LE¶		Trace	Trace	Trace	160	40	10		
	Water to 100 ml									
	Total‡	24·1	2·4	4·2	3·1	311	76	15·3	3·6	0·1

* By calculation renal solute load is the sum of sodium, potassium, chloride and (protein × 4) = mmol/100 ml. Because of the high renal solute content feeds 2 and 3 should be used with caution in infants.
† Essential fatty acid supplements may be necessary.
‡ Vitamin and trace mineral supplements as 6 to 12 Cow & Gate Supplementary Vitamin Tablets plus 5 ml Ketovite Liquid per day are recommended.
§ Three Ketovite Tablets plus 5 ml Ketovite Liquid per day is recommended. Other levels of protein can be provided by appropriately increasing the Maxipro.
¶ Other brands of glucose polymer can be used but contain higher quantities of sodium and potassium.
N/S Not specified.

and their use monitored biochemically and clinically. Extra fluid should be offered, especially if the child is unwell.

For older children the daily fat intake can be reduced to approximately 1 g fat per year of age by selecting foods from Table 7.4, but the diet is monotonous for the child and such a severe degree of restriction is seldom required. Its main uses are in the treatment of abetalipoproteinaemia, initially in fat-induced hypertriglyceridaemia while the serum is being cleared of accumulated fat, and in intestinal lymphangiectasia, chlyothorax and chyluria where reduction in chyle flow is desired. Most patients with these conditions can manage between 5 and 20 g fat

per day after the initial improvement, but the degree of fat restriction varies with the clinical condition and diagnosis (Lloyd 1982).

LOW-FAT DIETS

A fat intake in the range of 10 to 20% of energy from dietary fat, i.e. 2·5 to 6 g fat/1000 kJ or 10 to 25 g fat/1000 kcal, is usually tolerated by most patients with conditions requiring treatment with a low-fat diet, but must be assessed individually. Such a diet is used in patients with obstructive jaundice, steatorrhoea and in those patients with familial hypercholesterolaemia treated by diet. The individual diet is devised using the information in Table 7.5, which lists the fat and protein content of different groups of food, in conjunction with the basic minimal fat diet in Table 7.4. The occasional patient will tolerate a simple no-added-fat diet.

Protein intake in fat-restricted diets

Adequate protein must be provided in the diet. Skimmed milk, cottage cheese and low-fat yoghurt, white fish and egg-whites are excellent low-fat sources of protein, as are cereals and pulses, but not

Table 7.4   Basic minimal fat diet.

(a) Allowed and forbidden foods.

Foods allowed	Foods forbidden
Skimmed milk, low-fat yoghurt, cottage cheese, skimmed milk powder, non-fat milk powder	Whole milk, butter, cream, evaporated milks, all ice-creams
Casilan, Maxipro HBV Sweetened condensed skimmed milk	'Filled' milks, Five-Pints, Compliment, Coffee-mate Non-milk fat products Soya milks and milk substitutes containing ordinary fat
Egg-white	Fats, oils, margarines
*Lean meat (*see* Table 7.5). White low-fat fish	Fatty meats, oily fish: sausages, sardines, beefburgers, etc.
Fruit—fresh, frozen, tinned, dried fruits	Fruit pies, avocado pears, olives
Vegetables, including green salads: frozen, fresh, canned, unless cooked with added fat *Baked beans (canned) in moderation *Pulses, dried peas, beans, gram, mung, red kidney, lentils, dahl Textured vegetable protein (free of added fat)	Crisps, chips, roast potato, fried vegetables, canned vegetables and potato salad containing sauces Nuts and seeds including dry roast nuts
*Cereals: wheat, maize, barley, rice, rye, flour Rice Krispies, Cornflakes, Puffed Wheat, Sugar Puffs, Weetabix, baby rice type products *Bread: white, brown, wholemeal	Oats, Ready Brek, muesli-type cereals Farley's Rusks and similar cereals with added fat
Matzos, rye crispbread, water biscuits, meringue, fat-free chapatis	All cakes and all biscuits, cream crackers, starch-reduced crispbreads
*Pasta including wholemeal pasta, spaghetti, macaroni Cornflower, custard powder Instant Whip or jelly creams made with skimmed milk Table jellies, sago, tapioca	Whole-milk puddings, suet puddings, pies, pastries, Angel Delight, Dream Topping type desserts
Sugar, jam, jelly, syrup, honey, sweets, boiled sweets, fruit gums, pastilles, water ice-lollies and sorbet	Chocolate, nuts, toffees, peanut butter, lemon curd
Glucose, glucose polymers, Lucozade, fruit juices, squash, carbonated beverages	
Chutney, tomato ketchup, sauces, Worcestershire sauce, pickles	Salad cream, French dressings, oil mayonnaise
Marmite, Bovril, Oxo, Bisto, salt, pepper, herbs, spices, fat-free stock and soup Stock cubes* in moderation	Gravy made from meat fat and juices
Tea, coffee (made with skimmed milk) Essences and food colourings, milk-shake syrups and flavours	Milk-type beverages, e.g. Horlicks, Bournvita, malted milk, Ovaltine, drinking chocolate*

* These foods contain traces of fat and may need to be restricted in minimal fat diets.

Table 7.5 provides details of the fat and protein content of different foods which can be used in conjunction with this table as appropriate for the diet prescription.

Table 7.4 *continued*

(b) Low-fat diet menu: sample menu

Breakfast	Serve of cereal, e.g. Rice Krispies, Cornflakes
	Skimmed milk plus sugar or glucose polymer
	Bread and Outline* from allowance, may be toasted (no butter)
	Marmite, jam, honey, marmalade
	Fruit—fresh, stewed or tinned
	Egg-whites scrambled (*see* recipe)
	Grilled tomatoes or mushrooms
Mid-morning	Fruit drink or skimmed milk plus sugar or glucose polymer
	Fruit
Dinner	Meat from allowance or Mexican beans, *see* recipe, p. 186
	Potato, boiled or mashed with skimmed milk, jacket potatoes
	Vegetable cooked without fat
	Puddings made with skimmed milk, e.g. rice, custard, sago, blancmange
	Fruit or jelly, as desired
Tea	Fruit juice or skimmed milk plus sugar or glucose polymer
	Fat-free cake (*see* Recipes) or meringue
	Boiled sweets or water-ice, jelly
	Bread and Outline* from allowance
Supper	Cottage cheese or grilled white very low-fat fish, and/or fat-free lentil/pea soup
	Vegetables or salad or baked beans or red bean salad (*see* Recipes)
	Jelly or fruit or skimmed milk pudding or fruit meringue or fruit snow
	Skimmed milk or fruit plus sugar or glucose polymer
Bedtime	Bread and Outline* from allowance or fat-free cake
	Skimmed milk plus sugar or glucose polymer
Appropriate vitamin, mineral supplements	3 Ketovite Tablets plus 5 ml Ketovite Liquid (Paines & Byrne)
	Fluoride

*Outline is a low-fat spread and should be used in restricted quantity as appropriate for the diet prescriptions. Other brands may be equally suitable, *see* Table 7.5.

nuts or seeds. Vegetarian dishes are usually lower in fat than traditional meals and can be incorporated to reduce the fat intake, provide variety and energy intake and increase the protein content of the diet. To improve the quality of protein, cereals and pulses should be used in conjunction with each other or with some first-class protein, e.g. skimmed milk. Meat extenders and textured vegetable proteins are usually low in fat. Meat contains fat in addition to protein and must be limited in fat-restricted diets or chosen with care. Chicken or turkey breast, liver and kidney are lower in fat than other meats. All meat should be very lean, not 'marbled', trimmed of all visible fat and skin, and cooked without additional fat/oil, and by methods such as grilling which enables the fat to be drained away. Stews and casseroles should be cooked in advance and chilled so that the fat can be removed before thoroughly reheating to serve. Fatty minced meat should be avoided or it can be prepared from meat from which all the fat has first been removed. The latter can be used to prepare home-made low-fat beefburgers and similar popular dishes, but commercially prepared beefburgers, hamburgers and sausages are too high in fat for inclusion in minimal and very low-fat diets.

Essential fatty acids

Minimal and low-fat diets have a reduced content of

essential fatty acids. Although blood levels of $C_{18:2}$ may be low, clinical evidence of deficiency has rarely been reported, even in children on very low-fat diets for considerable periods, and growth and development have been normal (Tamir *et al.* 1969, Lloyd 1982), unless malabsorption is also present, as seen in children with CF (McCollum & Harries 1977). Low-fat diets using MCT supplements may reduce the requirement of $C_{18:2}$ (Kaunitz *et al.* 1958). Some polyunsaturated fat, for example 2 to 5 ml of corn or safflower oil per day, may be included in the diet and will increase the linoleic acid content of the diet, but this may reduce the allowance of other dietary fat. Alternatively, part of the permitted fat allowance can be selected from chicken, turkey and rabbit meats which are lower in total fat but richer in essential fatty acids than other meats.

Several MCT 'filled' milks (*see* Table 7.9) contain linoleic acid supplements in the form of corn or safflower oil. This can contribute greatly to the total dietary long-chain fat, and in cases requiring a minimal or very low-fat intake these products may therefore be contraindicated, unless an appropriate product is selected with care or given in limited quantity.

Mineral and vitamin supplements

Fat-soluble vitamin supplements, ideally in water-miscible form, are necessary with minimal and low-fat diets to provide adequate vitamins A, D, E and K. Vitamin E is particularly important in patients with abetalipoproteinaemia (Muller *et al.* 1977). Additional iron, vitamin B_{12} and possibly zinc are needed when the intake of meat is severely restricted. The choice of supplement depends on the conventional food intake, e.g. dark-green leafy vegetables contain vitamin K and iron; cereals and pulses contain some calcium, iron and zinc but it is poorly absorbed; some MCT 'filled' milks, e.g. Portagen, contain added vitamins, and if an adequate volume is used (at least 500 ml daily) additional vitamins may be unnecessary; polyunsaturated margarines contain added vitamins A and D which may eliminate the necessity

Table 7.5 Fat and protein content of different foods. These foods may need to be restricted when used in conjunction with a very low-fat diet.

(a) Selected foods

Food (100 g)	Fat (g)	Protein (g)
Skimmed milk powder, non-fat milk powders	0·8 to 1·3	35 to 36
Fresh liquid skimmed milk (separated)	0·1	3·4
Casilan	1·8	90
Maxipro HBV	Trace	88
Egg-white	Nil	9
Low-fat yoghurt: natural, flavoured, fruit	1·0‡	5·0
Flour: white, plain, self-raising, wholemeal	1·2‡	9·5
*Bread: average white, brown, wholemeal, Hovis	2·2	8·8
Rice and pasta/spaghetti (boiled)	0·3	2·2 to 4·2
Cereals: Rice Krispies, Cornflakes, Sugar Puffs, Puffed Wheat	1·4‡	8·7‡
Pulses: beans (boiled) and baked beans	0·5‡	5·7‡
Weetabix	3·4	11·4
Lean meat and fish (*see* Table 7.5(b) for further details of the quantity per serve)		
1 very low-fat	1·0 to 2·0	15 to 20
2 low-fat	4·0 to 6·0	18 to 27
3 moderate-fat	8·5 to 12	18 to 27
4 high-fat	18‡	18‡
Egg, 2 × size 3 or 4	11·0	12·2
Whole milk (not Channel Island/Jersey type)	3·8	3·3
Margarines†, only suitable on more generous diets	80	0·1
Low-fat spreads, e.g. Outline†, Gold†	40	Trace
Polyunsaturated margarine (*see* Table 7.11 for further details)	81	0·1

* The fat content of bread can be reduced by omitting added fat/oil in home-baked bread and cooking in a non-stick or silicone-lined tin.

† Not necessarily high in PUFA.

‡ Average values.

Table 7.5(b) Meat, cheeses and fish for use in low-fat diets.

All meats should be lean, trimmed of visible fat, not 'marbled', and weighed after cooking. No fat should be used in cooking, i.e. steam, grill, bake in foil or roast on a wire mesh tray, without fat. Appropriate selection from the following groups is suggested according to the diet prescription.

(i) *Very low-fat:* 100 g contains on average 1 to 2 g fat and 15 to 20 g protein

Cod	Hake
Haddock—smoked or fresh	Sole—lemon and Dover
Plaice	Mussels
Whiting	Oysters
Scallops	Cockles
Prawn*	Flounder
Shrimps*	Fillet
Turbot	

(ii) *Low-fat:* 100 g contains on average 4 to 6 g fat and 18 to 27 g protein

Chicken	Halibut
Turkey	Trout
Kidney	Lobster
Grouse	Crab
Heart*	Bass
Tripe*	Bream (red and sea)
Venison	Brill
Cottage cheese	

(iii) *Moderate fat:* 100 g contains on average 8·5 to 12 g fat and 18 to 27 g protein

Beef	Pilchards
Lamb—very lean only	Salmon, fresh or tinned
Mutton—very lean only	Rabbit
Ham—very lean only	Hare
Veal	Pheasant
Liver*	Low-fat cheeses* (Tendale and Shape)

(iv) *High fat:* 100 g contains on average 18 g fat and 18 g protein

Bacon, lean only, e.g. gammon, back	Cheeses*—other than low-fat and cottage cheeses
Pork	
Tongue	Bloaters
Duck	Herrings
Goose	Kippers
	Sardines

* Moderate to high in cholesterol.

for separate supplementation in the older child. The compositions of different vitamin and mineral supplements are given by Francis (1986).

Energy intake
Low-fat diets, because of the energy intake that fat normally contributes to the diet (37 kJ, 9 kcal/g fat), may require energy supplements (Francis 1979), though many children given a variety of 'fat-free' foods (Table 7.4) will obtain an adequate energy intake to promote growth. However, such a diet is low in energy density, and young children find it difficult to eat sufficient bulk of food to cover their energy needs (*see* Francis 1986).

(a) Carbohydrate.   In some patients on low-fat diets as much as 75 to 80% of dietary energy may need to be supplied from carbohydrate. The choice of carbo-

hydrate must be acceptable, practical and cheap. Many popular dishes and convenience foods are unsuitable for inclusion, e.g. crisps and chocolate, because of their fat content. The child's appetite usually ensures adequate energy intake, but it must be satisfied with appropriate low-fat foods. Wholegrain and refined cereals, pulses, low-fat pasta, white and wholemeal bread (no butter), and flour can be made into a wide variety of low-fat dishes and baked goods, e.g. savoury rice and vegetables, spaghetti and fat-free tomato sauce, beans on low-fat toasted bread, low-fat angel cake, custard or rice pudding made with skimmed milk, cottage cheese with chives or pineapple with crispbread and salad, chilli con carne made with beans (a low-fat vegetable textured protein can be used in place of meat), and jacket potato and cottage cheese. These foods together with fruit and vegetables are the basis of the older child's low-fat diet. Because the diet has a low energy density, young children should be offered 5 to 6 meals and/or snacks daily to ensure adequate opportunity to eat enough dietary energy. Refined carbohydrates such as fruit juices, drinks, carbonated beverages, sweets, sugar and meringues are popular and can be incorporated into the diet (see Table 7.6). Glucose polymers can be useful supplements, particularly for the infant and young child. As concentrated monosaccharides and disaccharides can precipitate osmotic diarrhoea, adequate fluid intake is necessary. An example of a very low-fat diet is given in Table 7.7.

Table 7.6   Fat-free energy supplements.

1600 kJ, 400 kcal are continued in approximately:

   100 g sugar, glucose, glucose polymer (Calonutrin, Caloreen, Maxijul and Maxijul LE, Polycose, etc.)
   115 g boiled sweets
   130 g honey
   145 g jam
   600 ml Lucozade
   1000 ml Coke, Pepsi (sweetened)
   1750 ml carbonated beverage (sweetened)
   ≃1 bottle Hycal*—dilute with at least an equal quantity of water for children
   500 ml 20% solution of carbohydrate, e.g. glucose polymer*
   1000 ml 10% solution of carbohydrate, e.g. glucose polymer*
   2000 ml 5% solution of carbohydrate, e.g. glucose polymer
   50 ml MCT oil
   100 ml MCT emulsion, Liquigen

---

* Various glucose polymer drinks are now available.

As the diet is high in carbohydrate, meticulous oral hygiene and fluoride supplements (where water supply is low in fluoride) are recommended in order to reduce the risk of dental caries.

(b)   *Medium-chain triglycerides* (MCT).   MCT can be used as an adjunct to a minimal or low-fat diet as it is absorbed and transported differently (Fig. 7.1). It can increase energy intake, provide variety and increase palatability of the diet. It has no specific therapeutic properties, and there is no indication for its use as a medicine. It does not contain, nor can it be metabolized to, essential fatty acids, being quickly metabolized to carbon dioxide in the liver.

MCT is synthesized from coconut oil by fractionation. It is a clear, oily liquid, partially water-soluble, with a melting point below 0°C. It has the advantage of being high in energy, 35 kJ (8·3 kcal) per g, compared to carbohydrate, 16 kJ (4 kcal) per g, and it is less cariogenic than sucrose. It is more ketogenic than ordinary dietary fat (Huttenlocher *et al.* 1971), but is relatively unpalatable and requires great care with cooking, especially frying, to prevent formation of a bitter taste, due to its low 'smoke' point. It has a higher osmolality than ordinary fat for a given concentration, which can lead to gastrointestinal side-effects such as diarrhoea, vomiting, abdominal distension and pain (Holt 1967). The latter may also be due to the metabolites formed on oxidation of MCT.

MCT is contraindicated in abetalipoproteinaemia. In other patients it is a matter of preference whether carbohydrate and/or MCT provides the additional energy needed with low-fat diets.

A number of MCT products are available (Tables 7.8 and 7.9) and include MCT oils, 'filled' milks, and an emulsion, Liquigen; margarine made from MCT oils is available from Germany.

The total quantity of fat (conventional fat and MCT) in the diet should not exceed a maximum of 35% of the energy requirement, unless a ketogenic diet is prescribed. However, it is not practically possible to give as much MCT as ordinary fat (which is commonly associated with protein foods). Usually no specific prescription for MCT is necessary and the patient can simply use MCT oils as a replacement of other fats in cooking and if necessary use an MCT 'filled' milk. However, Lloyd (1982) suggests that these milks are not essential beyond infancy, even in type I hyperlipidaemia which requires severe restriction of dietary fat, less than 10 g daily.

MCT oil must never be given undiluted and should always be incorporated in at least an equal volume

Table 7.7 An example of a very low-fat (7 to 8 g) diet. Suitable for 6- to 9-year-olds.

(a) Recommended daily intake.

	Fat (g)	Protein (g)	Energy	
			kJ	kcal
Basic minimal fat diet foods including fruit and vegetables	>1·0	5 to 10	840 to 2000	200 to 500
30 g cereal, Rice Krispies, Cornflakes or 1 Weetabix	0·4	2·6	470	110
500 ml fresh liquid skimmed milk (or 50 g skimmed milk powder)	0·5	17·0	710	165
200 g bread, preferably wholemeal. (no butter/margarine)	4·4	17·6	1916	450
100 g very low-fat fish (Table 7.5b)	1·5	17·5	408	96
50 g egg-white (fat-free scrambled)	Nil	4·5	77	18
100 g pulse beans or baked beans	0·5	5·7	350	85
180 g glucose polymer or equivalent	Nil	Nil	2880	720
Vitamin and mineral supplement and fluoride drops				
Total	7·3 to 8·3	69·9 to 74·7	7651 to 8811	1844 to 2144

(b) Sample menu incorporating the above diet prescription.

On waking	Fruit juice and glucose polymer
Breakfast	30 g Rice Krispies, Cornflakes and sugar Skimmed milk and glucose polymer for cereal 40 g bread (no butter/margarine) Marmite, Bovril or marmalade Grilled tomatoes and/or mushrooms) Scrambled egg-white (fat-free) Cup of tea with skimmed milk and sugar
Mid-morning	Fruit or fruit juice, etc.
Lunch (picnic box)	160 g bread (no butter/margarine) Potato, fat-free, mashed or jacket, and ketchup or mustard or Bovril/Marmite 100 g baked beans Salad vegetables, tomato, celery, etc. Dried fruit or sweets, e.g. fruit gums (optional) Fresh fruit
Tea	100 g smoked haddock or grilled cod, etc. Potato, jacket or fat-free mashed, or fat-free potato cakes Vegetables Fruit and custard made with skimmed milk and/or jelly
Bedtime	Skimmed milk and glucose polymer and/or milk-shake powder Fruit

of other fluid or food. Gastrointestinal side-effects are most likely to occur during the introduction of MCT, which should therefore be started slowly, e.g. only 25% of the final estimated amount of MCT is given on the first day, 50% on the second day, 75% on the third day and the full quantity on the fourth or fifth day. The MCT may replace the ordinary dietary fat, which is simultaneously reduced, or may be added to a low-fat diet. In infants, the time taken to introduce MCT should probably be extended considerably, increasing by only 1 or 2 g increments per day (whether from MCT emulsion or MCT milk powder). If gastrointestinal symptoms occur MCT should be introduced more slowly, the quantity reduced or discontinued. Food, fluids and made-up dishes containing MCT are tolerated better if consumed slowly and a small quantity is given at several meals, rather than all in one meal. Once the introduction of MCT

Table 7.8   Medium-chain triglyceride MCT preparations*. Fatty acid composition per 100 g. Based on information supplied by the manufacturer.

	$C_{6:0}$	$C_{8:0}$	$C_{10:0}$	$C_{12:0}$	$>C_{14:0}$
MCT oils (approximate values)					
Cow & Gate	2·0	56	40	1·5	n/s
Lovelock (Alembicol D)	0·4	56·8	32·6	9·8	0·3
Mead Johnson	<3·0	71	23	← <3 →	
Scientific Hospital Supplies	1·1	81·1	15·7	2·1	N/S
Margarine					
Ceres margarine†	—	17·9	73·3	1·4	6·9
MCT emulsion					
Liquigen (SHS)	1·1	81·1	15·7	2·1	N/S

* Some MCT preparations are available on prescription as borderline substances. Details of MCT 'filled' milks are given in Table 7.9.

† Contains vitamins A, D, E, and also skimmed milk powder. Energy value 2800 kJ, 670 kcal per 100 g. Includes approximately 5% as $C_{18:2}$ and $C_{18:4}$ which accounts for the high percentage of $>C_{14:0}$ fatty acids present. Only available direct from Margarine Union GMBH, Germany, by hospitals, for clinical and research purposes.

N/S Not specified.

Table 7.9   MCT 'filled' milks.

	g per 100 g fatty acids						g per 100 g powder					
	$C_{6:0}$	$C_{8:0}$	$C_{10:0}$	$C_{12:0}$	$>C_{14:0}$ other than $C_{18:2}$	$C_{18:2}$ and $C_{18:3}$	Total fat (g)	Carbo-hydrate (g)	Protein (g)	Energy		Comment
										kJ	kcal	
MCT Pepdite 0–2	N/S	44	39	N/S	5·15	11·8	18·9	62·6	13·8	1870	450	Complete formula for infants
MCT Pepdite 2+	N/S	44	39	N/S	5·15	11·8	18·8	62·4	13·9	1930	460	Complete formula for older children
					⎵17⎵							
MCT 1 (Cow & Gate)	<2·0	56	40	1·5	Trace	Nil	28	40·6	25·6	2038	487	Incomplete formula* Not suitable sole source nutrition
Portagen	2·5	62	20	2·5	7	6	22·5	54·3	16·5	1950	464	Adult formula high in vitamin A
					⎵13⎵							
Pregestimil	N/S	25·8	13·1	1·3	N/S	N/S	18·3	52·4	12·8	1940	462	Infant formula. High content of LCT fatty acids
					⎵59·7⎵							
Flexical	N/S	16·1	5·7	Trace	44·2	33·5	15	67·3	9·9	1850	441	Adult formula. High content of LCT fatty acids
					⎵77·7⎵							
Triosorbin	N/S	N/S	N/S	N/S	7	13	19	56	19	2000	420	Adult formula
		⎵Approx 80⎵			⎵20⎵							

Based on information supplied by the manufacturers 1984/5.

* Formula to be revised. This product requires supplementation with a full range of vitamins and trace minerals.

N/S Not specified.

is completed various foods incorporating MCT can be included, e.g. MCT-fried fish and chips, and soups, sauces, cakes and puddings made with MCT oil in place of other fats; or MCT emulsion can be added to drinks, desserts and low-fat ice-cream; and MCT margarine spread on bread. An example of a low-fat diet incorporating MCT is given in Table 7.10.

Table 7.10 Diet containing 10 g fat with added MCT suitable for 6- to 9-year-olds; extra energy can be added by increasing carbohydrate intake: sample menu.

	Carbohydrate (g)	Protein (g)	Fat (g)	MCT (g)
Daily				
60 g (2 oz) skimmed milk powder ⎫ 'MCT'	31	21·3	0·6	
60 ml (2 oz) Liquigen ⎬ milk				30·0
Water to 600 ml ⎭ mixture				
Vitamins				
3 Ketovite Tablets plus 5 ml Ketovite liquid				
Fluoride tablets				
Breakfast				
30 g (1 oz) cereal, e.g. Rice Krispies	20	2·6	0.4	Nil
10 g (⅓ oz) sugar	10	Nil	Nil	Nil
40 g (1½ oz) bread, toasted	20	3·6	0.8	Nil
100 g (3½ oz) baked beans	10·3	5·1	0·5	
'MCT' mixture for cereal and/or cup of tea				
Mid-morning				
1 piece of fruit	10·0	Trace	Nil	Nil
Lunch/supper				
60 g (2 oz) MCT chips	22	2·3	—	6·5
100 g (3½ oz) egg-whites, fat-free scramble, or MCT fried	Nil	9·0	Nil	0 to 2
Vegetables (no added fat)	—	Trace	—	—
100 g (3½ oz) custard made with skimmed milk and 10 ml Liquigen	17	3·8	0·2	5·0
1 piece fresh fruit or 60 g (2¼ oz) tinned fruit	10	Trace	Nil	Nil
Tea				
1 serve cake made with MCT	12	1·0	0·5	5·0
Fruit juice	20	Nil	Nil	Nil
'MCT' mixture (optional)				
Supper/lunch (can be adapted to a picnic box school lunch)				
40 g (1½ oz) bread	20	3·6	0·8	Nil
50 g (1⅔ oz) meat (low-fat list, Table 7.5b)	Nil*	11·0*	2·5*	Nil*
Salad vegetables—no added fat	Trace	Trace	Nil	Nil
150 g low-fat yoghurt, fruit-flavoured	21	7·5	1·4	Nil
Bedtime				
'MCT' mixture				
40 g (1½ oz) bread	20	3·6	0·8	Nil
10 g (⅓ oz) honey	8·0	Nil	Nil	Nil
Daily total	251·3	74·4	8·5	46·5
Energy 7385 kJ, 1965 kcal				
Distribution	57%	16·9%	4·3%	22%

*Average values.

(c) Polyunsaturated fatty acids in familial hypercholes- terolaemia. Supplements of PUFA (see Table 7.11) can be used in conjunction with the low-fat dietary treatment of familial hypercholesterolaemia (Lloyd 1982) to increase the P/S ratio, replace the energy deficit, improve palatability and partly reduce the carbohydrate intake (Segal et al. 1970). Patients treated with cholestyramine may not need a specific diet or a more generous fat intake may be permitted. Although it is uncertain whether PUFA has a specific hypocholesterolaemic action in familial hypercholes- terolaemia (Segal et al. 1970), oils rich in PUFA lower serum cholesterol in normal subjects (Gordon 1959) and therefore are the preferred type of fat supplement in these patients. Because of the saturated fat content of polyunsaturated oils, excessive use of these oils (by their contribution to the total amount of saturated fat present in the diet) may partially counteract the effect of the polyunsaturated fatty acids. A P/S ratio greater than one is not considered desirable (DHSS 1984), and therefore PUFA, dietary fat and total fat should be considered in the diet prescription. Saf- flower, sunflower and soya bean oils are the highest in polyunsaturated fatty acids and therefore are pre- ferable even to corn oil. Various brands of PUFA mar- garines are available (Table 7.11) but should be used sparingly as part of the prescribed diet, and care is

needed to select a suitable brand containing at least 50% of the fat as PUFA.

An example of a diet suitable for use in the treat- ment of a child with familial hypercholesterolaemia is given in Table 7.12 and excellent recipe books for use with this diet are available, e.g. Cooking for Your Heart's Content (Wanwright-Evans & Greenfield 1976). Many household and vegetarian recipes can be adapted by substitution of fat with suitable oils.

Dietary principles for patients with familial hypercholes- terolaemia treated by drugs such as cholestyramine. Although a specific diet prescription is not required, the following should be encouraged in conjunction with normal nutrition principles.

1 Avoid visible fats as far as possible, e.g. trim fat off meat.
2 Increase the intake of wholegrain cereals and pulses, and peas and beans; encourage pasta.
3 Use wholemeal bread from thick-sliced loaf to encourage dietary fibre and reduce fat intake.
4 Use PUFA margarines in place of butter and other margarines, but still use these sparingly.
5 Use vegetable oils high in PUFA, i.e. saf- flower, sunflower, soya or corn oil, for cooking rather than hard fats and other oils. Grill rather than fry foods.

Table 7.11 Fatty acid composition of fats, oils and margarines.

100 g fat contains	Saturated fatty acids (g)	Monounsaturated fatty acids (g)	Polyunsaturated fatty acids (g)
(a) *Oils*			
Coconut	90·5	7·0	1·8
Cottonseed	26·8	22·3	50·4
* Maize, corn	17·2	30·7	51·6
Olive	14·7	73	11·7
Palm	47·4	43·6	8·7
Peanut, groundnut, arachis	19·7	50·1	29·8
Rapeseed (high erucic acid)	5·6	67·3	26
Rapeseed (low erucic acid)	6·9	59·9	33
* Safflower seed	10·7	13·2	75·5
* Soya bean	14·7	25·4	59·4
* Sunflower seed	13·7	33·3	52·3
Lard	44·2	44	9·5
(b) *Margarine, composition varies†, average values*			
Hard, animal and vegetable oils	38·5	44·7	16
Hard, vegetable oils only	38·5	48·9	12·6
Soft, animal and vegetable oils	30·7	47·1	20·4
Soft, vegetable oils only	34·0	43·5	23·1
*Polyunsaturated vegetable oils only	24·7	20·5	54·6
Low-fat spread	28·2	39·9	31

* Contain more than 50% polyunsaturated fatty acids.
† Some manufacturers will supply compositional data.

Table 7.12 Diet containing 44 g total fat, low in saturated fatty acids suitable for a child with familial hypercholesterolaemia: sample menu.

		Protein (g)	Total fat (g)	Mono, saturated and *trans* fatty acids (approximate g)	PUFA (approximate g)
Daily	600 ml (1 pint) skimmed milk	21·3	0·5	0·5	0
Breakfast	30 g (1 oz) cereal, e.g. Puffed Wheat	2.6	0·3	0·1	0·2
	40 g (1⅓ oz) bread, wholemeal, toasted	3·6	0·9	0·5	0·4
	10 g (⅓ oz) PUFA margarine†	—	8·0	4·0	4·0
	Marmite, Bovril, marmalade	—	—	—	—
	Skimmed milk for cereal and or cup/tea	—	—	—	—
Mid-morning	Fruit juice or fruit	Trace	—	—	—
Lunch/supper (can be adapted to a picnic box or sandwich school lunch)	100 g (3½ oz) meat, e.g. lean lamb/pork, moderate fat list (Table 7.5b)	22·5*	10·0*	9·4*	0·6*
	60 g (2 oz) bread, wholemeal	5·4	1·3	0·7	0·6
	10 g (⅓ oz) PUFA margarine†	—	8·0	4·0	4·0
	Vegetables without added fat, e.g. salad	Trace	—	—	—
	Fruit	Trace	—	—	—
Tea	Fruit	Trace	—	—	—
	Skimmed milk or cup of tea	—	—	—	—
Supper/lunch	100 g (3½ oz) very low-fat fish, e.g. plaice	17·5	1·3	0·8	0·5
	Fried in oil‡	—	10·0	4·0	6·0
	60 g (2¼ oz) chips‡	2·3	2·3	1·0	1·3
	Pulses, pasta and vegetables	2·0	Trace	Trace	Trace
	150 g low-fat yoghurt	7·5	1·4	1·3	Trace
	Fruit (optional)	Trace	—	—	—
Bedtime	Fruit	Trace	—	—	—
	Skimmed milk				
	Daily total	84·7	44	26·3	17·6
				P/S = 0·67	

* Average values.
† Margarine containing at least 50% polyunsaturated fatty acids (*see* Table 7.11)
‡ Cooked in PUFA-type oil (*see* Table 7.11).

6 Encourage fish and poultry as an alternative to other meats. Select low-fat (Tendale or Shape) cheese or cottage cheese instead of high-fat cheeses. Limit eggs to three or four per week. Limit lean meat to one serve daily.

7 Encourage plenty of fruit and vegetables, and dried fruit and nuts.

8 For children over two years old use skimmed milk, 500 ml/day, in place of whole milk. Children under two years old need special consideration to ensure their diet is nutritionally adequate to promote normal growth.

9 Avoid added salt at the table if there is any suspicion of hypertension.

10 Children under five years should have vitamin A, D, and C supplements. All children on cholestyramine should have supplements of folic acid (5 mg/day).

Overweight should be corrected or avoided, exercise encouraged and smoking strongly discouraged. These principles are largely applicable to all members of the family in which familial hypercholesterolaemia has been identified in specific members, provided special attention is given to young children under five years in whom the energy density of the diet requires specific consideration (Francis 1986).

Social eating on a low-fat diet
The strictness of the diet varies according to the primary diagnosis and symptoms which may result from dietary indiscretion, or whether the diet is prophylatic treatment, as in familial hypercholesterolaemia.

A wider variety of low-fat convenience foods are becoming available. Practical advice on social eating should include ideas for packed lunches, as school meals are mostly unsuitable unless specially prepared.

Suitable items to include for school lunches:

A picnic box containing sandwiches or rolls filled with chicken, lean cold meat or ham, salad, Marmite or Bovril. Cottage cheese with herbs, chives, ketchup, pineapple, or peppers, bean salads, rice salads.
Low-fat yoghurt.
Low-fat cakes or meringues.
Fruit or dried fruits, e.g. sultanas, apricots.
Fruit juice (individual carton or in a plastic flask).

At cafes or restaurants the following can be selected:

Consommé or clear soup, fruit juice, or carbonated beverages. Fruit dishes such as melon, fruit cocktail, grapefruit, fruit salad.
Salads (omit dressing).
Roll or bread (omit butter); beans on toast (omit butter).
Water ice or sorbet; jelly.
Made-up savoury dishes, chips, roasts and gravy should be avoided, though home-prepared substitutes are permissible if cooked to appropriate recipes in which the permitted oil is substituted for other fats. Ice-cream including non-milk fat ice-cream, 'filled' milks containing non-milk fat and coffee creamers are unsuitable.

Invitations to friends should be accepted and the hostess informed to avoid fried and fatty foods, or a simple menu, e.g. beans on toast (no butter), can be tactfully suggested in advance.

Assessment
In malabsorption conditions the effect of treatment can be assessed by the clinical progress of the patient, linear growth and weight gain, and rarely by comparing faecal fats before and after introducing the diet. (The faecal fat estimation method should take into account that MCT is partially water-soluble.)

In the hyperlipoproteinaemias serum lipids before and after diet modification will give a guide to the effect the diet is having, e.g. clearing of serum, reduction of serum triglyceride and lipoprotein or cholesterol levels towards normal values.

REFERENCES

ANDERSON J. T., GRANDE F. & KEYS A. (1973) Cholesterol-lowering diets *J. Amer. diet. Ass.* **62**, 2, 133.
ANONYMOUS (1984) Lipid Research Clinic's coronary primary prevention trial results I and II. *J. Amer. med. Ass.* Vol. **251**, No. 3, 351–74.
BEAUMONT J. L., CARLSON L. A., COOPER G. R. *et al.* (1970) Classification of hyperlipidaemias and hyperlipoproteinaemias, *Bull. Wld Hlth Org.* **43**, 891.
BURKE V. & DANKS D. M. (1966) Medium chain triglyceride diet. Its use in treatment of liver disease. *Brit. med. J.* **2**, 1050–1.
DARMADY J. M., FOSBROOKE A. S. & LLOYD J. K. (1972) Diagnosis of familial hypercholesterolaemia in the first year of life. A prospective study of serum cholesterol concentration. *Brit. med. J.* **2**, 685.
DHSS (1974) Diet and coronary heart disease. *Report of Health and Social Subjects* No. 7. London: HMSO.
DHSS (1984) Diet and cardiovascular disease. *COMA Report on Health and Social Subjects* No. 28. London: HMSO.
FRANCIS D. E. M. (1979) Inborn errors of metabolism: the need for sugar. *J. hum. Nutr.* **33**, 146–54.
FRANCIS D. E. M. (1984) Should we be advising on low fat diets in U.K.? *Health Visitor* **57**, 145–6.
FRANCIS D.E.M. (1986) *Nutrition for Children.* Oxford: Blackwell Scientific Publications.
FREDRICKSON D. S. & LEVY R. I. (1970) Treatment of essential hyperlipidaemia. *Lancet* **1**, 191–2.
FREDRICKSON D. S., LEVY R. I., JONES E., BONNELL M. & ERNST N. (1970) *Dietary Management of Hyperlipoproteinaemia. A Handbook for Physicians.* Bethesda, Maryland: National Heart and Lung Institute (NIH), U.S. Dept Health Education and Welfare.
FREDRICKSON D. S., GOLDSTEIN J. L. & BROWN M. S. (1983) The familial hypercholesterolaemias. In *The Metabolic Basis of Inherited Disease*, 5th Edition (eds. Stanbury J. B., Wyngaarden J. B. & Fredrickson D. S.), Chapter 30. New York: McGraw-Hill.
FRIEDMAN G. & GOLDBERG S. J. (1975) Concurrent and subsequent serum cholesterols of breast and formula fed infants. *Amer. J. clin. Nutr.* **28**, 42.
GRACY M., BURKE V. & ANDERSON C. M. (1970) Medium chain triglycerides in paediatric practice. *Arch. Dis. Childh.* **45**, 445–52.
GORDON H. (1959) The regulation of the human serum cholesterol level. *Postgrad. med. J.* **35**, 186–96.

GURR M. I. (1984) *The Role of Fats in Food and Nutrition.* Amsterdam: Elsevier.

HASHIM S. A. (1967) Medium chain triglycerides—clinical and metabolic aspects. *J. Amer. diet. Ass.* **51**, 221–7.

HERBERT P. N., ASSMAN G., GOTTO A. M. & FREDRICKSON D. S. (1983) Familial lipoprotein deficiency. In *The Metabolic Basics of Inherited Disease*, 5th Edition, (eds. Stanbury J. B., Wyngaarden J. B., Fredrickson D. S., Goldstein J. & Brown M.), Chapter 29. New York: McGraw-Hill.

HILDITCH T. P. & WILLIAMS P. N. (1964) *The Chemical Constituents of Natural Fats*, 4th Edition. London: Chapman & Hall.

HOLT P. R. (1967) Medium chain triglycerides. *Gastroenterology* **53**, 961–6.

HUTTENLOCHER P. R., WILBOURN A. J. & SIGNORE J. M. (1971) Medium chain triglycerides as a therapy for intractable childhood epilepsy. *Neurology* **21**, 1097–103.

JAMES W. P. T. (Chairman) (1983) *A discussion paper on proposals for nutritional guidelines for health education in Britain.* Prepared for the Nutritional Advisory Committee on Nutrition Education. The Health Education Council.

KAUNITZ H., SLANETZ C. A. & JOHNSON R. E. (1958) Nutritional properties of the triglycerides of saturated fatty acids of medium chain length. *J. Amer. Oil Chem. Soc.* Vol. **35**, No. 1, 10–13.

KOCHHAR S. P. & MATSUI T. (1984) Essential fatty acids and *trans* contents of some oils, margarine and other food fats. *Food Chemistry* **13**, 84–101.

KWITEROVICH P. O., LEVY R. I. & FREDRICKSON D. S. (1973) Neonatal diagnosis of familial type II hyperlipoproteinaemia. *Lancet* **2**, 118.

LARCHER V. F., SHEPHERD R., FRANCIS D. E. M. & HARRIES J. T. (1977) Protracted diarrhoea in infancy. Analysis of 82 cases with particular reference to diagnosis and management. *Arch. Dis. Childh.* **52**, 597–605.

LEVY R. I., FREDRICKSON D. S., SHULMAN R. *et al.* (1972) Dietary and drug treatment of primary hyperlipoproteinaemia. *Ann. intern. Med.* **77**, 267.

LEYLAND F. C., FOSBROOKE A. S., LLOYD J. K., SEGALL M. M., TAMIR I., TONKINS R. & WOLF O. H. (1969) Use of medium chain triglyceride diets in children with malabsorption. *Arch. Dis. Childh.* **44**, 170–9.

LLOYD J. K. (1982) Disorders of lipid metabolism. In *Textbook of Paediatric Nutrition*, 2nd Edition (eds. Burman D. & McLaren D. S.), Chapter 5. Edinburgh: Churchill Livingstone.

LLOYD J. K. & MULLER D. P. R. (1972) Management of abetalipoproteinaemia in childhood. In *Protides of the Biological Fluids* (ed. Peeters H.), 19th Colloquim, p. 331. Oxford: Pergamon Press.

LLOYD J. K. & WOLF O. H. (1969) Disturbances of serum lipoproteins. In *Endocrine and Genetic Diseases of Childhood* (ed. Gardener L. I.), p. 937. Philadelphia: Saunders.

LLOYD J. K. & WOLF O. H. (1974) Abetalipoproteinaemia and familial alphalipoprotein deficiency. In *Hanbuch der Inneren Medizin* (ed. Linneweh F.) Vol. 7, 1, Part 3, 605, Berlin: Springer-Verlag.

McCOLLUM J. P. K. & HARRIES J. T. (1977) Disorder of the pancreas. In *Essentials of Paediatric Gastroenterology* (ed. Harries J. T.), Chapter 20. Edinburgh: Churchill Livingstone.

MOWAT A. P. (1979) Fulminant liver failure. In *Liver Disorders in Childhood* (ed. Mowat A.P.), pp. 126–37. London: Butterworth.

MULLER D. P. R., LLOYD J. K. & BIRD A. Ċ. (1977) Long-term management of abetalipoproteinaemia: possible role for vitamin E. *Arch. Dis. Childh.* **52**, 209.

MYANT N. B. (1982) Cholesterol transport through the plasma. *Clin. Sci.* **62**, 261–71.

MYANT N. B. & SLACK J. (1973) Type II hyperlipoproteinaemia. In *Clinics in Endocrinology and Metabolism*, Vol. 2, No. 1 (ed. Rifkind B. M.), p. 81. Philadelphia: Saunders.

OLIVER M. F. (1982) Risks of correcting the risks of coronary disease and stroke with drugs. *New Engl. J. Med.* **306**, 297–8.

OLIVER M. F. (1984) Hypercholesterolaemia and coronary heart disease: an answer. *Brit. med. J.* **288**, 423–4.

PARTIN J. C., PARTIN J. S. & SCHUBERT W. K. (1974) Micronodular cirrhosis in abetalipoproteinaemia: possible exacerbation by medium chain triglycerides (MCT) feeding. *Paediatric Research* **8**, 384/110.

PAUL A. A., SOUTHGATE D. A. T. & RUSSELL J. (1980) Amino acid composition mg per 100 g and fatty acid composition g per 100 g. 1st Supplement to McCance and Widdowson's *The Composition of Foods*. London: HMSO.

RIFKIND R. M. & LEVY R. I. (eds.) (1977) *Hyperlipidaemia: Diagnosis and Therapy.* New York: Grune & Stratton.

SEGAL M. M., FOSBROOKE A. S., LLOYD J. K. & WOLFF O. H. (1970) Treatment of familial hypercholesterolaemia in children. *Lancet* **1**, 641.

SCHLIERF G., HUECK C. C., OSTER P. *et al.* (1977) Dietary management of familial type II hyperlipoproteinaemia in children and adolescents—a feasibility study. In *Atherosclerosis* (eds. Manning G. W. & Hanst M. D.) New York: Plenum Press.

SLACK J. (1969) Risks of ischaemic heart disease in familial hyperlipoproteinaemia. *Lancet* **2**, 1380.

TAMIR I., GOULD S., FOSBROOKE A. S. & LLOYD J. K. (1969) Serum and adipose tissue lipids in children receiving medium chain triglycerides. *Arch. Dis. Childh.* **44**, 180–6.

THOMAS L. H., JONES P., WINTER J. A., & SMITH H. (1981) Hydrogenated oils and fats: the presence of chemically modified fatty acids in human adipose tissue. *Amer. J. clin. Nutr.* **34**, 877–86.

WANWRIGHT-EVANS D. & GREENFIELD M. A. M. (1976) *Cooking for your Heart's Content.* British Heart Foundation, 57 Gloucester Place London WIH 4DH.

WEST R. J. & LLOYD J. K. (1973) Use of cholestyramine in treatment of children with familial hypercholesterolaemia. *Arch. Dis. Childh.* **48**, 370.

WEST R. J. & LLOYD J. K. (1974) Adherence to treatment in children with familial hypercholesterolaemia. *Pediat. Res.* **8**, 911 (abstract).

WEST R. J. & LLOYD J. K. (1979) Hypercholesterolaemia in childhood. In *Advances in Pediatrics* (ed. Barnes L. A.), **26**, 1. Chicago: Year Book Medical Publishers.

Wheeler K. A. H., West R. J., Lloyd J. K. & Barley J. (1985)
   Double-blind trial of bezafibrate in familial hypercholesterolaemia. *Arch. Dis. Childh.* **60**, 34–7.

WHO (1982) Expert Committee. *Prevention of coronary heart
   disease.* Technical Report Series, No. 678. Geneva: World
   Health Organisation.

Recipes

FAT-FREE AND LOW-FAT RECIPES

White and wholemeal flour and white and
brown rice can be interchanged in these recipes but cooking time will need adjusting.

Red bean salad   (4 serves)

1 cup red kidney beans
1 onion
1 green pepper
1 tbsp vinegar
2 tbsp permitted oil (optional)
1 tsp salt
1 clove of garlic
1 tsp mustard
$\frac{1}{4}$ tsp black pepper or 1 pinch chilli powder

Soak beans overnight in water, drain, then
replace water (no salt). Bring to the boil and
drain off water a second time. Recover with
water and cook 1 to 1$\frac{1}{2}$ hours, until soft.
Drain. Make dressing with garlic, mustard,
salt and pepper, oil and vinegar. Mix well.
Check seasoning. Serve with green salad or
on a bed of lettuce.

Pea or lentil soup   (4 serves)

1 cup split peas or lentils
1 carrot
1 onion
1 stick celery (and or leek)
500 ml (1 pint) fat-free stock
Salt and pepper

Cover peas or lentils with water (no salt)
and boil for $\frac{1}{2}$ to $\frac{3}{4}$ hours until soft. Drain.
Add stock, dried vegetables and seasoning.
Simmer $\frac{1}{2}$ hour. Check seasoning. Serve.
Add bread or toast croutons crisply fried in
permitted oil, sprinkled with parsley if

desired. Alternatively, liquidize to a smooth
pureé and serve.

Scrambled egg-whites (fat-free)

2 egg-whites
30 ml water (1 oz)
2 drops Yolkline or yellow food colour
Salt and pepper

Whisk the egg-white and water. Add
colouring. Place in a non-stick pan or bowl
over boiling water. Cook slowly stirring all
the time until set. A little mustard, herbs or
tomato ketchup may be added if desired.

Broad beans in tomato sauce   (4 to 6 serves)

1 onion
500 g (1 lb) broad beans (shelled)
1 tbsp tomato purée
150 ml (5 oz) water
Salt, pepper, sugar

Chop onion and place in non-stick pan with
a little water and soften over a gentle heat
stirring all the time. Add shelled broad
beans, seasonings, tomato purée and water.
Simmer gently with lid on pan till beans are
tender. Remove lid and simmer a few
minutes longer to reduce liquid to a syrupy
glaze. Check seasonings. Serve. The bean
pods can be cooked separately as a green
vegetable.

Mexican beans   (4 to 6 serves)

1 cup red kidney beans
150 g (4 oz) textured vegetable protein
   (mince variety)
1 clove garlic, crushed

1 onion, chopped
1 tin condensed tomato soup
Salt and pepper
$\frac{1}{2}$ to 1 tsp chilli powder
Black pepper
Pinch orgeano

Soak beans overnight. Drain, then replace water (no salt). Bring to the boil and drain off water a second time. Recover with water and cook 1 to 1$\frac{1}{2}$ hours until soft. Drain. Soak and cook textured vegetable protein according to manufacturer's instructions until tender. Combine beans, 'mince', chopped onion, soup and seasonings, in an ovenproof dish. Cover and cook in a moderate oven for 45 minutes. Check seasoning. Serve.

Rice Krispie cakes

2 tbsp golden syrup
2 to 3 cups Rice Krispies
1 tbsp castor sugar

Heat syrup and sugar until the sugar dissolves; stir in the Rice Krisipies until the syrup is absorbed. Spoon into paper cases. Leave to cool and harden.

Rice Krispie macaroons (fat-free)

2 egg-whites
45 g (1$\frac{1}{2}$ oz) crushed Rice Krispies
1 drop almond essence
85 g (3 oz) sugar
Glacé cherries

Whisk egg-whites until very stiff. Add almond essence, and fold in sugar and Rice Krispies. Spoon onto rice paper, and top with a glacé cherry. Bake in a moderate oven. regulo 4 (375°F, 190°C) for 20 to 25 minutes. Remove from rice paper when nearly cool.

Penny-wise macaroons (low-fat)

55 g (2 oz) flour
110 g (4 oz) sugar

55 g (2 oz) quick-cooking rolled oats
1 to 2 egg-whites

Icing
55 g (2 oz) icing sugar
1 egg-white
Lemon juice

Mix flour, rolled oats and sugar and work in the egg white. Roll on a board sprinkled with sugar, to about $\frac{1}{4}$ inch thick. Cut into fingers or rounds. Prepare icing by mixing all ingredients in a bowl, and beating until smooth and thick. Cover pastry rounds with a thin layer of the icing, and transfer to a lightly greased and floured baking sheet. Bake in a cool oven, regulo 2 (300°F, 150°C) for 10 to 15 minutes. Cool before removing from the baking sheet.

Mirlitons (low-fat)

3 egg-whites
55 g (2 oz) plain flour
pinch of salt
55 g (2 oz) porridge oats
250 g (8$\frac{1}{2}$ oz) sugar

Mix all the ingredients together. Spread mixture thinly onto a lightly greased and floured baking tray. Bake in a hot oven, gas regulo 6 (425°F, 220°C) for 15 to 20 minutes, until a very pale brown. Cut into squares, and roll around the handle of a wooden spoon. If the mixture begins to harden before it can be rolled, return to the oven for a few minutes to soften.

Low-fat biscuits

170 g (6 oz) plain flour
or 140 g (5 oz) flour
plus 30 g (1 oz) ground rice
1 tsp baking powder
55 g (2 oz) sugar
5 dsp water
3 dsp golden syrup

Add sufficient water and syrup to the flour to bind to a dough. Roll out and cut into rounds. Bake in a moderately hot oven, regulo 5 (400°F, 200°C) for 15 minutes.

Angel cake (fat-free)

NB This is best eaten on the day it is made.

4 egg-whites
85 g (3 oz) flour
55 g (2 oz) castor sugar
Flavouring and colouring

Whisk egg-whites until stiff; add sugar and flavouring. Carefully fold in sieved flour. Divide into three tins, and colour each mixture differently. Cook for 10 to 15 minutes in a moderate oven. Bake at regulo 4 (375°F, 190°C). Cool on wire trays. Sandwich together with jam, or icing.

Brock (Irish tea bread) (fat-free)

140 g (5 oz) brown sugar
280 g (10 oz) dried fruit
280 g (10 oz) plain flour
2 egg-whites
Soak overnight in one cup of cold tea
1 rounded tsp baking powder

Mix the ingredients together. Place in a lightly greased and floured loaf tin. Bake at regulo 5 to 6 (400 to 425°F, 200 to 220°C), for 1 to 1½ hours.

Fruit buns (fat-free)

340 g (12 oz) plain flour
Pinch of salt
7 g (¼ oz) dried yeast
230 g (8 oz) warm water
110 g (4 oz) mixed dried fruit
55 g (2 oz) mixed peel
45 g (1½ oz) sugar

Mix water, sugar and yeast together, and leave in a warm place for 10 to 15 minutes until frothy. Mix the dry ingredients together, and work in the yeast mixture. Knead well. Place dough in a warm bowl, and leave in a warm place for about one hour, until the dough has doubled its size. Form into small buns, and leave to prove for 15 minutes on warm tray. Bake in a hot oven, regulo 8 (475°F, 240°C), for 10 to 15 minutes. Mix some sugar and water and glaze buns immediately they come out of the oven.

Fat-free pastry

170 g (6 oz) plain flour
1 tsp baking powder
Pinch of salt
2 egg-whites
Water

Mix together the sieved flour, baking powder and salt. Mix in the egg-whites, and add enough water to form a soft dough. Roll out in the usual manner. Bake in a hot oven, regulo 6 (425°F, 220°C) for about 20 minutes.

Sweet mincemeat (fat-free)

55 g (2 oz) currants
55 g (2 oz) sultanas
55 g (2 oz) raisins
55 g (2 oz) mixed peel
1 small grated apple
½ tsp mixed spice
½ tsp ground nutmeg
55 g (2 oz) brown sugar
Juice of 1 lemon

Mix all of the ingredients together. Use for mince pies and tarts with fat-free pastry.

Ice-cream (low-fat)

30 g* (1 oz) non-fat milk powder
230 g (8 oz) water
30 g (1 oz) sugar
15 g (½ oz) cornflour
2 egg-whites
Flavouring and colouring

Place non-fat milk powder, sugar, cornflour, flavouring and water into a pan, and cook, stirring the whole time. Whisk the egg-whites until stiff and fold into the mixture. Freeze.

* For high-protein–low-fat ice-cream use 60 g non-fat milk powder.

Fondant (fat-free)

7 g ($\frac{1}{4}$ oz) gelatine
340 g (12 oz) icing sugar
1$\frac{1}{2}$ tbsp water

Put gelatine and water into a small bowl over hot water, and heat until gelatine is dissolved. Sift half the icing sugar into a large bowl and pour on the gelatine. Beat until smooth. Knead in the rest of the sugar. Roll out and cut into shapes, leave to set and decorate with icing.

Sandwich fillings

Cottage cheese fillings

Use cottage cheese as a meat exchange together with:

Chopped chive	Cucumber
Spring onion	Sliced radishes
Gherkin	Parsley
Celery	Mint
Watercress	Marmite
Lettuce	Pineapple
Tomato	

Vegetable fillings

Vegetables may be chopped and combined using special mayonnaise or other sauces to bind them. Chopped fruits, hard-boiled egg-white, and Marmite also mix well with some vegetables.

Celery	Mustard and cress
Chive	Radishes
Watercress	Onion
Spring onion	Grated carrot
Green peas	Fried mushrooms
Cucumber	Gherkins
Lettuce	Crushed corn (tinned)
Tomato	French runner beans
Beetroot	and special
Chicory	mayonnaise
Mint	Parsley
	Dried fruit

Fruit fillings

Banana—mashed
  plus lemon juice and brown sugar
Apple—grated
  plus celery and beetroot
  or celery and walnuts*
  or dates or raisins
Dates—mashed
  plus lemon or orange juice
  or lemon juice and apple
  or lemon juice and nuts*
Raisins—chopped
  plus honey and lemon juice
  or grated apple
Pineapple—crushed
Special mayonnaise may be used to moisten.

* Nuts should only be used if allowed on the diet.

Miscellaneous fillings for sandwiches or to be served on toast

Baked beans in tomato sauce
Spaghetti in tomato sauce (no cheese)
Golden syrup
Permitted oil, brown sugar and cinnamon
Jam and marmalade
Honey
Mushrooms in permitted oil

Cooking with MCT oils

Medium-chain triglyceride oil can be used in place of other oils and fats in many recipes. The oil should not be overheated to blue smoke point or higher, as a bitter taste is formed. Therefore great care should be taken in its use.

Food such as potatoes should be par-boiled before frying or roasting and will take longer to cook than usual. MCT oil can be re-used only three or four times. Care should be taken not to mix it with other oils and fats. If foods containing fat, such as meat or bacon, are fried in MCT, fat will leak out into the MCT oil which should then be discarded.

MCT 'filled' milks and MCT emulsion, Liquigen, can be used to make sauces, or added to soups and baked goods. Recipe leaflets are available from the manufacturers.

MCT is expensive and should only be used for patients on a low-fat diet.

RECIPES INCORPORATING SPECIAL OILS

The appropriate oil should be selected for the diet prescribed.

Margarine spread

30 ml (1 fl oz) water
30 g (2 tbsp) dried skimmed milk powder
30 ml (2 tbsp, 1 fl oz) oil
1 to 2 drops yellow food colouring
Salt to taste or Marmite, Bovril to flavour

Add water to milk powder and mix well to a smooth cream. Add oil gradually, mixing in an electric mixer or using a rotary whisk. Add colouring and salt. Put into the refrigerator for 2 to 4 hours to allow to thicken before use as a spread in place of ordinary margarines. Not suitable for cooking. Use within 2 to 3 days of mixing.

Special French dressing

60 g (2 oz) oil
30 g (1 oz) vinegar or lemon juice
Seasoning such as salt and pepper
    and a $\frac{1}{4}$ tsp sugar

Variation.   Use either (1) celery salt, (2) chives, (3) garlic flavouring, (4) paprika, (5) mustard, (6) onion.

Place ingredients in a small screw-top bottle. Shake well before using. Sprinkle on salad, fish, etc.

Oil cream

120 ml (4 oz) water
15 g ($\frac{1}{2}$ oz) skimmed milk powder
30 ml (1 oz) oil emulsion
2 drops yellow colouring

Flavouring, e.g. vanilla
Sugar to taste

Beat together with a rotary beater or electric mixer. Serve with fruit, coffee, desserts or puddings.

Never-fail mayonnaise

$\frac{1}{4}$ level tsp sugar
$\frac{1}{2}$ level tsp dry mustard
$\frac{1}{2}$ level tsp salt
Pinch of red pepper
1 egg-white
115 ml (4 fl oz) oil
3 tsp vinegar

Combine sugar, mustard, salt and red pepper in a basin. Add the egg-white and beat well. Continue beating and add the oil a little at a time until half is used. Add 2 teaspoons of vinegar and continue beating adding the remainder of the oil. Beat in the remaining 1 teaspoon vinegar. Store in a covered jar in the refrigerator. Makes about $\frac{1}{4}$ pint. (Keeps 1 week.)

Tomato macaroni

45 ml (1$\frac{1}{2}$ oz) oil
$\frac{1}{2}$ medium green pepper
Salt and pepper
$\frac{1}{2}$ tsp mustard
55 g (2 oz) chopped onion
Small tin canned tomatoes
170 ml (6 oz) water
110 g (4 oz) macaroni

Cook onion and pepper in oil until tender. Add all other ingredients except macaroni. Bring water to boil, add macaroni, cover, lower heat and simmer 20 to 30 minutes until macaroni is tender. Stir occasionally to avoid sticking. 1 to 2 serves.

Rice pilaf

15 ml ($\frac{1}{2}$ oz) oil
1 cup water
Salt and pepper

½ tbsp chopped onion
½ cup rice (brown or white)
½ beef or chicken stock cubes
1 tsp chopped parsley

Cook onion in oil, add rice and brown. Add stock cube and water to rice. Bring to boil. Cover and simmer 12 to 40 minutes until rice is soft and all water absorbed. Garnish with parsley and serve. 1 to 2 serves.

Rice with vegetables

½ cup uncooked rice
115 g (¼ lb) chopped mushrooms
230 g (½ lb) tomatoes
1 cup water
1 chopped onion
1 tbsp chopped green pepper
2 tbsp oil
1 tsp salt

Heat oil in frying pan. Add mushrooms, onions and green pepper. Cook slowly until tender and browned. Add tomatoes and water and bring to the boil. Add rice. Turn to low heat when mixture boils and simmer 30 minutes with a cover over the pan until rice is tender. Stir occasionally during cooking.

Spanish rice

⅓ cup uncooked rice (brown or white)
⅓ cup oil
⅓ cup chopped onions
⅓ cup chopped green peppers
3 cups cooked tomatoes
2½ cups water
2 tsp salt
¼ tsp pepper
1 bayleaf
½ cup chopped celery

Heat oil in large frying pan. Add rice and fry until golden in colour. Add onion next, and cook for 1 minute, then add tomatoes, water, seasonings, green pepper and celery. Cover and cook over low heat until rice is tender (½ to ¾ hour) stirring occasionally.

Potato sticks

115 ml (4 fl oz) oil
115 g (4 oz) cooked mashed potato
Pinch salt and pepper
55 g (2 oz) flour
Little beaten egg-white

Mix the ingredients together and refrigerate for at least ½ hour (overnight preferably). Roll out between greaseproof paper, and cut into thin sticks. Brush with a little beaten egg. Bake in a moderate oven, regulo 2 to 3 (325°F, 160°C) until golden brown.

Haddock kedgeree

115 g (4 oz) rice (brown or white)
15 ml (½ oz) oil
1 hard-boiled egg-white
170 g (6 oz) smoked haddock (cooked)
½ tsp curry powder
Parsley

Cook rice, flake fish. Place oil in pan and curry powder and chopped egg-white, add rice and flaked fish. Heat thoroughly. Serve onto a dish, decorate with parsley.

Variations. (1) Use unsmoked haddock, add ½ cup cooked peas to the final dish. (2) ½ cup sweet corn kernels or diced vegetables can be added.

French toast

1 egg-white
Pinch salt
30 ml (1 oz) oil
30 g (1 oz) skimmed milk powder
2 to 3 drops of yellow colour
2 slices bread from allowance

Beat egg-white, milk powder and salt. Dip bread into the mixture. Fry lightly in oil until brown. Turn and brown the second side.

Sauces

Ginger sauce

$\frac{1}{4}$ onion
15 ml ($\frac{1}{2}$ oz) oil
Salt and pepper
1 tomato
$\frac{1}{4}$ tsp ground ginger
30 ml (1 oz) water

Fry onion and tomato in oil for 5 minutes.
Add ginger, salt, pepper and water. Simmer
15 minutes. Serve hot with baked or fried
fish and rice or baked potato. May also be
served with meat allowance.

Creole sauce

45 ml ($1\frac{1}{2}$ oz) oil
30 g (1 oz) chopped green pepper
2 tomatoes
1 tsp tomato ketchup
30 g (1 oz) chopped onion
55 g (2 oz) mushrooms
Salt and pepper

Cook onion, green pepper, and mushroom in
oil for 5 minutes. Add tomato and
seasoning. Simmer 20 minutes. Serve with
fish and rice or meat allowance, e.g.
chicken.

Sweet and sour sauce

1 dsp oil
1 level dsp sugar
300 ml ($\frac{1}{2}$ pint) tomato juice
$1\frac{1}{2}$ tsp cornflour
Salt
1 dsp lemon juice

Mix the oil, cornflour, sugar together and
cook 1 minute. Add tomato juice, cook a
further 2 minutes stirring constantly. Add
lemon juice and salt to taste. Serve with
baked fish, or meat allowance with savoury
rice.

Pastry

Savoury pastry

180 g ($1\frac{1}{2}$ cups) flour
60 ml ($\frac{1}{2}$ cup) oil
$\frac{1}{4}$ tsp salt
30 ml cold skimmed milk (or water) to mix

Sift flour and salt. Beat oil and milk together
until creamy. Pour all at once over flour and
mix to a dough. Roll out between
greaseproof or waxed paper. Bake for 15
minutes, regulo 3 (350°F, 180°C).

Sweet pastry (non-roll) for single shell pie

180 g ($1\frac{1}{2}$ cups) flour
5 g (2 tsp) sugar
Pinch of salt
60 ml ($\frac{1}{2}$ cup) oil
$\simeq$30 ml cold skimmed milk to mix

Sift flour, sugar and salt into pie dish. Beat
milk and oil together and pour over the
flour. Mix to a dough. Press dough with
fingers to form an even lining to the pie
dish. For baked shell, prick with fork and
bake at regulo 6 (425°F, 220°C), fill when
cool. For unbaked shell, fill and bake at
regulo 5 (400°F, 200°C) for 15 minutes,
then at regulo 3 (350°F, 180°C) until filling
is cooked.

Biscuits

Basic biscuits with oil

2 egg-whites
$\frac{1}{3}$ cup oil
1 tsp vanilla
$\frac{1}{2}$ cup soft brown sugar
1 cup plain flour
1 tsp baking powder

Beat egg-whites with a fork. Stir in oil and
vanilla then add sugar. Sift flour and baking
powder together and add to egg mixture.

Drop teaspoons of mixture on to oiled baking sheet 2 inches apart. Flatten with oily spoon. Bake for 10 minutes at regulo 5 (400°F, 200°C). Remove from baking sheet while still hot.

Variations. Use 1 teaspoon mixed spice or cinnamon or cocoa or instant coffee.

Shortbread

85 g (3 oz) flour
30 g (1 oz) sugar
2 tbsp oil
Flavouring, e.g. vanilla

Sieve the flour, mix in the sugar. Add the oil drop by drop, mixing all the time. When the mixture starts to bind remove from bowl and knead until smooth. Roll out and cut as usual. Bake at regulo 2 to 3 (325°F, 160°C) for approximately 20 minutes.

Flapjacks

4 tsp golden syrup
55 g (2 oz) demarara sugar
110 g (4 oz) quick-cooking oats*
Pinch of salt
85 ml (3 fl oz) oil

Melt the syrup in a saucepan. Add the sugar, oats and salt. Stir in the oil. Turn into an oiled tin and press mixture together. Bake at regulo 4 (350°F, 180°C) for 20 to 30 minutes. Cut and remove from tin whilst still hot. Cool on wire rack.

* Only if oats allowed in the diet.

Cakes

Feather sponge with oil

100 ml (3½ fluid oz) oil
100 ml (3½ fluid oz) skimmed milk
2 egg-whites
140 g (5 oz) plain flour
30 g (1 oz) cornflour

170 g (6 oz) castor sugar
2 level tsp baking powder
½ level tsp salt

Mix all ingredients except 55 g (2 oz) of the sugar and egg-whites. Make a stiff meringue mixture with these two and fold into the mixture. Place in 2 × 8 inch tins, cook at regulo 5 (400°4, 200°C) for 25 minutes.

Queen cakes

2 tbsps oil
55 g (2 oz) castor sugar
55 g (2 oz) flour
1 egg-white
¼ teaspoon baking powder
Flavouring

Mix the oil and the sugar. Add in the sieved flour and baking powder. Fold in the stiffly beaten egg white and flavouring. Put into cake cases or tins and bake for 15 to 20 minutes at regulo 3 (350°F, 180°C). Decorate with glacé icing and cherries.

Fruit cake

170 g (6 oz) self-raising flour
55 g (2 oz) brown sugar
140 g (5 oz) dried fruits (sultanas, raisins, glacé cherries, mixed peel, currants)
1 tsp mixed spice
55 g (2 oz) skimmed milk liquid
55 ml (2 oz) oil

Mix flour, sugar, fruits and spice together. Combine skimmed milk and oil. Mix flour to a stiff dough with skimmed milk and oil. Place in a small lined cake tin. Cook at regulo 3 (350°F, 180°C) for 1½ hours.

Gingerbread

115 g (4 oz) plain flour
Pinch salt
2 level tsps ground ginger
½ level tsp bicarbonate of soda

3 tbsps skimmed milk
2 tbsps oil
55 g (2 oz) demerara sugar
115 g (4 oz) syrup or treacle
1 egg-white

Mix dry ingredients. Beat in oil and milk. Fold in beaten egg-white. Place in 6 inch tins, cook at regulo 3 (350°F, 180°C) for 40 minutes.

Pancakes

115 g (4 oz) self-raising flour
Pinch of salt
40 ml (1½ tbsps) oil
300 ml (½ pint) skimmed milk

Sieve the flour and salt, make a well in the centre. Add the oil and half of the skimmed milk. Mix to a smooth consistency beating well. Then add the remainder of the skimmed milk. Leave to stand for ½ hour. Fry a tablespoon at a time in oil. Sprinkle with sugar and lemon juice, or serve with golden syrup. Note: The above recipes using only ¼ pint skimmed milk can be used for drop scones or fruit fritters.

Special 'ice-creams'

Frozen dessert

300 ml (10 oz) water
15 g (½ oz) cornflour
30 ml (1 oz) oil
55 g (2 oz) skimmed milk powder

30 g (1 oz) sugar
2 egg-whites

Flavouring and colouring, e.g. vanilla essence, milk-shake syrup or 'Nesquik', blackcurrant juice.

Mix the dry ingredients with the water and heat together in a saucepan. Bring to the boil and cook until thickened. Cool. Beat with a rotary whisk or electric mixer, to aerate. Slowly beat in the oil and flavouring. Stiffly beat the egg-whites in a separate basin. Carefully fold the egg-white into the mixture with a metal spoon. Pour into refrigerator tray and freeze. Serve when just set as a mousse or frozen as ice-cream.

Frozen strawberry dessert

1 tbsp gelatine
400 ml (14 oz) liquid skimmed milk
Pinch salt
55 ml (2 oz) oil
55 ml (2 oz) water
115 g (4 oz) sugar
115 g (4 oz) frozen strawberries or other
    suitable fruit

Dissolve gelatine in water. Warm skimmed milk and add the dissolved gelatine taking care not to curdle by having the milk at blood-heat. Add sugar, oil, salt. Allow to set. Beat to aerate. Fold in strawberries. Place in refrigerator tray and freeze.

Variations. Use 4 bananas in place of strawberries; use 4 oz drained diced tin fruit; or fresh crushed strawberries or raspberries.

Protein- and sodium-modified diets for renal, liver and other conditions in infants and children

A number of conditions, including various renal conditions and liver disease, require dietary modification of protein and sodium. The specific inborn errors of protein metabolism such as hereditary hyperammonaemia and the organic acidaemias are dealt with in Chapter 10.

Dietary protein is digested, and free amino acids and small peptides are absorbed into the mucosal cells of the small bowel where digestion is completed. Movement across the cell membranes involves many specific transport mechanisms. Unabsorbed amino acids are decomposed by lumen bacteria, producing a series of metabolites; some of these, e.g. ammonia, organic acids and amines, are potentially toxic and are subsequently absorbed and detoxified in the liver. Increased amounts of these metabolites occur in the blood, for example when liver function is impaired or production increased, as in bacterial overgrowth of the small intestine or in transport defects, e.g. hyperammonaemia is a feature of liver failure (*see* Smith & Francis 1982).

In the liver, amino acids are used in protein synthesis and other anabolic processes. Amino acids in excess of anabolic requirement are degraded for ATP production, gluconeogenesis and lipogenesis, and the amine groups are converted into urea (Fig. 8.1), which is excreted by the kidneys. The release of amino acids into the body's free amino acid pool depends on the rate of amino acid metabolism in the liver. Breakdown of body protein also contributes to this pool (Munro 1970). A dietary protein intake greater than that needed does not increase liver protein synthesis, but increases instead the proportion of amino acids available for degradation by the liver and thus increases urea production, as does any increase in gluconeogenesis caused by starvation, energy deficit, infections and catabolic states (*see* Smith & Francis 1982, Barratt 1985).

In children growth utilizes amino acids and enhances protein synthesis, thus decreasing amino acid degradation and urea production. Thus growth has been termed the third kidney (Barratt 1985).

Approximately 1 g protein/kg per day is used for growth and anabolism in infants, and less in older children and adults. Dietary protein in excess of the need for growth will form urea, which is excreted in the urine; 1 g protein is metabolized to 5 mmol of urea.

LIVER DISEASE

In hepatic failure, protein synthesis is affected and toxic metabolites cannot be metabolized adequately (Mowat 1979, Psacharopoulos *et al.* 1980). Dietary protein intake should be reduced. Hypoglycaemia, hypocalcaemia and hypokalaemia may occur and should be corrected with either intravenous or oral glucose (or glucose polymers), and added calcium and potassium as appropriate (Trey 1970). Treatment of the underlying cause and removal of the toxic metabolites (e.g. by the use of lactulose to decrease absorption from the intestine, dialysis, or, where appropriate, detoxification of ammonia by conjugation with sodium benzoate) is necessary, for example in Reye's syndrome and fulminant hepatic failure (Psacharopoulos *et al.* 1980). Blood ammonia monitoring with a controlled protein intake and adequate carbohydrate and energy intake is essential. Temporarily, a protein-free, high-energy regimen may be needed, e.g. 10 to 20% solution of glucose polymer with or without 2·5 to 5% solution of fat in the form of an oil emulsion. Table 8.7 gives further details. At least the minimal protein requirement for age and weight (discussed later, Table 8.2b) should be given once the child improves clinically, or ultimately growth failure will occur. As generous a protein intake as clinically tolerated should be given, together with a high energy intake. Practical details of protein-restricted diets are given later (p. 204). The presence of ascites requires dietary sodium restriction (*see* p. 210) and/or diuretic therapy (Conn 1973). Fluid restriction is not normally necessary.

Interference with bile salt metabolism may occur, e.g. in biliary atresia fat absorption is affected and

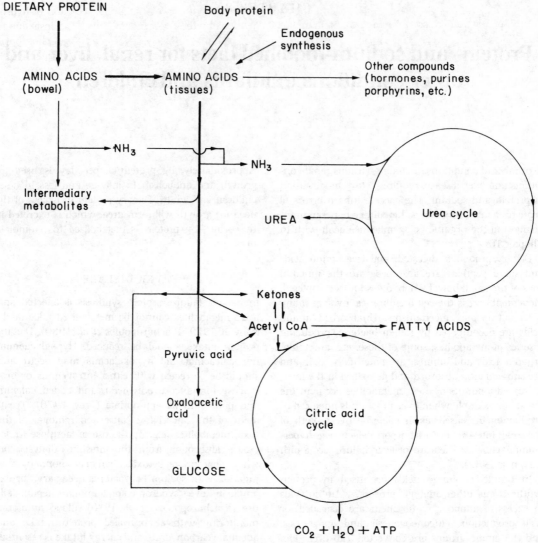

Fig. 8.1   Fate of dietary protein. From Smith and Francis (1982) with permission.

energy malnutrition and growth failure are common features. Deficiency of vitamins A, D, E and K can occur, and supplements, ideally in water-miscible form, should be prescribed. A reduced fat intake may be necessary to correct the steatorrhoea, but the depleted energy must be replaced with additional carbohydrate and/or MCT (*see* Chapter 7).

In chronic hepatic failure hypoalbuminaemia can occur, in which case a normal to high protein intake with no added salt in the diet is desirable, but blood ammonia must be monitored. High-protein diets should be used with caution because of the risk of hyperammonaemia and of hepatic encephalopathy

and coma (Burman *et al.* 1982, Crossley & Williams 1984).

RENAL FUNCTION

The kidney has the responsibility for the maintenance of volume and composition of the extracellular fluid, the 'internal environment' of Claude Bernard (Barratt 1985) in which the cells of the body live. The kidney is required to excrete those constituents of the diet which are not disposed of by catabolism to carbon dioxide and water, and which are not retained by growing tissues. The urine is thus composed of an aqueous solution of salts (sodium, potassium, chloride, phosphate) and the end-products of protein metabolism, principally urea and creatinine. The excretory load presented to the kidney is thus principally determined by the dietary intake (Barratt 1982, 1985).

The kidney functions by a system of ultrafiltration of plasma at the glomerulus followed by selective reabsorption and secretion of water and solutes by the renal tubules. The scale of filtration is huge, the amount of glomerular filtrate in two hours being approximately equal to the extracellular fluid volume itself. Tubular reabsorption has to equate approximately with this to maintain the glomerulotubular balance, and the majority of the energy consumed by the kidney is utilized by sodium transport systems which drive the reabsorptive mechanisms (Barratt 1985).

Pathophysiological consequences of renal disease

These are discussed fully by Barratt (1982, 1985) and can be summarized as follows:

1 Glomerular dysfunction
The glomeruli are filters and thus may become leaky, blocked, or both.

(a) *Glomerular leak* is manifested by haematuria or proteinuria. If the proteinuria is mild it may merely be a marker of renal disease and not cause symptoms, but if severe it may lead to protein depletion, hypoalbuminaemia and oedema, and may require a high protein intake to minimize the consequences of the protein loss (*see* later, p. 220).

(b) *Block.* A reduction in the glomerular filtration rate (GFR) leads to accumulation in the body of the water and solutes normally excreted in the urine. GFR may fall to 20% of normal without symptoms. However, a GFR of less than 40% of normal warrants a reduction in dietary protein (*see* p. 204); a GFR of between 10 and 20% means that dietary intakes of sodium, protein and phosphate should be reduced to decrease the excretory burden on the kidney; and with a GFR below 10% the need for dialysis or transplantation is imminent (Barratt & Williams 1979, Barratt 1985).

2 Tubular dysfunction
(a) *Reabsorptive failure* by the tubules may lead to losses of water, sodium, potassium, bicarbonate or phosphate, which may need replacement by dietary means or as mineral supplements.

(b) *Secretory failure.* Failure of secretion of hydrogen ions by the renal tubule leads to acidosis due to the retention in the body of sulphuric and phosphoric acids generated by the metabolism of organic sulphates and phosphates in the diet. Correction of the acidosis with bicarbonate is necessary.

MATCHING OF EXCRETORY LOAD WITH EXCRETORY CAPACITY

In health, the wide range of excretory capacity of the kidney creates a tolerance of an equivalently wide range of excretory loads and thus of dietary intakes. The effect of renal disease is to reduce the range of excretory capacity and thus generate a need to control dietary intake so that the excretory load lies within this capacity. In some circumstances this involves a reduction of dietary intake, in others it involves increasing intake to make up for obligatory losses.

Sodium provides a good example. In health, obligatory sodium losses are less than 0·1 mmol/kg per 24 hours, whereas over the short term at least, except in the young infant, excretion rates as high as 10 mmol/kg per 24 hours can be achieved; the range of sodium excretion is 100-fold or more (Rodriguez-Soriano *et al.* 1981). Sodium intake usually lies comfortably in the middle of this range, about 1·0 mmol/kg per day. In chronic renal failure with reduced GFR the ability to excrete sodium is reduced, and may approach dietary intake: in these circumstances sodium retention may occur, with extracellular fluid volume expansion, oedema and hypertension. With renal tubular damage, obligatory sodium losses may rise and approach dietary intake, so that sodium depletion occurs, with a reduced extracellular fluid volume, hypotension and further impairment of renal function.

In some children with both glomerular and tubular dysfunction both effects may occur, leading to a very narrow margin of tolerance and variation in intake, so that with one dietary intake sodium wasting may occur, but with only a modest increase in dietary intake there may be sodium overload. Further, as the disease progresses, sodium requirements may change, usually in the direction of a reduction of sodium tolerance.

FLUID REQUIREMENTS

Fluid intake is often about 150 ml per 420 kJ (100 kcal) when renal function is normal, which in babies is approximately 150 ml/kg per day. When renal function is compromised, fluid balance is crucial and may be maintained by an intake equivalent to insensible losses, in sweat, faeces and respiration, of 20 ml per 420 kJ (100 kcal) plus the total lost in urine, gastrointestinal fluid and by dialysis where applicable. If the child becomes fluid overloaded it may be necessary to prescribe, temporarily, an intake even less than this, which makes it difficult to ensure an adequate energy intake, especially in young children with poor appetites.

A high fluid intake is recommended for patients with high urine concentrations of calcium, oxalate or uric acid who form renal calculi. In patients with idiopathic hypercalciuria the dietary calcium intake should be limited to $\leqslant 20$ mmol (800 mg) per day and may require reduction to 7·5 mmol (300 mg) per day (*see* Low-calcium diets, Chapter 12). If the urine calcium concentration remains elevated ($>12\cdot5$ mmol/l), diet alone may not suffice and cellulose phosphate and/or benzofluorophosphate may be used to decrease calcium absorption. Oxalate intake should be monitored or appropriately reduced by avoidance of high-oxalate foods, such as rhubarb, cocoa/chocolate, spinach, beetroot, instant coffee and possibly parsley (Geigy Scientific Tables 1981) in patients who form oxalate stones. A high ascorbic acid intake

should also be avoided (Hughes *et al.* 1981). In cystinuria, alkaline urine, by the administration of bicarbonate, helps prevent cystine crystal formation, and penicillamine treatment is indicated. A low-methionine diet (400 mg per day in adults) has been suggested by some workers. Such a diet can be devised from the information given for the dietary treatment of homocystinuria but without cystine supplements (Chapter 10).

OSMOLAR LOAD

Defects of urinary concentrating capacity necessitate an increased fluid intake to compensate for the obligatory urinary losses necessary to excrete the osmolar load. The inability of the kidney to reabsorb water and concentrate urine is a feature of the immature kidney of the young infant (Rodriguez-Soriano *et al.* 1981). Plasma osmolality is about 280 mmol/l, and in the healthy individual is maintained constant in the face of a changing water intake by antidiuretic hormones, which control changes in the urine osmolality ranging from 50 to 1000 mmol/l. Renal disease has the effect of drawing in these limits. In some diseases there is a disproportionate loss of concentrating capacity, with the urine remaining dilute with

Table 8.1 Comparison of 150 ml human and cow's milk with a modified milk and the DHSS recommendations for artificial feeds for young infants (DHSS 1983).

	Cow's milk	Human milk (mature)	Example of one whey-based modified infant formula reconstituted*	Recommendations for artificial feeds for the young infant (DHSS 1983)
Protein (g)	5·0	2·0	2·3	Cow's milk-based 2·3 to 3 Whey-based 1·8 to 3
Energy				
kJ	410	434	413	405 to 473
kcal	98	104	98	98 to 113
Sodium (mmol)	3·3	0·9	1·0	0·9 to 2·2
Potassium (mmol)	5·9	2·3	2·1	1·9 to 3·8
Chloride (mmol)	4·0	1·8	1·5	1·7 to 3·4
Calcium (mmol)	4·5	1·4	1·7	1·1 to 4·5†
Phosphorus (mmol)	4·7	0·8	1·7	0·7 to 2·9†
Fluid (ml)	150	150	150	150
Renal solute (mmol)‡	33·2	13·0	13·8	N/S

* Gold Cap SMA (J. Wyeth Laboratories). Other modified whey-based formulae (Premium, Osterfeed and Aptamil) also comply with the DHSS 1983 recommendations, although Aptamil has a higher renal solute than the example given above.

† Ratio calcium (mg) to phosphorus (mg) not less 1·2:1·0 and not more than 2·2:1·0.

‡ By calculation (protein × 4) + sodium + potassium + chloride, mmol/150 ml.

N/S Not specified.

respect to plasma. For example, in nephrogenic diabetes insipidus, a male-linked inherited disease, the kidney is unresponsive to the action of antidiuretic hormone, and a high urine flow with an osmolality of 50 to 70 mmol/l persists whatever the plasma osmolality or state of hydration of the child (Barratt 1985).

When there is a major defect in urine concentration, the urine volume (and thus fluid intake) is determined by the maximum urine osmolality that can be achieved and the osmolar load presented for excretion. The principal urinary solutes are urea, sodium, and potassium with their attendant anions. The renal solute load may be estimated from the dietary intake as follows: each 1 mmol of dietary sodium, potassium and chloride or other anions contributes 1 mmol, and each 1 g of protein contributes 4 mmol. If details regarding the anion intake are not available, the solute content contributed by sodium and potassium should be doubled.

On average, the renal solute load for an infant fed on human milk or modified infant formulae is 12 to 15 mmol/kg per day and on cow's milk is 33 mmol/kg per day (Table 8.1). A water intake in an infant of 150 ml/kg per day, after insensible losses in sweat and faeces, means the residual water excreted in the urine is usually about 100 ml/kg per day. Under these circumstances the osmolar concentration in the urine of an infant fed on human or modified milk is 130 mmol/l, and in one fed on cow's milk is 330 mmol/l. If urine osmolality is restricted, as in nephrogenic diabetes insipidus, to 70 mmol/l, a urine volume of 170 ml/kg per day is necessary to excrete an osmolar load of 12 mmol/kg per day (including insensible losses), indicating a requirement for fluid intake in excess of 200 ml/kg per day. The principle of dietary management of these infants is therefore to provide a high fluid intake, adequate dietary energy intake, the minimum protein requirement for growth and as low a sodium and potassium intake as can be achieved. Failure to provide these patients with adequate fluid and a low osmolar diet will lead to hypernatraemic dehydration with the danger of brain damage and mental retardation. Even short periods without water can cause dehydration, and frequent fluids at two-hourly intervals in young infants and later three-hourly, during both the day and night, are essential. Until the child is old enough to satisfy his own thirst, he must be given fluids regularly.

Water supplied in several plastic-type baby bottles from which the child can help himself as required from the toddler age onwards is a practical way of providing fluid, especially at night. Sodium intake increases fluid needs. Excess protein and potassium-rich foods should also be avoided. 'The more salt the more fluid' is the rule, and for the older child it is a matter of choice as to which is preferable. The child craves water to such an extent that the appetite can be suppressed by the large fluid volumes consumed, and poor growth may result. Glucose polymer (low electrolyte) added to water is ideal to increase energy intake if the child can be coaxed to take it. Large quantities of fruit juice and milk which add to the renal solute should be discouraged.

PROTEIN REQUIREMENTS

Catabolism of protein surplus to the requirements for growth produces urea: 5 mmol of urea is formed from each gram of protein broken down. Protein retention by growth in infancy approximates 1 g/kg per day (Barratt 1982, 1985). In a baby consuming 2 g protein/kg per day net urea production will be approximately 5 mmol/kg per day. Urea production is reduced if protein intake is reduced, provided energy intake is adequate and the protein consumed is of high biological value (or some is given as an essential amino acid mixture).

Goals for dietary protein restriction in chronic renal failure are twofold:

1 *Correction of uraemia.* The accumulation of urea and other nitrogenous waste products is responsible for symptoms such as anorexia, vomiting, ill-health and anaemia, which can be alleviated by a reduction in protein intake. The plasma urea concentration should be kept below 25 mmol/l* by reduction of protein intake to minimum requirements for height and age (Table 8.2); further reduction is potentially dangerous as it may lead to protein malnutrition, particularly if continued for any length of time (Chantler *et al.* 1980).

2 *Preservation of renal function.* Recently there has been considerable interest in protein restriction as a means of preservation of renal function (Barratt 1985). It is a common experience that if a substantial proportion of kidney function is lost residual function inexorably declines over a period of years, known as 'remnant kidney nephropathy'. Two mechanisms have been put forward to explain this: phosphate nephrotoxicity (*see* below) and hyperfiltration (Barratt 1985).

---

* Urea: mg/100 ml × 0·166 = mmol/l
Creatinine: mg/100 ml × 88·4 = μmol/l.

Table 8.2 Protein and energy requirements.

(a)   Minimum requirements for protein and energy at different ages. (Adapted from DHSS 1973.)

Age range	Expected body weight (kg)	Energy requirement per day kJ	Energy requirement per day kcal	Minimum requirement for protein (NPU 70%) g/day	Minimum requirement for protein (NPU 70%) Percentage energy
Infants					
Birth–3 months	4·6	2300	550	13	9·5
3–6 months	6·6	3180	760	14	7·4
6–9 months	8·3	3800	910	15	6·6
9–12 months	9·5	4180	1000	16	6·4
Boys and girls					
1–2 years	11·4	5020	1200	19	6·3
2–3 years	13·5	5860	1400	21	6·1
3–5 years	16·5	6700	1600	25	6·1
5–7 years	20·5	7530	1800	28	6·1
7–9 years	25·1	8800	2100	30	5·7
Boys					
9–12 years	31·9	10460	2500	36	5·8
12–15 years	45·5	11720	2800	46	6·6
15–18 years	61·0	12550	3000	50	6·7
Girls					
9–12 years	33·0	9620	2300	35	6·1
12–15 years	48·6	9620	2300	44	7·6
15–18 years	56·1	9620	2300	40	7·0

(b)   Protein and energy intakes for age and actual weight* in low-protein diets.

Age	Minimal protein requirement for growth (g/kg per day)†	Energy for normal requirement (per kg per day) kJ	Energy for normal requirement (per kg per day) kcal	Energy for high-energy diets (per kg per day) kJ	Energy for high-energy diets (per kg per day) kcal
0–6 months	1·8	525 to 630	125 to 150	840	200
By 1 year	decreasing to 0·9	420 to 525	100 to 125	750	180
1–3 years	0·8 to 1·5	420 to 375	100 to 90	630	150
3–6 years	0·5 to 0·8	335	80	420	100
7–12 years	0·5 to 0·8	300	70	420	100
Teenage	0·3 to 0·5	300 to 200	70 to 45	335	80
Adult	0·2 to 0·3	200	45	300+	70+

* Weight should be corrected for oedema and/or dehydration.

† Based on information contained in FAO/WHO reports on protein requirements, 1973, 1975 and 1978. Protein should be of high biological value. Chantler and Holliday (1973) suggested not normally less 1 g protein/kg per day in children and 2 g protein/kg per day in infants, should be recommended. As generous a protein intake as clinically tolerated should be prescribed.

Loss of nephrons causes an increased filtration rate in each remaining functioning glomerulus (hyperfiltration), which is believed ultimately to be damaging to that glomerulus, leading to scarring and later deterioration of renal function. This hyperfiltration can be blocked by a reduction in protein intake, and recent controlled trials showed a beneficial effect on renal function of reduced protein intake in mild chronic renal failure (*see* Barratt 1985). It is therefore now recommended that any child with a GFR of less than 40% of normal should be on a minimum recommended dietary intake of protein for height and age (Table 8.2), even though they may be symptom-free on a normal intake.

Although some protein restriction is advised in chronic renal failure a common error has been unnecessary over-restriction of protein and an inadequate energy intake (Holliday 1978, Chantler *et al.* 1980, Barratt 1985).

ENERGY

The intake of dietary energy must be adequate in order to preserve protein for growth. Requirements are suggested in Table 8.2.

A difficulty arises in children who are growth-retarded. One way of overcoming the problem is to calculate dietary intakes for height age. The child's actual height is compared with the age for which such a height would be average and the diet calculated for this age rather than the child's chronological age.

Children, and particularly infants, with renal failure are notoriously difficult to feed, often vomit, and appear to dislike food. Factors responsible in addition to the usual feeding problems of childhood (Frances 1986) and those associated with a child on a special diet (*see* Chapter 9) include:

1 Uraemia.
2 A need to maintain a high fluid intake and thus a preference for fluid rather than solid intake.
3 Disordered taste perception, with a preference for salty or savoury rather than sweet foods.
4 An unsatisfactory weaning period.
5 Dietary deficiencies limiting growth with poor appetite as a consequence.

The diet must be continually assessed and modifications recommended to encourage the child to adhere to the prescribed diet. Sometimes, particularly in infants, an adequate intake is extremely difficult to achieve, and it is necessary to resort to enteral feeding via a nasogastric tube administering an appropriate feed or supplement to improve the child's nutrition (Chantler *et al.* 1980, Barratt 1985).

SODIUM

The principles of dietary sodium prescription have been outlined above.

A reduced dietary sodium intake is required with oedema or hypertension. Patients with liver disease accompanied by ascites and those with congestive cardiac failure also need to reduce salt intake. Severe dietary sodium restriction is difficult to achieve in children, and diuretic or antihypertensive therapy is often preferable. There is some concern that a high sodium intake in healthy children may exacerbate the tendency to hypertension in predisposed individuals, but hypertension in children is usually secondary to renal disease.

The sodium content of the diet, however, in patients with renal disease should not be altered unless there is good reason for doing so (James 1976). Sodium depletion can give rise to reversible decreased renal function (Barratt 1985, James 1976). Sodium supplementation may be required in salt-wasting renal disease, e.g. in cystinosis in the early stages of the disease (Schneider *et al.* 1978). As children with salt-losing tubular dysfunction are often acidotic, the sodium supplementation is usually best undertaken with sodium bicarbonate, rather than by dietary means alone. These children often crave salty foods. Sodium intake may need to exceed 100 mmol per day.

POTASSIUM

Potassium intake may need to be restricted in renal failure. Treatment with an exchange resin such as calcium resonium may be appropriate. Severe restriction is not usually necessary, for if renal function is impaired to that extent dialysis is usually required, as hyperkalaemia is potentially dangerous (Barratt 1985, James 1976). Some limitation of potassium intake is needed in conjunction with dialysis if hyperkalaemia continues.

Potassium supplementation may be required with renal potassium wasting in, for example, renal tubular disease.

CALCIUM, PHOSPHORUS AND VITAMIN D

A variety of disturbances of calcium, phosphorus and bone metabolism are associated with renal disease (Barratt 1985).

1 Uraemic osteodystrophy. Chronic renal failure may result in a bone disorder known as uraemic osteodystrophy, characterized by a mixture of rickets and secondary hyperparathyroidism. Two principal mechanisms are operative: (a) defective 1-hydroxylation of 25-hydroxycholecalciferol, and (b) phosphate retention. Accompanying hypocalcaemia also occurs.

The kidney is the only site of 1-hydroxylation of 25-hydroxycholecalciferol, forming 1,25-dihydroxycholecalciferol, the active metabolite, which promotes the absorption of calcium by the bowel (Lawson *et al.* 1971). This can be circumvented by the administration of the vitamin D analogue 1α-hydroxycholecalciferol (calcidiol) or minute doses (1 to 2 μg/day) of the active 1,25-dihydroxycholecalciferol (calcitriol) itself (Barratt 1985). A high calcium intake is also required, and dietary phosphate should be limited. The regimen must be monitored by measurement of plasma calcium and phosphorus, as hypercalcaemia can occur if excess vitamin D is prescribed.

Reduction in GFR tends to cause phosphate retention, which is counteracted by increased parathormone secretion, causing decreased renal tubular phosphate reabsorption and restoring phosphate balance. However, this is achieved at the expense ('trade-off') of hyperparathyroid bone disease. Phosphate retention is also one of the factors causing progressive renal damage in the 'remnant kidney nephropathy'. The therapeutic strategy is to reduce phosphate absorption *pari passu* with the decline in GFR. This may be achieved with dietary phosphate restriction or by phosphate binders, which block absorption of dietary phosphate from the bowel. The most commonly used phosphate binder was aluminium hydroxide (7.5 ml Aludrox binds 1·0 mmol phosphate), but there is concern about aluminium toxicity, which will probably lead to increased reliance on dietary phosphate restriction in the future (Barratt 1985).

2 Hypophosphataemic rickets. Familial vitamin D-resistant rickets is due to defective renal tubular reabsorption of phosphate, resulting in phosphate depletion with hypophosphataemia. Treatment consists of phosphate supplements, together with 1,25-dihydroxycholecalciferol (Barratt 1985).

3 Hypercalcaemia/hypercalciuria. Increased calcium absorption from the bowel, such as may occur in vitamin D intoxication or idiopathic hypercalcaemia, may cause nephrocalcinosis or urolithiasis, and needs a low-calcium diet. Restriction of dairy products may suffice, but with idiopathic hypercalciuria and recurrent stone formation, as already discussed, a high fluid intake and a more aggressive calcium restriction may be necessary, including using a water softener in hard water areas (*see* Chapter 12 for details of low-calcium diets).

Growth failure

The most important of the many consequences of chronic renal failure in children is growth failure (Barratt 1985, James 1976, Holliday 1978). It is most severe in those who have been in renal failure since infancy. The precise pathogenesis has not been elucidated, but many factors have been implicated:

1 Inadequate energy intake.
2 Uraemic osteodystrophy.
3 Electrolyte imbalance: salt and water depletion, acidosis, phosphate depletion, etc.
4 Uraemia.
5 Nutritional deficiencies.

Of these the most important is an inadequate energy intake. Many children with renal failure have a poor food intake, and if energy intake is inadequate, growth will be unsatisfactory; the converse is not necessarily true, as an adequate energy intake does not necessarily result in good growth as other factors may be operative. However, an adequate energy intake is of paramount importance and there is evidence that energy supplements can improve the growth of at least some children with chronic renal failure (Simmons *et al.* 1971, Chantler & Holliday 1973, Holliday 1978, Chantler *et al.* 1980, Barratt 1985).

Growth is frequently poor in children on dialysis and even after kidney transplant catch-up growth is rare, although growth velocity may return to normal for age depending on growth potential at the time of transplant (James 1976). The height pre-dialysis may determine the ultimate adult height of the patient, and therefore it is essential to aim at optimal growth throughout treatment by provision of all known dietary factors (Holliday 1978, Barratt 1985).

TRACE MINERALS AND VITAMINS

Deficiency of trace nutrients can have profound effects on growth and metabolism (*see* Francis 1986).

Anaemia due to decreased production of erythrocytes is common in chronic renal failure, due to a deficiency of erythropoietin. Blood transfusions are not normally appropriate. Iron supplements are required, especially as dietary iron is likely to be inadequate. Absorption of iron is improved if iron sulphate supplements are given with vitamin C.

The dietary intake of trace nutrients such as zinc, chromium, copper, folic acid and vitamin B_{12} may be inadequate, due to a self-selected diet or superimposed refined carbohydrates providing a large proportion of dietary energy (Underwood 1977, Aggett & Davies 1983). Dialysis also depletes vitamins, especially vitamin C, folic acid, B_6 and B_{12}. Supplements are needed if there is doubt regarding their adequacy. The following have been found useful preparations and an appropriate combination can be selected as a supplement: Ketovite Tablets plus Ketovite Liquid; Cow & Gate Supplementary Vitamin Tablets; Forceval capsules. Modified Seravit and Paediatric Seravit may also prove useful new preparations which combine a range of vitamins and minerals.

Acute renal failure: acute nephritis

A variety of causes can precipitate acute renal failure (Burman *et al.* 1982, Barratt 1985), which rarely lasts longer than two weeks. Oliguria is a feature, and accurate fluid balance and electrolyte control is essential. Insufficient circulating blood volume may occur, and requires immediate correction followed by restoration of normal hydration and electrolyte balance (Burman *et al.* 1982). Weight gain or hyponatraemia during oliguria suggests overhydration (James 1976). Circulatory overload is the commonest indication for dialysis, though biochemical disturbances are other indications (Counahan *et al.* 1977, Barratt 1985).

There is no evidence that protein restriction alters the prognosis or shortens the course of the disease (James 1976), but it may delay the need to dialyse in those with less severe illness (Barratt 1985). However, increased requirements, including protein, occur due to endogenous protein catabolism, which increases with infection and is present in the majority of patients. The protein is therefore only restricted (Table 8.2) if the blood urea exceeds 25 mmol/l and the patient is not being dialysed. Many patients self-limit intake due to anorexia, and energy supplements are essential (e.g. glucose polymers and fat emulsions, enteral or parenteral nutrition). The protein intake should be gradually increased during the recovery phase as blood urea returns to normal.

Restriction of protein to minimal levels or less for long periods, particularly if catabolism is present, results in weight loss and wasting, even if energy requirements are met. Adequate nutrition is therefore essential in order to prevent malnutrition with its consequences of increased risk of infection, sepsis and further catabolism. As soon as a diuresis occurs all dietary and fluid restrictions should be discontinued. In the majority of cases prognosis is good (Cameron 1970, Barratt 1985). A normal nutritionally adequate diet is resumed after recovery.

Chronic renal failure

A number of renal insults can cause long-standing and progressive loss of renal functions, and 3 to 5 children/million per year can be expected to reach 'end-stage' renal disease in the U.K. (Barratt 1985).

Dietary treatment of renal disease does not alter the basic defect of kidney function, but aims at control of the related symptoms (Table 8.3), prevention of 'remnant kidney nephropathy' and promotion of adequate growth. Alternative therapy is appropriate and available for a number of the symptoms; the most appropriate therapy for any patient must be decided in the light of clinical, physiological and psychological parameters. Ultimately kidney transplant with the back-up of dialysis facilities is desirable before 'end-stage' chronic renal failure is reached (Barratt 1985).

Most children with chronic renal failure can be identified by their lack of spontaneous movement, which may be a means of energy conservation. Those children who participate in active sports and exercise appear to have a better prognosis. Whether this is an indication of clinical status or a specific effect of exercise is still unknown.

Table 8.3 Clinical features of renal disease correlated with the dietary nutrient involved (after Barratt 1985).

Clinical feature	Dietary nutrient(s)
Uraemia	Protein
	Energy deficit
Blood pressure	Sodium
Osmolar balance	Water
Hyperkalaemia	Potassium
Acidosis	Bicarbonate
Bone disease and	Calcium
demineralization	Phosphorus
	Vitamin D
Anaemia	Iron
	Vitamin B_{12}
	Folic acid
	Other vitamins
Growth failure	Especially energy and protein plus all of the above

The dietary management of a child with chronic renal failure is very demanding for the child, his family and the dietitian, and is one of the most important aspects of his management. It is frequently frustrating and difficult to achieve the desired goals, causing anxiety and psychological problems. A sympathetic dietitian fully versed in the principles of the dietary management of the child with kidney disease is an essential member of the renal team. The psychosocial aspects of the dietary regimen described for phenylketonuria in Chapter 9 largely apply to the situation in renal failure, but frequently with the additional problem of a clinically ill child with poor prognosis.

Practical aspects of low-protein diets

PROTEIN

The source of protein should be of high biological value in order to meet the essential amino acid requirement for growth with a minimum of amines for degradation. Human milk and the whey-based modified infant formulae (*see* Table 8.1) have optimal amino acid profiles for infant nutrition: eggs and meat (Table 8.4a) are good sources of protein for the older child. Milk and cheese, although excellent sources of protein, are high in phosphorus, and in chronic renal failure should be used sparingly. A more generous protein prescription, if clinically appropriate, permits a wider range of foods to be incorporated into the diet. Pulses, bread and cereals (Table 8.4b) have lower biological values than egg and meat proteins, but contribute a higher energy value for protein intake. They are useful in combination with other foods, add variety to the diet and are particularly useful if the diet prescription can be more generous than minimal requirements. Approximately 70% of the protein should ideally come from high biological value sources for practical purposes. However, it is important that the diet is eaten happily and therefore patient food preferences must be taken into account in the dietary prescription. The daily protein intake, together with energy sources, should be distributed between the meals.

Supplements of essential amino acids (Dialamine or Hepatamine) can be prescribed to improve the amino acid profile in conjunction with a low-protein diet. Ketoacid analogues of essential amino acid have also occasionally been used as a replacement of part of the prescribed protein. They are metabolized to release essential amino acids with less nitrogen for urea (or ammonia) production. They are available from Scientific Hospital Supplies. Due to their extremely bitter taste they need to be strongly flavoured and introduced gradually as part of a praise and reward system; even so, many find them unpalatable and unacceptable. Their use in the diet of children with chronic renal failure is still under review, though the author has occasionally used them in conjunction with minimal protein diets and in the treatment of ornithine transcarbamylase deficiency (hereditary hyperammonaemia, *see* Chapter 10).

In order to provide variety in protein-restricted diets, protein intake is conveniently measured using an exchange system of foods containing 6 g protein for meat, milk, and egg (Table 8.4a) and foods containing 1 g protein for cereals, potato, bread, etc. (Table 8.4b). Selected fruit, vegetables and foods of negligible protein content (Table 8.4c and d) are permitted without measurement, as they contribute only small additional quantities of protein to the diet.

Most young infants are either breast-fed or given a modified and preferably a whey-based infant formula (DHSS 1983). The use of these milks, (Table 8.1) reduces protein, phosphate and electrolyte intake and solute load, and is particularly recommended for infants and young children requiring a low-protein diet. Additional energy intake and fluid may be required. Some formulae suitable for low-birthweight infants may be useful because of their higher nutrient density in comparison to their protein and fluid content, but they have higher protein to volume ratios and should be used only as individually calculated as part of low-protein diets.

It is only rarely that a specific low-protein intake is required, in which case a whey-based modified milk is used as the basic protein source. The diet must be calculated individually for protein, energy and, where applicable, other nutrients such as sodium or phosphate. Supplements should be prescribed to ensure the regimen is nutritionally adequate for growth and to correct any biochemical abnormalities.

Infants and toddlers with renal disease frequently require a high fluid intake. It is important that the extra fluid is given as dextrose, or glucose polymer in water or dilute fruit juice, and not as milk formulae, or the total protein intake and solute load may be too high. If the infant rejects the required volume of fluid, a more frequent feeding schedule should be given, or nasogastric feeding may be necessary.

Weaning solids should be encouraged at the appropriate age, and are normally introduced from 3 to 4 months, in order to establish good eating habits. The manufacturers of baby foods, milks and weaning solids will provide up-to-date lists with the composition of their products. Suitable foods should be carefully chosen according to the dietary prescription and the quantity in an appropriate-sized serving. Many commercially prepared infant foods are relatively high in protein of low biological value; some contain sodium, potassium or both. An egg, however, contains 6 g high biological value protein and 3 mmol sodium (Table 8.4), and thus increases the total intake dramatically in a small child.

Many toddlers will eat better if provided with three small meals and three snacks per day (Francis 1979). The change from modified milk to cow's milk or 'follow-on' milks should be delayed until a good range of solids is incorporated into the diet at about two years old. If the child rejects the modified milks, diluted full-fat cow's milk with supplementary energy from glucose polymer and/or cream can be substituted, and vitamins and iron given medicinally.

In children in whom a reduced intake of protein is required, the diet should be planned and calculated taking into account individual preferences and appetite. Alternatively, it can be planned using the exchange lists supplied in Table 8.4 and the suggested distribution given in Table 8.5.

ENERGY

Adequate energy intake is vitally important in all situations where protein intake is restricted, including renal and liver conditions. Endogenous protein catabolism contributes significantly to the raised blood ammonia or urea. Energy from carbohydrates and fats has a protein-sparing action (Holt 1960, Cameron & Hofvander 1983) and should be provided in increased amounts in low-protein diets. The energy requirement in renal and liver disease may be 25% higher than normal (Holliday 1978, Chantler *et al.* 1980), and for catch-up growth and in hypercatabolic states even higher energy intakes may be necessary (Table 8.2).

In some children energy supplements given before meals may decrease both appetite and protein intake (and sodium where applicable). This can be a practical means of providing a moderate reduction in protein with an adequate energy intake (Burman *et al.* 1982).

Table 8.4 Composition of different foods used in planning low-protein diets. Protein exchanges: quantity of food providing (a) 6 g protein, and (b) 1 g protein, (c) Low-protein foods, (d) Low-protein fruit and vegetables.

(a) 6 g protein exchanges (cooked weight). Weight of food (to nearest 5 g) containing 6 g protein.

	Sodium† to nearest		Potassium to nearest		Energy	
	0·1 mmol	5 mg	0·1 mmol	5 mg	kJ	kcal
50 g egg (1 only, size 3)	3·0	70	1·8	70	306	74
180 ml (6 oz) milk‡	3·9	90	6·9	270	490	117
20 g (¾ oz) beef, chicken, lamb, veal, pork (lean only), average	0·7	15	1·8	70	175	42
30 g (1 oz) cod, plaice, haddock	2·2	50	2·3	90	260	62
50 g (1¾ oz) fish fingers	7·6	175	3·3	130	488	116
25 g (¾ oz) cheese, Cheddar‡	6·5	150	0·8	30	420	102
30 g (1 oz) ham	16·3	375	2·2	85	150	36
25 g (1 oz) corned beef	10·4	240	0·9	35	226	54
50 g (2 oz) luncheon meat	22·8	525	1·8	70	650	156
45 g (1½ oz) sausages, pork or beef, average	20·6	475	2·2	85	547	130
30 g (1 oz) sardines in oil	7·0	160	2·8	110	415	100
25 g (1 oz) smoked haddock	13·3	305	1·8	70	107	25
40 g (1½ oz) tongue	18·3	420	1·0	40	353	85
20 g (¾ oz) bacon, lean only	19·6	450	1·8	70	244	58
25 g (1 oz) bacon, average	21·7	500	1·8	70	430	103
50 g (2 oz) liver sausage	18·7	430	2·2	85	642	155
25 g (1 oz) liver	1·7	40	1·9	75	130	53

† Cooked without salt.
‡ High in phosphorus.

Table 8.4 *continued*

(b) 1 g protein exchanges (cooked weight unless specified). Weight of food (to nearest 5 g) containing 1 g protein.

	Sodium† to nearest		Potassium to nearest		Energy	
	0·1 mmol	5 mg	0·1 mmol	5 mg	kJ	kcal
40 g baked potato (in skin), flesh only	Trace	Trace	6·9	270	180	42
75 g (2½ oz) boiled potato	Trace	Trace	6·3	247	257	60
30 g (1 oz) chips	0·2	5	7·8	306	320	76
40 g (1¼ oz) roast potato	0·2	5	7·7	300	265	63
45 g (1½ oz) raw potato or baked in jackets with skin	0·2	5	6·6	257	167	40
20 g (¾ oz) peas, fresh or frozen	Trace	Trace	0·6	25	35	8
20 g (¾ oz) baked beans, salted	4·1	95	1·5	60	54	13
45 g (1½ oz) boiled rice	Trace	Trace	0·4	17	235	55
30 ml (1 oz) milk	0·7	15	1·2	45	82	20
40 g (1½ oz) single cream	0·7	15	1·3	50	350	84
70 g (2½ oz) double cream	0·9	20	1·4	55	1288	313
20 g (¾ oz) yoghurt, natural and fruit, average‡	0·7	15	1·2	45	43 to 80	10 to 20
12 ml evaporated milk (unsweetened)‡	0·9	20	1·2	45	70	17
30 g (1 oz) custard made with cow's milk and powder‡	0·7	15	1·2	45	120	30
10 g (⅓ oz) white flour, plain	Trace	Trace	0·4	17	147	34
10 g (⅓ oz) white flour, self-raising	1·5	35	0·4	17	147	34
7 g (¼ oz) Puffed Wheat	Trace	Trace	0·8	30	97	22
20 g (¾ oz) Sugar Puffs	Trace	Trace	0·8	30	296	70
10 g (⅓ oz) Shredded Wheat	Trace	Trace	0·9	35	138	32
10 g (⅓ oz) porridge oats, raw	Trace	Trace	0·9	37	170	40
70 g (2½ oz) porridge (cooked with salt)	17·6	405	0·8	30	132	30
70 g (2½ oz) porridge (cooked without salt)	0·2	5	0·8	30	132	30
12 g (⅓ oz) bread, white, brown, wholemeal‡	2·8	65	0·3	10	114	27
10 g (⅓ oz) bread, Hovis	2·4	55	0·3	10	99	23
12 g (⅓ oz) chapati, with fat‡	0·7	16	0·5	19	170	40
25 g (¾ oz) sponge, jam-filled or Swiss roll	4·6	105	0·9	35	320	26
15 g (½ oz) semi-sweet and short biscuits, average	2·6	60	0·5	20	290	70
15 g (one rusk) Farley's Original Rusks	Trace	Trace	0·4	17	285	67
10 g (⅓ oz) Weetabix	1·5	35	1·0	40	144	34
15 g (½ oz) Rice Krispies	7·3	167	0·6	24	234	56
10 g (⅓ oz) Cornflakes	5·0	116	0·3	10	157	37
40 g (1½ oz) spaghetti, canned in tomato sauce, average	8·7	200	1·4	53	100	20
100 g (3½ oz) cream of tomato soup, canned, ready to serve, average	20·0	460	4·9	190	230	55
60 g (2 oz) vegetable soup, canned, ready to serve, average	13·0	300	2·2	86	95	22
15 g (½ oz) crisps (with salt)	3·7	85	4·6	180	334	80
15 g (½ oz) crisps, Salt & Shake (without salt)	0·2	5	4·6	180	334	80
30 g (1 oz) ice-cream (vanilla)	1·1	25	1·3	50	208	50
10 g (⅓ oz) dairy milk chocolate	0·5	12	1·1	42	221	53
20 g (¾ oz) plain chocolate	Trace	Trace	1·9	75	550	131
30 g (1 oz) Coffee-mate (Carnation)	1·9	44	7·1	275	672	160
60 ml (2 oz, 2 scoops) Gold Cap SMA*	0·4	10	0·8	35	165	39
60 ml (2 oz, 2 scoops) Premium*	0·5	10	0·9	35	170	41
70 ml (2½ oz, 2½ scoops) Osterfeed*	0·6	15	1·0	40	199	48

* Other brands of modified infant formulae may be equally suitable.

† Cooked without salt.

‡ High in phosphorous.

Table 8.4 *continued*

(c) Foods of negligible protein content.

	Sodium† to nearest		Potassium to nearest		Energy	
	0·1 mmol	5 mg	0·1 mmol	5 mg	kJ	kcal
100 g (3½ oz) boiled sweets and candy	1·1	25	0·3	10	1397	327
10 g (⅓ oz) salted butter or margarine	3·7	85	Trace	Trace	304	74
10 g (⅓ oz) unsalted butter	Trace	Trace	Trace	Trace	304	74
20 g (⅔ oz) Rite-Diet Low-Protein Bread (salt-free)	Trace	Trace	0·3	10	208	50
20 g (⅔ oz) Rite-Diet Low-Protein Bread (plus salt)	4·8	110	0·3	10	208	50
10 g (⅓ oz) tomato ketchup	4·8	110	1·5	60	40	10
10 g (⅓ oz) brown sauce	4·3	100	1·0	40	42	10
10 g (⅓ oz) salad cream	3·7	84	2·1	80	130	31
100 ml (3½ oz) Lucozade	1·3	30	Trace	Trace	288	68
100 ml (3½ oz) Coke (sweetened)	0·4	10	Trace	Trace	168	39
100 ml (3½ oz) lemonade (sweetened)	0·4	10	Trace	Trace	90	21
10 g (⅓ oz) Dietade Salt Free Ketchup	Trace	Trace	1·3	50	40	10
10 g (⅓ oz) Dietade Salt Free Salad Cream	Trace	Trace	1·3	50	40	10
14 g (1 only) Aminex	0·2	5	0·1	5	197	47
Glucose polymers						
100 g (3½ oz) Caloreen*	<1·7	<40	0·3	10	1674	400
100 g (3½ oz) Calonutrin	3·9	90	0·3	10	1720	410
100 g (3½ oz) Maxijul*	2·0	45	0·1	5	1570	375
100 g (3½ oz) Maxijul Low Electrolyte	Trace	Trace	Trace	Trace	1570	375
100 g (3½ oz) Polycal*	2·2	50	1·3	50	1610	380
100 ml (3½ oz) Fortical	≤0·3	5	0·1 to 0·2	5	1045	246
100 ml (3½ oz) Hycal	0·7	15	Trace	Trace	960	240
Fat emulsions						
100 ml (3½ oz) Prosparol	3·9	90	0·3	10	1880	450
100 ml (3½ oz) Calogen	0·9	20	0·5	20	1880	450
100 ml (3½ oz) Liquigen MCT Emulsion	1·7	40	0·8	30	1700	400

Additional special products are listed in Table 8·7.

* Also available as liquid concentrates.

† Cooked without salt.

(d) Fruit and vegetables suitable for inclusion in low-protein diets.* Contain less than 1% protein (fresh, frozen, canned, provided salt† or sugar only is added).

Fruit	Fruit	Fruit	Vegetables	Vegetables
Apple	Lemons	Peaches (not dried)	Aubergine	Marrow
Apricot (not dried)	Lychees	Pears	French beans	Onions
Cherries	Mandarin oranges	Pineapple	Carrots	Peppers
Damsons	Mangoes	Plums	Celery	Pumpkin
Fruit-pie filling	Melon	Quinces	Chicory	Radish
Fruit salad	Nectarines	Raspberries	Courgette	Swede
Grapes	Olives	Rhubarb	Cucumber	Tomato
Grapefruit	Oranges	Strawberries	Lettuce	Turnip
Greengages	Paw paw	Tangarine		
Guavas				

* Provide considerable quantities of potassium and small quantities of sodium.

† Omit salt in no-added-salt and low-sodium diets.

Table 8.5 Suggested distribution of protein in low-protein diets, using protein exchanges from Table 8.4a and b.

Protein (g/day)	6 g protein exchanges. Number per day from Table 8.4a	1 g protein exchanges. Number per day from Table 8.4b
10	1	4
15	1½	6
20	2	8
25	2½	10
30	3	12
35	3½	14
40	4	16
45	5	15
50	6	14

Selected fruit and vegetables (Table 8.4d) and foods of negligible protein content (Tables 8.4c and 8.8) are permitted in addition.

Hyperosmolar solutions from concentrated carbohydrates and fats can cause gastrointestinal side-effects such as osmotic diarrhoea. Table 8.6 gives guidelines for the concentrations tolerated by most children at different ages.

Glucose polymers (Caloreen, Calonutrin, Fortical, Hycal, Maxijul, Polycal), appropriately diluted, are useful for fortifying the energy content of drinks and meals, due to their lower osmolar contribution compared to other sugars.

Uraemia interferes with the utilization of both carbohydrate and fat. Hyperglycaemia and glucosuria occur due to insulin resistance and the hormonal changes associated with renal disease. This can be corrected by dialysis (Barratt 1985).

Fats in the form of vegetable oil emulsions (Prosparol, Calogen) or margarine, butter and cream are concentrated sources of energy which can be added to the diet and incorporated into drinks to make 'milk-shakes' with appropriate flavouring, Table 8.7 gives some examples. Fat supplements should preferably be high in polyunsaturated fatty acids in order to help correct the raised triglyceride levels which are associated with renal disease. Fat in any meal or drink should never exceed the carbohydrate content, due to the risk of ketosis, and high intakes may be contraindicated in patients with acidosis.

In liver disease steatorrhoea may occur due to abnormal bile salt metabolism (Mowat 1979). Dietary fat may need to be reduced and the energy deficit should be replaced with either MCT (oil or emulsion, Liquigen) and/or additional carbohydrate.

Gastrointestinal symptoms may also be related to increased gut ammonia produced by micro-organisms. This is particularly important in young children, in poorly nourished patients and when fluid intake has to be restricted. Hyperosmolar solutions should, however, be introduced gradually over several days and such solutions are better tolerated when given in small, frequent quantities. Anorexia and food refusal due to abdominal cramp and nausea as a result of concentrated supplements should be avoided. Excessive and unrealistic energy intakes are inappropriate, as food refusal can result. Synthetic energy supplements in children with anorexia may simply replace food intake of better nutritional content without actually achieving an increased total energy intake (Francis 1979). As a result of the poor conventional food intake the dietary content of vitamins and trace nutrients such as zinc, chromium and iron can be reduced, resulting in chronic nutritional deficiencies (*see* Francis 1986).

Various low-protein special products are available as energy supplements and add variety to the diet (Tables 8.4c and 8.8). These include low-protein breads with or without salt, various biscuits, pasta and low-protein flours from which low-protein recipes can be devised (some recipes given in Chapter

Table 8.6 Maximum concentration of solutions normally tolerated by children of different ages with renal conditions.

	Percentage solution (g/100ml)		
Age	Carbohydrate, ideally as glucose polymer	Fat, ideally as vegetable fat emulsion	Maximum osmolality (mmol/l)
Infants	10 to 15	4 to 5	≤ 500
Young children ≤ 5 years	15 to 25	5 to 10	≤ 500
Older children, 5–12 years	25 to 30	≤ 10	≤ 700
Teenagers	maximum 50 to 60	maximum 10	≤ 700

Table 8.7 Examples of protein-free energy supplements for children.

	Carbohydrate (g)	Fat (g)	Energy		Sodium (mmol)
			kJ	kcal	
Infants					
15 g glucose polymer* and fruit flavouring	15	Nil	240	60	*
10 ml Prosparol or Calogen	Nil	5	185	45	Trace
Water to 100 ml					
100 ml total	15	5	425	105	Trace
Older children					
(a) 30 g glucose polymer* and fruit flavouring	30	Nil	480	120	*
20 ml Prosparol or Calogen	Nil	10	370	90	Trace
Water to 100 ml					
100 ml total	30	10	850	210	Trace
(b) 1 bottle Hycal† (174·2 ml = 107 ml free fluid)	106	Nil	1778	425	1·1
Each 100 ml volume	60	Nil	1020	244	0·6
(c) 1 bottle Hycal†	106	Nil	1778	425	1·1
50 ml Prosparol or Calogen	Nil	25	925	225	Trace
Water to 500 ml					
Total	106	25	2703	650	1·1
Each 100 ml volume =	21	5	541	130	0·2
(d) 1 bottle Fortical† (200 ml = 123 ml free fluid)	123	Nil	2090	492	0·6
Each 100 ml volume =	61·5	Nil	1045	246	0·3

* Electrolyte content varies according to the brand of glucose polymer chosen. *See* Table 8.4c.
† Should be diluted for children under 12 years with at least an equal quantity of water. Unsuitable for children under two years old.

9 can be adapted).

Examples of various low-protein diets are given in Tables 8.9 to 8.11. These examples can be adjusted for energy intake by changing the prescription of the energy supplements, and the sodium intake adjusted by the omission or addition of salt or sodium bicarbonate.

Dental caries are less prevalent than expected in children with chronic renal failure and uraemia, despite diets containing a high intake of concentrated, refined sugars and carbohydrates. Meticulous oral hygiene should be encouraged and fluoride supplements may be desirable.

It is very important to review the diet frequently: in infants initially at one- to two-weekly intervals, and in older children one- to two-monthly. The diet must be modified in the light of clinical findings, growth, age and weight. This is absolutely essential where a minimum protein intake is used, since it should be outgrown and will then inhibit further growth.

The actual dietary intake should be assessed from time to time and compared with offered and recommended intakes. Advice should be given regarding the intake and manipulations needed to improve nutritional adequacy. Force-feeding should be avoided. Snacks as well as meals should be encouraged in order to achieve a better total dietary intake in children with a poor appetite. Encouragement, praise and reward schemes and ingenuity are required in achieving an optimal intake in the majority of patients with chronic renal and liver failure. Some patients may benefit from nasogastric tube feeding when growth failure is a major concern. A relaxed atmosphere at mealtimes encourages co-operation from mother and child, so preventing food refusal and reducing parental anxiety. Ample opportunity should be given to the parents to discuss problems and their anxiety relating to treatment and prognosis.

Table 8.8 Low-protein special manufactured products.

Product	Manufacturer
Biscuits	
Aglutella Gentili Azeta Cream-Filled Wafers (vanilla flavour)	GF Supplies Ltd
Aminex Low-Protein Biscuits	Liga, Cow & Gate
Aproten Low-Protein Biscuits	Ultrapharm (Carlo Erba) Ltd
dp Low-Protein (Chocolate-Flavoured) Chip Cookies	GF Supplies Ltd
dp Low-Protein (Butterscotch-Flavoured) Chip Cookies	GF Supplies Ltd
Rite-Diet Low-Protein Gluten-Free Crackers	Welfare Foods Ltd
Rite-Diet Low-Protein (Chocolate-Flavoured) Cream-Filled Biscuits	Welfare Foods Ltd
Rite-Diet Low-Protein Sweet Biscuits	Welfare Foods Ltd
Rite-Diet Low-Protein Filled Wafers (Vanilla Flavour)	Welfare Foods Ltd
Bread	
Aproten Crispbread	Ultrapharm (Carlo Erba) Ltd
Juvela Low-Protein Pre-baked Bread (loaf)	GF Supplies Ltd
Rite-Diet Gluten-Free Low-Protein Bread with or without salt (canned or pre-baked)	Welfare Foods
Rite-Diet Low-Protein Bread with Added Soya Bran (canned)	Welfare Foods
Flour	
Aproten Flour	Ultrapharm (Carlo Erba) Ltd
Juvela Low-Protein Mix	GF Supplies
Rite-Diet Low-Protein Flour-Mix	Welfare Foods
Tritamyl Low-Protein Flour 'PK'	Procea Branch of Odlum Group
Pasta	
Aglutella Gentili Low-Protein Spaghetti, Rings, Macaroni, Semolina	GF Supplies
Aproten Pasta: Anellini (small rings), Tagliatelle (flat noodles), Ditalini (small macaroni), Rigatini (macaroni)	Ultrapharm (Carlo Erba) Ltd
Rite-Diet Low-Protein Pasta: macaroni, spaghetti, short-cut spaghetti	Welfare Foods

1 A number of these items are available on prescription at NHS expense for treatment of renal conditions, liver failure and amino acid disorders
2 Gluten-free products are not necessarily low in protein or suitable for use in restricted-protein diets.

SODIUM AND SALT

The degree of salt or sodium restriction should be correlated to clinical findings (*see* pp. 197 & 201). In patients with renal conditions a change from a low to a high sodium intake, or the reverse, may be recommended for the same patient from time to time, or sodium restriction may be lifted once clinical improvement occurs, e.g. following remission in nephrotic syndrome. Sodium and protein intake may simultaneously need to be modified. Table 8.4 provides information regarding the content of different foods. Occasionally a relatively constant sodium intake is needed, in which case a 5 mmol sodium* exchange system can be helpful. Tablets containing 5 mmol sodium (300 mg sodium chloride) can be used to supplement the dietary intake to the desired level.

* Dietary sodium is prescribed in millimole (mmol); 23 mg sodium or 58·5 mg sodium chloride contains 1 mmol sodium.

Natural food contains some sodium, and this must be calculated in low-sodium diets. However, the major source of sodium is the salt used in cooking, or added in food manufacture by salting, curing, and smoking, or in prepared foods such as tinned and packet soups and savoury dishes. Prescribed supplements containing sodium must be taken into account in assessing the total sodium intake (James 1976). Low-protein diets tend to be low in sodium. Salt-losing is relatively common in children with renal failure, and, unless oedema or hypertension is present, an increased sodium intake should be tried to assess if renal function can be improved.

(*a*) *No-added-salt diets.* This is all that is required in the majority of cases requiring salt restriction, e.g. in nephrotic syndrome. The amount of sodium in a normal diet varies considerably, according to individual preference, due to added salt as well as the sodium content of natural foods used. This increases

Table 8.9 Example of a low-protein diet.
The sodium content of this diet can be modified by selection of appropriate foods.
Eggs, meat, cheese, fish, 6 g protein exchanges (Table 8.4a) × † daily.
Potatoes, bread, cereal; 1 g protein exchanges (Table 8.4b) × † daily.
Energy supplement, Table 8.7‡.
Foods allowed freely: Table 8.4c, d and Table 8.8.

Breakfast	† × 6 g exchanges protein, e.g. milk or egg
	† × 1 g exchanges protein, e.g. cereal
	Low-protein bread (with or without salt)
	Butter/margarine* (with or without salt)
	Jam, honey, marmalade, etc.
	Energy (high-calorie) supplement drink‡
Mid-morning	Low-protein biscuit or wafers or fruit
	Energy (high-calorie) supplement‡
Lunch	† × 6 g exchanges protein, e.g. meat
	† × 1 g exchanges protein, e.g. potato
	Low-protein vegetables
	Margarine*/butter (with or without salt) — Cooked with or without salt as appropriate
	1 tablespoon gravy
	Fruit or low-protein pudding
Tea	Low-protein bread, biscuit or wafer or fruit
	Energy (high-calorie) supplement‡
Supper	† × 6 g exchange protein, e.g. egg or meat
	† × 1 g exchange protein, e.g. bread
	Low-protein bread or vegetables — Cooked with or without salt as appropriate
	Butter/margarine (with or without salt)
	Fruit or low-protein pudding
Bedtime	Low-protein biscuit or wafer or fruit
	Energy (high-calorie) supplement‡

* The selected fats and margarine should ideally be high in PUFA.
† Prescribe as appropriate (*see* Table 8.5).
‡ Prescribe as appropriate (*see* Table 8.7).

considerably with age, as the quantity of protein foods, and bread, cake and biscuits increases.

Omitting added salt and very salty foods reduces the sodium content of the diet. A diet without added salt contains approximately 60 to 90 mmol (1·4 to 2 g) sodium daily according to the child's appetite and age; Table 8.12 gives a sample menu, and lists salty foods to avoid.

(b) *Low-sodium diets.* The sodium content of a diet can be reduced further by considering the contribution from natural foods, such as milk, and using salt-free bread and butter as well as omitting salty foods and all salt in cooking (Table 8.12). It is important that food is palatable e.g. by the use of herbs and spices, as energy intake is decreased if food is rejected, and energy intake may be of more conse-

quence than sodium restriction, and an alternative such as antihypertensive drugs or diuretics more appropriate. Where very low-sodium diets are essential energy supplements are frequently required, at least in young children.

In infants the use of or a change to a modified infant formula (*see* Table 8.1) will give adequate restriction in sodium in the majority of cases. If protein as well as sodium requires adjustment in the diet, the feed should be calculated individually. Lonalac (Mead Johnson) is a low-sodium milk substitute from the U.S.A. which could be used if a very low sodium intake is needed, but this is rarely required.

A number of baby weaning solids do not contain added salt and can be used to introduce solids in a normal way. Alternatively, home-prepared purées from which salt has been omitted can be used.

Table 8.10   Calculated sample menu for an 18 g protein diet for a school-age child. Based on information given in Tables 8.4 to 8.9.

		Sodium* (mg)	Protein (g)	Energy‡ kJ	Energy‡ kcal
Breakfast	1 × 6 g exchanges protein, e.g. 180 ml milk	90	6·0	490	117
	1 × 1 g exchange protein, e.g. 15 g Rice Krispies	167	1·0	234	56
	Sugar			80	20
	30 g low-protein bread (with salt)	165	Trace	312	75
	Butter/margarine† salted (10 g)	85	Trace	304	74
	1 teaspoon jam, honey, marmalade, etc.	Trace	—	125	30
	100 ml energy (high-calorie) supplement to drink‡				
Mid-morning	Low-protein biscuit (or wafers or fruit)	Trace	Trace	210	50
	100 ml energy (high-calorie) supplement‡				
Lunch	1 × 6 g exchange protein, e.g. 20 g chicken	15	6·0	175	42
	1 × 1 g exchange protein, e.g. 30 g chips cooked in vegetable oil†	5	1·0	320	76
	Low-protein vegetables	5	<0·5	80	20
	Margarine†/butter with or without salt		—	‡	‡
	Gravy (1 tablespoon)	45	—	20	5
	Fruit or low-protein pudding	Trace	<0·5	420	100
	100 ml energy (high-calorie) supplement‡				
Tea	1 × 1 g exchange protein, e.g. 15 g semi-sweet biscuits	60	1·0	290	70
	100 ml energy (high-calorie) supplement‡				
Supper	Nil × 6 g exchange protein				
	3 × 1 g exchange protein, e.g. 60 g baked beans canned with salt	285	3·0	162	39
	60 g low-protein bread (with salt)	330	Trace	624	150
	and 20 g butter/margarine† (and jam)	170	Trace	608	148
	Fruit or low-protein pudding	Trace	Trace	420	100
	Boiled sweets	Trace	Nil	‡	‡
Bedtime	Low-protein biscuits (or wafer or fruit)	Trace	Trace	210	50
	100 ml energy (high-calorie) supplement‡				
	Sub-total	1422 = 62 mmol*	18 to 19	5064	1222
	Daily energy supplement‡ (Recipe, Table 8.7) 150 g glucose polymer and Nesquik 100 ml Prosparol/Calogen Water to 500 ml	Trace	Nil	4250	1050
	Total	1422 = 62 mmol*	18 to 19	9314‡	2272‡

In the Lunch section, the exchanges "1 × 6 g exchange protein... chicken", "1 × 1 g exchange protein... chips cooked in vegetable oil†", "Low-protein vegetables", and "Margarine†/butter with or without salt" are bracketed together as "No added salt".

* mg sodium ÷ 23 = mmol.

  The sodium content of this diet can be increased by using salt in cooking and selecting salty foods or reduced by selecting salt-free alternatives.

† The selected ‚margarine and fats used in cooking should be high in polyunsaturated fatty acids.

‡ The quantity of energy supplement should be adjusted for energy needs as over-prescription can cause food refusal, under-prescription growth failure.

Table 8.11 Example of a moderate-protein diet (= 50 g protein) for an older child, based on information given in Tables 8.4 to 8.9.

		Protein (g)	Energy† kJ	Energy† kcal
Breakfast				
	1 × 6 g exchange protein, e.g. 180 ml milk = allowance	6	490	117
	1 × 1 g exchange protein, e.g. 20 g Sugar Puffs	1	296	70
	Sugar (5 g)		80	20
	2 × 1 g exchanges protein, e.g. 24 g bread	2	228	54
	Butter/margarine* (10 g)	Trace	304	70
	1 × 6 g exchange protein, e.g. 1 egg	6	306	74
	Tea or coffee with milk from allowance			
Mid-morning	1 piece fruit	1	200	50
	†Energy supplement			
Lunch	2 × 6 g exchanges protein, e.g. 100 g fish fingers	12	976	232
	10 g oil*/margarine*/butter for cooking	Trace	304 to 378	70 to 90
	3 × 1 g exchanges protein, e.g. 90 g chips	3	960	228
	Low-protein vegetables (100 g)	<1	80	20
	1 tablespoon gravy	Trace	20	5
	Tinned fruit or low-protein pudding	<1	600	150
	†Energy supplement			
Mid-afternoon	1 × 1 g exchanges protein, e.g. 15 g semi-sweet biscuits	1	290	70
	1 piece fruit (optional)		Trace	Trace
Supper	2 × 6 g exchanges protein, e.g. 90 g sausages	12	547	130
	6 × 1 g exchanges protein, e.g. 72 g bread	6	684	162
	Low-protein vegetables (100 g)	<1	80	20
	Butter/margarine* 10 g	Trace	304	70
	Fruit and/or jelly (vegetarian-type)	Trace	400	100
	†Energy supplement			
	Sub-total	50	7149 to 7223	1712 to 1732
	†Daily energy supplement (1 bottle Hycal diluted with water)	Nil	1778	425
	Total	50	8927 to 9000	2137 to 2157

*The selected margarine and fats used in cooking should be high in polyunsaturated fatty acids.

† Alternative energy supplements could be selected and the quantity should be adjusted for energy needs. Over-prescription can cause food refusal, under-prescription growth failure.

In children the diet rarely has to be as strict as the basic low-sodium diet given in Table 8.13, which contains only 5 to 15 mmol (115 to 345 mg) of sodium, according to age and appetite. The amount of dietary salt or sodium can be adjusted by adding restricted quantities of natural foods which contain sodium (Table 8.14a) or their salt-free substitutes (Table 8.14b) to the basic low-sodium diet. Table 8.15 gives details of a diet which contains 44 mmol (1 g) sodium. Table 8.4a, b and c provides information from which a diet for an individual patient can be devised.

In some areas bakeries make salt-free bread. Alternatively, home-made salt-free bread can be made by omitting salt from a household recipe. Cakes, biscuits, and puddings can be made from household recipes using plain flour, salt-free baking powder, salt-free butter and other permitted ingredients. Salt substitutes containing potassium in place of sodium are available to add to savoury foods in place of salt, e.g. Selora, Ruthmol. They and salt-free baking powder are contraindicated if potassium has to be restricted. Herbs and spices can be used to increase the palatability of low-sodium and no-added-salt savoury foods,

Table 8.12 No-added-salt diet.

This is a completely normal diet, except that:

(a) No salt is used at table.

(b) Salt in cooking is omitted or kept to a minimum, e.g. $\frac{1}{4} \times 5$ ml level teaspoon salt to 1 litre (2 pints) of water for cooking vegetables or added to stews and casseroles.

(c) The following salty foods should be avoided:

Salt, monosodium glutamate.

Bicarbonate of soda (unless prescribed medicinally).

Bacon, ham, sausages, salt beef, corned beef, other salted meats.

Tinned meats, e.g. luncheon meat, paté and continental sausages, meat paste, fish paste.

Tinned and packet soups, stock cubes, savoury sauces, tinned vegetables, baked beans, spaghetti and similar savoury dishes.

Marmite, Bovril, Yeastril, gravy mixes, soup and stock cubes, e.g. Oxo, Bisto.

Tomato ketchup, pickles and sauces.

Kippers, sardines, smoked fish, salted fish, tinned fish.

Salted savoury biscuits, e.g. Ritz, Twiglets, etc.

Salted and flavoured crisps, salted peanuts, dry roast peanuts, savoury snack foods.

(d) Milk, regular salted breads and butter/margarines are permitted. Cheese should be used sparingly.

Sample menu.

Breakfast	Cereal, all varieties are permitted
	Milk and sugar
	Bread, toast, roll and butter/margarine*
	Egg(s), boiled, poached, scrambled or plain omelette, fried*
	Milk, tea, coffee or fruit juice
Mid-morning	Milk or fruit juice
Lunch and supper	Meat, roast, grilled, casserole, or fish or egg(s)
	Potato, rice, chips, bread and butter/ margarine*
	Vegetables or salad, salad cream or oil* and vinegar
	1 tablespoon gravy if appropriate to type of food may be permitted
	Fruit, custard, milk pudding, ice-cream, sponge pudding
	Fruit pie or tart, yoghurt, mousse
	Cake or biscuits
Tea	Milk, tea, fruit juice
	Fruit
	Bread and butter/margarine*

Include 500 ml (1 pint) milk daily unless the dietary protein intake is restricted.

_____

* The selected margarine and fats used in cooking should be high in polyunsaturated fatty acids.

but monosodium glutamate should be avoided. An increasing range of low-sodium foods is available for use in conjunction with low and minimal sodium diets: these include: Rite-Diet Salt-Free Bread, Rite-Diet Low-Protein Salt-Free Bread, Life low-sodium condiments (with no added potassium chloride) including ketchups and sauces, Dietade unsalted baked beans, processed peas, tomato ketchup and salad cream, Nistria tinned and monocup meat products.

Baking powder and self-raising flours contain sodium. Salt-free baking powder can be made from the following recipe and used as a substitute, provided potassium is not restricted:

20 g (1 oz) starch, e.g. cornflour

5 g ($\frac{1}{4}$ oz) potassium bicarbonate

40 g (2 oz) potassium bitartrate

Using dry utensils weigh ingredients and sieve two or three times to mix well. Store in an airtight jar. Use a dry spoon to measure. This baking powder is used with plain flour in the normal quantity, that is 1×5 ml spoon to 230 g (8 oz) plain flour for cakes, puddings, sponges; $\frac{1}{2}$ teaspoon to 230 g (8 oz) plain flour for biscuits, batter, pastry.

POTASSIUM

Low-potassium diets. The potassium intake of children's diets varies from about 50 to 180 mmol/day*.

(a) Simple restriction to approximately 26 mmol (1 g) potassium daily requires a limited intake of milk, meat, all types of potato, citrus and soft fruits, especially apricots and bananas, nuts and dried fruits, fruit juice, vegetables, meat and yeast extracts (Bovril and Marmite), treacle, tea and coffee. Rice can be substituted for potato, and stewed apple, tinned pear or pineapple can replace other fruit. A small quantity of diluted lemon juice or blackcurrant juice may be given as a source of vitamin C.

(b) Dietary potassium can be reduced to a minimum of about 1 mmol/kg per day if necessary but is rarely required (*see* p. 201). This degree of dietary restriction of potassium requires individual calculation and prescription. Low-protein diets benefit from a more generous potassium intake and allow a larger food bulk from fruit, vegetables and potato. The potassium content of various foods is given in Table 8.4a, b and c.

_____

* Dietary potassium is prescribed in millimole (mmol); 39 mg potassium or 74 mg potassium chloride contains 1 mmol potassium.

High-potassium diets. To increase dietary potassium intake a normal diet with generous quantities of the foods restricted above should be given. Supplements of potassium are necessary if the child's appetite is poor and/or unreliable. Fresh fruit juice and bananas can be used to increase the potassium intake, or potassium supplements prescribed medicinally.

100 ml orange juice	4·6 mmol	180 mg
100 g pineapple—canned	2·4 mmol	94 mg
100 g bananas	9·0 mmol	350 mg
100 g apricots—canned	6·7 mmol	260 mg
15 g crisps with or without salt	4·6 mmol	180 mg

LOW-PROTEIN DIETS WITH RESTRICTED SODIUM WITH OR WITHOUT POTASSIUM AND FLUID RESTRICTIONS

Low-protein diets are lower in sodium than the normal diet for a child of the same age, because protein foods are rich in sodium. To reduce the sodium intake further 'salt-free' low-protein bread is available and can replace regular bread; salt-free butter can be used and salt omitted at the table and in cooking. A diet of appropriate protein and sodium content can be devised from the information in Table 8.4 and the patient's personal food preferences. An example is given in Table 8.16, or the information given in Table 8.9 can be adapted. Appropriate energy, vitamin and mineral supplements should be prescribed.

Table 8.13 Basic low-sodium diet (5 to 15 mmol sodium). No salt should be used in cooking or at table.

(a) Allowed and forbidden foods.

Foods allowed	Foods forbidden
All fresh meat, poultry, offal	Bacon, ham, salt-beef, tongue, sausages, tinned meats, meat pastes, prepared foods, e.g. beefburgers, frozen meals, etc.
All fresh fish	Smoked and salted fish, tinned fish, fish pastes, fish fingers, cooked shellfish
Milk allowance or Lonalac (Mead Johnson) as appropriate	Cheese, evaporated, condensed and dried milks, yoghurt
Fresh and frozen vegetables, unsalted nuts and salad	Tinned vegetables, baked beans, salted crisps, tinned and packet soups, salted nuts, salted and flavoured crisps
Fresh fruit, stewed fruit, tinned fruit, fruit juice, prunes	Dried fruits
Shredded Wheat, Puffed Wheat, Farley's Rusk, Ready Brek, porridge oats, Sugar Puffs	Other breakfast cereals, e.g. Rice Krispies, Cornflakes
Matzos biscuits, Salt-free bread	Cream Crackers, crispbread. Salted breads.
Home-made salt-free biscuits and cakes	Ordinary cakes, biscuits, pastry
Plain flour, cornflour, custard powder, arrowroot, barley, sago, rice, macaroni, spaghetti, semolina, other pasta	Self-raising flour, baking powder, rennet, canned spaghetti, bicarbonate of soda
Salt-free baking powder	
Jam, honey, marmalade, sugar, jelly	Golden syrup, treacle, sweet mincemeat
Boiled sweets, ice-lollies, fruit gums	Chocolate, toffee, fudge, ice-cream, sherbet
Tea, coffee, natural fruit juice	Cocoa, drinking chocolate, Ovaltine, Horlicks
Fruit drinks without sodium preservatives	Lucozade, soda water, fizzy drinks, fruit squashes with sodium preservatives
Fruit-flavoured Nesquik, milk-shake syrup	
Cooking oils,* salt-free butter, salt-free margarine*	Salted butter, margarine
Vinegar, herbs, spices, pepper, curry powder, parsley, mint	Bovril, Oxo, Marmite, Bisto, pickles, bottled sauces and ketchup, chutney, salad cream, mayonnaise

Table 8.13 *continued*

(b)   Low-sodium diet menu (5 to 15 mmol sodium†): sample menu.

Breakfast	'Salt-free' cereal and sugar, e.g. Sugar Puffs, Farley's Rusk
	Milk or substitute
	White fish or egg if permitted
	Salt-free bread
	Unsalted butter/margarine*
	Jam, honey, marmalade
	Natural fruit juice
Mid-morning	Fruit juice
Dinner	Meat or fish
	Rice, pasta
	Potatoes/pulses } Cooked without salt
	Vegetables/salad
	Fruit or jelly
Tea	Natural fruit juice
	Salt-free bread
	Unsalted butter/margarine*
	Jam, honey, marmalade
Supper	Meat, fish, vegetables—cooked without salt
	Salt-free bread
	Unsalted butter/margarine*
	Fruit or jelly
	Natural fruit juice

* The selected margarine and fats used in cooking should be high in polyunsaturated fatty acids but contain no added salt.
† Selected items from Table 8.14 can be incorporated to derive the permitted sodium intake prescribed.

The fluid prescription should state the volume (ml) per 24 hours, and whether this is total or free fluid, or the range of fluid within which to keep the intake.

DIALYSIS

Dialysis is being increasingly used in acute renal failure (Barratt 1985), and dialysis with the chance of a kidney transplant should be considered and planned in chronic renal failure before 'end-stage' renal disease is reached. Not all patients will be suitable for dialysis. Experience, however, with both techniques in children is continually increasing, and 80% of children treated by home dialysis or transplant achieve full school activity and life expectancy is improving (Chantler & Barratt 1976, Barratt 1985).

Protein, amino acid, iron, magnesium, phosphate, vitamin C, folic acid, B_6 and B_{12} losses occur in the dialysate unless the latter contains these as additives. Trace mineral losses are less frequently reported but

almost certainly occur (Aggett & Davies 1983). To compensate for dialysis previous dietary restrictions apart from fluid should normally be lifted (Booth 1973), and at least 10 g of protein per day above normal requirement and an adequate nutrient intake should be encouraged. Energy supplements have been suggested to ensure an adequate intake for growth (Simmons *et al.* 1971, James 1976, Chantler *et al.* 1980). Vitamin and mineral losses should be replaced with supplements (Parsons 1974). Nutrition can be given at the same time as dialysis by adding appropriate supplements to the dialysate or as enteral or parenteral nutrition. During dialysis in the acutely ill patient who is hypercatabolic parenteral nutrition is indicated to provide adequate nutrition.

Fluid and electrolyte balance is critical in children on dialysis, but this is normally controlled by more frequent dialysis rather than by rigid dietary measures, although some sodium restriction may be imposed if the blood pressure is raised, and a fluid restriction is usually advised (Booth 1973).

Table 8.14 Sodium content of foods used in conjunction with low-sodium and low-salt diets. The appropriate quantities of these foods are incorporated into the basic low-sodium diet (Table 8.13) according to prescribed sodium intake.

	Sodium	
Restricted food items	mg	mmol
(a) *Moderate sodium*		
Milk		
100 ml (3½ oz)	50	2·2
560 ml (1 pint)	280	12·2
Milk puddings, custard 100 g	77*	3·3*
Gold Cap SMA (J. Wyeth Labs)†		
100 ml reconstituted	15	0·7
Bread		
100 g (3½ oz) wholemeal, brown or white	540*	23·6*
30 g (1 oz = 1 thin slice)	162	7·0
40 g (1⅓ oz = 1 large slice)	216	9·4
Egg 50 g (1 only, size 3)	70	3·0
Ice-cream 40 g (1 small brickette)	30*	1·3*
Weetabix 20 g (1 only)	72	3·1
Cornflakes 15 g (½ oz)	174	7·6
Rice Krispies 15 g (½ oz)	166	7·2
Butter (salted) 10 g (3 teaspoons)	87	3·8
Rite-Diet Low-Protein Bread with salt (canned) 100 g	540	23·5
Crisps salted (20 g)	110	4·8
(b) *Minimal sodium*		
Lonalac (Mead Johnson USA) milk substitute 100 ml (3½ oz)	4·2	0·2
Salt-free bread		
100 g (3½ oz)	3	Trace
30 g (1 oz = 1 thin slice)	0·9	Trace
40 g (1⅓ oz = 1 large slice)	1·2	Trace
Salt-free butter 10 g (3 teaspoons)	Trace	Trace
Rite-Diet Low-Protein Bread without salt (canned) 100 g	9·0	0·4
Crisps—'salt-free', e.g. Salt & Shake type omitting the salt sachet 20 g	1·4	Trace
(c) *Controlled or high-sodium*		
300 mg sodium chloride salt tablets (1 tablet)	115	5
'Normal' saline 100 ml (3½ oz)	354·2	15·4
Sodium bicarbonate 84 mg powder	23	1·0
Sodium chloride 58·5 mg powder	23	1·0

* Average value.
† Other modified infant formulae may be equally appropriate, but they vary slightly in sodium content.

NEPHROTIC SYNDROME

This is characterized by proteinuria in excess of 50 mg/kg per day or 1 g/m² body surface per day, a plasma albumin of less than 3 g/100 mg and a reduced plasma volume, which requires immediate intervention as it can be life-threatening: oedema and sodium retention result. Blood urea and blood pressure are usually normal (James 1976, Barratt 1985). The commonest type is the idiopathic form related to an immunological problem: there is also an inherited (Finnish) type which occurs from birth with poor prognosis, and a type secondary to conditions such as malaria or congenital syphilis (Hallman & Rapola 1978). The majority of patients with idiopathic nephrotic syndrome respond to steroids and dietary therapy. Relapse occurs in some. A small group of patients are steroid-resistant and may require cyclophosphamide therapy.

To replenish 1 g plasma albumin in adults it has been estimated that 10 g dietary protein is used. Protein supplementation may be required when there is excessive protein loss, as in the nephrotic syndrome. In general, the limiting factor in the ability of the liver to synthesize albumin is not the availability of dietary protein, provided the intake is of the usual generous affluent western-style diet, but it is a major factor in the management of malnourished children with nephrotic syndrome, especially in the Third World. James (1976) suggests that 2 to 3 g protein/kg per day should be given to children with nephrotic syndrome, calculated on the child's own non-oedematous weight. In oedematous patients sodium intake should also be reduced, as far as is compatible with the maintenance of protein intake. A no-added-salt diet (Table 8.12) with the provision of 500 ml of cow's milk and three serves of meat, egg or fish per day provides an adequate protein intake for the majority of children. Sometimes, however, particularly with the nephrotic syndrome due to focal segmental glomerulosclerosis or of congenital onset, protein losses may be very heavy and protein supplements up to ≃5 g/kg per day may be necessary. Because of the increased filtration rate with high protein intakes some workers consider high protein intakes are contraindicated (*see* p. 201).

Table 8.18 lists a number of protein supplements which can be incorporated into high-protein diets (*see* p. 220) for older children, for example as fortified drinks.

Infants and toddlers are normally breast-fed or given a modified whey-based milk (*see* Table 8.1). These are low in protein as well as sodium and solute.

Table 8.15 Example of a 44-mmol sodium (1 g sodium) diet for a school-age child. No salt should be used in cooking or at table.

		Sodium	
		mg	mmol
Daily	500 ml milk	250	11·0
Breakfast	20 g (¾ oz) Puffed Wheat or porridge plus sugar	Trace	Trace
	50 g (1 only) egg	70	3·0
	30 g (1 oz) ordinary bread	163	7·0
	Salt-free butter/margarine*	Trace	Trace
	15 g (½ oz) marmalade or jam or honey	Trace	Trace
Mid-morning	Fruit juice	Trace	Trace
Dinner	60 g (2 oz) meat or fish or chicken	45	2·0
	115 g (4 oz) potato boiled, mashed or roasted	5	0·2
	Vegetables	Trace	Trace
	85 g (3 oz) 'unsalted' fruit tart or sponge pudding *plus*	5	0·2
	100 g (3½ oz) custard	77	3·3
Tea	60 g (2 oz) chicken or fish or meat	45	2·0
	Salad or vegetables	10	0·4
	60 g (2 oz) ordinary bread	326	14·0
	Salt-free butter/margarine*	Trace	Trace
	15 g (½ oz) jam or honey	Trace	Trace
	30 g (1 oz) 'unsalted' biscuits *or*		
	30 g (1 oz) 'unsalted' sponge cake	5	0·2
	Apple or orange or pear	Trace	Trace
Bedtime	Milk from allowance with tea or coffee		
	Fresh fruit *or* 15 g (½ oz) unsalted biscuits		
		5	Trace
	Total	1006	43·3

This diet provides approximately 75 g protein, 245 g carbohydrate, 84 g fat and 8473 kJ (2025 kcal)
* The selected margarine and fats used in cooking should be high in polyunsaturated fatty acids but contain no added salt.

Small calculated quantities, 1·5 to 3 g per 100 ml feed of high biological protein (Maxipro HBV or Casilan) can be added to increase the protein content of the feed to 3 to 4 g per 100 ml without significantly increasing the sodium.

Energy intake should be adequate or protein will not be available for liver protein synthesis. Initially the child has a poor appetite and will need encouragement to eat; later steroid therapy usually increases appetite, and excess energy intake, particularly from low nutrient density foods, should be avoided, but 'slimming' is inappropriate. The diet should be nutritionally adequate in all respects and may require vitamin supplements.

The occasional patient becomes grossly malnourished and benefits from nutritional supplements (*see* Table 8.18) or appropriate nutrition given by nasogastric tube to help break the vicious circle of hypoalbuminaemia, ascites, reduced intake and even further reduction of plasma albumin concentration.

Gross oedema, hypertension and/or ascites require a further restriction of sodium and restricted fluid intake until response to drug therapy occurs (James 1976, Barratt 1985). An accurate fluid balance should be kept. Large quantities of protein in low fluid volumes should be avoided, and where used of necessity the child should be regularly monitored biochemically and clinically.

Table 8.16 Example of combined protein-, sodium-, potassium-restricted diet containing approximately 21 g protein, 10 mmol sodium, 21 mmol potassium, 1000 ml fluid. Suitable for a pre-school-age child. Based on information given in Tables 8.4 to 8.9. No salt should be used in cooking or at table.

	Energy		Protein	Sodium	Potassium
	kJ	kcal	(g)	(mg*)	(mg†)
Daily: Energy supplements					
(i) 'Protein-free milk shake'					
100 g glucose polymer, e.g. Maxijul	1570	375	Nil	45	5
Flavouring				Trace	Trace
50 ml Calogen	940	225	Nil	10	10
Water to 500 ml					
(ii) 500 ml Coca Cola (sweetened)	840	225	Nil	40	5
Breakfast					
20 g slice Rite-Diet Low-Protein Bread, no salt	208	50	Trace	Trace	10
Unsalted margarine‡/butter (10 g)	304	74	Trace	Trace	Trace
Jam, honey	+	+	Trace	Trace	Trace
1 egg (50 g)	306	74	6·0	70	70
Energy supplement					
Mid-morning					
25 g boiled sweets	349	82	Nil	6	3
Energy supplement					
Lunch					
20 g meat or 1 × 6 g protein exchange	175	42	6·0	15	70
30 g chips or 1 × 1 g protein exchange	320	76	1·0	5	306
100 mg potassium from vegetable, e.g. 50 g carrots					
or cauliflower	42	10	Trace	5	100
Oil for cooking‡	+	+	Nil	–	–
Tea					
Energy supplement					
Supper					
20 g meat or 1 × 6 g protein exchange	175	42	6·0	15	70
45 g boiled rice or 1 × 1 g protein exchange	235	55	1·0	Trace	17
100 mg potassium from fruit, e.g. 120 g stewed					
apple	210	50	Trace	Trace	100
70 g double cream and sugar	1288	313	1·0	20	55
Total				231 = 10	821 = 21
	6962	1663	21	mmol*	mmol†

Supplements

3 Ketovite Tablets + 5 ml Ketovite Liquid (Paines & Byrne) *plus* calcium, iron, zinc supplements

or 6 to 12 Cow & Gate Supplementary Vitamin Tablets + 5 ml Ketovite Liquid *plus* calcium supplement

* mg sodium ÷ 23 = mmol.

† mg potassium ÷ 39 = mmol.

‡ The selected margarine and fats used in cooking should be high in polyunsaturated fatty acids but contain no added salt.

Chapter 8

Table 8.17 Suggested protein and energy intakes per kg actual weight* per day in high-protein diets.

Age in years	High-protein diets (g)	Recommended energy intake		Recommended high-energy intakes	
		kJ	kcal	kJ	kcal
0–1	4 to 6†	540 to 420	130 to 100	840	200
1–3	4·5 to 3	420 to 375	100 to 90	630	150
3–6	3 to 2·5	335	80	420	100
7–12	3 to 2·5	300	70	420	100
Teenagers	2·5 to 2	300 to 200	70 to 45	335	80
Adults	2 to 1·5	200	45	300+	80+

* The child's weight should be corrected for oedema before calculating dietary nutrients.

† Use with caution in infants under six months of age.

Once remission occurs, proteinuria is reduced and the child is no longer oedematous, a normal diet can be resumed.

High-protein diets

High-protein diets are prescribed for conditions in which there is a marked increase in the breakdown of endogenous protein, or increased requirement for, or increased excretion of, nitrogen, e.g. malabsorption, protein-losing enteropathy, and ulcerative colitis, and in patients with hypercatabolic states such as extensive burns and protein–energy malnutrition. A high-protein diet should not be used if the blood urea exceeds 17 mmol/l ($\simeq$100 mg/100 ml) and is contra-indicated in liver failure because of the risk of hepatic encephalopathy and hyperammonaemia (Crossley & Williams 1984) and certain renal conditions, e.g. chronic renal failure (*see* p. 199).

The level of protein at which to aim is $1\frac{1}{2}$ to 2 times the normal requirement. Table 8.17 gives suggested intakes for high-protein diets. The child's actual weight used in the dietary calculations should first be corrected for any oedema. The blood urea should be checked from time to time. The energy intake must be adequate to cover any increased requirements, so that protein is not used to supply energy needs, and to reduce endogenous nitrogen catabolism to a minimum. High energy intakes as well as an increased protein are required in some conditions, such as protein–energy malnutrition and hypercatabolic states, and suggested intakes are given in Table 8.17. Dietary management of catabolism and the chronically ill child are dealt with by Francis (1986) where enteral feeds and supplements are dealt with in greater detail.

High-protein feeds for infants should be used with caution, particularly in the first six months of life because of the immaturity of the kidney excretory and liver degradation systems. Protein increases the solute load of the feed, and therefore blood urea, electrolytes and plasma proteins should be monitored and, at least from time to time, plasma amino acids should be estimated to ensure that elevated levels are avoided. When clinically necessary Maxipro HBV or Casilan can be used to supplement the protein content of the modified infant formulae, as suggested above for infants with nephrotic syndrome, but skimmed milk powder, Complan and adult enteral feeds are not recommended, as they will increase solute and other nutrients inappropriately for infant nutrition and some products contain ingredients which are not recommended for infants.

In children the inclusion of two to three serves of meat, egg, cheese or fish plus at least 500 ml (1 pint) of milk each day will normally provide a high-protein intake. In a child who is anorexic and not eating adequately, protein supplements (Table 8.18) can be incorporated into the diet. High-protein milk-shakes are popular (Francis 1986), especially if chilled and served in a milk-shake container with lid and straw, similar to several commercial snack meal cafeterias. Fortified soups or savoury Complan are useful if milk is disliked, provided sodium is not restricted. Other recipes are given by Grant and Todd (1982). Adequate fluid intake is usually recommended with high-protein diets in order to avoid a high solute for the kidney to handle, especially in some patients with kidney conditions and those with burns.

Hyperosmolar solutions can cause malabsorption, nausea, vomiting and abdominal cramp, and should be avoided. The osmolality of any feed used in paediatrics should not normally exceed 550 mmol/l.

Table 8.18 Protein supplements*.

		Protein (g)	Energy kJ	Energy kcal	Sodium (mmol)	Potassium (mmol)
Milk, cow's		3·3	272	65	2·2	3·8
Clinifeed Protein rich†		6·0	420	100	2·6	4·3
Clinifeed Select†		4·5	420	100	1·4	2·9
Ensure Plus†	per 100 ml	5·5	600	145	4·8	4·9
Fortimel (High Protein)‡		9·7	420	100	2·2	5·1
Fortison Low Sodium†		4·0	420	100	<1·1	3·8
Lonalac (Mead Johnson USA)		5·6	441	105	§0·2	5·3
Whole-protein foods						
Build-Up, vanilla‡		22·4	1447	350	14·5	26·2
Casilan = calcium caseinate		90	1573	376	<4·3	N/S
Complan, natural‡		20	1870	444	15·2	21·8
Comminuted Chicken ¶	per 100 g	7·5	251	60	0·4	1·2
Forceval Protein = calcium caseinate		55	1506	360	5	1
Maxipro HBV = whey protein isolate		88	1623	388	10	11·5
Skimmed milk powder (various)¶		36·4	1512	355	23·9	42·3
Egg (2 eggs)		12·3	612	147	6	3·6
Hydrolysates and amino acids						
Albumaid Complete = beef serum (SHS)		89.4 amino acids 75 protein§	1496	358	43·5	5·1
Dialamine essential amino acids (SHS)	per 100 g	30 amino acids	1500	360	7·3	0·2
Hepatamine essential amino acids high in arginine (SHS)		30 amino acids	1500	360	7·3	0·2
Ketoamino acid analogues (SHS)		83 amino acids and ketoacids	1411	352	N/S	N/S

N/S: not specified.

* Unsuitable for infants and as a sole source of nutrition in children. If a high-protein formula is needed for an infant, 1·5 to 2 g Maxipro HBV or Casilan can be added to each 100 ml of a modified infant feed.

† Other varieties are available by the same companies and an increasing range of different products are becoming available continually from different manufacturers.

‡ Various flavours available.

§ Approximate values.

¶ Average values.

HIGH-PROTEIN, SALT/SODIUM-RESTRICTED DIETS

A high-protein, salt/sodium-restricted diet may be prescribed for conditions such as oedema with hypoproteinaemia or cirrhosis of the liver with ascites. The protein intake can be increased with minimal effect on the sodium intake by incorporating high-protein, low-sodium supplements (Table 8.18) to the selected no-added-salt or low-sodium diet (Tables 8.12 to 14).

As all the naturally occurring high-protein foods also contain some sodium, this diet may present problems in raising the protein intake to the required level without exceeding the level of sodium permitted. The diet must be as palatable as possible to avoid food refusal with resultant poor nutrient and protein intake. The diet should be monitored clinically and biochemically; frequently such a diet is only a temporary regimen.

REFERENCES

AGGETT P.J. & DAVIES N.T. (1983) Some nutritional aspects of trace metals *J. inher. metab. Dis.* **6**, Suppl. I, 22–30.

BARRATT T.M. (1982) Renal disease in the first year of life. In *Recent Advances in Renal Medicine II* (eds. Jones N.F. & Peters D.K.), pp. 197–212. Edinburgh: Churchill Livingstone.

BARRATT T.M. (1985) The kidney in childhood. In *Postgraduate Nephrology* (ed. Marsh F.), pp. 459–98. London: William Heinemann Medical Books Ltd.

BARRATT T.M. & WILLIAMS D.I. (1979) Obstructive uropathy in childhood. In *Renal Diseases*, 4th Edition (eds. Black D. & Jones N.F.), pp. 804–24. Oxford: Blackwell Scientific Publications.

BOOTH E.M. (1973) The dietary treatment of renal disease. *Nutrition* **27**, 375.

BURMAN D., PERHAM T.G.M. & CLOTHIER C. (1982) Nutrition in systemic disease. In *Textbook of Paediatric Nutrition*, 2nd Edition (eds. McLaran D.S. & Burman D.), pp. 353–66. Edinburgh: Churchill Livingstone.

CAMERON J.S. (1970) Glomerulonephritis and the nephrotic syndrome. *Brit. med. J.* **IV**, 285 and 350.

CAMERON M. & HOFVANDER Y. (1983) *Manual on Feeding Infants and Young Children*, 3rd Edition. Protein Advisory Group of United Nations I. Oxford Medical Publications.

CHANTLER C. & BARRATT T.M. (1976) Letter to Editor. *Lancet* **1**, 583.

CHANTLER C. & HOLLIDAY M.A. (1973) Growth in children with renal disease with particular reference to the effect of calorie malnutrition: a review. *Clinical Nephrology* **1**, 4, 230.

CHANTLER C., BISHTI E.I. & COUNAHAN R. (1980) Nutritional therapy in children with chronic renal failure. *Amer. J. clin. Nutr.* **33**, 168–9.

CONN H.C. (1973) The rational management of ascites. In *Progress in Liver Disease* (eds. Popper H. & Schaffner F.), Vol. 4, p. 269. New York: Grune & Stratton.

COUNAHAN R., CAMERON J.S., OGG C.S. *et al.* (1977) Presentation, management, complications and outcome of acute renal failure in childhood: 5 years experience. *Brit. med. J.* **1**, 599.

CROSSLEY I.R. & WILLIAMS R. (1984) Progress in the treatment of portasystemic encephalopathy. *Gut* **25**, 85–98.

DHSS (1973) *Recommended intakes of nutrients for the United Kingdom*. Report on Public Health and Medical Subjects, No. 120, first published 1969. London: HMSO.

DHSS (1980) *Artificial feeds for the young infant*. Report No. 18. London: HMSO.

DHSS (1983) (revision) *Present day practice in infant feeding*. Report No. 20 (1980). London: HMSO.

DHSS (1985) (revision) *Recommended daily amounts of food energy and nutrients for groups of people in the UK*. Report No. 15, London: HMSO.

FAO/WHO (1978) *An examination of current recommendation on requirements of protein and energy*. Report of consultants meeting in Rome, 15–17 Oct. 1979. Also 1973 and 1975 reports.

FRANCIS D.E.M. (1979) Inborn errors of metabolism. The need for sugar. *J. hum. Nutr.* **33**, 146–54.

FRANCIS D.E.M. (1986) *Nutrition for Children*. Oxford: Blackwell Scientific Publications.

GEIGY SCIENTIFIC TABLES (1981) Vol. 1 *Units of Measurement, Body Fluids, Composition of the Body, Nutrition*, 8th Edition (ed. Lentner C.). Basle: Ciba-Geigy Ltd.

GRANT A. & TODD E. (1982) *Enteral and Parenteral Nutrition*. Oxford: Blackwell Scientific Publications.

HALLMAN N. & RAPOLA J. (1978) Congenital nephrotic syndrome. In *Pediatric Kidney Disease* (ed. Edelmann C.M.), pp. 711–8. Boston: Little, Brown.

HOLLIDAY M.A. (1978) Growth retardation in children with kidney disease. In *Pediatric Kidney Disease* (ed. Edelmann C.M.), pp. 331–41. Boston: Little, Brown.

HOLT E. (1960) *Protein and Amino Acid Requirements in Early Life*. New York: University Press.

HUGHES C., DUTTON S. & TRUSWELL A.S. (1981) High intakes of ascorbic acid and urinary oxalate. *J. hum. Nutr.* **35**, 274–80.

JAMES J. (1976) *Renal Disease in Childhood*, 3rd Edition. St Louis: C.V. Mosby.

LAWSON D.E.M., FRASER D.R., KODICEK E., MORRIS H.R. & WILLIAMS D.H. (1971) Identification of 1,25 dihydroxycholecalciferol, a new kidney hormone controlling calcium balance. *Nature* (Lond.) **230**, 228–30.

MOWAT A.P. (1979) Fulminant liver failure. In *Liver Disorders in Childhood* (ed. Mowat A.P.), pp. 126–37. London: Butterworth.

MOWAT A.P. (1982) Hepatic disorders. In *Clinics in Gastroenterology* (ed. Harries J.T.), pp. 171–205. Philadelphia: W.B. Saunders.

MUNRO H.N. (1970) Free amino acid pools and their role in regulation. In *Mammalian Protein Metabolism* (ed. Munro H.N.), Vol. IV, p. 299. London: Academic Press.

PARSONS V. (1974) Renal aspects of intensive care. *Brit. J. Hosp. Med.* **11**, 843.

PSACHAROUPOULOS H.T., MOWAT A.P., DAVIES M., PORTMANN B., SILK D.B.A. & WILLIAMS R. (1980) Fulminant hepatic failure in childhood. An analysis of 31 cases. *Arch. Dis. Childh.* **55**, 252–8.

RODRIGUEZ-SORIANO J., VALLO A., CASTILLO G. & OLIVEROS R. (1981) Renal handling of water and sodium in infancy and childhood: a study using clearance methods during hypotonic saline diuresis. *Kidney Int.* **20**, 700–4.

SCHNEIDER J.A., SCHULMAN J.D. & SEEGMILLER J.E. (1978) Cystinosis and the Fanconi syndrome. In *Metabolic Basis of Inherited Disease*, 4th Edition (eds. Stanbury J.B., Wyngaarden J.B. & Fredrickson D.S.), pp. 1660–82. New York: McGraw-Hill.

SIMMONS J.M., WILSON C.J., POTTER D.E. & HOLLIDAY M.A. (1971) Relation of calorie deficiency to growth failure in children on haemodialysis and the growth response to calorie supplementation. *New Engl. J. Med* **285**, 653.

SMITH I. & FRANCIS D.E.M. (1982) Disorders of amino acid metabolism. In *Textbook of Paediatric Nutrition*, 2nd Edition (eds. McLaren D.S. & Burman D.), pp. 295–323. Edinburgh: Churchill Livingstone.

TREY C. (1970) The critically ill child: acute hepatic failure. *Pediatrics* **45**, 93.

UNDERWOOD E.J. (1977) Trace elements. In *Human and Animal Nutrition*, 4th Edition. New York: Academic Press.

WEST C.D. & SMITH W.C. (1956) An attempt to elucidate the cause of growth retardation in renal disease. *Amer. J. Dis. Child.* **91**, 460.

CHAPTER 9

Phenylketonuria

Phenylketonuria is a group of recessively inherited metabolic disorders in which the conversion of phenylalanine to tyrosine is impaired. The most severe form of the condition, often termed 'classical' phenylketonuria, was first described by Fölling (1934). In all forms of the condition both parents are heterozygote carriers, and the risk of other children being affected is one in four. The incidence varies in Caucasian populations, usually being between 1 in 12 000 and 1 in 30 000 newborns, but it is more common in Ireland (1 in 4000) and rarer in Finland (1 in 50 000).

Biochemistry

Phenylketonuria (PKU) is characterized by accumulation of phenylalalnine in the blood and tissues (upper limit of normal, 240 μmol/l*) and an excessive production of phenylketones. In 'classical' phenylketonuria hepatic phenylalanine hydroxylase activity is very low or absent (Bartholomé *et al.* 1979), and blood phenylalanine levels on a normal diet usually exceed 1200 μmol/l and tyrosine levels are low or normal (Fig. 9.1). In the majority of untreated patients developmental progress is retarded, although as many as 1 in 6 patients escape severe intellectual impairment and have an IQ above 70 (Smith & Wolff 1974). Comprehensive reviews of the clinical and biochemical features are available in *The Metabolic Basis of Inherited Disease* (Stanbury *et al.* 1983), and in *Amino Acid Metabolism and its Disorders* (Scriver & Rosenberg 1973). The cause of the mental subnormality in 'classical' phenylketonuria is far from understood. There is incomplete myelination of the central nervous system (Clayton 1971). Work with experimental animals has shown that high phenylalanine levels early in life can produce changes in the brain's composition (Agrawal *et al.* 1969, Chase & O'Brien 1970) and the metabolism of other amino

acids may be inhibited by high phenylalanine levels and the abnormal metabolites (Davidson 1973).

'Atypical' forms of the disease, in which the enzyme block is less complete than in the 'classical' condition, occur in approximately 1 in 6 cases in the south-east of England, and in certain populations (for example Ashkenazi Jews in Israel) greatly outnumber the classical cases (Smith & Francis 1982). Siblings usually have a similar biochemical abnormality. Blood phenylalanine levels are usually less than 1200 μmol/l, although a high dietary protein intake or an acute catabolic episode may raise levels above this figure. Phenylketones are detectable with the standard methods of testing (ferric chloride, paper chromotagraphy) only when the blood phenylalanine exceeds 600 to 900 μmol/l. In general, patients with 'atypical' PKU have a higher tolerance of dietary phenylalanine, managing 2 to 3 times the quantity of natural protein tolerated by those with the 'classical' form when phenylalanine levels are in a safe range. It is generally agreed that the mildest forms of PKU with blood levels consistently below 600μmol/l do not need treatment, although the natural history of 'atypical' forms is not well documented. Some untreated patients are reported to have some mental retardation (Smith & Wolff 1974, Berry *et al.* 1979).

Some 1 to 2% of patients with PKU have a defect of pterin metabolism rather than phenylalanine hydroxylase deficiency (Smith *et al.* 1975a, Hase *et al.* 1982) and this requires very different management (Danks *et al.* 1978, Smith 1985, Smith *et al.* 1985). Three hydroxylases (phenylalanine, tyrosine and tryptophan hydroxylases) require a specific cofactor, biopterin, in its 'active' tetrahydro form (Fig. 9.2), as the donor hydrogen ions. Tetrahydrobiopterin (BH₄) is converted to dihydrobiopterin (BH₂) during the hydroxylation, and must be recycled by the action of dihydrobiopterin reductase (Fig. 9.3). If BH₄ is deficient, production of dihydroxyphenylalanine (dopa) and 5-hydroxytryptophan, which are the precursors of the neurotransmitters dopamine, noradrenaline, adrenaline and serotonin, cannot be synthesized in normal

---

* 60 μmol/l = approximately 1 mg/100 ml blood phenylalanine.

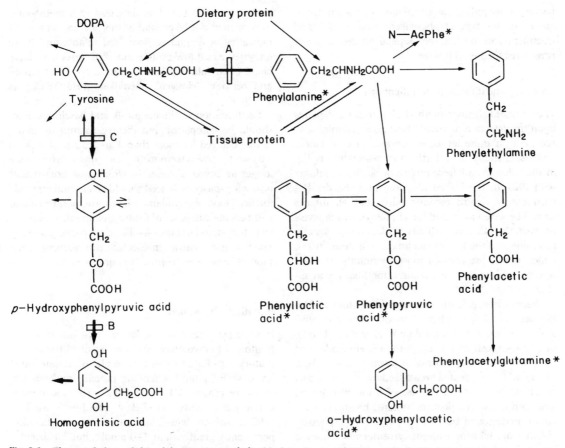

Fig. 9.1 The metabolism of phenylalanine. A, metabolic block in classical PKU; B, metabolic block in tyrosinosis; (C) + B, metabolic block in neonatal hypertyrosinosis; ➝ main degradative pathway; *excreted in classical PKU.

Fig. 9.2 Biopterin in the dihydro- (BH₂) and tetrahydro-(BH₄) forms. From Smith *et al.* (1975a) with permission.

7,8 –Dihydrobiopterin (BH₂)   *3,4,7,8 –Tetrahydrobiopterin (BH₄)*

non-tetrahydrobiopterin species. These patients require supplements of folinic acid (5-formyl tetrahydrofolate) (Smith 1985, Smith *et al.* 1985). Experience is still limited however, and longer follow-up is

amounts. Because of the neurotransmitter deficiency patients with disorders of biopterin metabolism develop a characteristic progressive neurological illness which is unresponsive to dietary phenylalanine restriction alone (Smith *et al.* 1975a, Niederweisser *et al.* 1979, Smith 1985, Smith *et al.* 1985). Therapy is with a combination of tetrahydrobiopterin, 5-hydroxytryptophan, L-dopa and carbidopa, which is effective in controlling both the symptoms and the phenylalanine accumulation. In patients with the dihydrobiopterin reductase problem there appears to be an interference with folate metabolism by accumulating

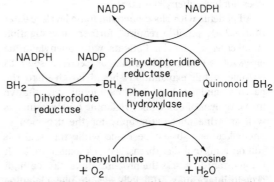

Fig. 9.3 Hydroxylation of phenylalanine to tyrosine and role of biopterin (after Kaufman). BH₂, dihydrobiopterin; BH₄, tetrahydrobiopterin. From Smith *et al.* (1975a) with permission.

necessary to judge the effectiveness of such treatment. As this type of phenylketonuria is rare and treatment does not entirely depend on diet it is not considered further in this text.

Screening and diagnostic investigations

The most satisfactory method of screening depends upon the detection of raised blood phenylalanine levels. Phenylalanine levels are normal in cord blood, and rise steadily after birth, and especially on the introduction of milk feeds (breast or bottle), in infants with PKU. In the United Kingdom in 1968 the Department of Health recommended that all infants should be tested for raised blood phenylalanine levels between the 6th and 14th day of life, and specifically recommended the Guthrie technique (Guthrie 1961), which is still the method most commonly used for screening, although other suitable methods are available.

The experience of the screening laboratory at The Hospital for Sick Children, London, between 1969 and 1978 has been described by Walker *et al.* (1981). One change seen as a result of the recommendations given in *Present Day Practice in Infant Feeding* (DHSS 1974), which advocated breast-feeding or, where this could not be achieved, the use of a modified infant feed with a reduced protein content, has been a reduced incidence of transient neonatal hyperphenylalaninaemia with or without tyrosinaemia amongst infants being tested for raised phenylalanine levels.

New siblings of known patients with phenylketonuria should, ideally, be breast-fed, or given a whey-based modified milk, until this diagnosis has been excluded. In the event of an initial normal phenylalanine level in a sibling, one repeat test is recommended about two weeks later to confirm the child does not have phenylketonuria.

All patients with blood phenylalanine levels greater than 240 μmol/l require further investigation (Walker *et al.* 1981). Patients with phenylalanine levels of $\geqslant 600\,\mu$mol/l should be seen as soon as possible, a full explanation should be given to the parents, and at least one additional quantitative measurement of blood phenylalanine and tyrosine, as well as urine chromatography for the detection of phenylketones, should be made while the infant is still on a normal diet (breast-fed or modified milk). It is important to assess the protein intake, since a high protein intake may artificially elevate phenylalanine levels.

It is becoming usual to test all infants with a raised blood phenylalanine on the screening test for the presence of the pteridine defects. Urine metabolites may or may not be present at this age and so are not indicative of diagnosis. Breast-fed infants and those on whey-based low-protein modified milks may have blood phenylalanine levels lower than 1200 μmol/l and yet have 'classical' phenylketonuria (Walker *et al.* 1981).

Confirmation of the diagnosis and baseline studies should be completed, but dietary treatment should not be delayed for more than 1 to 2 days, at least in 'classical' phenylketonuria. Diagnosis may take longer in 'atypical' cases, in which case breast feeds or a whey-based milk feed should be continued, while further blood phenylalanine levels are monitored and will become the basis of future treatment. Prolonged elevated phenylalanine blood levels especially in early infancy may cause intellectual impairment even though subsequent control is maintained.

Initiation of treatment

It is our practice to initiate low-phenylalanine dietary treatment immediately after the result of the confirmatory tests for all patients with phenylalanine blood levels $\geqslant 900\,\mu$mol/l when the protein intake is not excessive (Smith & Francis 1982). This recommendation agrees with that of Berry and her co-workers (1979). Infants with blood levels of phenylalanine persistently greater than 240 μmol/l, but consistently below 900 μmol/l, should be monitored closely, by a paediatrician with expertise in phenylketonuria (Walker *et al.* 1981), even if dietary treatment is not given, at least until the child is established on a full toddler diet. Mildly elevated blood phenylalanine levels seen in patients with variant forms of phenylketonuria receiving human milk or whey-based modified formulae may increase sharply if a higher protein and phenylalanine intake occurs subsequently, e.g. when weaning solids are introduced. Particularly where phenylalanine levels are $\geqslant 600\,\mu$mol/l, advice concerning the avoidance of excess dietary protein should be given, but adequate protein and energy, usually from conventional foods, are essential for the maintenance of normal growth. Continued breast-feeding or prolonged use of a whey-based modified infant formula, the avoidance of cow's milk and 'follow-on' milks, especially in bottle-fed infants, and careful introduction of appropriate weaning solids for age should be advised. Such an approach is likely to prevent any possible effects of the hyperphenylalaninaemia on intellectual function (Smith & Francis 1982).

Assessment of 'atypical' forms of the disorder

It is not always possible to differentiate between 'classical' and 'atypical' phenylketonuria in the neonatal period, and it is important to keep under review the need for continued dietary treatment. Exceptionally 'good' control or persistently low phenylalanine levels may suggest the presence of an 'atypical' defect. The tolerance to phenylalanine once the patient is well established on dietary treatment is also a good guide to the chemical severity of the disease. Once the phase of rapid growth during the first 6 to 9 months of life is over, patients with 'classical' phenylketonuria rarely tolerate more than 400 mg dietary phenylalanine per day when blood phenylalanine levels are controlled between 180 and 480 μmol/l. It is customary to challenge patients who have an above-average phenylalanine tolerance with an increase in natural protein intake sometime during the latter part of the first year of life.

A protocol for a high-protein, three-day challenge was described by Blaskovics *et al.* (1974). At The Hospital for Sick Children, London, a milk load which avoids very high phenylalanine levels is normally given, as follows, as an out-patient at approximately one year of age.

Cow's milk (90 ml) or evaporated milk (30 ml) per day is divided and given with the three main meals to provide an extra 450 mg phenylalanine in each 24 hours. The child's normal dietary regimen is continued unchanged. Blood phenylalanine levels are taken 3 to 4 hours after meals, before the start of the test, at 48 hours, and at one week. (It is essential the child is well at the time of the test, as intercurrent infections and energy deficit can cause a rapid rise in phenylalanine levels, making interpretation of the test impossible.) When the blood phenylalanine levels rise above 1200 μmol/l the test is terminated and the child resumes his normal low-phenylalanine diet. The test rarely raises the blood phenylalanine level above 1500 μmol/l, and causes little disturbance to feeding. The mother must fully understand the aim of the test and be able to measure the diet accurately, and arrangements for blood collection must be made appropriately. Approximately one quarter of all cases have phenylalanine levels over 1200 μmol/l at 48 hours, and three-quarters at the end of one week (Francis & Smith 1982), in which case a low-phenylalanine diet must be continued. In patients in whom phenylalanine levels remain below 1200 μmol/l the test is continued with gradual increases of milk and natural protein (and a decreased dose of the low-phenylalanine protein substitute) until either a normal protein intake (2 g protein per kg per day at one year) is reached with levels still below 1200 μmol/l (and a diagnosis of 'atypical' phenylketonuria is made), or levels rise to $\geqslant$ 1200 μmol/l, when the test is terminated. Patients with levels persistently below 600 μmol/l are placed on a 'free' diet. Patients with levels between 600 and 1200 μmol/l are continued on a diet which will maintain blood phenylalanine levels below 600 μmol/l. Follow-up is essential, even in patients in whom the diet has been stopped, and the possible implications of maternal hyperphenylalaninaemia should be discussed with the parents.

Principles of dietary treatment

Treatment of phenylketonuria is by a controlled low-phenylalanine diet, started as early in life as possible. The phenylalanine intake is lowered to a safe level, monitored by regular estimation of blood phenylalanine concentration. The diet must be nutritionally adequate in all respects. The recommended intake of nutrients is similar to that of other infants and children, except for phenylalanine and tyrosine. Because of the severe restriction of conventional foods, supplements of amino acids (other than phenylalanine), protein-free energy, all vitamins, and macro and trace minerals are necessary to ensure the adequacy of the diet. These may be given together in the low-phenylalanine protein substitute or as separate modules.

PHENYLALANINE AND PROTEIN REQUIREMENT

Phenylalanine comprises 4 to 6% of all dietary protein and is an essential amino acid which must not be completely removed from the diet for more than short periods, as without it the patient cannot grow or indeed survive (Irwin & Hegsted 1971). Dietary restriction of natural protein to the degree needed to control blood phenylalanine levels within a safe range (between 180 and 480 μmol/l) requires between 1/3 and 1/10 of the normal protein and phenylalanine intake, and therefore necessitates the use of a low-phenylalanine protein substitute (*see* below and Tables 9.5 and 9.6) to ensure that protein requirements for growth are supplied, adequate amounts of tyrosine (an essential amino acid in patients with phenylketonuria) are given and the imbalance of amino acids corrected (Berry *et al.* 1971, Kindt *et al.* 1983). The effect of high tissue levels of phenylalanine on amino acid transport in bowel, kidney and brain (Davidson 1973) can, in theory, be counteracted by the administration of amino acids.

This, together with the synthetic nature of the protein substitutes and their theoretically low biological value, leads most units to prescribe a generous total protein intake along with adequate energy (Table 9.1), vitamins and minerals to ensure optimal growth. In order to achieve smooth control of blood phenylalanine and other amino acid levels it is important that both the daily phenylalanine allowance and the low-phenylalanine protein substitute be divided as equally as is practical over the day, and a proportion is given at each feed or main meal, at least in young children. The low-phenylalanine protein substitute cannot be utilized for growth in the absence of phenylalanine, and once phenylalanine levels have been controlled it is dangerous to give it without a regular supply of phenylalanine, since this can readily precipitate a state of phenylalanine deficiency. Holt and Snyderman (1967) suggested that children with phenylketonuria require the same essential minimum quantity of phenylalanine for growth and tissue repair as normal children of the same age. Adequate amounts of all other nutrients necessary for growth must be provided.

The theoretical requirements of phenylalanine for groups of children at different ages, adapted from the findings of Holt and Synderman (1967) and the recommendations of Berry *et al.* (1971), are given in Table 9.1. The requirement for phenylalanine varies from child to child and from time to time in the same child due to the natural fluctuations in growth rate. Catabolism for whatever cause (energy deficit, protein deficit, infection) temporarily reduces growth rate, and phenylalanine tolerance declines, leading to a rise in blood phenylalanine concentration; during subsequent catch-up growth phenylalanine tolerance increases. An insufficient phenylalanine intake, especially in an infant, results in growth failure, and a rash develops and other symptoms of protein deficiency occur (*see* Table 9.20). Death from chronic phenylalanine deficiency has been reported (Rousse 1966).

Table 9.1 Guide to requirements in the dietary management of 'classical' phenylketonuria per kg actual body weight per day.

Age in years	Energy	Supplement of amino acids or protein equivalent from hydrolysate* (g)	Total protein and amino acids* (g)	Theoretical initial intake of phenylalanine from natural protein†‡ (mg)
0 to 1	420 to 550 kJ (100 to 130 kcal)	3	3 to maximum 4	50 to 60
1 to 2	380 to 420 kJ (90 to 100 kcal)	2 to 3	2·5 to 3·5	30 to 40
2 to 4	330 to 420 kJ (80 to 100 kcal)	2	2 to 3	25 to 40
4 to 6	330 to 420 kJ (80 to 100 kcal)	2§	2 to 3	25
6 to 8	290 to 380 kJ (70 to 90 kcal)	1 to 2§	2 to 2·5	15 to 25
8 to 14	230 to 310 kJ (55 to 75 kcal)	§	1 to 1·5	As tolerance
Over 14	190 kJ (45 kcal)	§	1	As tolerance
Pre-conception and pregnancy		§	Minimum 1 (⩾ 50 g/day)	As tolerance, increasing with the demands of the fetus in the second half of pregnancy

* Low-phenylalanine protein substitutes vary in composition. *See* Table 9.5.
† 1 g natural protein contains approximately 50 mg phenylalanine.
‡ This suggested intake of phenylalanine must be adjusted according to the results of initially very frequent then regular blood phenylalanine estimations (*see* p. 237). Infants usually tolerate 70 to 90 mg/kg per day in the first month of life and during rapid growth periods may tolerate up to 110 mg/kg per day.
§ As appropriate according to natural protein intake to provide recommended total protein plus amino acids intake.

SOURCES OF PHENYLALANINE

Various tables give the amino acid content of conventional foods. The most helpful are *McCance and Widdowson—The Composition of Food* (Paul & Southgate 1978) and its supplement (Paul *et al.* 1980). When the phenylalanine analysis is not available, as in the case of most manufactured products, 1 g protein is assumed to contain 50 mg phenylalanine. The estimated phenylalanine content of food will vary according to the method of calculation and accuracy of the original protein and/or phenylalanine analyses and the protein content of the sample examined. This is well illustrated by the varying phenylalanine content of human milk (*see* Table 9.13) as recorded by different workers.

A system of 50 mg phenylalanine exchanges has

Table 9.2 Quantity of food supplying 50 mg phenylalanine (exchanges). Food should be weighed after cooking unless otherwise stated.

Gold Cap SMA (reconstituted) (J. Wyeth Laboratories)	60 ml
Milk	30 ml
Single cream	40 ml
Double cream	60 ml
Potatoes	
Mashed and milk-free	75 g
Boiled	75 g
Roast	40 g
Chips	30 g
Canned, new (drained contents)	100 g
Jacket weighed without skin	45 g
Jacket weighed with skin	55 g
Crisps (Smiths) plain or salt & vinegar	15 g
Peas—fresh or frozen only	20 g
Sweetcorn kernels	25 g
Sweetcorn kernels, canned	35 g
Brussel sprouts—fresh or frozen	50 g
Broccoli tops—fresh or frozen	45 g
Cornflakes	15 g
Frosties	20 g
Rice Krispies	15 g
Sugar Puffs/Smacks	15 g
Weetabix/Weetflakes	10 g
Shredded Wheat	10 g
Ready Brek (Lyons)	7·5 g
Oatmeal (raw)	7·5 g
Porridge, cooked with water	65 g
Rice (raw), white or brown	15 g
Rice (boiled), white or brown	45 g
Farley's Rusk (Farley) one rusk (original or low-sugar)	≃15 g
Farex Weaning Food (Farley)	10 g
Baked Beans in Tomato Sauce (Heinz)	20 g
Cream of Tomato Soup (Heinz)	110 g

been found to be a practical approach to dietary management for the majority of parents of children with phenylketonuria. A list of basic foods and the quantity required to provide 50 mg phenylalanine is given in Table 9.2. Figures for the weight of foods are rounded off to the nearest 5 g, 7·5 g, 10 g, 15 g, etc. It is recognized that the smaller the weight of food measured the greater the percentage error in the phenylalanine content. Supplementary lists of appropriate manufactured products are available, but because of frequent changes in their content they need continual revision and are not suitable for publication in a book.

The foods with a higher phenylalanine content (Table 9.3) are not permitted for patients with 'classical' phenylketonuria in the younger age group. Older patients on a more generous phenylalanine intake, and younger ones with 'atypical' phenylketonuria can usually incorporate some of these foods in their diet. The 1 g and 6 g protein exchange lists given for low-protein diets, Table 8.4, p. 205, can be adapted, and contain approximately 50 mg and 300 mg phenylalanine respectively. Aspartame (Canderel and Nutrasweet), the artificial sweetener which contains phenylalanine and aspartic acid, should *never* be used by patients with phenylketonuria. It is also widely used to sweeten low-calorie drinks and other low-sugar foods such as desserts and yoghurt.

The analysis of fruit and many vegetables has shown them to have a very low protein content, and

Table 9.3 High-phenylalanine foods. Usually not permitted in the diet of patients with 'classical' phenylketonuria.

Meat, all types: lamb, beef, pork, mutton, ham, bacon, poultry, chicken, game, sausages, pies, luncheon meats.
Fish, all varieties: fresh, frozen, smoked, shellfish
Textured vegetable proteins and meat extenders
Cheese
Eggs
Bread*, biscuits*, cakes*, flour* and wheat products
Soya and other pulses. Bran.
Nuts, spinach, pod beans e.g. red kidney beans, butter beans etc.
Yeast and meat extracts: Bovril, Oxo, Marmite, Yeastril, Barmene
Gravy mixes and powders: Bisto, gravy granules
Chocolate beverages, chocolate vermicelli
Ordinary table jellies and gelatine
Marzipan, royal icing; sweets, fudge, toffee containing gelatine, whey sugar, etc.
Peanut butter, lemon curd made with egg
Aspartame and artificial sweeteners and foods containing it, e.g. Canderel, Nutrasweet

* Low-protein alternatives are available.

Table 9.4 Fruit and vegetables permitted in low-phenylalanine diets.

(a) Fruit and vegetables which can be taken freely, as a normal helping will not exceed 50 mg phenylalanine.
Fresh, frozen, raw, cooked provided sugar or salt only are added, canned in syrup or salt brine.

Fruit	Apple	Melon and watermelon	Angelica
	Apricots (not dried)	Medlars	Glacé cherries
	Bilberries	Mulberries	Ginger
	Blackberries	Nectarines	
	Cherries	Olives	
	Cranberries	Oranges	
	Currants, black and red and dried	Passionfruit	
	Damsons	Paw paw	
	Figs, fresh (not dried)	Peaches (not dried)	
	Fruit-pie filling	Pears	
	Fruit salad	Pineapple	
	Gooseberries	Plums	
	Grapes	Pomegranate	
	Grapefruit	Quince	
	Greengages	Raisins	
	Guavas	Raspberries	
	Lemons	Rhubarb	
	Loganberries	Strawberries	
	Lychees	Sultanas	
	Mandarins	Tangerines	
	Mangoes	Mixed peel	
Vegetables	Artichoke, globe and Jerusalem	Marrow	
	Aubergine	Mushrooms	
	Beans, French and green beans (avoid seeds)	Mustard and cress	
	Cabbage	Onion and pickled onions	
	Carrots	Parsley	
	Cauliflower	Parsnip	
	Celeriac	Peppers, green and red	
	Celery	Pumpkin	
	Chicory	Radish	
	Cucumber	Spring greens	
	Endive	Swede	
	Gherkin	Tomato	
	Lady's fingers	Turnip	
	Leek	Watercress	
	Lettuce		

(b) Fruit and vegetables which if taken in large quantities add a significant amount of phenylalanine to the day's intake. They should be restricted to one serve per day of any one item. These foods may be used freely in small quantities such as in vegetable stews, sauces, and fruit salad.

Fruit	Banana, e.g. $\frac{1}{2}$ per day in babies;	Figs, dried
	1 per day in children	Peaches, dried
	Apricots, dried	Prunes, dried or stewed
	Dates	Fruit mince
Vegetables	Asparagus	Plantain
	Beans, runner	Salsify
	Beansprouts	Seakale
	Beetroot	

less phenylalanine than expected, and therefore for many years The Hospital for Sick Children, London, has permitted those listed in Table 9.4 to be used in the diet without measurement. Satisfactory biochemical control is achieved by monitoring blood phenylalanine levels and adjusting the number of 50 mg phenylalanine exchanges in the diet. A dietary assessment of total phenylalanine intake, including the contribution from fruit and vegetables, can be made from time to time.

LOW-PHENYLALANINE PROTEIN SUBSTITUTES

A variety of products (Table 9.5) are available. They differ not only in their protein source and content, but also in the presence or absence of carbohydrate, fat, minerals and vitamins. They are based either on hydrolysed proteins from which phenylalanine is removed or on a mixture of synthetic amino acids free of phenylalanine; Table 9.6 compares their amino acid profile. None of the amino acid-based products contains taurine which is now considered important (Geggal *et al.* 1985), and many are not optimal compared to reference protein and human milk profiles. Several new products are currently being evaluated and others reformulated.

The acid-hydrolysed protein products (e.g. Minafen) contain some D-amino acids (approximately 2 to 3%), which causes some degree of hyperaminoaciduria (Clayton *et al.* 1970). Enzyme hydrolysates (e.g. Lofenalac) do not contain D-amino acids, but more phenylalanine remains bound to the protein.

Some low-phenylalanine protein substitutes such as Lofenalac and Minafen are almost complete foods containing carbohydrate, fat, minerals and, in the case of Lofenalac, relatively large amounts of phenyl-

Table 9.5 Low-phenylalanine protein substitutes. Composition per 100 g.

	Protein (g) equivalent (N × 6·25)	Phenylalanine (mg)	Energy kcal	Energy kJ	Carbohydrate (g)	Fat (g)
(a) Hydrolysed protein-based preparations						
Infants						
Lofenalac (Mead Johnson)*	15	80	460	1930	59·6	18
Minafen (Cow & Gate)†‡	12·5	≤20	509	2130	47·9	31
Older children						
Albumaid XP (Scientific Hospital Supplies)†§	33·8	<10	324	1350	50	Nil
Albumaid XP Concentrate (Scientific Hospital Supplies)†§‖	73·4	<25	291	1222	Nil	Nil
(b) Amino acid-based preparations	Amino acid (g)					
Aminogran Food Supplement *plus* Aminogran Minerals (Allen & Hanburys)†§	100	Nil	400	1675	Nil	Nil
PK Aid 1 *plus* Metabolic Mineral Mixture (Scientific Hospital Supplies)†§‖	100	Nil	400	1675	Nil	Nil
Maxamaid XP (Scientific Hospital Supplies)*§‖	30	Nil	335	1500	62	Nil
Milupa PKU 1§¶	50	Nil	272	1138	17·6	Nil
Milupa PKU 2§‖¶	67	Nil	295	1234	7·1	Nil

* Minerals, trace elements and vitamins included.
† Comprehensive range of vitamins, e.g. three Ketovite Tablets plus 5 ml Ketovite Liquid, daily is recommended.
‡ Formula under review.
§ Essential fatty acids must be supplied.
‖ Not recommended for infants.
¶ Contain only some vitamins and minerals and must be supplemented together with essential fatty acids and additional energy.

The dose of the protein substitute required depends on age and nutritional needs. In young children and infants it should always be given with each meal together with a proportion of the daily phenylalanine intake to ensure best utilization for growth.

Some low-phenylalanine protein substitutes are available on prescription as borderline substances for treatment of patients with phenylketonuria.

Table 9.6 Amino acid comparison of low-phenylalanine protein substitutes, g per 100 g product.

| | Amino acid-based preparations | | | | | Hydrolysed protein-based preparations | | |
	Aminogran* (Allen & Hanburys)	PK Aid 1* (SHS)	Maxamaid XP† (SHS)	Milupa PKU 1†	Milupa PKU 2†	Lofenalac‡ (Mead Johnson)	Minafen§ (Cow & Gate)	Albumaid XP‖ (SHS)
L-Phenylalanine	Nil	Nil	Nil	Nil	Nil	0·08	<0·02	<0·01
L-Alanine	2·4	8·0	1·08	2·4	3·1	0·64	N/S	2·1
L-Arginine	4·2¶	6·0	2·33	2·0	2·7	0·34	0·45	1·7
L-Aspartic acid	6·1	14·0	1·95	5·7	7·6	1·34	N/S	4·2
L-Cystine	1·5	5·0	0·75	1·4	1·8	0·025	N/S	1·7
L-Glutamic acid	12·2	16·0	2·53	12·0	16·0	3·78	N/S	4·8
Glycine	6·1	8·0	1·86	1·4	1·8	0·35	N/S	1·6
L-Histidine	3·4**	3·0	1·34	1·4	1·8	0·26	0·26	1·0
L-Isoleucine	8·5	3·0	1·79	3·4	4·5	0·75	1·12	2·0
L-Leucine	10·0	5·0	3·06	5·7	7·6	1·41	1·36	3·4
L-Lysine	6·6¶	9·5**	2·34	4·0	5·4	1·57	1·67	3·3
L-Methionine	3·0	2·0	0·5	1·4	1·8	0·45	0·21	1·0
L-Proline	4·3	2·5	2·16	5·4	7·1	1·15	N/S	1·9
L-Serine	8·4	2·5	1·33	3·0	4·0	1·02	N/S	2·6
L-Taurine	Nil	Nil	Nil	N/S	N/S	N/S	N/S	N/S
L-Threonine	5·7	4·0	1·5	2·7	3·6	0·77	0·88	2·6
L-Tryptophan	1·5	1·5	0·6	1·0	1·4	0·19	0·21	0·4
L-Tyrosine	6·4	6·0	2·7	3·4	4·5	0·81	0·81	3·2
L-Valine	7·0	4·0	1·95	4·0	5·4	1·2	0·96	2·5
L-Glutamine	—	—	0·23	—	—	—		
Total amino acids	97·2	100·0	30·00	60·3	80·1	16·14	12·5	40·0
Protein equivalent			50		67	15	12·5	33·8

* A mixture of L-amino acids. Vitamins, minerals and essential fatty acids and energy must be supplied separately.
† A mixture of L-amino acids plus some carbohydrate, vitamins and minerals. Fat-free.
‡ Specially processed enzymatic casein hydrolysate plus amino acids, carbohydrate, fat, vitamins and minerals.
§ Specially processed enzymatic casein plus tyrosine, tryptophan, carbohydrate, fat, minerals and some vitamins. Formula under review 1986.
‖ Bovine serum acid hydrolysate plus amino acids, carbohydrate, fat, minerals and some vitamins. Fat-free.
¶ As glutamate.
** As HCl.
N/S Not specified.

alanine together with vitamins. This type of product is ideal for bottle-fed infants and they are nutritionally 'safe' providing sufficient quantity is consumed. They can be used as the basis of a relatively simple dietary regime for any age group. It can be difficult or even impossible, however, to get the older child to take an adequate amount and diets based on these products can contain little natural food or variety.

Lofenalac and Minafen have many practical advantages for the mother, especially in the initial period after diagnosis. Only two foods need to be given (milk plus Lofenalac or Minafen) and they are made up similarly to other infant feeds using:

One level unpacked scoop of Lofenalac powder to each 2 oz (55 ml) water, i.e. approximately a 15% solution.

or

One level slightly packed scoop of Minafen powder to each 1 oz (30 ml) water, i.e. approximately a 15% solution.

For older children they can be mixed to a drink or given as a paste, and if necessary can be supplemented with PK Aid 1 or Aminogran Food Supplement to boost the protein content (*see below*)

Albumaid XP is an hydrolysate of beef serum with a higher protein, lower energy content. As it is fat-free, essential fatty acids, ideally from vegetable fats, together with additional carbohydrate, vitamins and a source of phenylalanine, must be provided. This necessitates the use of multi-ingredients when it is used as an infant feed (Table 9.12) which is less practical for the mother at a time when she is coming to terms with the child's diagnosis. It is more suited to the needs of the older infant or child who is on a range of solids. Albumaid XP concentrate has an even higher protein, lower energy content, which is more suited to older children. Both products have been widely and successfully used by some units.

The amino acid-based preparations, Aminogran and PK Aid 1, contain no added carbohydrate or fat and have a much smaller bulk. They are particularly useful for the older child (Bentovim *et al.* 1970) since, except in the young infant, they can be given in a small volume as a 'medicine' so that feeding difficulties are fewer and easier to manage. In addition, since they are phenylalanine-free and low in energy, a wide range of measured and low-protein foods can be given, which makes the diet appear more like that of the rest of the family. Minerals and vitamins must be added separately and it is essential to ensure that

essential fatty acids and adequate energy are provided from protein-free sources.

The appropriate dose of Aminogran Food Supplements or PK Aid 1 is calculated for weight and age (Table 9.2), taking into account the contribution from natural protein and phenylalanine intake. The prescribed dose is measured to the nearest half-scoop, using the scoop supplied by the manufacturer. Eight gram of Aminogran or Metabolic Mineral Mixture is added and the amino acids plus minerals are flavoured and mixed with water. A third of the resultant mixture is given within 20 to 30 minutes of each of the three main meals, or half is given twice daily to the school-age and older child. Vitamins are supplied as three Ketovite tablets plus 5 ml Ketovite Liquid.

Some of the amino acids and minerals are insoluble in water, and the most acceptable way to mix the amino acids and minerals is to add flavouring and sufficient water to make a thick 'paste' with the consistency of custard. Alternatively, a 'creamier' mixture can be made by mixing with one of the permitted non-dairy creams or oil emulsions, Calogen (SHS) or Prosparol (Duncan Flockhart). The quantity of fat should not exceed that of the carbohydrate in any meal. The resultant mixture can be given neat, diluted with water, heated and/or flavoured with synthetic fruit flavours, or added to fruit juices or carbonated beverages. The latter is the most popular as it causes the mixture to effervesce profusely as the mixture is added, and if taken in this form leaves no bitter taste and the slight grittiness of the mixture is not noticed. Adequate fluid must be offered to satisfy thirst if Aminogran or PK Aid 1 is given as a 'paste'. These mixtures should always be given with praise and reward, as should any of the low-phenylalanine protein substitute mixtures.

Aminogran, as the supplementary protein, has been used from the start of treatment as a modular feed in infants with phenylketonuria (Smith *et al.* 1975b). Satisfactory growth and biochemical parameters, including control of phenylalanine, was achieved. The practical difficulties of preparing and calculating the modular feed, however, for both the mother and dietitian, especially during the bottle-feeding phase of treatment, were a definite disadvantage compared with the ease of regimens based on Minafen or Lofenalac. During weaning, and particularly once a three meal per day diet has been achieved, Aminogran (Food Supplement and Minerals) has many advantages and is usually the author's regimen of preference, unless there are practical reasons for keeping to a simplified regimen.

Maxamaid XP, another amino acid preparation

with added carbohydrate, vitamins and minerals, has
recently become available. It has a larger bulk and
energy content than Aminogran or PK Aid 1 and
contains no fat, but has the advantage of a better
amino acid profile and a good flavouring. Preliminary
observations (Sardharwalla 1982, personal communication) suggest it is more palatable than other products and is mostly accepted well. It may relieve dietary difficulties in some cases where the taste of other
products has become a problem. Dietary difficulties
are often related to parental anxiety, depression or
peer group pressures, rather than the taste of the
products used in treatment.

Milupa PKU 1 and 2 have also recently become
available in the U.K. These products are comparable
with Albumaid XP and Albumaid XP concentrate in
their nutritional role in the diet. They rely extensively
on natural food intake to provide phenylalanine, supplementary essential fatty acids, vitamins, minerals
and energy, are no less unpalatable than other products and do not therefore appear to have advantages
over the range of products already available in the
U.K.

Both hydrolysate and amino acid types of product
have been used with success and allow for normal
growth and good biochemical control. It is necessary
to understand their individual nutritional role in the
diet if they are to be used safely. All products have
unusual tastes.

Energy
Adequate dietary energy must be available for
growth needs. A guide to energy needs for different
age groups is given in Table 9.2, but the child's appetite is the best guide to the individual's need provided free access to suitable foods is permitted, the
child is clinically well and there are no emotionally
determined disturbances of food intake.

Minafen and Lofenalac, as 15% solutions, provide,
respectively, 320 and 290 kJ (75 and 70 kcal) per
100 ml. When fed to appetite after the prescribed
phenylalanine given as milk or formula they will provide adequate energy, minerals and protein for
growth needs of the infant so long as the child is well
and feeding normally.

Mixtures of amino acids, Aminogran and PK Aid 1,
provide little energy in the dose required for
protein needs. Albumaid XP, Maxamaid XP and Milupa PKU 1 and 2 contain some energy but no fat.
Patients treated with these products require a source
of the essential fatty acid $C_{18:2}$ and suitable additional
energy sources. These are partly provided by the
measured conventional foods which supply the

Table 9.7 Foods containing negligible phenylalanine.

Water
Sugar: white, brown, icing, castor, glucose
Jam, honey, marmalade, golden syrup, treacle
Hard-boiled sweets, rock, candy, sherbet, barley sugar,
    candy floss
Soda water, mineral water, Coca Cola*, Lucozade,
    lemonade*, Pepsi*, and similar carbonated beverages*
Black tea, instant tea, lemon tea, black coffee, instant
    coffee and coffee powders
Fruit cordial*, squash*
Food essences and colourings, e.g. vanilla, cochineal,
    peppermint, almond essence
Cornflour
Custard powder (not instant custards)
Blancmange powder—vanilla and fruit-flavoured (not
    blancmange mix)
Sago, tapioca (not ready-to-serve milk puddings)
Baking powder, bicarbonate of soda, cream of tartar
Vegetarian jellies without gelatine, agar agar
Solid vegetable oils, lard, Trex, Cookeen
Oil—cooking, salad, vegetable edible oils, Crisp & Dry
Salt, pepper, herbs, spices, monosodium glutamate, curry
    powder, mustard, vinegar
Butter—all brands
Margarine—all brands except with buttermilk

* Those containing aspartame, Canderel or Nutrasweet are
  contraindicated.

natural protein and phenylalanine intake (50 mg
phenylalanine exchanges, Table 9.2), such as milk,
cereals, potatoes, chips and crisps, and by the low-
protein foods which contain negligible phenylalanine,
such as some vegetables, many fruits (Table 9.4) and
fruit drinks, cornflour, sago, tapioca, sugar, jam,
honey, butter, margarine, vegetable oils and some
sweets and candy such as barley sugar (Table 9.7).
A range of proprietary low-protein flours, breads, biscuits, pasta, glucose polymers and fat emulsions
(Table 9.8) are available and can be prescribed at
NHS expense in the U.K. for patients with phenylketonuria. Patients need careful instruction about the
preparation and use of these foods. Some basic recipes
are given at the end of this chapter. Additional recipes and lists of manufacturers' products used in
family meals and by peer groups as popular treats are
available to dietitians from The National Society for
Phenylketonuria and Allied Disorders Limited, but
need continual revision, at least annually.

Energy deficiency leads to increased gluconeogenesis, and breakdown of body protein leads to impaired growth, loss of biochemical control and hungry, bad-tempered children: when old enough they
demand or pilfer food in order to satisfy their appe-

Table 9.8 Proprietary low-protein foods of negligible phenylalanine content.

Product	Manufacturer or U.K. distributor
Biscuits	
Aminex	Cow & Gate
Aproten Low-Protein Biscuits	Ultrapharm (Carlo Erba) Ltd
Aproten Crispbread	Ultrapharm (Carlo Erba) Ltd
Aglutella Gentili Azeta Cream-Filled Wafers (vanilla flavour)	GF Dietary Supplies Ltd
dp Low-Protein Chocolate Flavoured Chip Cookies (and Butterscotch)	GF Dietary Supplies Ltd
Rite-Diet Low-Protein Sweet Biscuits	Welfare Foods Ltd
Rite-Diet Low-Protein Cream-Filled Wafers (vanilla and chocolate flavoured)	Welfare Foods Ltd
Rite-Diet Low-Protein Chocolate Cream-Filled Biscuits	Welfare Foods Ltd
Rite-Diet Low-Protein Gluten-Free Crackers	Welfare Foods Ltd
Pasta	
Aglutella Gentili Low-Protein Pasta	GF Dietary Supplies Ltd
Spaghetti	
Spaghetti rings	
Macaroni	
Semolina	
Aproten Pasta	Ultrapharm (Carlo Erba) Ltd
Small rings (anellini)	
Macaroni (rigatini)	
Flat noodles (tagliatelle)	
Small macaroni (ditalini)	
Rite-Diet Low-Protein Pasta	Welfare Foods Ltd
Macaroni	
Spaghetti—short-cut	
Spaghetti rings	
Bread, flour and mixes	
Rite-Diet Gluten-Free Low-Protein Bread	Welfare Foods Ltd
with or without salt (canned) (Low-Protein Soya Bran Bread is not suitable for most PKUs)	
Rite-Diet Low-Protein Flour Mix	Welfare Foods Ltd
Rite-Diet Low-Protein Pre-baked Loaf	Welfare Foods Ltd
Juvela Low-Protein Mix	GF Dietary Supplies
Juvela Low-Protein Prebaked Bread Loaf	GF Dietary Supplies
Aproten Flour	Ultrapharm (Carlo Erba) Ltd
Tritamyl Low-Protein PK Flour	Procea branch of Odlum Group
Glucose polymers	
Caloreen	Roussel
Calonutrin	Geistlich
Maxijul and Maxijul LE	Scientific Hospital Supplies
Fat emulsions	
Calogen (Liquigen if MCT is indicated)	Scientific Hospital Supplies
Prosparol	Duncan Flockhart
Non-dairy (imitation) cream (check ingredients)	Various brands
Miscellaneous	
Ener-G Egg Replacer	GF Dietary Supplies Ltd
Edifas Fibrous Methyl Ethyl Cellulose	ICI
Edifas Fibrous Methyl Ethyl Cellulose	Bow Produce Ltd

tites. This is a common cause of undernutrition, behaviour problems and premature lapse of diet. The toddler and child's meals should always conclude with low-protein foods with which the child can satisfy his appetite, and two or three snacks should be offered each day which contain a variety of low-protein foods, e.g. fruit, fruit juice and low-protein biscuits, or 'milk-shake' made from non-dairy cream, milk-shake flavouring and water. Infants should be demand-fed. In the low phenylalanine breast-feeding regimen the child can breast-feed on demand (p. 239). Lofenalac or Minafen used during the bottle-feeding and the weaning phase of treatment can be fed to appetite.

Food energy in excess of the individual child's need can cause food refusal or overweight. An exact prescription based on theoretical requirement of protein, phenylalanine and energy which is expected to be totally consumed every feed, or even every day, does not take into account individual requirements and the natural fluctuations of appetite and intake. For example, 100 ml of a 15% solution of Lofenalac plus 30 ml cow's milk per kg per day may be adequate energy and phenylalanine for normal growth in an individual infant, but this is slightly low compared to the theoretical requirements. To encourage additional Lofenalac may cause feeding problems, maternal anxiety and further rejection of feeds. Older children usually refuse the least desirable part of the diet which is usually the low-phenylalanine protein substitute.

A strict low-energy 'reduction' diet for secondary obesity in patients with phenylketonuria is not normally appropriate, as it can cause loss of biochemical control. A moderate reduction in energy intake, e.g. aspartame-free low-energy (low-calorie) drinks instead of sweetened varieties, to reduce weight gain with careful biochemical monitoring may be necessary in some instances.

Vitamins

Some of the low-phenylalanine protein substitutes contain an adequate range of vitamins (e.g. Lofenalac, Maxamaid XP), and provided an adequate quantity of the product is taken supplements are not necessary. However, most do not contain vitamins; others contain only an incomplete range of vitamins, in which case it is recommended that supplements are taken of the comprehensive range of all known vitamins, e.g. Ketovite Tablets, three per day, plus Ketovite Liquid, 5 ml per day. Severe vitamin deficiencies will occur in patients on synthetic diets (*see* Francis 1986) unless adequate vitamin supplemen-

tation is given (Royston & Parry 1962, Mann *et al.* 1965); however, an excess intake, particularly of vitamins A and D, should also be avoided. An intake of $\geqslant 100$ g Lofenalac or $\geqslant 70$ g Maxamaid XP per day does not necessitate separate vitamin supplements, and > 200 g Lofenalac or $\geqslant 150$ g Maxamaid XP is not advised because of their high content of vitamins A and D as well as some minerals.

The child receiving a more generous natural protein diet may not always obtain a sufficient intake of some vitamins; B_{12} is difficult to obtain on a restricted intake of meat and other first-class proteins. Folic acid and possibly vitamin K can be inadequate when vegetables are disliked and milk intake limited. Appropriate supplements should be prescribed in accordance with the potential and actual intake.

Minerals

The essential requirement of macrominerals, calcium, magnesium, phosphorus, potassium, sodium and trace minerals must be provided for optimal growth. Recommended dietary allowances (iron and zinc) and estimated safe and adequate intakes of other trace minerals (copper, manganese, chromium, selenium and molybdenum) have recently been suggested by Aggett and Davies (1983). These trace minerals, together with iodine, nickel and cobalt, are essential, though the need for cobalt may be met by vitamin B_{12}.

The macro and some trace minerals are present as an integral part of the low-phenylalanine protein substitutes Lofenalac, Minafen, Albumaid XP, Maxamaid XP and Milupa PKU 1 and 2. Others require separately prescribed minerals; Aminogran Mineral Mixture is intended to be used in conjunction with Aminogran Food Supplement and Metabolic Mineral Mixture with PK Aid 1. These comprehensive mineral mixtures are given as a standard dose of 8 g per day for children over 5·5 kg weight. Natural protein-containing foods, fruit, vegetables and other low-protein foods incorporated into the diet can contribute significantly to the mineral content of the total diet. Children on a more generous natural protein intake may only require a reduced dose, or an alternative mineral supplement may be more appropriate.

Metabolic balance studies by Alexander *et al.* (1974) showed that the original formulations of Aminogran and of Metabolic Mineral Mixtures were inadequate in certain respects. Subsequently a reformulation of Aminogran Mineral Mixture was tested by Lawson *et al.* (1977) and appeared to be an adequate supplement to the prescribed diet for the minerals tested, i.e. calcium, cobalt, copper, iron, magnesium, manganese, molybdenum, phosphorus, potassium, sodium and zinc. The other trace minerals were not extensively investigated.

At the time of writing none of the low-phenylalanine protein substitutes discussed contains selenium, chromium or nickel, though some mineral mixtures now contain selenium and chromium, together with other trace minerals with or without macrominerals (Francis 1986). Serum selenium concentrations in dietetically treated patients with phenylketonuria and maple syrup urine disease have been shown to be much lower than those of healthy children of the same age group (Lombeck *et al.* 1978, 1984). These workers have now made recommendations for selenium intakes in these patients as they found that within 8 to 12 weeks selenium levels decreased from normal to very low levels under diet therapy, despite the fact that the patients were in a good clinical state and thriving. Further investigation is needed to determine the significance of these findings and to establish the appropriate supplement of this and other trace minerals in patients with phenylketonuria.

Practical management

The prescribed phenylalanine allowance should be divided between the infant's feeds, and in the older child between the main meals, in a practical manner, to the nearest 5 ml of milk in infants or half or one 50 mg phenylalanine exchange once the child has been weaned. Normally at least three 50 mg phenylalanine exchanges per day are prescribed for the child over one year of age; one 50 mg exchange is given with each main meal, together with a proportion of the low-phenylalanine protein substitute.

The range of foods which are suitable for any one patient will vary, but as great a variety as practical is an advantage in order to give a wide range of additional amino acids, vitamins and minerals from natural sources. In infants, the phenylalanine is provided by breast-feeding, milk or a modified whey-based infant formula. The older child will delight in a range of snack foods which are used in family meals and by peer groups. Some parents can only cope with one or two simple set menus, while others can manage a choice of numerous food items from which to select meals. There are advantages in introducing additional variety, according to age, bearing in mind the child's phenylalanine tolerance and the parents' ability to manage the previously given information. It boosts the older child's morale when he is permitted new foods, particularly when it makes his diet more similar to family meals and that of his peers.

Regular monitoring of blood phenylalanine levels is undertaken to ensure that phenylalanine restriction is adequate and to avoid phenylalanine deficiency. A fall in plasma phenylalanine level to below normal is the first indication of amino acid deficiency, the dangers of which have led most clinics to aim at phenylalanine levels a little above the normal range (Rouse 1966, Sutherland *et al.* 1966). Application of micro-methods for amino acid analysis, allowing specimens to be collected by heel- or finger-prick thus avoiding repeated venepunctures, enables specimens to be sent by post for analysis. Many parents can be taught to collect blood specimens, which greatly reduces the inconvenience for patients, parents and the hospital, and this has become an essential part of routine at The Hospital for Sick Children, London. Receipt of the specimen by the laboratory must be followed by a rapid result and early communication of any dietary manipulation and/or reassurance to the parents: otherwise measurements become meaningless. There is little justification in continuing an expensive, potentially dangerous diet if biochemical control is unimportant (Smith & Francis 1982).

Practice with regard to the frequency of blood tests varies in different units. In the author's clinic, after diagnosis and initial stabilization, the blood specimen is collected on Guthrie cards. A non-fasting specimen, $3\frac{1}{2}$ to 4 hours after a feed or main meal, is taken at the following intervals:

Weekly in infants during the first months of life.
Every two weeks after the infant is weaned, during the toddler age and after dietary changes.
Three- to four-weekly in the pre-school age child.
Four-weekly thereafter while the child is on strict diet aimed at controlling blood phenylalanine levels between 180 and 480 μmol/l.

The blood test is repeated in 1 to 2 weeks if control is inadequate and following infections or pilfering.

Once the older child is established on a relaxed diet allowing blood phenylalanine levels between 900 and 1200 μmol/l blood specimens are taken every two or three months, provided control is satisfactory.

A variety of methods are available for measuring phenylalanine levels. In the author's clinic the blood spots from the Guthrie cards are analysed either by a semi-quantitative phenylalanine assay on whole-blood spots adapted from the method described by

Guthrie and Susi (1963) or by using thin-layer chromatography after elution of the blood spot (Walker *et al.* 1981). The latter is used when the patient (or the mother, if the child is breast-feeding) is on antibiotics which interfere with the bacterial inhibition assay of the Guthrie method. From time to time a full plasma amino acid profile is useful in assessing the protein and tyrosine status of the patient and hence the adequacy of the low-phenylalanine protein substitute prescription and its intake.

Blood phenylalanine levels must be interpreted in the light of clinical findings. After initial stabilization, providing the patient is well and eating his full prescribed diet, no dietary indiscretion has been noted, and investigation of any relevant cause(s) has been undertaken, the diet is adjusted according to blood phenylalanine levels (Table 9.9).

The commonest cause of a low phenylalanine level is underprescription of phenylalanine, often due to a rise in requirements associated with increased growth

Table 9.9   Blood phenylalanine monitoring in young children. Adjustment of daily dietary phenylalanine according to blood phenylalanine levels (after initial stabilization) in children under eight years to maintain blood phenylalanine between 180 and 480 μmol/l*.

(a)   Phenylalanine levels of $\leqslant 60 \mu$mol/l require an additional 50 to 150 mg dietary phenylalanine per day, irrespective of cause, and a repeat blood phenylalanine estimation is recommended in one week to ensure adequate diet adjustment has been made.

(b)   Phenylalanine levels of $\leqslant 180 \mu$mol/l require an increase in the dietary phenylalanine content by 50 mg phenylalanine per day. A repeat blood phenylalanine estimation is recommended in 1 to 2 weeks.

(c)   Phenylalanine levels of 180 to 480 μmol/l require no dietary change in phenylalanine prescription. Subsequent blood phenylalanine estimation appropriate for age in 1 to 4 weeks is recommended.

*(d)   Phenylalanine levels of 540 to 900 μmol/l indicate 25 mg dietary phenylalanine per day should be omitted from the diet. A repeat blood phenylalanine estimation is recommended in 1 to 2 weeks.

*(e)   Phenylalanine levels of 900 to 1200 μmol/l or more, omit 50 mg dietary phenylalanine per day. A repeat blood phenylalanine estimation is indicated in 1 to 2 weeks.

Never omit all phenylalanine and usually do not decrease to less than three 50 mg phenylalanine exchanges a day plus low-protein fruit and vegetables permitted to appetite.

* The patient should be well, eating his full prescribed diet and no dietary indiscretion noted. 60 μmol/l phenylalanine = 1 mg/100 ml.

rate following an infection or period of energy deficit. Inadequate consumption of phenylalanine due to food refusal or misunderstandings, or vomiting or other illness, especially if supplements of the low-phenylalanine protein substitute are continued, may also cause low phenylalanine blood levels. In the breast-fed infant, inadequate maternal lactation, for example as a result of insufficient suckling by the infant, may also be the cause of low levels and a slow growth rate.

If the dietary phenylalanine intake needed to maintain phenylalanine blood levels in the selected range regularly exceeds the expected requirements, 'atypical' phenylketonuria should be suspected and reassessment should be undertaken.

If phenylalanine blood levels are low, or if deficiency is suspected (skin rash, weight loss or low phenylalanine intake), and delay due to post and/or distance is inevitable, immediate action should be taken to increase the dietary phenylalanine without waiting for confirmation. The phenylalanine deficiency rash is commonly seen on buttocks and face and is hard to distinguish from other nappy rash and *Candida* infection (thrush). A temporary increase in dietary phenylalanine prescription allows healing and does no harm, even if the rash is due to other causes. An increase of 50 to 100 mg phenylalanine (30 to 60 ml cow's milk) per day is usually adequate in mild deficiency; one or two whole feeds of normal cow's milk formula may be indicated in severe deficiency.

High blood phenylalanine levels are most commonly due to:

1   Catabolism due to infections, poor food intake and undernutrition (inadequate total protein and/or energy).
2   Dietary indiscretion and food pilfering.
3   Overprescription, especially as growth diminishes and phenylalanine tolerance decreases after early infancy and after a period of catch-up growth.

Temporary high levels, for example due to an intercurrent infection (*see* p. 247), do no clinical harm, and normally no dietary phenylalanine adjustment is indicated, although a high energy and fluid intake helps to limit catabolism and therefore reduces phenylalanine accumulation. Pilfering is commonly due to hunger, and attention to the supply of acceptable low-protein energy foods, which the child is encouraged to eat to appetite, is often helpful in restoring phenylalanine blood levels to an acceptable range. Parental anxiety and peer group pressure for the child can be the underlying cause of pilfering and should be dealt with appropriately and not normally by reprimand (*see* p. 250).

(*see* p. 250)

DIETARY MANAGEMENT IN INFANCY

(a) Breast-feeding combined with Lofenalac, Minafen or similar low-phenylalanine protein substitutes
The incidence of breast-feeding has increased in the U.K. In 1980 some 67% of mothers were breast-feeding their infants, so that a number of infants with phenylketonuria are now being breast-fed at the time of diagnosis. Human milk is lower in phenylalanine per unit of nitrogen than cow's milk and provides less protein for the proportion of other nutrients including energy. Whey-based modified milks most closely resemble the amino acid profile of human milk.

During exclusive demand breast-feeding the quantity of milk produced is largely dependent on the stimulation of successful suckling. Complement feeds lead to less stimulation of the breast and therefore less milk production. In infants with phenylketonuria who are given a measured volume of Lofenalac or Minafen before feeds suppression of lactation in proportion to Lofenalac or Minafen volume occurs, thus lowering the intake of human milk, and therefore the protein and phenylalanine intake, and subsequently the infant's blood phenylalanine level (Francis & Smith 1981). Minafen and Lofenalac have been selected as the most practical low-phenylalanine protein substitutes to combine with breast-feeding because of their appropriate protein, low phenylalanine and high energy content. Other low-phenylalanine protein substitute products can be made up to a similar protein energy density (*see* Table 9.12) and could be used just as effectively to suppress lactation.

At the start of dietary treatment in a breast-fed infant human milk is withdrawn for a period of 48 to 72 hours if the phenylalanine blood level is $\geqslant 1200$ $\mu mol/l$ (*see* Table 9.10). The mother expresses milk at least five times per 24 hours to maintain lactation during the period when the infant is not breast-fed, and she should be reassured that the baby will be able to suckle again once the blood phenylalanine level has fallen. Lofenalac or Minafen is demand-fed, offering approximately 540 kJ (120 kcal) per kg per day during these 2 to 3 days while the initial blood phenylalanine level falls. Thereafter, prescribed quantities of Lofenalac or Minafen are given five times per day, according to the blood phenylalanine level, before demand breast-feeds (Tables 9.10 and 9.11). Blood phenylalanine levels are monitored three times per week until they have stabilized, and thereafter weekly.

Breast-feeds are permitted *ad libitum* and no attempt is made to measure or limit breast-milk intake directly. If the blood phenylalanine level is low a reduction of Lofenalac or Minafen intake is prescribed and the mother is advised that the baby will be more hungry and will probably suckle more often. Likewise if the phenylalanine level is higher than the recommended range the Lofenalac or Minafen prescription is increased; breast fullness may occur but the mother should not express. Water and fruit juice, and even a dummy, are discouraged unless the child is unwell, as they will reduce suckling by the infant and lactation performance of the mother.

Clinical progress is monitored by phenylalanine levels and weight gain, just as with a bottle-fed infant. If the infant or mother is unwell the family doctor should be contacted for advice in the normal

Table 9.10 Initial breast-feeding regimen for infants with phenylketonuria (adapted from Francis & Smith 1981).

Initial blood phenylalanine ($\mu mol/l$)	Lofenalac or Minafen (15% solution)*	Breast-feeds
>2000	(a) 150 to 200 ml per kg wt per day fed on demand *then* (b) 60 ml × 5 feeds	Nil for 3 days† On demand, 5 + times per day
1200 to 2000	(a) 150 to 200 ml per kg wt per day fed on demand *then* (b) 45 ml × 5 feeds	Nil for 2 days† On demand, 5 + times per day
<1200	30 ml × 5 feeds	On demand, 5 + times per day
< 900	‡	On demand, 5 + times per day

* Alternative low-phenylalanine protein substitutes with similar protein energy density (Table 9.12) can be used.
† Mother expresses to maintain lactation.
‡ As appropriate on clinical judgement.

Table 9.11   Blood phenylalanine monitoring with breast-feeding and Lofenalac or Minafen* (adapted from Francis & Smith 1981).

Blood phenylalanine (μmol/l)	Lofenalac or Minafen volume per day compared to previous intake	Breast-feeds
>480	+75 ml (+15 ml × 5 feeds)	On demand: babe will be expected to demand fewer feeds
<180	−75 ml (−15 ml × 5 feeds)	On demand: babe will be expected to demand more feeds
180 to 480	No change	On demand

The prescribed Lofenalac or Minafen is altered according to blood phenylalanine results provided the infant is gaining weight satisfactorily and is not unwell.

* Alternative low-phenylalanine protein substitutes with similar protein energy density (Table 9.12) can be used.

way. The diet is offered to appetite, continuing breast-feeds, if possible, on demand. The specialist PKU clinic should be contacted if the baby refuses the prescribed Lofenalac or Minafen feed for more than a day or two.

Solids can be started in the breast-fed infant with phenylketonuria at the usual time, from 3 to 6 months. Initially one 50 mg phenylalanine exchange of cereal (10 g Farex Weaning Food or one Farley's Rusk, *see* Table 9.2) is introduced, mixed with boiled water; this is given at the beginning of a feed before the Lofenalac or Minafen and breast-feeds. Fruit and low-protein vegetable puṙees (*see* Table 9.4) are introduced next, but in a limited quantity until a wider range of solid measured foods are incorporated into the diet. The higher energy low-protein solids are not given until breast-feeds no longer provide a major part of the diet. Measured 50 mg phenylalanine exchange solid foods are gradually introduced at a third and fourth feed as appropriate, and Lofenalac or Minafen is given at only four, and then three, feeds per day, while breast-feeds are continued on demand. The selected measured foods should have an appropriate energy:protein density (165 to 210 kJ, 40 to 50 kcal:1 g protein) in order to suppress breast-milk intake appropriately.

At approximately six months of age additional protein is required and is usually given as Aminogran (Food Supplement and Minerals) which is started as a well-flavoured 'paste' given as a medicine. Initially one teaspoon per day is given from a spoon before one feed, mixed in the proportion of:

5 g Aminogran Food Supplement (1 scoop) *plus*
1·3 g Aminogran Minerals ($\frac{1}{2}$ scoop)
flavoured with a concentrated fruit juice or fruit flavouring and mixed with water to a paste of custard consistency.

The infant is encouraged, praised but never forced

with the Aminogran mixture. The quantity is not increased until it is accepted willingly. It is then gradually increased to one teaspoon three times per day, then eventually, but not before the infant is at least 5·5 kg in weight, to the full dose of 3 g Aminogran Food Supplement per kg weight per day, plus 8 g Aminogran Minerals (three scoops) per day. Breast-feeds and Lofenalac or Minafen feeds are proportionally reduced and finally omitted. Thereafter the range of solids is increased appropriately for age and phenylalanine tolerance, according to blood level control.

Breast-feeding can continue as long as mother and baby desire, providing growth and biochemical control is satisfactory. If breast-feeding is discontinued before the infant is fully weaned, it is possible to transfer to a bottle-feeding regimen by initially prescribing 50 mg phenylalanine as milk or formula (Table 9.13) in place of each full breast-feed normally given, i.e. three to a maximum of five × 30 ml cow's milk per 24 hours. This is given before each of a similar number of demand Lofenalac or Minafen feeds, and the previous weaning solids are continued for 2 to 3 weeks, while the prescribed milk is adjusted according to blood phenylalanine levels taken once or twice weekly, and the diet adjusted according to Table 9.9. Occasional suckling at the breast is permitted for comfort.

Infants manage the combined breast and bottle-feeding regimen well. Control of phenylalanine blood levels is good, and the cost of treatment is considerably less than the traditional bottle-feeding regimens. The author's experience so far suggests that bonding between mother and child is made secure as a result of their breast-feeding experience (Francis & Smith 1981). The problems encountered in normal breast-feeding occur just as frequently in infants with phenylketonuria, and lactation failure leading to poor weight gain and low phenylalanine levels can occur.

(b) Bottle-feeding using milk and Lofenalac, Minafen or similar low-phenylalanine protein substitute

At the start of treatment Lofenalac, Minafen or an alternative low-phenylalanine protein substitute, adapted to meet infant nutritional requirements (Table 9.12), is given alone for three to a maximum of five days if phenylalanine levels are $\geqslant 1200$ μmol/l, provided that daily phenylalanine levels are obtainable. If blood phenylalanine levels cannot be obtained daily, or the biochemical service is delayed, milk is given, as suggested below, from the beginning of treatment.

Homogenized, TB-tested, pasteurized, fresh milk is generally used as the source of phenylalanine because it is easy to measure and convenient. It is not normally boiled, as boiling denatures and partially precipitates the protein, which results in a less constant source of phenylalanine. Diluted evaporated milk (unsweetened) has occasionally been used when a reliable source of cow's milk is not available.

An alternative approach, which in the light of modern trends in infant feeding has many advantages, especially for the pre-term or small-for-date infant, is to use a whey-based modified milk as the source of phenylalanine (Table 9.13) during the neonatal period. More of the nutrient intake is pro-vided from natural sources with this approach, and the nutrient content of these milks, e.g. a higher cystine and essential fatty acid content, may be advantageous. The total protein intake of such a regimen may be a little lower than the guide to requirement suggests, but will be similar to that provided for normal infants on modified feeds. The tyrosine which is an essential amino acid in phenylketonuria may become the limiting amino acid, but the intake will depend on the choice of low-phenylalanine protein substitute and its tyrosine content.

Cow's milk is prescribed and measured in 5 ml increments using a medicine glass. The whey-based modified milk must be correctly reconstituted and prescribed, either to the nearest 5 ml, as for cow's milk, or to the nearest level scoop for the daily prescription, using the scoop provided with the product. The daily milk intake is divided between the feeds and given separately before the Lofenalac or Minafen. These can be given on demand, with an additional night feed if necessary. The total volume of feeds should not normally exceed 150 to 200 ml/kg per day or 1000 to 1200 ml maximum total per day. Calculated examples of two different feed regimens are given in Table 9.14. The mother should be instructed regarding the dietary prescription and practical de-

Table 9.12 Alternative low-phenylalanine protein substitute feeds for infants.

	Carbohydrate (g)	Amino acid or protein (g)	Fat (g)	Energy kcal	Energy kJ	Phenylalanine (mg)
(a) 100 ml 15% solution Lofenalac	8·9	2·3	2·7	69	290	12
(b) 100 ml 15% solution Minafen*	7·2	1·9	4·7	76	320	3
(c) Aminogran Feed*						
2 g Aminogran Food Supplement	Nil	2	Nil	8	32	Nil
7 g sugar or glucose polymer	7	Nil	Nil	28	112	Nil
8 ml Prosparol (Duncan Flockhart) or Calogen (SHS)	Nil	Nil	4	36	148	Nil
†Aminogran Mineral Mixture						
Water to 100 ml						
Total 100 ml	7	2	4	72	292	Nil
(d) Albumaid XP Feed*						
6 g Albumaid XP	3	2	Nil	22	88	0·6
4 g sugar	4	Nil	Nil	16	64	Nil
8 ml Calogen (SHS) or Prosparol (Duncan Flockhart)	Nil	Nil	4	36	148	Nil
Water to 100 ml						
Total 100 ml	7	2	4	74	300	0·6

*These regimes require supplements of vitamins as three Ketovite Tablets plus 5 ml Ketovite Liquid.

† 1·5 g Aminogran Mineral Mixture/kg per day up to a full dose of 8 g daily.

Table 9.13 Phenylalanine content of different milks, 100 ml reconstituted.

	Phenylalanine (mg)	Tyrosine (mg)	Protein (g)
Human milk	48*		
	64†		
First 5 days colostrum	70‖	N/S	2·3
Post 15 days mature	46‡	36	N/S
Post 15 days mature	40‖	46 to 52	1·1
6 to 10 days transitional	71‡	56	2·0
	62‖	N/S	1·6
Cow's milk	180‡	150	3·3
	180‖	N/S	3·1
Channel Island milk	190‡	160	3·6
Evaporated unsweetened milk	460‡	380	8·6
Double cream	82‡	67	1·5
Aptamil (Milupa)	65§	52	1·5
Premium (Cow & Gate)	65§	62	1·5
SMA Gold Cap (Wyeth Laboratories)	80§	81	1·5
Osterfeed (Farley)	62§	N/S	1·45
Pregestimil (Mead Johnson) (hydrolysed casein)	87§	48	1·9
Prosobee (Mead Johnson) Soya	97§	75	2·0
Cow & Gate S Formula Soya	90§	67	1·8
Wysoy (Wyeth Laboratories) Soya	110§	82	2·1

* DHSS (1977).

† Macy and Kelly in Kon and Cowie (1961).

‡ Amino acid composition/100 g food (Paul *et al.* 1980).

§ Calculated from manufacturers' data. Other products may be equally suitable.

‖ Geigy Scientific Tables Vol. I (1981). *Units of measurement, body fluids, Composition of the body.*

N/S Not specified.

tails of the feed preparation. The diet is adjusted during stabilization according to frequent (three per week) blood phenylalanine estimations as follows:

Until the blood phenylalanine level falls to ≤480 μmol/l the selected feeding regimen is continued, providing the infant is taking the feed adequately, is well and is gaining weight.

A blood phenylalanine ≤480 μmol/l indicates the dietary phenylalanine should be increased to 70 to 75 mg per kg actual body weight per day. A subsequent blood phenylalanine of ≤180 μmol/l indicates an increase of dietary phenylalanine to 90 to 100 mg phenylalanine per kg actual body weight per day.

Thereafter the diet is monitored by regular (weekly) blood phenylalanine estimations, as suggested in Table 9.9, adjusting the diet by increments *per day* and not on a weight basis.

A comprehensive range of vitamins (three Ketovite Tablets plus 5 ml Ketovite Liquid) is always required in conjunction with Minafen, but only if less than 100 g Lofenalac is taken per day.

Weaning solids are started at the normal age, from about 3 to 4 months in the bottle-fed infant. The low-protein foods containing negligible phenylalanine selected from Tables 9.4, 9.7 and 9.8 are given after the bottle-feeds and fed to appetite, e.g. fruit purées, or Aminex or Aproten biscuits crushed and mixed with boiled water as a smooth cereal, and later suitable vegetable purées, are offered. The 50 mg phenylalanine exchange foods (Table 9.2), which are given before the bottle feeds, are gradually introduced in place of part or all of the prescribed milk at three feeds, e.g. one Farley's Rusk or 10 g Farex Weaning Food mixed with boiled water equals 50 mg phenylalanine. Gradually the range and quantity of weaning solids is increased. A guide regarding a realistic intake of solids for the child's age and the type of feeding regimen should be given to parents.

At about eight months of age, finger foods should be introduced, initially as foods containing negligible phenylalanine, such as Aminex, pieces of fruit, low-protein bread plus butter/margarine and Aproten biscuits (Table 9.8). The range of phenylalanine exchanges should also be increased appropriately, e.g.

Table 9.14 Examples of low-phenylalanine feeds for a 4 kg infant based on Lofenalac and different milks.

	Protein (g)	Energy kcal	Energy kJ	Phenylalanine (mg)
A (i) 100 ml cow's milk, 20 ml each at 5 feeds. Given before each Lofenalac feed. Replace if rejected or vomited.	3·3	65	272	180
(ii) 75 g Lofenalac (≃8 scoops) } 15% solution Boiled water, 500 ml / Lofenalac Offer 100 ml at 5 feeds Give after cow's milk on demand*	11·5	345	1450	60
Total	14·8	411	1725	240
This provides (per kg per day)	3·7	103	431	60
Theoretical requirement (per kg per day)	3 to 4	100 to 130	420 to 550	Initially 50 to 60 then as tolerated
or:				
B (i) 10 scoops Premium } 60 ml each at 5 feeds 300 ml water / Given before each Lofenalac feed Replace if rejected or vomited	4·5	204	852	195
(ii) 45 g Lofenalac (≃5 scoops) } 15% solution Boiled water, 300 ml / Lofenalac Offer 60 ml at 5 feeds Give after Premium feeds on demand*	6·9	207	870	36
Total	11·4	411	1722	231
This provides (per kg per day)	2·9	103	431	58
Comparison with theoretical guide to requirement (per kg per day)	3 to 4	100 to 130	420 to 550	Initially 50 to 60 then as tolerated

*Lofenalac can be given on demand. Fruit juice feed or 5% dextrose can be given in addition in small quantities.

potatoes, chips, and the child encouraged to help feed himself and to drink from a cup.

Tolerance of phenylalanine can be expected to decrease after the initial growth spurt of early infancy.

(c) Combined Lofenalac or Minafen plus Aminogran regimen for infants and toddlers
As the child takes more solids, bottle-feeds will decrease and the protein intake will fall unless a more concentrated source of protein is introduced. A mixture of L-amino acids and minerals such as Aminogran, given as a 'paste' or a drink, can be introduced. Initially just one teaspoon of such a 'paste' (p.240) is given before one, then each of the three, main feeds, with praise, reward and a drink or bottle-feed to follow, similar to the recommendations for breast-fed

infants. A calculated example of such a regimen is given in Table 9.15 and a sample menu in Table 9.16.

Alternatively or simultaneously in the infant who is gaining excessive weight for height, or in whom feeds have reduced in number, e.g. to four daily, the protein intake can be maintained by gradually adding small quantities of Aminogran Food Supplement (no minerals initially) into the Lofenalac or Minafen feeds. As the quantity of Lofenalac or Minafen decreases the appropriate dose of Aminogran Mineral Mixture, and Ketovite Tablets and Liquid should be introduced (taking into account any contribution from the Aminogran 'paste') to ensure adequate intake of calcium, iron, trace minerals and vitamins, for example:

Table 9.15 Calculated example of a Lofenalac plus Aminogran weaning regimen suitable for an 8 kg infant of about eight months.

	Protein plus amino acid (g)	Energy kcal	Energy kJ	Phenylalanine (mg)
Daily				
(i) 100 g Lofenalac ($\simeq$10 scoops)	15·0	460	1930	80
600 ml (20 oz) water divided into 4 feeds				
(ii) 2 scoops 10 g Aminogran Food Supplement	10·0	40	160	Nil
1 scoop 2·7 g Mineral Mixture (Allen & Hanburys)	Nil	Nil	Nil	Nil
Flavouring, e.g. blackcurrant juice.	Trace	20	80	Trace
Water to mix to a 'paste'				
Give 1 teaspoon before each main meal				
(iii) 3 Ketovite Tablets plus 5 ml Ketovite Liquid				
(iv) Solids including 50 mg phenylalanine exchanges				
First feed Aminogran 'paste'				
30 ml milk	1·0	20	80	50
1 Farley's Rusk = 1 × 50 mg phenylalanine	1·0	50	200	50
exchange				
Lofenalac feed				
1 Aminex biscuit to chew	Trace	50	200	Trace
Second feed Aminogran 'paste'				
35 g boiled potato = $\frac{1}{2}$ × 50 mg phenylalanine	0·5	25	100	25
exchange)				
Purée vegetable	Trace	10	40	Trace
45 ml milk or custard = $1\frac{1}{2}$ × 50 mg	1·5	50	200	75
phenylalanine exchange)				
Lofenalac feed				
'Snack' Fruit juice	Trace	20	80	Trace
1 Aproten biscuit to chew	Trace	25	100	Trace
Third feed Aminogran 'paste'				
60 g chips = 2 × 50 mg phenylalanine	2·0	100	400	100
exchanges				
Tomato	Trace	10	40	Trace
Lofenalac feed				
Fruit purée or $\frac{1}{2}$ banana	Trace	50	200	Trace
Fourth Feed 60 ml milk	2·0	40	160	100
Lofenalac feed				
Total	33·0	870	3970	480
Provides (per kg per day)	4·1	109	496	60
Comparison with guide to requirements (per kg per day)	3 to 4	100 to 130	420 to 550	According to tolerance

Table 9.16 Sample weaning diet menu for an infant with phenylketonuria. Suitable for a 6- to 10-month-old child. The order of foods offered is important and will be different in the breast-fed and bottle-fed infant.

First feed	Aminogran paste from a spoon as instructed
	... g cereal, e.g. Farley's Rusk and/or milk in measured quantity to supply phenylalanine allowance
	Lofenalac with or without Aminogran feed
	Low-protein bread (toast) and butter (and/or honey or jam) to chew as a finger food
Second feed	Aminogran paste from a spoon as instructed
	... g potato and/or milk in measured quantity to supply phenylalanine allowance
	Lofenalac with or without Aminogran feed
	Vegetable (purée or mashed)
Snack time	Aminex or Aproten biscuit, or piece of apple, to chew as a finger food
	Fruit juice
Third feed	Aminogran paste from a spoon as instructed
	Milk in measured quantity or measured cereal to supply phenylalanine allowance
	Lofenalac with or without Aminogran feed
	Fruit purée, mashed or small pieces and/or Quick Jel and/or no-protein custard
Fourth feed (*bedtime*)	Milk in measured quantity
	Lofenalac with or without Aminogran feed

No minerals are required when ⩾ 100 g Lofenalac or Minafen is taken per day.

2·7 g (1 scoop) of Aminogran Mineral Mixture is needed when 80 to 100 g Lofenalac or Minafen is taken per day.

5·4 g (2 scoops) Aminogran Mineral Mixture is needed when 30 to 80 g Lofenalac or Minafen is taken per day.

And a full dose of 8 g (3 scoops) Aminogran Mineral Mixture is needed if less than 30 g Lofenalac or Minafen is taken per day.

The gradual change from Lofenalac or Minafen to all Aminogran can be timed to coincide with the change from bottle to cup. However, Lofenalac can continue indefinitely as the protein substitute if that seems appropriate for the particular child. The quantity should never exceed 200 g per day because of the mineral and vitamin content. It can be concentrated gradually to as much as one scoop Lofenalac to each 30 ml water after the infant is six months old, and it can be given by cup or spoon as appropriate. Alternatively, another low-phenylalanine protein

Table 9.17 Quantity (approximate) of powder contained in various scoops.

1 level scoop supplied of Aminogran Food Supplement (Allen & Hanburys) = 5 g powder
1 level yellow scoop supplied of Aminogran Mineral Mix (Allen & Hanburys) = 2·7 g powder
1 level Aminogran Food Supplement scoop ≃ 8 g glucose
1 level Aminogran Food Supplement scoop ≃ 8 g sugar (castor)
1 level Aminogran Food Supplement scoop ≃ 5·5 g Caloreen (Roussel)
1 level yellow Aminogran Mineral Mixture scoop ≃ 4·5 g glucose
1 level yellow Aminogran Mineral Mixture scoop ≃ 4·5 g sugar (castor)
1 level scoop Lofenalac (Mead Johnson) scoop supplied = 9·5 g powder
1 level Lofenalac scoop ≃ 8 g Caloreen (Roussel)
1 level scoop Metabolic Mineral Mixture (SHS) size 3 scoop supplied = 4·5 g powder
1 level scoop Albumaid XP (SHS) size 3 scoop supplied = 4·5 g powder
1 level scoop Maxamaid XP (SHS) size 3 scoop supplied = 7·2 g powder
1 level scoop PK Aid I (SHS) size 2 scoop supplied = 5·7 g powder
1 level scoop Milumil PKU I scoop supplied on request = 10 g powder
1 level scoop Milumil PKU II scoop supplied on request = 10 g powder

Table 9.18 Sample menu for a child with phenylketonuria.

Daily

1   ... large scoops Aminogran Food Supplement/PK Aid 1

Three small yellow scoops Aminogran Mineral Mixture/four scoops Metabolic Mineral Mix   } Or ... scoops Maxamaid XP

Flavouring is optional, e.g. fruit Nesquik, milk-shake syrup or fruit concentrate, tomato ketchup, etc.

Water to mix to a paste or drink as preferred

Mix and give at each main meal. Always offer a drink to follow and give within 20 to 30 minutes of the meal.

2   ... 50 mg phenylalanine exchanges (Table 9.2). Divide between meals. Breakfast ... exchanges; lunch ... exchanges; supper ... exchanges; ... exchanges for snacks.

3   Unlimited fruit and vegetables from Table 9.4.

4   Unlimited special low-protein bread, biscuits, pasta, Prosparol/Calogen and 'free foods' (Tables 9.7 and 9.8).

5   Vitamins: three Ketovite Tablets plus 5 ml Ketovite Liquid except with Maxamaid XP.

Sample diet for day

Breakfast   1/3 Aminogran, PK Aid 1, or Maxamaid XP mixture; fruit juice or drink or cup of tea with no-protein milk

... exchange breakfast cereal   } See list of 50 mg phenylalanine exchanges (Table 9.2)
... ml/oz milk = ... exchanges

Permitted low-protein bread (Table 9.8)

Butter or margarine, jam or honey or marmalade (Table 9.7)

Fruit, tomato or mushrooms (Table 9.4)

Mid-morning   Fruit juice or squash or no-protein 'milk'-shake

Aproten or Aminex or low-protein special biscuits or permitted sweets

Piece of fruit to clean teeth

Dinner   1/3 Aminogran, PK Aid 1, or Maxamaid XP mixture; fruit juice or drink

... exchanges of potato, rice, chips (Table 9.2)

Salad or vegetables allowed freely. Do not give ordinary gravy

Aproten or Aglutella spaghetti or pasta

Permitted low-protein special bread or biscuits

Butter or margarine and jam or honey

... exchanges ordinary custard, crisps (Table 9.2)

Tea   Fruit juice or squash or cup of tea with no-protein 'milk'

Permitted low-protein special bread or biscuits

Butter or margarine and jam or honey

Permitted sweets, e.g. barley sugar, Jelly Tots

... exchanges chocolates or crisps (Table 9.2)

Piece of fruit to clean teeth

Supper   1/3 Aminogran, PK Aid 1, or Maxamaid XP Mixture; fruit juice, squash or cup of tea with no-protein 'milk'

... exchange potato, rice (Table 9.2)

Low-protein vegetables allowed freely; tomato ketchup (permitted brands)

Fruit and/or protein-free pudding, e.g. Snowcrest Jelly

... exchange ordinary custard, crisps (Table 9.2)

Permitted low-protein bread and butter or margarine

Special low-protein pasta, pizza, biscuits (*see* Recipes)

Bedtime   Cup of tea with no-protein 'milk', fruit juice or squash

Aproten or Aminex or low-protein special biscuits

Fruit

As the diet is high in refined carbohydrate dental care is essential, and fluoride supplements are advised if the local water supply is low in fluoride. Regular dental check-ups are recommended.

substitute can be introduced, such as Albumaid XP or Maxamaid XP, which have the advantage of a lower energy content. Maxamaid XP also has the added advantage of good flavour and contains adequate vitamins, provided ⩾70 g is taken per day, but the quantity should never exceed 150 g per day because of its high mineral and vitamin content. It can be given as a drink or as a concentrate mixed to a 'paste' with a little water.

PK Aid 1 plus Metabolic Mineral Mixture can be used in a similar way to Aminogran, but the scoops supplied contain different quantities of the products (Table 9.17). Both Aminogran and PK Aid 1 should be well flavoured and not mixed with other food. The older child finds milk-shake flavourings, coffee, essences (vanilla, almond) and fruit concentrates and powders, or savoury sauces containing only permitted ingredients, acceptable flavourings, and the majority of patients accept them well.

(d) Low-phenylalanine diet for one-year-olds onwards

Once bottle-feeds are omitted from the diet, and three main meals with two to three snacks per day have been established, the main change in the diet will be increased variety and quantity of food for weight and age. Although the requirement for protein on a weight basis decreases with age (Table 9.2) total protein intake in normal children generally increases with age. The child with PKU is no different and therefore is usually allowed to grow into the dose rather than the prescription of the low-phenylalanine protein sustitute being decreased at any stage, unless the natural protein intake is markedly increased. Measurement of blood phenylalanine levels is continued at two- to three-weekly intervals, with appropriate dietary adjustment (Table 9.9). A range of manufactured foods (both those classified as 'free' foods and exchanges) and suitable recipes are introduced as the child demands more variety, e.g. a birthday cake at one year old is much appreciated by family and friends if not the child. A sample menu used as a guide for parents of the child over one year old is given in Table 9.18 and a calculated sample diet is given in Table 9.19.

Nutritional deficiencies and difficulties

Growth failure occurs less often than in the past with modern treatment of phenylketonuria, but undernutrition and food refusal still occur, with or without loss of biochemical control, as a result of deficiency of essential nutrients such as phenylalanine, protein and/or energy. Vitamin and mineral deficiencies (*see* Francis 1986) may also be involved, particularly if the low-phenylalanine protein substitute, which is the major source, is rejected or supplements omitted. Underprescription of nutrients for the individual's needs, misunderstandings about the dietary regimen, food refusal and pilfering are the commonest problems; a less frequent, but not uncommon, problem is overprescription of food, causing refusal, usually of the least palatable part of the diet.

(a) Phenylalanine deficiency

The main features of phenylalanine deficiency (Rouse 1966) are summarized in Table 9.20. The first sign of deficiency is a fall in blood phenylalanine to below normal. Phenylalanine levels are low unless accompanied by total protein and/or energy deficiency, when levels may rise above normal. The commonest cause of low phenylalanine levels is underprescription of phenylalanine, often in association with increased requirement during a period of rapid growth, or inadequate intake (*see* p. 237).

The very severe malnutrition documented by Hanley *et al.* (1970) was attributed to phenylalanine deficiency; however, their data suggest that the patients also suffered general nutritional deficiencies, probably secondary to inadequate consumption of Lofenalac (Smith & Francis 1982).

(b) Infections and minor illness in children with phenylketonuria

Loss of appetite is common with intercurrent infections, and blood phenylalanine levels rise as a result of catabolism. Illness should be treated as for any other child, with additional advice as follows:

1   Never force feed.
2   Carbohydrate-containing fluids should be offered, a little and often, to prevent thirst and dehydration. Fruit juices, and squash, and lemonade, Coke, etc., or in the more severe illness 5% dextrose, Dioralyte or Rehydrat, are appropriate.
3   The phenylalanine exchanges in the most acceptable form should be offered to appetite, but can be omitted for a few days if necessary, e.g. with diarrhoea and vomiting.
4   Protein substitutes, vitamins and minerals should be omitted temporarily, especially if vomiting and/or diarrhoea occur, restarting as halfstrength or half-dose. They should *never* be given without phenylalanine exchanges.
5   Regrade back onto the full diet as the child improves clinically and appetite returns. With a

Table 9.19   Calculated example of a diet for a school-age child of 20 to 25 kg with phenylketonuria.

		Protein and amino acids (g)	Energy kcal	Energy kJ	Phenylalanine (mg)
Daily	40 g Aminogran Food Supplement	40	160	640	Nil
	8 g Aminogran Minerals	Nil	Nil	Nil	Nil
	Flavouring, e.g. fruit juice concentrate (30 ml)	Trace	69	293	Trace
	Water to mix				
	Divide in two and give before or with meals				
	Three Ketovite Tablets plus 5 ml Ketovite Liquid				
	100 ml no-protein 'milk' for cereal, drinks and cooking	Nil	65	273	Nil
Breakfast	½ Aminogran mixture				
	Cup of tea with no-protein 'milk'				
	30 g Rice Krispies, 2 × 50 mg phenylalanine exchanges	1·8	110	475	100
	Sugar (5 g)	Nil	20	80	Nil
	No-protein 'milk'				
	40 g low-protein bread (toasted)	0·2	90	380	10
	10 g butter	Trace	74	304	2
	15 g marmalade	Trace	39	167	Trace
Snack	Fruit juice	Trace	30	137	Trace
	1 Aminex or 2 Aproten biscuits	0·1	47	197	3
	1 piece fruit (100 g apple)	0·2	46	196	6
Lunch	30 g Smith's Plain Crisps, 2 × 50 mg phenylalanine exchanges	1·9	160	667	100
	120 g low-protein bread ⎱ Sandwiches	0·7	270	1140	30
	30 g butter ⎰	Trace	222	912	7
	1 to 2 tomatoes (60 g)	0·5	8	36	9
	Fruit ⎰ 100 g orange	0·8	35	150	30
	⎱ 30 g sultanas	0·5	75	320	11
Snack	Fruit (50 g banana)	0·6	40	169	24
Tea/supper	½ Aminogran mixture				
	Fruit juice	Trace	30	137	Trace
	60 g chips, 2 × 50 mg phenylalanine exchanges	2·2	152	639	100
	20 g Heinz Baked Beans, 1 × 50 mg phenylalanine exchange	1·0	13	54	50
	Vegetables ⎰ 30 g onion fried	0·5	104	427	15
	⎱ 50 g carrot	0·4	12	49	7
	⎱ 50 g French beans	0·4	4	16	16
	Stewed/tinned fruit (100 g peaches)	0·4	87	373	8
	Daily total	52·2	1962	8231	528
	At 20 to 25 kg this provides (per kg per day)	2·6 to 2·1	98 to 78	412 to 329	26 to 21
	4- to 6-year-old comparison with theoretical guide to requirement (per kg per day)	2 to 3	80 to 100	420 to 330	According to tolerance

Table 9.20 Deficiency of an essential amino acid: phenylalanine (from Smith & Francis 1982).

	Symptoms and signs	Plasma phenylalanine	Other investigations
Early	Reduced weight gain Feeding difficulties Skin rash	< 1 mg/100 ml (60 μmol/l) (first abnormality detectable)	Some plasma amino acids raised Aminoaciduria
Late	Weight loss Growth rate reduced Dystrophic changes of skin, hair, nails Lethargy Gastrointestinal upset Frequent infections Oedema	< 1 mg/100 ml (60 μmol/l) (unless energy and/or total protein deficiency occur when levels may rise above normal)	As above *plus* Anaemia Hypoproteinaemia Low alkaline phosphatase Bone changes on X-ray
Terminal	Convulsion Mental retardation Death	< 1 mg/100 ml (60 μmol/l)	As above

prolonged illness, such as whooping cough, this may take weeks.

6 Blood phenylalanine levels should be monitored as recovery occurs, since catch-up growth following infection may require an increase in phenylalanine intake.

7 Medicines should be prescribed as needed, but if antibiotics are used the phenylalanine should be estimated by a chemical and not a bacteriological method.

(c) Feeding problems

Infection is the commonest cause of feeding problems and should be managed as above. Food refusal in a well child requires a supportive and calm attitude by the professionals involved with the family, and force-feeding should *never* be advised. Those supervising management should not direct their anxiety at the parents who are already under pressure. Critical comments are almost always out of place. A careful history of day-to-day food intake and associated behaviour and feelings is the first step towards helping the family. This cannot be done hurriedly. Along with a review of the child's growth, general health and phenylalanine control, and general 'mood' of the family members, the history will usually reveal the nature of the problem and dictate treatment. Overgenerous prescription of food or overgenerous provision of energy by the parents is a not uncommon cause of food refusal. Major food refusal, with weight loss and high phenylalanine levels, does occur from time to time, and is almost always due to extreme parental anxiety or conflict with the child. Practical and clear guidance should be given on the priority of

different items in the diet, e.g. low-phenylalanine protein substitutes first, phenylalanine allowance second, and other foods to appetite. The child's food preferences should be taken into account, and an effort is made to reduce tensions associated with food and eating by allowing the child to eat to appetite and, if necessary, little and often rather than giving main meals. Any rejected phenylalanine allowance should be replaced with an alternative such as milk or incorporated into a later meal in the same day, but should not be carried over into subsequent days. The parents need frequent reassurance and contact with the clinic (visit and/or telephone), initially at least weekly, until the child is eating properly.

Toddlers can be very conservative regarding food, and may demand a very monotonous diet, e.g. chocolate and chips for the natural protein intake and energy from drinks, low-protein biscuits and sweets. Such a diet is considered unsatisfactory by parents (and many professionals) with 'idealistic' ideas of nutrition, but provided it meets the dietary prescription and the child is well, growing and under biochemical control it is perfectly adequate when supplemented with the appropriate low-phenylalanine protein substitute, vitamins and minerals. In this situation reassurance is all that is required. Supplements such as glucose polymers should be used with caution as they may simply decrease appetite for other foods of better nutritional content and not achieve an overall increased intake.

Refusal of the low-phenylalanine protein substitute is a frequent problem. Full plasma amino acids are useful in identifying the problem. Inadequate intake leads to protein deficiency identified by low plasma amino acids, particularly tyrosine, and often coin-cides with energy, vitamin and mineral deficiency, unless appropriate supplements or natural foods re-place the substitute, in which case plasma amino acids will be normal and phenylalanine elevated. This is an important cause of undernutrition in children with phenylketonuria and may result in poor growth and/or loss of biochemical control of the blood phenylalanine.

A small-bulk amino acid preparation such as Ami-nogran or PK Aid 1, mixed to a 'paste' and given as a medicine, is useful in these situations (Smith *et al.* 1975b, Smith & Francis 1982). The child, even a toddler, should be told he is going to be given his 'medicine', then further comment should be resisted until praise and reward is given at the end. One tea-spoon of the low-phenylalanine protein substitute, e.g. Aminogran, mixed as a paste (*see* p. 250) is given as a 'medicine' once daily 20 to 30 minutes before a meal with a drink to follow; then twice daily; then three times daily, gradually increasing to the full dose for age over several weeks, but only moving onto the next step as the previous quantity is taken willingly. Some phenylalanine (one 50 mg phenylalanine ex-change) is given with each meal, even though high blood levels may occur as a result of the energy and/ or protein deficiency. This approach, combined with a praise and reward scheme appropriate for the child's age, is usually successful in overcoming rejec-tion of the protein substitute. The temporary period with less than optimal nutrition due to the reduced intake of the low-phenylalanine protein substitutes, although not ideal, is preferable to force feeding (which should *never* be advised), subsequent major dietary refusal, and the psychological problems these can cause.

Hospitalization can be useful when persistent feed-ing problems are present. The mother should accom-pany the child so that the help, encouragement and supervision from the hospital team can interact directly with mother and child. On rare occasions when the dietary problems are likely to lead to ser-ious malnutrition if prolonged further, or where in-tervention continually fails to control blood phenyl-alanine levels at a time in the child's life when dietary lapse is likely to cause serious harm, an approach similar to that used in cases of child abuse is appropriate.

(d)   Dietary indiscretion
Persistently elevated phenylalanine levels in a child who is growing normally and is healthy is due to an excessive phenylalanine intake. In the child over one year old, even with 'classical' phenylketonuria, it is most unusual to need to reduce the prescription of phenylalanine to less than three 50 mg phenylalan-ine exchanges per day, or to have to restrict the in-take of the fruits and vegetables listed in Table 9.5 to control phenylalanine blood levels. When phenyl-alanine has been reduced to the minimum described above and levels are still high then dietary indiscre-tion, with or without the knowledge of the parents, is the likely explanation.

In the young child indiscretion is frequently due to the child's normal exploration, and the occasional dietary indiscretion of this type is easily dealt with and does no permanent harm. When a young child has high phenylalanine levels repeatedly, the par-ent(s) as well as the child are likely to be involved in breaking the diet, and this can be a difficult situation to handle and may require the expert help of other professionals.

If a child is hungry he is more likely to demand or take forbidden food. Attention to energy intake by offering ample low-protein, acceptable foods at meals and as snacks does much to help overcome tempta-tion. A generous snack before going to tea with friends or a party can be a useful way of preventing pilfering. Encouragement of fruit, low-protein bis-cuits, cakes, drinks and permitted sweets and similar popular snack foods, and their easy availability when friends are sharing their 'goodies', also helps, espe-cially when the child is first becoming independent. Guidance to the parents to remain (at least out-wardly) calm, to explain to the child why he cannot indulge, in language which the child can understand, is needed. The child should be given good reasons as to why he is different and cannot have the same food as his siblings and peer group. A simple but truthful explanation is best, given with a warm and loving attitude and pride in the child and his achievements. Even a young child can quickly understand that it displeases his parents when he takes the wrong food, and that toddler tantrums do not succeed.

The diet prescription should not be altered follow-ing minor dietary indiscretion, though a decreased phenylalanine intake at the next meal is appropriate. The blood phenylalanine should be checked once the diet has been corrected.

Management of repeated high blood phenylalanine levels which do not respond to the above measures requires a full review of the diet, and of both the parents' and siblings' attitude to the diet and the diagnosis, by the paediatrician and, if necessary, other professionals.

PSYCHOSOCIAL ASPECTS OF TREATMENT

The strain put on a family when first informed that their child has a potentially handicapping condition even if treatable is considerable. In-patient admissions should be kept to a minimum and may be unnecessary if local facilities permit out-patient management. The initial contact between parents, paediatrician and dietitian is of prime importance, as the experience during the first weeks of treatment can determine success or failure of the diet. Misunderstandings about the treatment frequently have their origins in these early weeks, and feeding problems can be the result of unresolved anxiety surrounding the diagnosis. Parents need a full explanation about the disease, its genetics, the rationale of treatment and prognosis. Thorough instruction in the practical management of the diet is essential, and should be given by the dietitian, who will continue to keep contact with the family and instruct about dietary changes. All this is time-consuming but is beneficial to the parents' self-confidence and their subsequent ability to co-operate and manage the regimen. *The Child with Phenylketonuria* (Holten & Tyfield 1980) is a useful supplement to one-to-one counselling of parents, as well as for medical, nursing and dietetic staff less familiar with the condition. A society has been set up in the United Kingdom (The National Society for Phenylketonuria and Allied Disorders Ltd) which aims, amongst other things, to help parents with the practical and social aspects of dietary treatment. Similar groups exist in other countries.

Marino (1980) has developed a programmed instruction unit for phenylketonuria in Boston, U.S.A., and suggests such instructional units are more effective than traditional teaching methods for both higher and lower learning abilities. Such programmes deserve further evaluation. Individual instruction which can be adapted, without loss of essentials, to the intelligence and educational level of the family (Smith & Francis 1982) remains the basis for long-term management. A few mothers who are perfectly capable of adequately caring for and loving their children are unable to weigh, measure, use exchange lists or even to read and/or comprehend diet sheets. Local support of a well-instructed health visitor can be of great assistance. Regular review, by a dietitian and paediatrician every few weeks in the early months of treatment, of growth, food intake, changing nutritional requirements, biochemical control and general progress will help avoid feeding problems, and give the mother opportunity for discussion of any difficulties. Anxiety is common and can be overwhelming. Once the child is established onto three meals a day (plus snacks), and the parents are confident about the diet, visits to the hospital clinic can be infrequent. Dietary modification in accordance with the clinical situation, including weight gain, food intake, intercurrent infections and blood phenylalanine results, can be made in regular contacts by telephone (or letter if the former is not available) between parents and dietitian (or other designated member of the specialist treatment team).

Children with phenylketonuria should ideally be treated in centres with an interest in the nutritional management of metabolic disease (DHSS 1969). In this way the staff gain experience in caring for these children, laboratory facilities can be geared to their needs, and proper dietary supervision provided. It is more difficult to ensure that facilities are available for a single patient and parents gain comfort and confidence from meeting other parents and patients with similar problems.

The family doctor will also require extra information and support, since he may meet only one patient with this rare disorder. Usually he will be required to prescribe the special dietary items needed for treatment (such as the low-phenylalanine protein substitute, vitamins and special low-protein breads and biscuits classified by the Advisory Committee on Borderline Substances as prescribable at NHS expense for phenylketonuria) and will need to know what advice to give for common childhood illness.

A low-phenylalanine diet disturbs the normal cultural eating pattern and is a factor in the aetiology of feeding difficulties (*see* above). Parents knowing the consequences of failure are anxious, and this is reinforced by the normal ups and downs in the child's intake and biochemical control. They may experience hostile feelings towards the child and his treatment, and to the team, particularly when the diagnosis has been made by routine screening. Such reactions are commoner when family relationships show long-standing disturbance, but also occur due to the stress of a difficult diet even in stable, loving families. Many mothers pass through a phase of deep anxiety and depression when informed of the diagnosis. This may prevent normal 'mothering'. Given a nutritionally satisfactory diet this is the commonest cause of feeding difficulties in the infant and young child (Smith & Francis 1982).

During the toddler stage, when children normally explore new foods, problems can arise because of the restricted nature of the diet; food refusal with resultant tension and anxiety in the family may occur, needing practical advice and support (*see* above).

During the early years a special diet can be a status symbol to the child, but this is reversed as the child becomes older, is aware of the diet limitations, and seeks peer group conformity. Practical advice about school meals and social eating (p. 255) is of utmost importance. The use of as wide a variety of foods as possible, even if in restricted quantity, including the popular snack foods indulged in by the peer group, is helpful to both the child and his family.

Result of treatment

The early detection and subsequent treatment of 'classical' phenylketonuria with a low-phenylalanine diet can prevent mental retardation (Koch *et al.* 1973, Smith *et al.* 1973, Berry *et al.* 1979). Many reports have, however, suggested a difference of 10 to 15 points in the intelligence quotient of the patient in comparison with his parents and siblings, even when the diet is started in the first weeks of life (Smith *et al.* 1973, Berry *et al.* 1979). Malnutrition (Hanley *et al.* 1970), delayed diagnosis (Kang *et al.* 1970) and quality of dietary control (Dobson *et al.* 1977, Berry *et al.* 1979) probably all affect intellectual outcome. In the U.K. there has been a steady improvement in the average IQ at four and eight years of age, so that children with phenylketonuria from 1973–74 onwards have a mean IQ above 100, with the expected numbers of children of superior intelligence present in the groups, suggesting that patients are now reaching the optimal potential (MRC/DHSS Phenylketonuria Register Newsletter 1984).

The effect of treatment on patients who are already mentally retarded at diagnosis is more difficult to evaluate, but improvement in progress has been reported by various authors, expecially when the diet is introduced in the first years of life (e.g. Koch *et al.* 1967).

Treated patients with 'atypical' phenylketonuria do as well as 'classical' cases, although it is not possible to say how many would have made normal progress without treatment.

Duration and discontinuation of diet

Medical opinion varies about if and when it is safe to stop diet in patients with 'classical' phenylketonuria. Intellectual deterioration following elective discontinuation of diet at four years was reported by Cabalska *et al.* (1977). Smith and her colleagues (1978) reported a fall in mean IQ of eight points when a normal diet was introduced at eight years in both early- and late-treated patients. Other studies have failed to find evidence of a fall in IQ (Johnson 1972, Holtzman *et al.* 1975). However, follow-up in these studies has been over a relatively short period, and in some cases biochemical control had already been lost before formal diet discontinuation (*see* Smith & Francis 1982 and MRC/DHSS 1984).

Because the diet becomes increasingly irksome as patients reach mid and later childhood, many clinics allow some diet relaxation in older children.

As a result of the findings in patients in whom diet was stopped at eight years it became the policy at The Hospital for Sick Children, London, in 1975 to relax rather than stop the diet at that age, aiming to maintain blood phenylalanine levels between 900 and 1200 μmol/l whenever possible, *at least* until 12 years of age. Follow-up of patients on such a regimen (details below) shows no fall in IQ at 10 or 12 years of age, i.e. two and four years follow-up (MRC/DHSS 1984). The age at which it is safe to discontinue the relaxed diet is unknown, and as yet no hard and fast policy can be made, though continuation of the relaxed diet is advised indefinitely. However, many adolescents and their families find it increasingly difficult to comply with the diet limitations and must therefore share in the decisions regarding the diet's discontinuation or continuation. Reintroduction of a stricter diet is advised only rarely for fall-off in performance and IQ. The trauma of the diet must be balanced by the expected advantages.

Relaxed diet

A diet for the child over eight years old permitting phenylalanine blood levels to be maintained between 900 and 1200 μmol/l allows a more normal diet, usually of 7 to 20 g natural protein per day according to tolerance.

(a) Initially twice the number of previously tolerated 50 mg phenylalanine exchanges are prescribed. The range of permitted foods is increased and may include ordinary bread, biscuits and cake, together with ice-cream and cereals and a wide range of manufactured foods. If practical, and if the phenylalanine allowance is generous enough, limited quantities of meat, egg, cheese and fish may be permitted. Aspartame, Canderel and Nutrasweet artificial sweeteners should not be used by PKUs at any age. The range of low-protein foods can also be widened, e.g. to permit a little ordinary gravy, etc. The phenylalanine intake should be divided throughout the day's meals, but occasionally, e.g. at parties or Sunday lunch, a greater proportion of phenylalanine exchanges can be given at one meal, and in some cases this may make school dinners permissible. The phenylalanine intake is monitored and adjusted to maintain blood phenylalanine levels between 900 and 1200 μmol/l. Blood phenylalanine levels are estimated at two-week intervals until the child is stabilized on the new regimen; thereafter levels are usually estimated two-monthly.

(b) The low-phenylalanine protein substitute is still required to supplement dietary protein, correct amino acid imbalance and provide essential tyrosine, but the prescription can be reduced to compensate the increased intake of natural protein and because the total protein requirement for weight decreases with age.

(c) Appropriate vitamin and mineral supplements are prescribed to ensure the nutritional adequacy of the diet, including calcium, essential vitamin B_{12} and folic acid, which are difficult to obtain adequately on a low-protein diet.

If a near-normal diet is ultimately tolerated, supplements may be unnecessary.

(d) Adequate but not excessive energy intake is provided by selecting the higher and lower energy phenylalanine exchange foods appropriately, whilst continuing some low-protein bread and biscuit products to ensure the child does not 'lose the taste' for these items.

'Atypical' phenylketonuria

In those patients with 'atypical' phenylketonuria who require treatment the diet is based on the same principles as those for patients with 'classical' phenylketonuria, but more natural protein can be given, a wider selection of foods included and appropriately less low-phenylalanine protein substitute (vitamins and minerals) prescribed.

It is important that patients suspected of having 'atypical' phenylketonuria are reassessed at one year old, to determine whether the child can tolerate a more generous or normal diet. At eight years of age, and occasionally even earlier, a normal or near-normal diet can often be tolerated without causing high phenylalanine levels, except possibly during intercurrent infections.

Patients with 'atypical' phenylketonuria treated for varying lengths of time, aiming to maintain blood phenylalanine levels below 600 μmol/l, usually show no evidence of deterioration of intelligence when the diet is withdrawn (Cabalska *et al.* 1977), although Berry *et al.* (1979) reported reduced intellectual

achievement in such cases when treatment was withdrawn early in life.

Follow-up is important, particularly for females. The genetics of phenylketonuria, and particularly the risks of maternal phenylketonuria, should be discussed with parents and patient once old enough to appreciate their significance.

Alternative forms of therapy

Enzyme replacement, both orally and with ghost red blood cells filled with synthetic enzymes, is receiving preliminary investigation (Hoskins *et al.* 1980); phenylalanine antagonists have been administered but are potentially toxic (Krips & Lines 1972); the impaired catecholamine and serotonin production of phenylketonuria could be overcome by administration of dopa and 5-hydroxytryptophan; and the competitive effect of high phenylalanine levels on brain uptake of other amino acids could perhaps be overcome by appropriate amino acid administration (Smith & Francis 1982). Genetic engineering is a possibility for the future, and pre-natal screening will probably become available in the next few years. Alternative forms of therapy will have to prove themselves as effective and as safe as current dietary treatment before they are given trials in young children but may be a practical solution to the limitations of the dietary regimen for the older patient if treatment proves to be required indefinitely or lifelong.

Maternal phenylketonuria

The offspring of mothers who have phenylketonuria and who are on a normal diet during pregnancy may show a variety of congenital abnormalities, including microcephaly and mental retardation (Fisch *et al.* 1969, Bickel 1980, Lenke & Levy 1980, Levy 1982, Levy *et al.* 1982). These children, who do not have phenylketonuria unless the father is a carrier, are damaged *in utero* by the high circulating levels of phenylalanine and its metabolites. The ratio of fetal to maternal phenylalanine levels is approximately 1·7:1, and therefore the fetus is exposed to even higher phenylalanine levels than the mother. Probably at least two-thirds of women with 'classical' phenylketonuria are likely to have a baby with some abnormality unless preventive treatment is given. The effect of 'atypical' maternal phenylketonuria is still uncertain (Hansen 1970, Komrower *et al.* 1979), but fetal damage has been reported in some cases.

The greatest risk to the fetus from the structural anomalies is during the first 8 to 10 weeks of preg-

nancy. Diet initiated in the first trimester of pregnancy has failed to prevent fetal abnormalities in
three reported cases (Smith *et al.* 1979).

Recent experience suggests that a diet which is
introduced pre-conception, and which controls blood

phenylalanine levels in an optimal range (180 to
500 μmol/l), prevents damage of the fetus (Neilsen
& Warnberg 1979). A woman with phenylketonuria
who wishes to have children of her own should therefore be advised to start an appropriate low-phenyl-

Table 9.21   Menu suggestions for children's teas and parties.

Child with phenylketonuria	Child without phenylketonuria
Crisps and/or chocolate from phenylalanine allowance.	Unlimited crisps and chocolate.
Diced tomatoes on sticks. Serve with chips or crisps from allowance.	Diced tomato and sausages on sticks. Serve with chips or crisps.
A 'hedgehog' made from an orange or plasticine covered with foil in which are placed sticks with cubes of pineapple, cucumber, tomato, red and green pepper, celery. Sultanas can be used for 'eyes'.	A similar 'hedgehog' but with cheese and/or sausage cubes. Alternatively for older children a joint hedgehog can be used and each child helps himself to selected items.
Low-protein tomato sandwiches cut into interesting shapes, e.g. with a biscuit animal shape or hearts and diamonds.	Tomato sandwiches, with or without egg.
Jacket potato from phenylalanine allowance and butter, chives and/or permitted salad cream. Grated carrot.	Jacket potato and butter, grated cheese and/or salad cream. Grated carrot.
Baked beans from phenylalanine allowance on low-protein toast.	Beans on toast.
Chips from phenylalanine allowance. Spaghetti either from phenylalanine allowance or low-protein type with tomato ketchup.	Chips and spaghetti and cheese.
Low-protein spaghetti with fried onion, tomato, and mushrooms.	Spaghetti with onion, tomato and mushrooms.
Open low-protein sandwiches using low-protein bread or crispbread and a selection of toppings.	Open sandwiches using bread or crispbread with similar toppings.
Kebabs of mushroom, tomato, apple, and other fruits and vegetables (dip apple in low-protein flour or lemon juice to stop it going brown). Serve raw or grill at the last minute. May be served with chips or crisps from phenylalanine allowance.	Kebabs of vegetables, fruits, plus bacon and sausage (cooked). Serve with chips or crisps similarly to the child with phenylketonuria.
Omelette or savoury pancakes made from Ener G egg substitute and low-protein flour. Serve with chips from phenylalanine allowance.	Real omelette or savoury pancakes served with chips.
Soup (free recipe) or from phenylalanine allowance served with low-protein toast.	Soup and toast
Low-protein cauliflower without cheese (serve with low-protein sauce).	Cauliflower cheese.
Low-protein macaroni without cheese (served with low-protein sauce) and tinned tomatoes.	Macaroni cheese and tinned tomatoes.
Fruit set in vegetarian jelly or Quick-jel.	Fruit set in vegetarian or ordinary jelly.
Ice-cream as phenylalanine allowance or special low-protein recipe may be served with fruit sauce.	Ice cream. May be served with fruit sauce.
Permitted low-protein biscuits or cake may be iced with glacé icing and glacé fruit and/or hundreds-and-thousands sugar decorations.	Biscuits or cake similarly decorated.

alanine diet whilst still practising effective contraception. Any necessary weight reduction is preferable before the introduction of the low-phenylalanine diet (Kromrower *et al.* 1979, Bickel 1980). In the event of a pregnancy starting before the reintroduction of a low-phenylalanine diet, or in a woman in whom phenylketonuria has not been diagnosed before the start of pregnancy, careful consideration of all the facts must be weighed and discussed with the couple concerned. Should termination be ruled out, a low-phenylalanine diet should be started as a matter of urgency. The maternal diet must be nutritionally adequate for optimal fetal growth and should be monitored just as carefully as in the infant with phenylketonuria. Several centres now have experience with maternal phenylketonuria and their advice should be sought before devising the diet.

SUGGESTIONS FOR SCHOOL MEALS AND SOCIAL EATING

Social eating, such as mixing with other children at school dinner time, is very important for children on a diet. The majority of children requiring a low-phenylalanine diet will require a packed lunch at school, unless they can come home. The change in school lunch provision has reduced the difference between the child with phenylketonuria and his peer group, as many children take a packed lunch, and school canteens provide more snack foods and frequently a selective menu. It is important that the child gets enough of his own food to eat to ensure that he is not hungry. The child should be trusted to know his own diet, though supervision is helpful.

The low-phenylalanine protein substitute is usually omitted from the school meal, and given either with part of the phenylalanine allowance as a snack after school, or as two doses given at breakfast and the evening meal.

School milk is unsuitable and should be replaced with either no-protein 'milk' (*see* Recipes), fruit juice or water. Sandwiches can be made using low-protein bread or crispbread, margarine or butter and suitable fillings such as salad, tomato, jam, honey, fruit, permitted tomato ketchup, salad cream, or mustard. Crisps, chocolate and similar snack foods or soup in a child's flask can supply the phenylalanine allowance. Low-protein biscuits, permitted sweets, and fresh or dried fruits provide extra energy. Alternatively, a vegetable meal can be supplied by the school or sent in a plastic container for re-heating. Potato, chips or baked beans can supply the phenylalanine allowance. The school should be supplied with high-energy, low-protein foods such as low-protein bread and biscuits to supplement the meal.

A party or tea out with friends can pose quite a problem unless there is careful liaison between the parents in advance. The child can take along some of his own low-protein foods and/or can be given a snack before going so that he is less hungry at the meal time. The low-phenylalanine protein substitute is given at home, either before or after the outing. A larger proportion of the day's phenylalanine allowance can be reserved for the meal out. Inclusion of permitted fizzy pop or Coke, and sweets, with measured crisps or similar snack foods which can be enjoyed by all the children with or without phenylketonuria, makes the child on the diet feel included with his peers. The birthday cake can be brought home and substituted for a low-protein alternative.

Inviting friends to tea is somewhat easier, as plenty of low-protein foods can be included for the child with phenylketonuria and friends alike. Some suggestions are given in Table 9.21. The low-phenylalanine protein substitute can be given discreetly in the kitchen or after friends have departed. Birthday cakes made in novelty shapes can include a low-protein cake area, the rest being an ordinary recipe for friends, or of course all can on such occasions share the low-protein cake.

REFERENCES

AGGETT P.J. & DAVIES N.T. (1983) Some nutritional aspects of trace metals. *J. inher. metab. Dis.* Suppl. I, 22–30.

AGRAWAL H.C., BONE A.H. & DAVIDSON A.N. (1969) Inhibition of brain protein synthesis by phenylalanine. *Biochem. J.* 112, 27.

ALEXANDER F.W., CLAYTON B.E. & DELVES H.T. (1974) Mineral and trace metal balances in children receiving normal and synthetic diets. *Quart. J. Med.* 43, 89–111.

BARTHOLOMÉ K., SCHMIDT H. & LUTZ P. (1979) Phenylalanine hydroxlase and protein loading tests in phenylketonuria and hyperphenylalaninaemia. *Europ. J. Paediat.* 130, 206.

BENTOVIM A., CLAYTON B.E., FRANCIS D., SHEPHERD J. & WOLFF O.H. (1970) Use of an amino acid mixture in treatment of phenylketonuria. *Arch. Dis. Childh.* 45, 640.

BERRY H.K., HUNT M.M. & SUTHERLAND B.K. (1971) Amino acid balance in the treatment of phenylketonuria. *J. Amer. diet. Ass.* 58, 3, 210–14.

BERRY H.K., O'GRADY D.J., PERLMUTTER L.J. & BAFINGER M.K. (1979) Intellectual development of children treated early for phenylketonuria. *Development of Medicine and Child Neurology* 21, 311.

BICKEL H. DIRECTOR (1980) *The International Workshop Maternal PKU. Problems–Experiences–Recommendations.* Frankfurt: Main.

BLASKOVICS M.E., SCHAEFFLER G.E. & HACK S. (1974) Phenylalanainaemia: differential diagnosis. *Arch. Dis. Childh.* **49**, 835–43.

CABALSKA B., DUCEZYŃSKA N., BORZYMOWSKA J., ZORSKA K., KÓSLACZ-FOLGA A. & BÓZKOWA K. (1977) Termination of dietary treatment in phenylketonuria. *Europ. J. Paediat.* **126**, 253–62.

CHASE H.P. & O'BRIEN D. (1970) Effects of excess phenylalanine and other amino acids on brain development in the infant rat. *Pediat. Res.* **4**, 96–102.

CLAYTON B.E. (1971) Phenylketonuria. *J. med. Genet.* **8**, 37–40.

CLAYTON B.E. (1975) The principles of treatment by dietary restriction as illustrated by phenylketonuria. In *Treatment of Inherited Metabolic Disease* (ed. Raine D.W.), pp. 1–32. Lancaster: MTP Ltd.

CLAYTON B.E., HEELEY A.F. & HEELEY M. (1970) An investigation of the hyperaminoaciduria in phenylketonuria associated with the feeding of certain commercial low phenylalanine preparations. *Brit. J. Nutr.* **24**, 573.

DANKS D.M., BARTHOLOMÉ K., CLAYTON B.E., CURTIUS H., GROBE H., KAUFMAN S., LEEMING R., PFLEIDERER W., REMBOLD H. & REY F. (1978) Malignant hyperphenylalaninaemia. Current status June 1977. *J. inher. metab. Dis.* **1**, 49–53.

DAVIDSON A.N. (1973) Inborn errors of amino acid metabolism affecting myelination of the central nervous system. In *Inborn Errors of Metabolism* (eds. Hommes F.A. & can den Berg C.J.), p. 55. London: Academic Press.

DHSS (1969) *Screening for Early Detection of Phenylketonuria* (69), 72. London: HMSO.

DHSS (1974) *Present Day Practice in Infant Feeding*, Committee on Medical Aspects of Food Policy, Report 9. London: HMSO.

DHSS (1977) *The Composition of Mature Human Milk*. London: HMSO.

DHSS (1983) (Revision) *Present Day Practice in Infant Feeding* Report 20, 1980. London: HMSO.

DOBSON J.C., WILLIAMSON M.L., AZEN C. & KOCH R. (1977) Intellectual assessment of 111 four-year-old children with phenylketonuria. *Pediatrics* **60**, 822.

FEINBERG S.B. & FISCH R.O. (1972) Bone changes in untreated neonatal PKU patients: A new radiographic observation and interpretation. *J. Pediat.* **81**, 2, 540.

FISCH R.O., DOEDER D., LARSKY L.L. & ANDERSON J.A. (1969) Maternal phenylketonuria. Detrimental effects on embryogenesis and fetal development. *Amer. J. Dis. Child.* **118**, 847.

FÖLLING A. (1934) Uber ausscheidung von Phenylbrentraubersaure In der Harnals Stoffwech Selanomalie in Verbindüng mit Imbezillitat. *Hoppe-Seylers Z. physiol. Chem.* **227**, 169.

FRANCIS D.E.M. (1986) *Nutrition for Children*. Oxford: Blackwell Scientific Publications.

FRANCIS D.E.M. & SMITH I. (1981) Breastfeeding regime for the treatment of infants with phenylketonuria. In *Applied Nutrition* (ed. Bateman C.), pp. 82–3. London: John Libbey.

GARROD A.E. (1909) *Inborn Errors of Metabolism* (ed. Frowde H.). London: Hodder & Stoughton.

GEGGAL H.S., AMENT M.E., HECKERLIVELY J.R., MARTIN D.A. & KOPPLE J.D. (1985) Nutritional requirements for taurine in patients receiving long-term parenteral nutrition. *New Engl. J. Med.* **312**, 142–6.

GEIGY SCIENTIFIC TABLES (1981) Vol. I, *Units of Measurement, Body Fluids, Composition of the Body, Nutrition*, 8th Revised Edition (ed. Lentner C.), p. 214. Basle: Ciba-Geigy.

GUTHRIE R. (1961) Letter: Blood screening for phenylketonuria. *J. Amer. med. Ass.* **178**, 863.

GUTHRIE R. & SUSI A. (1963) A simple phenylalanine method for detecting phenylketonuria in large populations of newborn infants. *Pediatrics* **32**, 338–43.

HANLEY W.B., LINSAO L., DAVIDSON W. & MOES C.A.F. (1970) Malnutrition with early treatment of phenylketonuria. *Pediat. Res.* **4**, 318–27.

HANSEN H. (1970) Epidemiological considerations on maternal hyperphenylalaninaemia. *Amer. J. ment. Defic.* **75**, 22.

HASE Y., SHINTAKU H., TURUHARA T., OURA T., KOBASHI M. & IWAI K. (1982) A case of tetrahydrobiopterin deficiency due to a defective synthesis of dihydrobiopterin. *J. inher. metab. Dis.* **5**, 81–2.

HOLT L.E. JR. & SNYDERMAN S.E. (1967) Amino acid requirement of children. In *Amino Acid Metabolism and Genetic Variation* (ed. Nylan W.L), p. 381. New York: McGraw-Hill.

HOLTEN J. & TYFIELD L. (1980) *The Child with Phenylketonuria*, 2nd Edition. National Society for Mentally Handicapped Children and The National Society of Phenylketonura and Allied Disorders Ltd.

HOLTZMAN N.A., WELCHER D.W. & MELLITS E.D. (1975) Termination of restricted diet in children with phenylketonuria. A randomized controlled study. *New Engl. J. Med.* **292**, 1121.

HOSKINS J.A., JACK G., WADE H., PEIRIS R., WRIGHT E., STARR D. & STERN J. (1980) Enzymatic control of phenylalanine intake in phenylketonuria. *Lancet* **1**, 8165, 392–4.

IRWIN M.I. & HEGSTED D.M. (1971) A conspectus of research on amino acid requirements of man. *J Nutr.* **101**, 539.

JOHNSON C.F. (1972) What is the best age to discontinue the low phenylalanine diet in phenylketonuria? *Clin. Pediat.* **11**, 148.

KANG E.S., SOLEE N.D. & GERALD P.S. (1970) Results of treatment and termination of the diet of phenylketonuria. *Pediatrics* **46**, 881.

KAUFMAN S. (1971) The phenylalanine hydroxylating system from mammalian liver. *Advanc. Enzymol.* **35**, 245.

KINDT E., MOTZFELDT K., HALVORSEN S. & LIE S.O. (1983) Protein requirements in infants and children: a longitudinal study of children treated for PKU. *Amer. J. clin. Nutr.* **37** (5) 778–85.

KOCH R., ACOSTA P., FISHLER K., SCHAEFFLER G. & WOHLERS A. (1967) Clinical observations on phenylketonuria. *Amer. J. Dis. Child.* **113**, 6.

KOCH R., DOBSON J.C., BLASKOVICS M., WILLIAMSON M.L., ERNEST A.E., FRIEDMAN E.G. & PARKER C.E. (1973) Collaborative study of children treated for phenylketonuria. In *Treatment of Inborn Errors of Metabolism* (eds. Seakins J.W.T., Saunders R.A. & Toothill C.), pp. 3–18. Proceedings of 10th Symposium of the Society for the Study of Inborn Errors of Metabolism, Edinburgh: Churchill Livingstone.

KOMROWER G.M., SARDHARWALLA I.B., COUTTS J.M. & INGHAM D. (1979) Management of maternal phenylketonuria: an emerging clinical problem. *Brit. med. J.* **1**, 1382.

KON S.K. & COWIE A.T. (1961) *Milk: The Mammary Gland and its Secretion*, Vol. II. London: Academic Press.

KRIPS C. & LINES D.R. (1972) Phenylketonuria: reduction of serum levels of phenylalanine following oral administration of β-2 thienylalanine. *Aust. Paediat. J.* **8**, 318.

LAWSON M.S., CLAYTON B.E., DELVES H.T. & MITCHELL J.D. (1977) Evaluation of a new mineral and trace metal supplement for use with synthetic diets. *Arch. Dis. Childh.* **52**. 62–7.

LENKE R.R. & LEVY H. (1980) Maternal phenylketonuria and hyperphenylalaninaemia. *New Engl. J. Med.* **303**, 21, 1202–8.

LEVY H.L. (1982) Maternal PKU: control of an emerging problem. *Amer. J. publ. Hlth* **72** (12), 1320–1.

LEVY H.L., KAPLAN G.N. & ERICKSON A.N. (1982) Comparison of treated and untreated pregnancies in a mother with PKU. *J. Pediat.* **100** (6), 876–80.

LOMBECK I., KASPEREK K., FEINENDEGEN L.E. & BREMER H.J. (1978) Trace element disturbance in dietetically treated patients with phenylketonuria and maple syrup urine disease. *Monogr. hum. Genet.* **9**, 114–117.

LOMBECK I., EBERT K., KASPEREK K., FEINDENGEN L.E. & BREMEN H.J. (1984) Selenium intake of infants and young children, healthy children and dietetically treated patients with PKU. (1984) *Europ. J. Paediat.*, **143**, 99–102.

MACY I.G. & KELLY J.H. (1961) Human and cow's milk in infant nutrition. In *Milk: The Mammary Glands and its Secretion*, Vol. II (eds. Kon S.K. & Cowie A.T.), p. 265. New York: Academic Press.

MANN T.P., WILSON K.M. & CLAYTON B.E. (1965) A deficiency state arising in infants on synthetic foods. *Arch. Dis. Childh.* **40**, 364.

MARINO M.A. (1980) Developing and testing a programmed instruction unit on phenylketonuria. *J Amer. diet. Ass.* **76**, 1, 29.

MRC/DHSS (1978) *Phenylketonuria Register* (U.K.), Newsletter No. 5.

MRC/DHSS (1984) *Phenylketonuria Register* (U.K.), Newsletter No. 9.

NEAME K.D. (1961) Phenylalanine as inhibitor of transport of amino acids in brain. *Nature* (Lond.) **192**, 173–14.

NEILSON K.B. & WAMBERG E. (1979) Successful outcome of pregnancy in a PKU woman after low phenylalanine diet introduced before conception. *Lancet* **i**, 1245.

NIEDERWIESSER A., CURTIUS H-CH., BETTONI O., BIERI J., SCHIRCHS B., VISCOUNTINI M. & SCHAUB J. (1979) Atypical phenylketonuria caused by 7, 8-dihydrobiopterin synthetase deficiency. *Lancet* **i**, 131.

PAUL A.A. & SOUTHGATE D.A.T. (eds.) (1978) *McCance &*

Widdowson–The Composition of Food, 4th Edition. London: HMSO.

PAUL A.A., SOUTHGATE D.A.T. & RUSSELL J. (1980) *Amino acid composition, mg per 100 g food*. First supplement to *McCance & Widdowson—The Composition of Food*. London: HMSO.

ROUSE B.M. (1966) Phenylalanine deficiency syndrome. *J. Pediat.* **69**, 246–9.

ROYSTON N.J.W. & PARRY T.E. (1962) Megaloblastic anaemia complicating dietary treatment of phenylketonuria in infancy. *Arch. Dis. Childh.* **37**, 430.

SCRIVER C.R. & ROSENBERG L.E. (eds.) (1973) *Amino Acid Metabolism and its Disorders*, p. 453. Philadelphia: Saunders.

SMITH I. (1985) The hyperphenylalaninaemias. In *Genetic and Metabolic Disease in Paediatrics* (eds. Lloyd J. & Scriver C.), pp. 166–210. International Medical Reviews. London: Butterworth.

SMITH I. & FRANCIS D.E.M. (1982) Amino acid disorders. In *Textbook of Paediatric Nutrition*, 2nd Edition (eds. McLaren D. & Burman D.), pp. 295–323. Edinburgh: Churchill Livingstone.

SMITH I. & WOLFF O.H. (1974) Natural history of phenylketonuria and influence of early treatment. *Lancet* **ii**, 540.

SMITH I., LOBASCHER M. & WOLFF O.H. (1973) Factors influencing outcome in early treated phenylketonuria. In *Treatment of Inborn Errors of Metabolism*, Proceedings of the 10th Symposium of the Society for the Study of Inborn Errors of Metabolism, (eds. Seakins J.W.T., Saunders R.A. & Toothill C.), p. 41. Edinburgh: Churchill Livingstone.

SMITH I., CLAYTON B.E. & WOLFF O.H. (1975a) New variant of phenylketonuria with a progressive neurological illness unresponsive to phenylalanine restriction. *Lancet*, **i**, 1108.

SMITH I., FRANCIS D.E.M., CLAYTON B. & WOLFF O.H. (1975b) Comparison of an amino acid mixture and protein hydrolysates in treatment of infants with phenylketonuria. *Arch Dis. Childh.* **50**, 864.

SMITH I., LOBASCHER M.K., STEVENSON J. & WOLFF O.H. (1978) Effect of stopping low-phenylalanine diet on intellectual progress of children with phenylketonuria. *Brit. med. J.* **2**, 723.

SMITH I., ERDOHAZI M., MCCARTNEY J.F., PINCOTT J.R., WOLFF O.H., BRENTON D.P., BIDDLE S.A., FAIRWEATHER D.V.I. & DOBBING J. (1979) Fetal damage despite low phenylalanine diet after conception in a phenylketonuric woman. *Lancet* **i**, 17–19.

SMITH I., HYLAND K., KENDALL B. & LEEMING R. (1985) The clinical role of pteridin therapy in the treatment of tetrahydrobiopterin deficiency. *J. inher. metab. Dis.* **8**, Suppl. I, 39–45.

STANBURY J.B., WYNGARDEN J.B., FREDRICKSON D.S., GOLDSTEIN J.L. & BROWN M.S. (1983) *The Metabolic Basis of Inherited Disease*, 5th edition. New York: McGraw-Hill.

SUTHERLAND B.S., UMBARGER B. & BERRY H.K. (1966) The treatment of phenylketonuria: a decade of results. *Amer. J Dis. Child.* **111**, 505.

TASHIAN R.E. (1961) Inhibition of brain glutamic acid decarboxylase by phenalanine, valine and leucine derivatives: a suggestion concerning the etiology of the neurological defect in phenylketonuria and branched chain ketonuria. *Metabolism* 10, 393–402.

WALKER V., CLAYTON B.E., ERSSER R.S., FRANCIS D.E.M., LILLY P., SEAKINS J.W.T., SMITH I. & WHITEMAN P.D. (1981) Hyperphenylalaninaemia of various types among three quarters of a million neonates tested in a screening programme. *Arch. Dis. Childh.* 56, 10, 759–64.

Recipes

LOW-PHENYLALANINE COOKING HINTS

Low-phenylalanine recipes can be used to add variety to the diet and to increase the energy content from fat and carbohydrate. Foods containing protein must be excluded; those recipes which contain potato, rice or cream, etc. should be used as part of the phenylalanine allowance in the diet. Recipe booklets are available from the National Society for Phenylketonuria and Allied Disorders and from The Hospital for Sick Children, Phenylketonuria Clinic, for a small fee. The following give guidance in developing suitable recipes and a few examples of recipes are given:

(a)   In place of ordinary flour use a low-protein flour or mix (Table 9.8), most of which can be interchanged in the various recipes. Pure cornflour, arrowroot and custard powder are also suitable. NB Gluten-free flours are not necessarily suitable.

Low-protein mixes and flours are not self-raising, so baking powder or a suitable raising agent is needed in the recipes. Yeast contains phenylalanine so must be measured with care. Low-protein mixes and flours do not brown easily and so care must be taken not to overcook recipes.

To give a better colour add one teaspoon of custard powder, or use brown sugar in place of white in the recipes.

To prevent crumbling of biscuits and pastry it is helpful to knead the mixture well, then refrigerate for 20 minutes before rolling and cutting into shapes.

Yeast bread mixtures are made as a batter and do not require kneading.

(b)   Butter, or any margarine, lard, Shorteen or Trex can be used. Low-fat spreads ('margarines') are not suitable as they contain water, which affects the consistency of most recipes.

All cooking, vegetable and salad oils are suitable for frying or recipes containing oil.

(c)   In place of egg in recipes an egg replacer can be used.

(i)   Ener-G Egg Replacer by Ener-G Foods Inc. is available on mail order from GF Dietary Supplies Limited.

1 teaspoon Ener-G Egg Replacer / 2 tablespoons water } Mix and substitute for each 1 egg in recipe

If a recipe calls for unbeaten eggs, stir Ener-G Egg Replacer into water (do not beat). If a recipe calls for stiffly beaten egg-whites whisk the egg replacer and water with an electric beater until stiff (5 to 15 minutes). If a recipe calls for egg-yolks only, use half the amount of water with the egg replacer for each egg. Other liquids may be substituted for water if preferred.

(ii)   Edifas A (methylethylcellulose) is an alternative egg substitute and is obtainable from ICI Ltd or Bow Products Ltd. Soak 5 g (1/6 oz) Edifas A in 45 ml (1½ oz) hot water; stir. When cold add a further 45 ml (1½ oz) cold water to make 90 ml (3 oz) of Edifas solution.

Use 45 ml, half of the solution, to replace one egg in recipes. If the recipe calls for stiffly beaten egg-whites, whisk the Edifas solution with an electric beater until stiff (5 to 15 minutes).

(d) Low-phenylalanine cakes and biscuits stale quickly. One teaspoon of glycerine per recipe helps them to stay soft longer. Biscuits should be stored in an air-tight tin, cakes in a plastic bag in the refrigerator or air-tight tin or plastic container. Small quantities can be made frequently, e.g. each time the oven is on for other purposes a batch of low-pheny-lalanine cakes or biscuits can be cooked. Low-phenylalanine cakes, biscuits and other dishes can be deep-frozen in small individual packs and used as needed. Biscuits and cookies can be softened by storing in a tin with a few slices of fresh apple.

Low-phenylalanine cakes and biscuits which have become dry can be used to make crumbs for other recipes or in low-phenyla-lanine trifle (low-phenylalanine cake, vege-tarian jelly, fruit and no-protein custard). Low-phenylalanine bread, when dry, can be toasted, fried or used as crumbs for coating in other recipes.

(e) Quick Jel (Greens), Super Cook Jelly Glaze or Vegetarian Jelly (Snowcrest) can be given instead of jelly. The Quick Jel or Jelly Glaze can be made with diluted fruit juice concentrate or natural fruit juices and a little sugar to sweeten.

RECIPES

'No-protein milk' is permitted freely in the diet.

100 ml (3½ oz) water
10 ml (1/3 oz) Prosparol or Calogen or permitted brand non-dairy imitation cream
2 level (5 ml) tsp sugar

This 'milk' can be used on cereals, for custard and for drinks, milk-shakes and in tea or coffee.

To make custard use 1 to 2 teaspoons ordinary custard powder, e.g. Bird's, to the above recipe and cook in the usual way. Sweeten and flavour to taste.

Some brands of instant whips (vanilla and fruit flavours) are permitted but should usually be made with half the suggested quantity of no-protein milk to ensure a better final consistency of the recipe.

Soda bread—basic recipe

480 g (16 oz) Rite-Diet Low-Protein Flour
90 g (3 oz) margarine or butter
1 tsp sugar
1 tsp salt
1 level tbsp baking powder
½ pint water, approximately

Sift all dry ingredients together. Rub in the butter or margarine. Mix to a soft dough with water—soft enough to handle. Turn on to a floured table, knead very lightly, cut into three. Cook each third in a small log tin for 30 minutes. Oven temperature 160° C (325° F, regulo 3).

Basic recipe for bread

450 g (1 packet) Juvela Low-Protein Mix
30 g (1 oz) fresh baker's yeast or 1 sachet yeast from Juvela Mix or 7 g (¼ oz) dried yeast
400 ml (14 oz) water
55 g (2 oz) permited margarine or butter
½ to 1 tsp salt

The 'Mix' and margarine should be at room temperature. Place crumbled fresh yeast or dried yeast into a mixing bowl. Warm the water to about 40° C (105° F), 'blood' heat. Pour the water over the yeast. Stir until the yeast dissolves. Add 'Mix', margarine and salt. Beat for 1 minute with an electric mixer if using dried yeast, for 3 to 4 minutes for fresh yeast. Overbeating can cause a 'holey' dough. If salt is omitted from the dough, beat at a low speed. Divide the dough into two greased (with oil) loaf tins, tin size 9" × 4½" × 2½" or 25 cm × 12 cm × 6 cm. Cover tin with a clean cloth and let the dough rise in a warm, draughtproof place for 20 to 30 minutes (i.e. double in size). Bake in a hot oven, 220° C (425° F, regulo 9), for about 20 minutes for the two loaves, 25 minutes for the double loaf. Brush with hot water immediately after baking, let the bread cool under a baking cloth. To bake only one loaf, the ingredients may be halved. The bread can also be frozen.

Chapatis (unleaven bread cooked on griddle)

125 g (4 oz) Juvela Low-Protein Mix
30 g (1 oz) margarine or butter or ghee
Water to make a dough

Knead into dough as for ordinary chapatis. Divide into balls and roll into chapatis. Cook as for ordinary chapatis. Other low-protein flour or mix may be used instead of Juvela.

Sponge buns using Rite-Diet Low-Protein Flour or Mix

150 g (6 oz) granulated sugar
300 g (11 oz) Rite-Diet Low-Protein Flour or Mix
50 g (2 oz) butter or margarine
$\frac{1}{4}$ tsp vanilla essence or grated lemon or orange rind
2 tsp baking powder
Water to mix
Additions. 50 g (2 oz) candied peel, glacé icing or jam and permitted 'imitation' whipped cream.

Cream butter and sugar together until light. Blend together the water and half the flour, and add to the creamed mixture. Add the flavouring. Sift the rest of the flour with the baking powder, add to the batter. Place half the mixture in big heaped teaspoons in 12 paper baking cases. Add candied peel to the rest of the mixture and spoon into 12 more paper cases. Bake for 15 to 20 minutes in oven, 190° C (375° F, regulo 5).

To serve. Mix 150 g (6 oz) icing sugar with a little water or lemon or orange juice. Cover

buns with icing and decorate with a glacé cherry. The plain buns can have a 'lid' removed with a teaspoon when cold. Place a small teaspoon of jam inside and top with a spoonful of permitted 'imitation' whipped non-dairy cream. Replace 'lid' lightly, dust with castor sugar.

Apple cake

$\frac{1}{2}$ large cup sugar
60 g (2 oz) Trex or margarine
180 g (6 oz) Low-Protein Flour or Mix
$\frac{1}{2}$ cup cold tea
2 large cooking apples
$1\frac{1}{2}$ tsp baking powder
$\frac{1}{2}$ tsp bicarbonate of soda

Put sugar, tea and Trex or margarine into pan and heat until boiling. Cool. Stir in dry ingredients, sifted, and add the peeled and chopped apples (chopped not grated). Put in greased $6\frac{1}{2}$" tin. Cook in slow to moderate oven, 160° C (325° F, regulo 3), for 1 to $1\frac{1}{2}$ hours.

Fruit cake (Christmas and birthdays)

120 g Juvela Low-Protein Mix
100 g margarine or butter
2 tsp mixed spice
100 g brown sugar
75 g sultanas, raisins, mixed peel
20 g glacé cherries (no nuts) chopped
2 tsp Ener-G Egg Replacer
4 tbsp (120 ml) water
2 tsp baking powder

Cream margarine, or butter, and sugar. Mix Ener-G Egg Replacer with water; add to margarine and sugar. Add other ingredients. Mix well. Cook for approximately 1 hour at 190° C (375° F, regulo 5).

Ice with 'butter icing' using margarine and icing sugar, or water icing. A little almond essence may be added to the icing. Decorate with appropriate motif.

Meringues (an electric beater is essential)

30 ml (1 oz) Edifas A solution (*see* cooking
   hints, p. 258)
plus 30 ml (1 oz) cold water
90 g (3 oz) castor sugar
Pinch of salt
1 to 2 drops vanilla essence and/or food
   colouring

Mix together the extra-cold water, salt and
Edifas A solution. Beat in an electric mixer
to form a very stiff foam (about 15 to 20
minutes). Gradually add half castor sugar
and whisk to a peak. Fold in rest of sugar.
Pipe onto greaseproof paper, dust with a
little castor sugar. Dry in a slow oven,
140° C (275° F, regulo 1), until crisp and dry
(1 to 2 hours). Lift off the paper and store
in an airtight tin. They will keep for weeks if
really dry before storing. They can be left in
an airing cupboard overnight to dry out
thoroughly.

Rice Krispies cake*

4 level tbsps honey or syrup
15 g ($\frac{1}{2}$ oz) castor sugar
15 g ($\frac{1}{2}$ oz) margarine or butter
90 g (3 oz) Rice Krispies

Melt honey or syrup, sugar and margarine or
butter in a saucepan. Bring to boil and boil
for 2 minutes. Remove saucepan from the
heat source and add Rice Krispies. Mix well.
Turn into 7" square tin and then press down
firmly with the hand. Allow to cool and then
cut into 12 equal bars. Alternatively, divide
equally between 12 paper cases.

* *Important note.* Each one cake (1/12th) or 7 g ($\frac{1}{4}$ oz)
Rice Krispies is approximately equal to 25 mg
phenylalanine or half a 50 mg phenylalanine exchange.

Ice-cream

150 mg (5 oz) permitted non-dairy
   'imitation' cream
120 ml (4 oz) Edifas A solution (*see* cooking
   hints, p. 258)

120 g (4 oz) granulated sugar
180 ml (6 oz) water
Flavouring, e.g. vanilla, lemon juice, fruit
   Nesquik, blackcurrant juice, etc.

Boil granulated sugar in water to form sugar
syrup of thin thread consistency, but which
is still colourless. Cool. Whisk the Edifas
solution to a thick foam and add to the
sugar mixture, then freeze. When soft-frozen
place in the bowl of an electric mixer and
whisk until white, thick and frothy. Add
cream and whisk well until thick. Add
flavouring. Freeze in freezing compartment
of refrigerator on maximum cold, or in a
freezer until set.

Gravy

150 ml (5 oz) vegetable stock or tomato
   juice
1 to 2 tsp cornflour
1 to 2 drops gravy browning* or $\frac{1}{4}$ teaspoon
   tomato paste
Salt, pepper, herbs to season

Mix cornflour to a paste with a little cold
water. Add to stock and bring to the boil.
Season.
Variations. (i) Slightly brown cornflour on
a tray in the oven and use to give a better
colour. (ii) Make a browned roux with
permitted vegetable margarine or oil and
cornflour, then add vegetable stock and
seasoning and boil for 1 to 2 minutes. Strain
and serve.

* *Note.* Gravy mixes and granules are not suitable.

Savoury sauce

150 ml (5 oz) water
15 ml ($\frac{1}{2}$ oz) Prosparol or Calogen
15 g ($\frac{1}{2}$ oz) cornflour
30 ml (1 oz) vegetable oil
2 peppercorns
1 bay leaf
1 tsp chopped onion
Salt to season

Put the water in a pan with the onion, peppercorns and bay leaf. Heat gently for about 5 minutes. Mix Prosparol/Calogen with the oil and cornflour. Strain heated water into the cornflour mixture, stirring all the time. Return to the heat and stir until thick. A small pinch of mustard or turmeric will colour the sauce slightly. Herbs or other spices may be added as appropriate.

Macaroni without cheese

Savoury sauce as recipe above
60 g (2 oz) raw low-protein macaroni

(Aproten or Aglutella or Rite Diet)
1 to 2 tomatoes, or $\frac{1}{2}$ small tin of tomatoes
Low-protein breadcrumbs or biscuit crumbs
Salt and pepper to season

Cook macaroni in boiling water and salt for 6 to 8 minutes. Drain. Mix with savoury sauce. Put half in the bottom of a small greased dish. Cover with a layer of sliced tomato. Put remainder of macaroni on top. Sprinkle with low-protein breadcrumbs and sliced tomato. Bake for about 15 minutes at 190° C (375° F, regulo 5).

CHAPTER 10

Dietary management of disorders of amino acid metabolism, organic acidaemias and urea cycle defects

INTRODUCTION

An increasing number of inborn errors of metabolism, and variants of the disorders associated with protein, amino acids, and their degradation, have been recognized. Tremendous progress has been made in the understanding and diagnosis of this rare group of disorders, but new variants and treatment are continually being described (Scriver & Rosenburg 1973, Stanbury *et al.* 1983) and have recently been reviewed by Collins and Leonard (1985), and Lloyd and Scriver (1985).

Concentrations of amino acids and their metabolites in blood, tissues, brain, urine and faeces remain within well-defined physiological limits in healthy individuals (Clayton *et al.* 1980). They are disturbed by inherited enzyme defects, membrane transport mechanisms specifically concerned with amino acid metabolism or by secondary disturbances due to other disorders, e.g. liver disease or transient defects in early infancy. Abnormal accumulation of compounds does not usually occur until their intake or production after birth exceeds the infant's capacity to metabolize or excrete them. This usually takes several days, depending upon the type and severity of the defect and also upon the volume and composition of the diet, particularly the intake of the dietary substrate of the abnormal metabolite(s).

The clinical features of each inborn error are usually very variable and rarely specific. There are many causes for this variation. Each phenotype is commonly caused by a number of genetically distinct variants (Lloyd & Scriver 1985). The residual activity of the enzyme also varies; those with more enzyme activity have milder disease than those with low enzyme activity, who have the severe disease. The disorders are transmitted, with few exceptions, by Mendelian recessive inheritance. All are rare, though their incidence varies with the disease and from one population to another.

These disorders commonly present in the neonatal period with acute clinical deterioration due to accumulation of toxic metabolites, though some patients with milder or variant forms of the same disorder may not present until later in childhood (Leonard *et al.* 1984, Collins & Leonard 1985). Clinical emergencies often arise due to intercurrent infections and catabolism causing metabolic relapse.

The true incidence of these disorders, apart from phenylketonuria (*see* Chapter 9), is largely unknown. Although at present only a few institutionalized, retarded patients can be shown to have a definite biochemical abnormality, it is possible that further advances may lead to diagnosis and preventive therapy in a percentage of infants with biochemical disorders which, if untreated, would lead to mental retardation (Efron 1967).

Enzyme replacement therapy is largely not available for the inborn errors of protein metabolism, bone marrow and liver transplantation is not yet feasible for the majority of patients, and genetic engineering is still in its infancy (Hobbs 1981, Whiteman *et al.* 1983, Lloyd & Scriver 1985). Prenatal diagnosis, with the chance of a medical abortion, is now possible for a number of disorders, once the index case has been identified in a family (Stanbury *et al.* 1983).

Treatment requires an understanding of both normal nutrition requirements and the biochemistry of the defect. The principal strategies are:

1 Dietary reduction of substrate(s), frequently protein or specific amino acids, associated with the formation of the toxic metabolite(s).

2 Replacement of essential nutrients that are deficient as a result of the metabolic block, e.g. arginine in ornithine carbamyltransferase deficiency.

3 Cofactor therapy: pharmacological doses (up to 100 times the nutrient requirement) of specific vitamins to induce non-functional enzyme activity (Scriver & Rosenberg 1973, Collins & Leonard 1985).

4 Enhancement of excretion or product utilization to form non-toxic metabolite, e.g. sodium

benzoate and/or phenylacetate, to conjugate and enhance removal of ammonia in the urea cycle defects, arginine to enhance citrulline production in citrullinaemia, thus removing the more toxic ammonia (Brusilow 1985) and glycine in isovaleric acidaemia (Velazquez & Prieto 1980). 5 Essential amino acids and their analogues have been used to induce waste nitrogen utilization in conjunction with protein restriction in renal failure and the urea cycle defects with varying success (Close 1974, Batshaw *et al.* 1976, Brusilow 1985).

Treatment may be effective in reversing or preventing the consequences of the abnormality if started early enough. The choice of therapy depends on the enzyme defect and its consequences, but must be constructed to allow the infant to grow and develop normally. The main disorders and their current dietary treatments are summarized in Table 10.1. Only the disorders with dietary implications are discussed in this text. The important lessons learnt from the experience gained in the dietary treatment of phenylketonuria should be applied to the dietary treatment of the other amino acid disorders to prevent the nutritional and sociopsychological complications which can arise from treatment. These aspects are already dealt with in Chapter 9 and should be referred to as appropriate and used in conjunction with the information in this chapter.

Table 10.1 Summary of amino acid and urea cycle disorders.

Disorder	Amino acid(s) involved	Typical clinical features of untreated classical disorders*	Dietary regimen to correct biochemical abnormality—details in text
Phenylketonuria (*see* Chapter 9)			
(a) Phenylalanine hydroxylase deficiency	Phenylalanine	Mental retardation, fair hair, eczema, convulsions, tremor	Low phenylalanine; tyrosine supplements.
(b) Defects of tetrahydrobiopterin	Phenylalanine and neurotransmitter amines	Neurological abnormalities	As above plus tetrahydrobiopterin†, neurotransmitter precursors: dopa and 5-hydroxytryptophan.
Tyrosinaemia—hereditary type I	Tyrosine, phenylalanine ± methionine	Liver and renal dysfunction, rickets, chronic 'Fanconi' syndrome	Low tyrosine, phenylalanine ± methionine; cyst(e)ine supplements.
Tyrosinaemia—tyrosine amino transferase deficiency	Tyrosine, phenylalanine	Skin and eye disorders with or without mental retardation	Low tyrosine, phenylalanine.
Hawkinsinuria	Tyrosine	Dominant abnormality giving acute illness in infants	Vitamin C (1 g/day).
Maple syrup urine disease (MSUD) (several variants also occur—*see* text)	Leucine, isoleucine, valine and their ketoacids	Neurological abnormalities, feeding problems, ketoacidosis Smell of maple syrup in urine Episodic encephalopathy particularly with infections Mental retardation	Low leucine, isoleucine and valine. Emergency protein-free high-energy regimen during infections.

Table 10.1 *continued*

Disorder	Amino acid(s) involved	Typical clinical features of untreated classical disorders*	Dietary regimen to correct biochemical abnormality—details in text
Organic acidaemias Commonest (a) Propionic acidaemia (b) Methylmalonic acidaemia	Degradation of isoleucine, valine, theonine and methionine	May present: 1 Neonate—overwhelming illness, neurological abnormalities, acidosis 2 Infancy—failure to thrive, vomiting and retardation. 3 Older—intermittent acidosis 4 Mental retardation	Low-protein diet. Emergency protein-free high-energy regimen during infections.

There are many other organic acidaemias: *see* Table 10.3 for specific disorders and their treatment.

Disorder	Amino acid(s) involved	Typical clinical features of untreated classical disorders*	Dietary regimen to correct biochemical abnormality—details in text
Urea cycle disorders (i) Carbamyl phosphate synthetase deficiency—type I hyperammonaemia (ii) Ornithine carbamyltransferase (OCT)—type II hyper-ammonaemia (iii) Citrullinaemia—arginosuccinic acid synthetase deficiency (iv) Arginosuccinic acid lyase deficiency—arginosuccinic aciduria	Protein degradation Hyperammonaemia	May present: 1 Neonate—often lethal due to ammonia intoxication 2 Infancy—vomiting, anorexia with particularly protein intolerance 3 Older—intermittent drowsiness, behaviour problems, neurological abnormalities 4 Chronic—mental retardation, neurological abnormalities	Low-protein diet; arginine supplements. Sodium benzoate (*see* text). Emergency protein-free high-energy regimen during infections.
(v) Argininaemia—arginase deficiency	Arginine Protein degradation, hyperammonaemia	Spasticity and developmental regression	Very low-arginine and protein diet. Supplements of essential amino acids without arginine. Sodium benzoate (*see* text). Emergency protein-free high-energy regimen during infections.
(vi) Ornithine ketoacid transferase deficiency (vii) *N*-acetylglutamate synthetase deficiency		Similar to urea cycle disorders (i)–(iv) above	

Table 10.1 *continued*

Disorder	Amino acid(s) involved	Typical clinical features of untreated classical disorders*	Dietary regimen to correct biochemical abnormality—details in text
Hyperornithinaemia	Ornithine	Gyrate atrophy of the choroid and retina. Blindness	Low-arginine diet and/or proline supplements (*see* text).
Congenital lysine intolerance	Lysine and arginine	Ammonia intoxication, growth failure, neutropenia Mental retardation	Low-protein diet; citrulline supplements.
Hartnup disease	Normal blood amino acids Defective transport of the neutral amino acids, including tryptophan Neutral aminoaciduria	Pellagra-type rash, ataxia in some patients	Large doses of nictonamide (niacin) in those with pellagra-like complication.
Homocystinuria—cystathionine synthetase deficiency	Homocystine in blood and urine Methionine	Dislocated lenses Skeletal abnormalities Thrombosis Mental retardation	(i) Pyridoxine and folic acid in vitamin-responsive disorder. (ii) Low-methionine; cyst(e)ine supplements plus vitamin B_6 and folic acid.
Cystathioninuria (inherited and neonatal)	Low cystine, high methionine	Probably harmless	Large doses of vitamin B_6 and adequate dietary cystine.
Neonatal transient hypermethioninaemia	Methionine $\pm$ generalized hyperaminoacidaemia	No clinical symptoms May indicate underlying liver disease	Breast-feeds or whey-based modified milk, i.e. normal protein intake with adequate cystine.
Histidinaemia	Histidine	Enormous variation from 'normal' to mental retardation	Histidine restriction‡ (diet may in fact not be indicated—*see* text).

* Clinical features are very variable and rarely specific; *see* further details in text.
† Role in treatment still being evaluated (Smith 1985); *see also* Table 10.3.
‡ Effect of diet still unproven.

Dietary protein

Protein is digested, then absorbed, as either free amino acids or small peptides, into the mucosal cells where digestion is completed. Specific transport mechanisms are involved in the movement of free L-amino acids across cell membranes both in the bowel and similarly in the renal tubules. Impaired transport can lead to increased faecal and urinary amino acid losses, but these relatively small losses are not usually of nutritional importance, e.g. in cystinuria and Hartnup disease. The high tissue levels of one amino acid can inhibit the transport of other amino acids sharing the same transport system, e.g.

in phenylketonuria. Bacterial action on unabsorbed amino acids produces various metabolites, including ammonia, organic acids and amines, which are absorbed and then detoxified by the liver. Increased production, as for example in amino acid transport defects and various malabsorption syndromes, can lead to an increase of these products in the blood and subsequently they can contribute to clinical symptoms, for example ammonia in urea cycle defects or liver failure.

After absorption, amino acids reach the liver and are either used for protein synthesis, or are degraded for ATP production, gluconeogenesis or lipogenesis (Fig. 10.1). Urea represents the main end product of

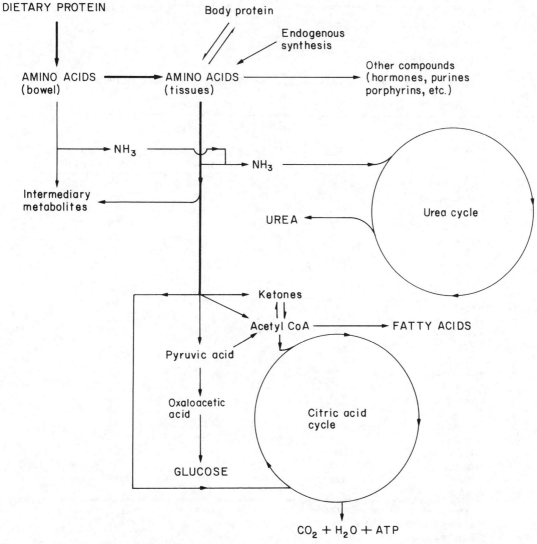

Fig. 10.1 Fate of dietary protein. From Smith & Francis (1982).

nitrogen metabolism. The urea cycle defects and amino acid disorders are due to a deficiency of the specific enzyme(s) or their cofactors needed for amino acid degradation.

Starvation, infections and catabolic states generally stimulate gluconeogenesis and increase the proportion of amino acids for degradation in the liver. In amino acid disorders this gives rise to a further, sometimes dangerous, increase in compounds, which may be toxic. Acute clinical deterioration can follow.

Blood amino acids

Values for plasma and urine amino acids for infants and children are given in Table 10.2 from Clayton *et al.* (1980). These are influenced by hormones such as insulin and glucagon and reflect the balance between absorption, utilization, endogenous production and degradation (Munro 1970). Ingestion of protein on its own causes a two- to three-fold rise in fasting levels, with a peak at 3 to 4 hours and return to baseline in 6 to 8 hours in normal individuals. A smaller rise occurs if protein and carbohydrate are given simultaneously. Liver failure results in an elevation of amino acids, with the exception of leucine, isoleucine and valine, which are predominantly degraded in striated muscle.

Amino acids in fetal and cord blood are slightly elevated by a factor of 1·5 to 3 (Lindblad 1976). These levels are maintained for several weeks in the infant who is breast-fed *ad libitum* (Pohlandt 1978). A fast after delivery causes a fall in essential amino

Table 10.2   Reference range of plasma and urine amino acids. From Clayton *et al.* (1980).

(a) Plasma amino acids (μmol/l)*.

	Molecular weight	Birth to 3 months. Maximum concentration	3 months to 14 years Non-fasting Mean	1 SD	Fasting Mean	1 SD
Taurine‡	125	256	78	31	59	12
Aspartic acid	133	100	81	46	25	6
Threonine†	119	336	149	34	138	31
Serine	105	324	188	50	99	19
Asparagine	132	52	60	15	56	15
Glutamic acid	147	142	68	31	34	15
Glutamine	146	960	690	73	640	58
Proline	115	435	185	48	183	39
Glycine	75	515	243	73	234	44
Alanine	89	675	328	76	320	71
Citrulline	175	63	45	12	35	8
α-Aminobutyric	103	40	25	8	20	6
Valine†	117	370	213	57	225	40
Cystine‡	240	92	67	20	49	9
Methionine†	149	96	41	18	21	4
Isoleucine†	131	105	59	18	60	12
Leucine†	131	230	141	41	115	23
Tyrosine	181	196	67	16	54	11
Phenylalanine†	165	182	77	28	48	7
Histidine‡	155	195	109	59	88	16
Tryptophan†‡	204	70	53	23	31	6
Ornithine	132	214	65	19	58	14
Lysine†	146	316	196	43	186	36
Arginine‡	174	155	80	24	82	17

All other amino acids—concentration less than 25 μmol/l.

* Plasma μmol/l × molecular weight ÷ 10^4 = mg/100 ml.

† Essential amino acids.

‡ Semi-essential amino acids in infants and young children.

Table 10.2 *continued*

(b)   Urine amino acids (μmol/mmol creatinine)*

	Molecular weight	Birth to 3 months. Maximum value	3 months to 2 years. Maximum value	2 to 14 years range
Taurine	125	54	106	37 to 162
Aspartic acid	133	46	36	7 to 30
Threonine	119	45	46	11 to 25
Serine	105	95	97	25 to 51
Asparagine	132	25	15	0 to 6
Glutamic acid	147	14	3	0 to 3
Glutamine	146	118	120	34 to 89
Proline	115	110	0	0
Glycine	75	950	617	113 to 542
Alanine	89	127	78	23 to 71
Citrulline	175	16	8	1 to 7
α-Aminobutyric	103	21	8	2 to 8
Valine	117	12	7	1 to 7
Cystine	240	36	24	4 to 15
Methionine	149	30	12	2 to 9
Isoleucine	131	39	8·6	1 to 6
Leucine	131	18	9·1	2 to 11
Tyrosine	181	31	16	5 to 15
Phenylalanine	165	19	15	4 to 17
Histidine	155	156	299	47 to 328
Tryptophan	204	15	4·6	1 to 8
Ornithine	132	12	10	2 to 8
Lysine	146	18	30	7 to 29
Arginine	174	16	10	3 to 11
α-Aminoadipic	161	12	8.7	1 to 8
β-Aminoisobutyric	103	60	47	2 to 50
Ethanolamine	61	80	20	2 to 25

* Urine μmol/24 hours $\times$ molecular weight $\div$ 10^3 = mg/24 hours.

Notes

1   In the newborn, and particularly in the premature infant, excessively high protein intake or immaturity of the enzymes in the liver may cause elevated concentrations of plasma amino acids. For this reason, a maximum value for the age group birth to 0·25 years is given in the table.

2   In premature infants a generalized amino aciduria (up to five times that of the adult) is physiological and in full-term infants the excretion of amino acids is more pronounced than in adults. For this reason, it is not unusual for laboratories working mainly with specimens from adults to report an amino aciduria in an infant when in fact the excretion and pattern are normal for its age.

acids, but glycine rises, and after a prolonged fast or where there has been placental insufficiency the amino acid pattern simulates that seen in protein–energy malnutrition. The introduction of feeds causes the essential amino acid levels to rise, but in infants fed low-protein formulae or pooled breast milk the blood amino acid levels never reach those of cord blood (Smith & Francis 1982). A high protein intake can elevate amino acid levels to many times normal, particularly in the neonate, and such levels may persist for weeks or months (Snyderman *et al.* 1968). The increased incidence, in recent years, of breast-feeding, and the use of modified milks, with their lower protein content, have considerably reduced the number of infants identified in the screening programme with transient neonatal amino acid disorders associated with enzyme immaturity (Walker *et al.* 1981). Elevated amino acids may be transient, due to an enzyme defect or underlying liver disease, and should be investigated. Because of the possible significance of elevated amino acids on the ultimate intelligence of the child (Menkes *et al.* 1972, Goldman *et al.* 1974, Mamumes *et al.* 1976) it is important to prevent and correct transient amino acid disorders by appropriate infant feeding practice (Francis 1986). The more severe transient disorders may require temporary treatment with a low-protein diet and/or relevant co-factor therapy, e.g. vitamin C in transient neonatal tyrosinaemia, arginine in transient hyperammon-aemia.

Clinical presentation and diagnosis

Screening programmes used for the detection of phenylketonuria and congenital hypothyroidism have been extended to include various amino acid disorders in some centres (Buist & Jhaveri 1973, Bickel *et al.* 1980, Naylor 1981). In other cases, clinical presentation, frequently in the first few days of life, will initiate investigation. Poor feeding, drow-siness, acidosis, and respiratory distress leading to coma and death may occur if immediate medical in-tervention is not taken. An unusual or characteristic smell, such as occurs in maple syrup urine disease, or the smell of sweaty feet in isovaleric acidaemia, can be a useful indicator and is often strongest first thing in the morning following the overnight 'fast'. A urine test, although not specific, can be useful, e.g. ferric chloride gives a colour change in a number of amino acid disorders, including phenylketonuria and maple syrup urine disease, and 2, 4-dinitrophenylhydra-zones can be used to test for ketoacids. Biochemical estimation of amino acids and their metabolites in serum and urine is essential, as is an acute rapid service, in establishing the diagnosis and thus start-ing treatment.

In the organic acidaemias the clinical presentation is not specific, the amino acids in plasma are not diagnostic as those involved in the metabolic block are not always elevated, depending on the position of the enzyme defect, and the metabolic pattern in the plasma and urine does not necessarily show whether the defect is in the enzyme or coenzyme.

Infants with amino acid disorders who are breast-fed tend to have a lower elevation of the amino acid(s) or metabolite(s) concerned than those fed higher protein feeds, because human milk provides the correct proportion and quantity of the amino acids for the infant's needs. Breast-feeding may there-fore delay the onset of symptoms (Smith & Francis 1982). Children who present with these disorders

after the neonatal period commonly have develop-mental delay, neurological abnormalities, failure to thrive or intermittent symptoms secondary to meta-bolic derangement (metabolic acidosis, hypoglyc-aemia or hyperammonaemia) (Leonard *et al.* 1984).

Some children have a variant or intermittent form of their disease and may present as late as school age, e.g. the variant form of maple syrup urine disease. These children may develop with normal intelligence, on a normal diet, as long as they survive the acute episodes which frequently accompany infections or other catabolic states. In certain of these disorders, episodes of metabolic acidosis require accurate, rapid diagnosis in the acute phase in order to initiate life-saving therapy (Gretter *et al.* 1972, Brusilow 1985).

NUTRITIONAL MANAGEMENT

Cofactor therapy

Some vitamins are the precursors or specific cofactors required by the enzymes concerned with amino acid degradation (Scriver & Rosenberg 1973). An inher-ited defect in the conversion of a vitamin to the active cofactor can cause a vitamin-dependent disorder. Structural abnormalities in the protein or apoenzyme portion of the holoenzyme can impair its ability to bind with its coenzyme required for functional ac-tivity. Often the binding defect is not absolute, and the apoenzyme retains some binding capacity at ab-normally high tissue levels of the coenzyme. How-ever, it is not clear by what mechanism other vitamin-dependent disorders respond to pharmacol-ogical doses of the appropriate vitamin. Primary de-ficiency of such a vitamin can lead to an amino acid disturbance which is corrected by normal doses of the appropriate vitamin, e.g. biotin deficiency can si-mulate propionic acidaemia (Mock *et al.* 1981).

Identification of the increased or abnormal meta-bolite(s) may indicate the possibility of vitamin or cofactor therapy. Table 10.3 summarizes the well-recognized vitamin-responsive disorders. Of the nutri-tional strategies available for the treatment of meta-bolic disease, cofactor therapy is by far the safest and simplest for the patient; when the disorder is fully responsive it is also the most effective treatment (Pul-lon 1980, Batshaw *et al.* 1981) and diet is unneces-sary. In other patients it allows a more generous dietary intake of protein. Newly diagnosed patients should always be given a trial of cofactor therapy if the condition is known to have a cofactor-responsive variant (Gompertz 1972, Collins & Leonard 1985). It

Table 10.3 Amino acid and urea cycle disorders.
    (a) Vitamin/cofactor.
    (b) Essential amino acid supplement(s) required in the classical disorder.

Disorder	(a) * Vitamin/cofactor	Dose (mg per day)	(b) † Amino acid supplement
Phenylketonuria	—	—	Tyrosine†
(a) Phenylalanine hydroxy-lase deficiency			
(b) Tetrahydrobiopterin defects			
(i) Defects of synthesis of tetrahydrobiopterin	Tetrahydrobiopterin‡	1 to 2 mg/kg per day	Tyrosine† plus neuro-transmitter precursors: dopa and 5-hydroxytryptophan
(ii) Dihydrobiopterin reductase deficiency	Tetrahydrobiopterin‡ plus tetrahydrofolates as folinic acid‡	5 to 6 mg kg per day	
Neonatal tyrosinaemia	Vitamin C	50 to 100	—
Hawkinsinuria	Vitamin C	1000	—
Homocystinuria (classical)	Pyridoxine (usually given with folic acid)	100 to 500 B$_6$ *plus* 10 to 20 folic acid	Cyst(e)ine† in those requiring a low-methionine diet
Cystathioninuria			—
Hyperoxaluria	Pyridoxine	50 to 500	
Xanthurenic aciduria			
Hartnup disease with pellagra	Niacin	100 to 250	—
Maple syrup urine disease (variant)	Thiamine	10 to 20	
Methylmalonic acidaemia			Bicarbonate§
	B$_{12}$	1 to 3	
Congenital B$_{12}$ malabsorption			—
β-methylcrotonylglycinuria			
Multiple carboxylase deficiency (biotinidase deficiency)	Biotin		
		10	—
Holocarboxylase synthetase deficiency			
Dicarboxylic aciduria	Riboflavin	300	—
Ornithine carbamyltransferase deficiency	—	—	Arginine† in those requiring protein restriction. Sodium benzoate§
Citrullinaemia	—	—	Arginine† in large doses§. Sodium benzoate§
Arginosuccinic aciduria	—	—	
Neonatal hyperammonaemia	—	—	Arginine temporarily†
Isovaleric acidaemia	—	—	Glycine§, L-carnitine

* These supplements are in excess of normal nutritional requirements.
† Amino acid which becomes essential due to the specific metabolic block.
‡ Still being evaluated.
§ Aids removal of toxic metabolites by conversion to a less toxic metabolite or by enhancing excretion (*see* text).

can be difficult to distinguish the effect of cofactor response from other therapeutic measures given simultaneously and therefore cofactor therapy should be reassessed subsequently when the patient is in a stable metabolic state (Collins & Leonard 1985). It may be found that a combination of cofactor therapy and dietary modification is required to maintain the patient in metabolic balance. The best index of cofactor effectiveness is the tolerance of the subject to the offending nutrients on and off cofactor therapy (Collins & Leonard 1985, Leonard & Daish 1985).

General principles of dietary treatment

A block in amino acid degradation leads to accumulation of the substrate amino acid and/or its metabolites if there is a continued supply of amino acid to the abnormal pathway. Dietary protein provides the essential, and is the major source of non-essential, amino acids for protein synthesis; those in excess of growth and metabolic needs are degraded primarily by the liver. A small irreducible quantity of nitrogen is produced from normal metabolism and increases during catabolism (Fig. 10.1).

A reduction in dietary protein or restriction of the specific amino acid(s) concerned can often prevent accumulation of the metabolite(s) and forms the basis of treatment, together with supplements of appropriate amino acids that become essential as a result of the metabolic block (Table 10.3). Diet will only benefit symptoms secondary to accumulation of compounds caused by the biochemical abnormality; it will not correct disorders in which the compound is mainly or totally produced by endogenous synthesis, e.g. hydroxyproline in hydroxyprolinaemia (Smith & Francis 1982). Diets in which protein intake is limited are potentially hazardous, and their use must be carefully weighed against the seriousness of the untreated disease.

The treatment of enzyme deficiency disorders of the amino acids mostly has to be continued for life, and therefore the prescribed diet must be adequate in all nutrients for growth and development whilst the nutrient(s) the child has limited ability to metabolize must be restricted. These patients may have different requirements of nutrients to normal individuals and require different nutrients which become essential (Acosta 1982, 1985). The degree of dietary protein restriction necessary will depend on both the particular inborn error and the severity of the metabolic block. It may be necessary to combine the reduction in dietary protein with modification of the amino acid profile.

When growth and nutrition are optimal, tolerance will be maximal for protein or the specific amino acid(s) concerned with the metabolic block. Any deficiency of an essential nutrient will limit growth and increase the load on the degradation pathways, and thus protein tolerance will decrease. Growth rate is at a maximum in early infancy and therefore protein tolerance for weight is at its greatest at that age. It varies from time to time in the same child according to natural variation in growth rate, due to increased growth velocity at different ages, and decreased growth or weight loss associated with infections and other catabolic states. Variation in tolerance also depends on residual enzyme activity and the contribution of cofactor(s), particularly in those with the variant disorders. It is therefore essential to modify the diet for each patient and monitor the intake regularly so that growth, clinical status and biochemical findings are satisfactory.

The intake of protein tolerated is determined not only by the need for protein synthesis and essential anabolic processes, but by the biological value of the protein, determined by the adequacy of its essential amino acid content and the total nitrogen supplied. The non-essential amino acids or their synthesis from an alternative nitrogen source may even be the limiting nutrient(s) for growth (Holt 1967, Bessman 1979, Acosta 1982). The requirement of protein (see Table 8.2) and essential amino acids (Table 10.4) must normally be provided in the diet. Total nitrogen requirement may be lower than normal for infants with organic acidaemias and urea cycle defects. Recommendations for non-essential amino acid intakes have not been firmly established. However, some infants cannot synthesize specific non-essential amino acids, or the rate of synthesis may not be rapid enough for normal growth, therefore at least in infancy all the major dietary amino acids should be provided in diets based on crystalline amino acids, ideally in the same proportions in which they are found in human milk (Table 10.5), as this profile is considered optimal for infant nutrition. In diets in which the nitrogen moiety is supplied only as essential amino acids, amounts greater than generally recommended are necessary to supply nitrogen for the synthesis of the non-essential amino acids. In addition to the eight amino acids considered essential, cyst(e)ine and taurine are at least semi-essential for the neonate, especially when delivered prematurely, and for an unknown period after birth (Pohlandt 1974, Gaull et al. 1977). Histidine is essential for the human infant until about six months of age, at which time the capability to metabolize this amino acid de-

Table 10.4 Amino acid requirement in mg/kg body weight per day.

	Infants		2 to 3		5 to 6		8 to 9		11 to 12		
	(i)	(ii)	(iii)	(iv)	(iii)	(iv)	(iii)	(iv)	(iii)	(iv)	(v)
(a) *Essential amino acids*											
L-Histidine	16 to 34	16 to 34	6·6	0	6	0	3·6	0	4·5	0	0
L-Isoleucine	79 to 110	102 to 119	48·7	88·6	42	80	37·5	71·4	31·5	60	30
L-Leucine	76 to 150	76 to 229*	81·9	155	72	140	64·3	125	54	105	45
L-Lysine	90 to 120	88 to 103	64·2	121·8	56	110	50	98·2	42	82·5	60
L-Methionine	20 to 45	33 to 45	55·4	77·5	50	70	44·6	62·5	37·5	52·5	27
L-Cystine	15 to 50										
L-Phenylalanine	40 to 80	47 to 90	73·1	132·9	66	120	58·9	107·1	49·5	90	27
L-Tyrosine	60 to 80										
L-Threonine	45 to 87	45 to 87	44·3	88·6	38	80	33·9	71·4	28·5	60	35
L-Tryptophan	13 to 22	15 to 22	15·5	22.1	14	20	12·5	17·9	10·5	15	3·3
L-Valine	65 to 105	80 to 105	53·1	110·7	48	100	42·9	89·3	36	75	33
(b) *Probably essential amino acids*											
L-Arginine		50 to 75†									

(i) Acosta (1982).
(ii) Holt (1967).
(iii) Lozy and Hegsted (1975).
(iv) FAO/WHO (1973).
(v) Nakagawa *et al.* (1971).

* Only one infant had a requirement in excess of 150 mg/kg per day (Holt 1967).

† Average content of 100 to 150 ml mature human milk. *See* Table 10.5.

velops (Holt & Snyderman 1965). Proline may be essential in infants on synthetic diets (Harries *et al.* 1971). Arginine may be essential for infants, in patients with urea cycle disorders (except arginase deficiency) and in end-stage liver disease. Arginine and histidine, previously considered non-essential for adults, have been shown to be necessary for long-term feeding on synthetic regimens, due to the limit of biosynthesis in such circumstances (*Nutrition Review* 1970). More recently taurine has received attention, particularly in patients on taurine-free total parenteral nutrition in whom low plasma levels have been documented and deficiency symptoms reported (Cooper *et al.* 1984, Geggel *et al.* 1985), and thus taurine is now considered an essential nutrient, at least in children receiving long-term parenteral nutrition, as well as in neonates.

(A) ALTERATION OF AMINO ACID PATTERN OF DIET

This type of diet is used when the plasma amino acid pattern is specifically altered by the inborn error. The elevated amino acid(s) involved is restricted in relationship to total protein intake, e.g. low-phenylalanine diet used in the treatment of classical phenylketonuria (Chapter 9); low-leucine, -isoleucine and -valine diet in maple syrup urine disease (*see* Table 10.1).

Dietary protein, in small measured quantities, is prescribed to supply the amount of the limiting amino acid(s). Where more than one amino acid is involved, e.g. in maple syrup urine disease, dietary protein supplies the most limiting amino acid, usually leucine, and pure L-amino acids of isoleucine and/or valine are added so that all three can be varied independently, according to biochemical monitoring of the plasma amino acids. Foods naturally low in a specific amino acid may be incorporated in the appropriate diet, e.g. pulses and soya are low in methionine. The prescribed diet should provide the individual's requirement of the restricted essential amino acid(s) for growth and any additional amount the patient can tolerate. The dietary intake of protein is thus titrated against the plasma amino acid levels. However, in some disorders the diet does not prevent continuing

Table 10.5 Amino acid composition of cow's milk, human milk and modified infant formulae (mg/100 ml).

	Cow's milk			Human milk		Modified infant formulae*						
	(i)	(ii)	(iii)	Mature (i)	Transitional (i)	Aptamil	Gold Cap SMA	White Cap SMA	Oster-feed	Prem-ium	Prosobee Soya	Pregestimil, hydrolysed casein and amino acids
(a) Essential amino acids												
L-Histidine	99	23	31	30	47	39	38	42	33	57	42	55
L-Isoleucine	180	86	67	64	99	65	103	80	87	74	84	112
L-Leucine	330	161	120	120	180	156	185	166	143	123	147	188
L-Lysine	270	79	90	86	130	130	156	137	123	104	109	158
L-Methionine	94	23	19	18	28	39	34	29 } 57		36	33†	57
L-Cystine	31	29	25	24	37	39	28	15		24	20	30†
L-Phenylalanine	180	64	48	46	71	65	80	88	62	65	97	87
L-Threonine	160	62	58	54	84	78	105	76	84	80	68	91
L-Tryptophan	47	22	30	28	43	26	27	21	30	18	23	29†
L-Valine	240	90	87	82	130	78	109	101	94	99	84	139
(b) Probably essential amino acids												
L-Arginine	130	51	49	46	71	52	53	66	N/S	43·5	118	74
(c) Non-essential amino acids												
L-Alanine	130	35	52	50	78	65	77	54	N/S	60	N/S	67
L-Aspartic acid	280	116	110	110	170	143	177	137	N/S	128	N/S	148
L-Glutamic acid	750	230	225	210	330	273	344	352	N/S	267	N/S	429
Glycine	73	N/S	32	30	47	39	36	33	N/S	26	N/S	44
L-Proline	310	80	120	120	180	117	150	172	N/S	99	N/S	200
L-Serine	190	69	54	52	81	78	102	104	N/S	83	N/S	116
L-Tyrosine	150	62	38	36	56	52	81	97	N/S	62	75	48†
Protein (g)	3·3	1·2	1·3	1·3	2·0	1·5	1·5	1·5	1·45	1·5	2·0	1·9
kcal	65	65	70	69	67	65	65	65	68	68	67	67
kJ	272	273	296	289	281	273	275	275	284	284	281	282

(i) Paul *et al.* (1980).

(ii) Kan and Cowie (1961).

(iii) *The Composition of Mature Human Milk* (DHSS 1977).

*Calculated from manufacturers' data (1984). Other products may be equally suitable. They must be assessed appropriately for the situation in which they are to be used.

† Fortified with synthetic L-amino acid. Most soya formulae are fortified with methionine.

N/S = not specified.

16 g nitrogen is taken as 100 g protein.

illness, e.g. in hereditary tyrosinaemia type I, restriction of phenylalanine, tyrosine and methionine will correct the plasma amino acids, but the liver damage continues.

The dietary protein is supplemented with amino acids in the form of a protein substitute specific for the disorder being treated, and has a reduced content of the amino acid which cannot be metabolized (Table 10.6). The total nitrogen intake is ideally maintained at an intake sufficient for growth needs. The supplementary amino acids correct the imbalance of amino acids caused by the metabolic block, and should supply any essential products of the degradation pathway.

As the dietary intake is severely reduced the diet may become unbalanced and essential amino acid deficiency can result (*see* p. 275). It is essential to ensure that the diet is nutritionally adequate with respect to energy, vitamins, minerals and essential fatty acids (Table 10.7).

(B) LOW-PROTEIN DIETS

Inborn errors of the catabolism of amino acids which lead to the accumulation not of a specific amino acid but of toxic metabolites such as ammonia require restriction of total protein and a high energy intake, usually provided by supplements. Those patients with the classical form of the disorder tolerate only sufficient protein for growth needs (Nyhan *et al.* 1973) so that there is ideally no excess to be degraded to form the toxic metabolite(s), e.g. propionate in propionic acidaemia. A very low intake of protein or the substrate amino acids concerned in the metabolic block will not only reduce the formation of the toxic metabolite, but will also rapidly lower plasma and tissue concentrations of the precursor amino acid, leading to deficiency and growth failure (Collins & Leonard 1985). An arbitrary protein intake therefore has to be prescribed, as fine control is not possible in most of these disorders. Alternative means of removing the toxic metabolites should be considered (Brusilow 1985). Recommended intakes for minimal and low-protein diet regimes are given in Chapter 8 (Table 8.2) and can be used to devise diets for the treatment of disorders of amino acid degradation. Protein intake and variety, especially of conventional foods, should be as generous as possible, and care must be taken to ensure a balance of essential amino acids and other nutrients. Protein should normally provide ⩾6% of total dietary energy, except temporarily during periods of metabolic relapse. In those who are severely affected, the protein restriction necessary to achieve biochemical control may be too low to support normal growth, e.g. the severely affected male with ornithine carbamyltransferase deficiency, in whom the condition has been invariably fatal to date with present treatment regimens.

(ç) COMBINED LOW-PROTEIN DIET WITH SUPPLEMENTARY AMINO ACIDS

Replacement of part of the conventional protein prescription with essential amino acids, and/or their keto analogues (Table 10.6), a proportion of which are transaminated *in vivo* to form the respective amino acid, permits provision of essential amino acids necessary for growth with a reduced total nitrogen intake. This has proved useful in some children with orni-

thine carbamyltransferase deficiency (Batshaw *et al.* 1976, Brusilow 1985; *see* later).

Certain disorders require limitation of total nitrogen intake, but need supplementation with specific amino acids which become essential or semi-essential as a result of the metabolic block (Table 10.3), e.g. arginine in the urea cycle defects (except for arginase deficiency): thus the low-protein diet is supplemented with arginine (*see* later under the specific disorder).

The value of amino acid supplements (omitting the offending amino acids) in conjunction with a limited total nitrogen intake in the treatment of the organic acidaemias (Satoh *et al.* 1981) requires further evaluation (Collins & Leonard 1985).

Deficiency of amino acids and biochemical monitoring

A fall in plasma amino acid(s) is the first indication of deficiency, and a much reduced amino acid profile in plasma, similar to that observed in protein–energy malnutrition, indicates an inadequate protein intake. Chronic deficiency leads to growth failure and subsequent poor tolerance of protein. Clinicians usually accept slightly higher than normal plasma amino acid and metabolite levels during treatment in most of the amino acid disorders, except in hereditary tyrosinaemia type I (Gagné 1983), and homocystinuria (Collins & Leonard 1985), in order to avoid the devastating effect of deficiency, as illustrated by phenylalanine deficiency (*see* p. 247). Deficiency of other essential amino acids has the same general effect, although abnormalities specific to the amino acid involved may occur (Smith & Francis 1982). Occasional episodes of deficiency occur even in the most carefully managed patients, and must be dealt with urgently, if necessary by hospitalization, or appropriate enteral feeding if associated with food refusal. An immediate increase in natural protein is essential, though caution regarding quantity is necessary in disorders such as maple syrup urine disease, tyrosinaemia, organic acidaemias and urea cycle defects, where acute clinical deterioration can occur following a sudden increase in dietary protein. The borderline between deficiency and excess is narrow.

Frequent measurement of plasma amino acids and abnormal metabolites is essential to monitor the dietary manipulations. A careful evaluation of the essential amino acid dietary intake and total nutrient intake is necessary to ensure that growth is not retarded by a limiting amino acid, other essential nutrient or total nitrogen intake (Acosta 1982, 1985). Not only the specific metabolite should be analysed,

Table 10.6   Protein substitutes and amino acid supplements. All require supplements of dietary protein or L-amino acids, essential fatty acids, energy; additional sources of vitamins and minerals are necessary for most products.

Amino acids: lowered or omitted	Name of product(s)	Quantity of amino acid/ protein equivalent in 100 g	Protein source	Disorders in which the product is mostly used
Branched chain amino acids (leucine, isoleucine, valine)	MSUD Aid*	98·2 g amino acids	L-amino acids	Maple syrup urine disease (classical, mild, some intermittent variants in relapse)
	MSUD 1†	40·9 g protein equivalent		
	MSUD 2†	54·3 g protein equivalent		
Methionine	Albumaid Methionine Low*	40 g amino acids	Beef serum hydrolysate	Homocystinuria, cystathionine synthetase deficiency unresponsive to pyridoxine
	Methionine Free Amino Acids RVHB*	100 g amino acids	L-amino acids enriched with cystine	
	HOM 1†	51·5 g protein equivalent		
	HOM 2†	68·8 g protein equivalent		
Phenylalanine and tyrosine ± methionine	Albumaid Phenylalanine/ Tyrosine/Methionine Low*	39·4 g amino acids	Beef serum hydrolysate	Inherited tyrosinaemia, types I and II
	Albumaid Phenylalanine/ Tyrosine Free*	40 g amino acids	Beef serum hydrolysate	
	TYR 1†	47·4 g protein equivalent	L-amino acids	
	TYR 2†	63·0 g protein equivalent		
Histidine	Albumaid Histidine Low*	40 g amino acids	Beef serum hydrolysate	Histidinaemia
	HIST 1†	50·7 g protein equivalent	L-amino acids	
	HIST 2†	64·4 g protein equivalent		

	Product	Amount	Composition	Indications
Isoleucine, valine, threonine, methionine	Code 105 Amino Acid Mixture* OS 1† OS 2†	96·3 g amino acids 42·3 g protein equivalent 56·2 g protein equivalent	L-amino acids	Methylmalonic acidaemia and propionic acidaemia requiring severe restriction of natural protein
Lysine	LYS 1† LYS 2†	48·5 g protein equivalent 64·4 g protein equivalent	L-amino acids	Hyperlysinaemia requiring lysine restriction
Essential amino acids	Dialamine*	30 g amino acids	Essential L-amino acids	Urea cycle defects. Chronic renal failure requiring severe restriction of natural protein.
	Hepatamine*	30 g amino acids	Essential amino acids high in arginine and branched chain amino acids	Urea cycle defects / Liver failure } Where arginine is essential
Ketoacid analogues	Alpha keto/Alpha Amino Acids 122* Alpha keto/Alpha Amino Acids 064*	41·5 g keto amino acids and L-amino acids 8·09 g keto amino acids and L-amino acids	Keto amino acids and L-amino acids	Usefulness in treatment of urea cycle disorders and chronic renal failure still being evaluated.

* Scientific Hospital Supplies. A new Maxamaid (SHS) product range is being developed.
† Milupa.

Full composition available from the manufacturer (*see* Chapter 17).

Table 10.7 Requirements of diets used in amino acid disorders.

1   At least the minimum requirement of essential amino acids and total nitrogen for growth needs must be supplied, ideally from conventional foods of high biological protein with or without supplementary amino acids in the form of a protein substitute.

2   Adequate energy to spare protein from gluconeogenesis, prevent catabolism associated with malnutrition and starvation and allow for growth. Replacement of energy normally provided from protein foods is essential.

3   Vitamins, minerals, trace metals and essential fatty acids to cover essential requirements and to supply those normally supplied from restricted foods.

4   The normal products of the degradation pathway which have an essential function must be provided, e.g. cystine in homocystinuria, arginine in ornithine carbamyltransferase deficiency become essential amino acids. *See* Table 10.3.

5   Restriction of essential amino acids, e.g. leucine, isoleucine and valine, in MSUD requires close supervision and biochemical monitoring to ensure that sufficient amounts are provided for growth without exceeding the individual patient's limited but changing capacity to utilize these amino acids (Snyderman 1976, Acosta 1985).

but also other relevant amino acids, e.g. cystine and methionine, as well as homocystine in homocystinuria. Parents can frequently be taught how to take blood samples which may then be posted to the treatment centre.

A full amino acid profile is useful, at least from time to time, in determining the state of nutrition, and is particularly useful to ensure that prescribed amino acid supplements are being taken, and that their content and dose are appropriate. Even though specific amino acids relevant to diagnosis and dietary treatment are not elevated in the urea cycle defects and the organic acidaemias due to irreversible metabolic reaction(s) in the amino acid(s) degradation, the blood amino acid profile, in conjunction with the abnormal metabolite, is necessary to monitor the nutritional adequacy of the diet, e.g. ammonia, arginine and full blood amino acids in ornithine carbamyltransferase deficiency; methylmalonate, isoleucine, valine, threonine, methionine and full blood amino acids in methylmalonic acidaemia.

In patients on diets limiting total protein intake, measurement of plasma albumin, transferrin and/or retinol binding protein are also useful in assessing nutritional status and protein needs.

Micromethods and a prompt laboratory service are essential; in a sick child even two or three hours may

be critical. In the well child it is recommended that levels should be monitored regularly, e.g. initially weekly and thereafter monthly in children with the classical form of the disorder in whom natural protein intake is severely limited. Relevant clinical details regarding dietary intake and clinical state are essential for appropriate interpretation of the results. Elevated levels of the toxic metabolite(s) may be due to infections, undernutrition and poor growth (including deficiency of an essential amino acid in conjunction with energy and/or protein deficiency), overgenerous dietary prescription, or pilfering.

During acute illness and metabolic relapse dietary protein is withdrawn temporarily and at least daily clinical observation and frequent biochemical monitoring is essential. The toxic metabolite(s) may be removed by dialysis (Sallan & Cottom 1969, Brusilow 1985) and/or by repeated exchange transfusion (Hammersen *et al.* 1978). This requires very frequent and careful biochemical monitoring of amino acids, electrolytes and acid–base balance.

PRACTICAL ASPECTS OF DIET CONSTRUCTION

Dietary protein/amino acid allowance

The restricted protein/amino acid intake is best provided by conventional foods which simultaneously provide some trace nutrients, thus helping to avoid 'unknown factor deficiency' (Synderman 1976), which can occur on synthetic diets containing only the known essential nutrients and which leads to growth failure. The protein, particularly in low-protein diets, should ideally be of high biological value, but practical aspects of measurement, dietary variety and protein to energy density must be considered. Human milk or a whey-based modified infant milk formula (Table 10.5) is ideal as the source of protein in infancy, (Forsum & Hambraeus 1972, Smith & Francis 1982, Francis 1986). Thereafter, a variety of foods, including cereals, potato, pulses, chocolate and milk, is normally introduced. If the protein prescription is generous enough it may be practical to include small measured quantities of high-protein relatively low-energy foods such as eggs, meat, cheese and fish. An exchange system of foods with the amino acid or protein content equivalent to one 'unit' is useful and allows variety. The same consideration regarding accuracy and application of such a system applies to that described for phenylalanine (Table 9.2, p. 229). Protein exchanges are given in

Table 8.4(a) and (b). Exchange lists for leucine, methionine and histidine are given with the details of the relevant amino acid disorders. The arithmetic is simple, most parents can understand without difficulty, and replacement of the refused protein by milk ensures that the intake matches the prescription and may be important for nutrition and growth. The daily intake of conventional food should be divided between feeds or main meals.

Analytical figures for amino acids in basic foods are given in *First Amino Acid Supplement to the Composition of Foods* (Paul *et al.* 1980). Manufactured foods are harder to assess for their amino acid content as analytical values are rarely available. Where the protein content is available and predominantly from one source, the amino acid content can be calculated. This is difficult for the many multi-ingredient convenience foods available, unless an assumption is made for the amino acid contribution from a range of proteins; for example, a simplified phenylalanine exchange system is based on the assumption that 1 g protein = 50 mg phenylalanine, apart from low-protein fruit and vegetables.

Protein substitutes

A variety of protein substitutes are available (Table 10.6) for specific inborn errors of amino acid catabolism. They are either hydrolysates from which amino acids have been removed chemically and/or a mixture of synthetic amino acids. The end product varies considerably in the content of protein, energy, vitamins and minerals. None is a complete diet and all of them require supplements of essential fatty acids, and energy, as well as conventional food, to meet the requirement of the limiting essential amino acid(s). Additional sources of minerals and vitamins are usually necessary. It is important to understand each product's specific nutritional role in the diet if they are to be used safely. It is possible to calculate and prepare from synthetic amino acids a protein substitute for individual requirements when none exists commercially. Such a preparation should provide the essential amino acid requirements and have an amino acid profile similar to human milk (Table 10.5).

Observations on the composition of available protein substitutes used for the treatment of inborn errors of amino acid catabolism have been made by Nyman *et al.* (1979), who has proposed rationalization of their nutrient content compared to human milk. New products are continually being developed and evaluated.

There are a few situations in which L-amino acids would, on theoretical grounds, be unsuitable. Patients with amino acid transport defects are probably dependent upon peptide uptake in the small bowel for maintenance of nutrition, e.g. Hartnup disease, cystinuria, but such patients do not normally require synthetic diets.

The prescription for the intake of dietary protein plus amino acid supplement will depend on the metabolic block and should cover the requirement for growth. Where the plasma amino acids are altered by an inborn error, for example homocystinuria and maple syrup urine disease, the principles given for the construction of the low-phenylalanine diet can be adapted (*see* Chapter 9).

The protein substitute(s) are often unpalatable and in the case of the analogues of the keto amino acids are extremely bitter. They are best given with praise and reward, in a way similar to that described for amino acid preparations used in the treatment of phyenylketonuria (p. 240). Their high osmolar load, together with that of the necessary mineral and energy supplements, can lead to osmotic malabsorption. The osmolality of the feed for infants should be continually monitored and modified to keep it under 500 mmol/l. Older children, in whom the protein substitute is given in a concentrate form or paste, should be offered extra drinks with each dose of protein substitute, in order to satisfy thirst.

Some of the dietary protein prescription should be given at the same meal time as the protein substitute, and both should be distributed as evenly as practically possible between feeds and main meals.

Fruit and vegetables

Most low-protein fruits and vegetables are permitted without measurement, similar to the protocol for low-phenylalanine diets (Table 9.2b), subject to any specific exception related to a particular disorder. For example, patients with the classical form of maple syrup urine disease need a more restricted list of fruit and vegetables (*see* later) and occasionally may have such a low tolerance of natural protein that fruit and vegetables have to be limited or included in the leucine prescription.

Energy

Protein cannot be utilized for growth unless adequate dietary energy is supplied. Energy deficiency leads to increased gluconeogenesis, accumulation of amino acids and metabolites, loss of biochemical control, poor growth and hungry bad-tempered children.

When they are old enough they demand or pilfer forbidden foods with which to satisfy their appetite.

Protein-restricted diets are frequently low in energy due to the restricted intake of many foods. Mixtures of amino acids and a number of the protein substitutes (Table 10.6), in the dose prescribed, provide relatively little dietary energy. Patients treated with such diets are particularly dependent upon other energy sources. A guide to recommended intakes of energy at different ages is given in Table 8.2 and Table 9.4, and can be adapted to the needs of children with amino acid disorders.

Although dietary energy is provided by:

1 measured quantities of natural protein foods, e.g. chips, crisps
2 low-protein or negligible protein foods (Table 9.2a and Table 8.2c), sugar, fats, butter
3 permitted fruits and vegetables (Table 9.2b and Table 8.2d)
4 a variety of proprietary low-protein bread, biscuit and pasta products (Table 9.9 and Table 8.7)

frequently glucose polymers and fat emulsions are necessary and useful high-energy protein-free supplements. In infancy they can be added to the protein substitute to provide a suitable bottle-feeding regimen; in older children they are used in drinks and other recipes (*see* Chapter 8, Table 8.7). Glucose polymers are particularly useful in the emergency treatment of metabolic relapse (*see* later) as the major source of carbohydrate and energy. The high refined carbohydrate intake and frequent feeding regimens required by these patients predisposes to dental caries and therefore meticulous oral hygiene and, where appropriate, fluoride supplements are recommended.

Hyperosmolar and overconcentrated solutions, however, should be avoided, as they can cause diarrhoea; excess intake of energy supplements can suppress the child's appetite for more important foods and/or cause obesity. Children commonly refuse the least desirable part of the diet, which is usually the protein substitute; feeding difficulties may arise and/or force-feeding may be resorted to by parents who know the importance of the dietary regimen. It is ideal to devise a diet which permits the child, when clinically well, to demand feed to appetite or have access to unlimited quantities of foods of negligible protein content with which to satisfy his/her appetite. Such a regime is described in Chapter 9.

Force-feeding should be avoided. Careful instructions are essential regarding the priority of each type of food within the diet or meal and will vary in different conditions and in the same child according to the changing clinical state.

Feeding problems are relatively common in children with the classical forms of the organic acidaemias and urea cycle defects, as the toxic metabolite(s) cause anorexia. Parental support and advice should be given and problems dealt with as early as possible. Long-term bolus enteral feeding of an appropriately devised formula or supplement can relieve these problems and should be considered if nutritional problems, or poor growth with poor metabolic control occur, or if the feeding problems are seriously interfering with the mother–child relationship. Careful and continued supervision of the diet, together with parental support, is essential.

Vitamins

Due to the restricted amount of natural foods in these diets, it is essential to ensure an adequate intake of all known vitamins to prevent deficiencies, rashes and growth failure, which can occur with synthetic and restricted diets (Royston & Parry 1962, Mann *et al.* 1965, Clayton 1975). Correct supplementation with vitamins becomes essential, especially in infants and toddlers. Some protein substitutes contain vitamins, but in the dose prescribed for treatment in the infant and young child the quantity is frequently inadequate, and for the older children excessive, or the full range of vitamins is not included. A complete supplement of all known essential vitamins can be given as Ketovite Tablets (three per day) plus Ketovite Liquid (5 ml per day). Alternatives such as the Cow & Gate Supplementary Vitamin Tablets, which include vitamins and trace elements, are useful. Table 10.8 suggests various vitamin–mineral supplements. A more comprehensive description of vitamins and minerals and their role in synthetic diets is given by Francis (1986), and new comprehensive vitamin–mineral supplements are being developed and evaluated.

In the vitamin-responsive amino acid disorders (Table 10.3) pharmaceutical doses of a specific cofactor vitamin alleviate the need for dietary treatment or allow a more generous diet (Scriver 1973, Smith & Francis 1982, Collins & Leonard 1985).

Minerals

Sodium bicarbonate may be required to correct accompanying metabolic acidosis and has a specific role in some conditions, e.g. methylmalonic acidaemia and uric acid defects, as excretion of the metabolite is increased in alkaline urine.

Table 10.8 Vitamin–mineral supplements for use in protein-restricted diets.

(a) Aminogran or Metabolic Mineral Mixture (1·5 g/kg per day to 8 g/day)	Macro and trace minerals
3 Ketovite Tablets 5 ml Ketovite Liquid }	Comprehensive range of vitamins
Fluoride drops*	
(b) 12 Cow & Gate Supplementary Vitamin Tablets	Comprehensive range of water-soluble vitamins and trace minerals
5 ml Ketovite Liquid Fluoride drops*	Vitamins A, D, B$_{12}$, choline chloride
(c) Ped-el may possibly be given orally	Macro and trace minerals
3 Ketovite Tablets 5 ml Ketovite Liquid }	Comprehensive range of vitamins
Fluoride drops*	
(d) 1 Forceval Capsule	Some vitamins and iron and a few trace minerals
1 Sandocal Tablet Fluoride drops*	Calcium

* Provided local water does not contain fluoride a supplement is recommended to protect teeth from the relatively high carbohydrate content of low-protein diets.

(i) The vitamins and minerals content of the supplementary protein substitutes or amino acid product must be taken into account.
(ii) Full composition available from the manufacturer (*see* Chapter 17).

Sodium benzoate can be used to conjugate ammonia with glycine in the liver to form hippuric acid, which is rapidly excreted in the urine, e.g. in the hyperammonaemias (*see* specific disorders).

A number of macro minerals and trace metals are essential nutrients. Their role in nutrition, interactions and dietary supplements has recently been reviewed by Aggett and Davies (1983) and by Francis (1986). The composition of foods for trace minerals is not always available. The synthetic nature and restricted intake of conventional food can result in a lack of essential minerals (Alexander *et al.* 1974, Lombeck *et al.* 1978, Lombeck *et al.* 1984). Some of the protein substitutes contain the macro minerals and some trace metals, but the complete range is rarely included, which may contribute to the 'unknown factor deficiency' described by Snyderman (1976). Symptoms of a deficiency of trace metals include growth failure, skin rashes and hair loss. The

quantity of the protein substitute, plus permitted dietary intake, determines the range and quantity of minerals. A careful assessment of the minerals provided by the diet must be made and appropriate supplements should be prescribed; Table 10.8 gives some suggestions. Mineral interactions and bioavailability should be borne in mind (Aggett & Davies 1983), as should the fact that infants and young children have a low tolerance of both deficiency and excess.

A relatively comprehensive range of macro and some trace minerals is contained in Aminogran Mineral Mixture* and Metabolic Mineral Mixture, which have been modified to incorporate the findings of Alexander *et al.* (1974). A dose of 1·5 g/kg per day to a full dose of 8 g daily of either Metabolic or Aminogran Mineral Mixture has been found appropriate when the protein supplement contains little or no mineral content. Permitted fruit, vegetables and low-protein foods, together with the prescribed conventional foods providing the permitted protein intake, are an important additional source of minerals (Lawson *et al.* 1977). A proportionally smaller dose of mineral supplement is prescribed when the diet contains a more generous quantity of natural food.

Alternatively, if it is only the intake of trace metals which is deficient, they are available with a comprehensive range of vitamins (without A and D) as the Cow & Gate Supplementary Vitamin Tablets.

In the young infant the contribution of the protein substitute, mineral supplements, medicinal bicarbonate and/or sodium benzoate to osmolality and renal solute load must be taken into account and carefully monitored. It is therefore recommended that each 1 g of mineral mixture should normally be diluted with at least 100 ml fluid in infant feeds, fluid diets or enteral feeds, and the osmolality of such formulae should be assessed and kept below 500 mmol/l.

Low levels of selenium have been found in dietetically treated patients with phenylketonuria and maple syrup urine disease (Lombeck *et al.* 1978, Lombeck *et al.* 1984). The significance of these findings in relation to the long-term outcome of treatment is unknown. Work in the field of trace metals can be expected to change rapidly as requirements and toxicity levels are established, particularly regarding selenium, nickel and chromium, and appropriate supplements become available for use in synthetic diets.

---

* Aminogran Food supplement is contraindicated, as it contains phenylalanine-free amino acids (*see* Chapter 17 and Table 9.5).

Fat and essential fatty acids

Fat intake should be at least sufficient to meet the essential fatty acid (EFA) requirement and prevent deficiency (Hansen *et al.* 1962).

To provide the minimum requirement of EFA at least 1 to 2% of dietary energy should come from linoleic acid; i.e. 1 to 2 g linoleic acid should be provided in every 4200 kJ/1000 kcal. Human milk contains approximately 4% of energy as linoleic acid, and this higher EFA content may be important for the development of the young infant.

The protein substitutes used in amino acid disorders (Table 10.6) are fat-free and must be supplemented with a source of EFA. The requirement of EFA can be provided by incorporating vegetable oils, PUFA margarines, or arachis oil emulsions such as Prosparol and Calogen into the diet. Each 10 ml Proparol/Calogen contains 5 g fat, of which approximately 1·4 g is linoleic acid. Medium-chain triglycerides (MCT) do not contain, nor can they be metabolized to, essential fatty acids, and MCT is therefore normally not appropriate or necessary in the diets used in amino acid disorders.

In the young infant, human milk or a whey-based modified milk containing vegetable fat is optimal as the source of dietary protein and provides additional EFA intake. Cow's milk, however, is not ideal for infant nutrition (Francis 1986) as the fat is poorly absorbed; it is not a good source of essential fatty acids and the protein has a poor amino acid profile (Table 10.5).

Fat contributes 35 to 50% of the energy of the young child's normal diet, and can continue to do so in the dietary regimens used in the treatment of the majority of amino acid disorders, except temporarily in some organic acidaemias during intercurrent infections and metabolic relapse (*see* below) and in patients with the disorders of fatty acid oxidation discussed on p. 300. The fat content of any infant feed, fluid diet or total dietary intake should not normally exceed the carbohydrate content, in order to avoid ketosis, except in ketogenic diets, used in the treatment of epilepsy (Chapter 11), and in pyruvate dehydrogenase deficiency (*see* p. 361), in which condition carbohydrate is contraindicated.

ACUTE ILLNESS AND METABOLIC RELAPSE

The emergency treatment required during metabolic stress in many of the disorders described is quite distinct from their long-term management.

Starvation, infection, surgery and other illness, particularly if accompanied by vomiting and/or diarrhoea, increase gluconeogenesis and endogenous protein catabolism with the release of large quantities of amino acids which become fuel for energy metabolism. Fat is also oxidized and converted to ketone bodies, which are themselves metabolized (Fig. 10.1). This leads to biochemical deterioration, irrespective of age, in patients with amino acid disorders, due to the accumulation of the 'toxic' amino acid and/or metabolite(s) and, in many patients, acute illness results. There may be accompanying drowsiness, metabolic acidosis, hypoglycaemia, hypokalaemia and acute clinical deterioration which is potentially life-threatening (Dickinson *et al.* 1969, Naughten *et al.* 1982, Leonard *et al.* 1984, Brusilow 1985), particularly in patients with maple syrup urine disease, inherited tyrosinaemia, the organic acidaemias and the various hyperammonaemias. This is in contrast to the relatively harmless rise in serum phenylalanine seen with infections in patients with phenylketonuria.

Infections should be sought carefully and treated rigorously; accompanying hypoglycaemia, acidosis and hypokalaemia should be corrected. A generous intake of energy with the temporary omission of protein (or reduction to less than 0·5 g protein/kg per day) is recommended and will help limit accumulation of the amino acid and/or metabolite(s). Suggested oral 'emergency' regimens for different age groups are given in Table 10.9. Most commonly the energy is given as frequent drinks of concentrated carbohydrate solutions. Fat is optional and can be omitted on the grounds that it could add a further burden to the citric acid cycle (Fig. 10.1), which may already be abnormal during metabolic relapse, and fat must be omitted temporarily at such times, in the disorders of fat metabolism and some organic acidaemias. Without fat the energy intake will be reduced but at least 168 kJ (40 kcal)/kg per day from carbohydrate should be provided (Brusilow 1985). If the oral feeds are refused they can be administered via a nasogastric tube. If vomiting persists hospital admission and intravenous therapy are indicated. The high osmolality of the feed may cause malabsorption in some patients, and hence glucose polymers are preferable to other carbohydrates and vegetable fat emulsions are preferable to MCT emulsion. The osmolality of the feed should not exceed 500 mmol/l.

Alternatively, where the age and clinical state of the child permits, frequent drinks and snacks of popular drinks such as sweetened fruit juice, 'Coke', or Lucozade, and sugar cubes, boiled sweets and low-protein biscuits can be given as energy sources. Li-

Table 10.9 High-energy protein-free temporary regimen for use during metabolic relapse.

Age	Optimal energy (per kg actual weight per day)		Fluid (ml/kg)	Carbohydrate* (g/100 ml)	Optional 50% fat emulsion† (ml/100 ml)	Sodium bicarbonate‡ (mmol/kg per day)	Potassium chloride‡ (mmol/kg per day)
	kJ	kcal					
0 to 6 months	525 to 540	125 to 150	160 to 200	15 (240 kJ/60 kcal)	4 = 2 g fat (74 kJ/18 kcal)	2 to 3	2 to 3
6 to 12 months	420 to 525	100 to 125	130 to 160	15 (240 kJ/60 kcal)	4 = 2 g fat (74 kJ/18 kcal)	2 to 3	2 to 3
1 to 3 years	420 to 380	100 to 90	90 to 100	20 (320 kJ/80 kcal)	6 = 3 g fat (111 kJ/27 kcal)	2	2
3 to 6 years	340	80	80 to 90	20 (320 kJ/80 kcal)	8 = 4 g fat (148 kJ/36 kcal)	2	2
7 to 12 years	330	70	70	20 (320 kJ/80 kcal)	8 = 4 g fat (148 kJ/36 kcal)	2	2
Teenage	330 to 190	70 to 45	60 to 40	20 (320 kJ/80 kcal)	8 = 4 g fat (148 kJ/36 kcal)	1 to 2	1 to 2

* Caloreen, Maxijul, Calonutrin are suitable glucose polymer powders. Figures in brackets refer to energy supplied by carbohydrate. Liquid glucose polymers, suitably diluted, can replace the glucose polymer powders (30 ml Hycal = 20 g carbohydrate). Older children may prefer carbonated beverages (Lucozade, Coke, etc.) or fruit juices appropriately supplemented with glucose polymer.
† Prosparol, Calogen are 50% fat emulsions. If double cream replaces these it will contribute traces of protein (1·7 g protein/100 ml). Figures in brackets refer to energy supplied by fat. Fat should be omitted in the disorders of fat metabolism and some organic acidaemias (*see* text).
‡ Blood gases and electrolytes should be monitored and intake adjusted accordingly.

quid glucose polymers, Hycal, Maxijul or Fortical, appropriately diluted, can replace the glucose polymer powders. Parents of patients at risk should be instructed in an appropriate individual regimen which they can initiate when their child is unwell at home, but they should keep in close contact with the treatment team, including during the reintroduction of the child's normal dietary protein prescription.

If the illness is mild and symptoms resolve quickly the child's normal diet should be reintroduced without delay over 3 to 4 days to minimize periods of inadequate nutrition.

If vomiting persists or further clinical deterioration occurs, hospitalization is necessary to observe the child's clinical state and to instigate vigorous treatment with intravenous fluids to maintain energy intake and correct blood gases and electrolytes. Insulin may be temporarily necessary to ensure utilization of the high carbohydrate intake and reduce catabolism. However, hypoglycaemia is not an uncommon feature of some organic acidaemias and maple syrup urine disease. The latter is probably due to the high leucine and isoleucine blood levels stimulating insulin secretion.

On the rare occasions when a patient requires an anaesthetic, energy intake must be maintained by the intravenous route until oral intake can be reintrod-

uced and is adequate to meet energy needs. The toxic amino acids or metabolite(s) can be removed if necessary by dialysis or repeated exchange blood transfusions (Harris 1971, Snyderman 1976, Hammersen *et al.* 1978, Brusilow 1985).

In some conditions specific treatment may be used in order to remove the abnormal metabolite(s), both as part of the emergency regimen and as regular treatment, e.g. arginine in citrullinaemia, and sodium benzoate, citrulline and/or phenylacetate in other urea cycle defects (Brusilow 1985); *see* details in the section on specific disorders. Cofactor vitamins should be continued with the emergency regimen in vitamin-responsive patients.

The above emergency measures are also necessary in the intermittent and variant forms of the amino acid disorders if infection or catabolism is accompanied by biochemical and clinical deterioration. In some instances this is the only time dietary treatment is required or any clue is given of the disorder's existence (Gretter *et al.* 1972, Zaleski *et al* 1973). Not all the amino acid disorders require an emergency regimen during infections and catabolism, though extra energy at such times is useful, e.g. in phenylketonuria, homocystinuria, histidinaemia.

Immunizations are normally recommended as they provide protection against certain diseases, but as they may have a similar, although milder, effect as infections in these children, it may be wise for them to be carried out under careful supervision when the child is clinically well, and with appropriate precautions, such as hospitalization.

Emergency protein-free high-energy regimens are not nutritionally adequate and will not permit growth. They should be used for as short a time as possible, e.g. 2 to 3 days maximum, and thereafter small quantities of natural protein are gradually reintroduced as recovery begins, e.g. $\frac{1}{4}$, $\frac{1}{2}$, $\frac{3}{4}$ the full normal protein prescription as chemically and clinically tolerated. The protein substitute, vitamins and minerals are reintroduced either simultaneously with the protein intake, e.g. in maple syrup urine disease, or when clinically appropriate, e.g. in homocystinuria their introduction can be delayed until the full dietary protein intake has been reintroduced as described in phenylketonuria (Chapter 9). Biochemical monitoring during the infection, and restabilization afterwards, is essential.

INFANT AND WEANING DIET

Infants may be diagnosed following an acute illness in the neonatal period or by routine screening programmes. Other patients, particularly those with variant or milder forms of the amino acid disorders, may not be diagnosed till later in childhood with failure to thrive, neurological abnormalities or episodes of metabolic acidosis.

Prolonged breast-feeding, appropriately supplemented, is the treatment of choice in some amino acid disorders, especially for patients with milder disease.

Those patients presenting with metabolic acidosis and/or an acute illness are initially treated with an emergency regimen as described above. The infant is then stabilized onto a frequent feed-bottle regimen incorporating the appropriate protein substitute (Table 10.6) and/or small daily increments of dietary protein are introduced as tolerated; for example, usually between 0·75 and 1·5 g protein/kg per day is tolerated in the severe variants of the organic acidaemias. The devised feed must be nutritionally adequate. Subsequent biochemical monitoring and dietary adjustment is essential. Once the infant is tolerating feeds by bottle at three- to four-hourly intervals, a two-bottle-per-feed schedule has been found useful (*see* protocol for phenylketonuria, Chapter 9). One bottle contains the most essential nutrients, e.g. the natural protein, usually human milk or the appropriate modified milk, which is given first, and the other contains the protein substitute/amino acid supplement, minerals and energy sources (glucose polymer and Prosparol/Calogen), made up to an energy density of approximately 300 to 315 kJ (70 to 75 kcal) per 100 ml feed. The latter is fed in appropriate volume to ensure adequate energy intake and total nutrients. The vitamin supplements are given medicinally as necessary. Once the infant is feeding well, a demandfeeding regimen may be permitted, and this has the advantage of lessening the likelihood of feeding problems. A guide to the minimum intake needed to provide the essential nutrients must be specified to parents and/or nursing staff.

A partial breast-feeding regimen may be appropriate where prescribed supplements of a protein substitute feed of appropriate energy density are used to suppress lactation in order to achieve biochemical control in the infant (*see* Breastfeeding regimen for infants with phenylketonuria, Chapter 9). Such a regimen has been used successfully in an infant with a mild variant of maple syrup urine disease but it is probably not possible to achieve biochemical control in classical maple syrup urine disease (personal observation). The initial emergency regimen and treatment period, during which time breast-feeding is contraindicated, and the relatively low tolerance of leucine may result in breast-feeding failure. The partial breast-feeding regimen could possibly be adapted for use in other amino acid disorders. Alternatively, the mother's expressed (breast) milk could be pooled from one day and a measured aliquot calculated and given the following day.

As soon as the infant is well enough, and the parents understand the essentials of treatment and the feeding regimen, the infant should be treated at home, but regular support, biochemical monitoring and dietary adjustment must continue. The mother should have ample opportunity to discuss any problems or feeding difficulties. Growth and clinical progress must be reviewed every few weeks. Once the child is established on a regimen and the parents are confident about the diet and treatment, visits to the treatment centre can be less often, and regular contact kept by letter/telephone between parents and dietitian for alterations of the diet according to the blood results and the clinical situation.

At about 3 to 6 months, if the child is well enough, appropriate solids can be introduced as spoon foods. The priority order of items in each meal should be specified but will vary in the different disorders, and according to whether the infant is bottle or breast-fed. The low-protein energy foods may be permitted to be fed to appetite so long as they do not oversuppress lactation in the mother of the breast-fed infant. In the bottle-fed infant for example, the natural protein feed is offered first, the protein substitute feed second, and low-protein fruit purées are offered at the end of the feed. Gradually, other low-protein foods and permitted fruit and vegetables purées are introduced. Finger foods, such as low-protein biscuits or peeled fruit, are offered to encourage chewing. The protein substitute and mineral supplement could be offered as a 'paste', if appropriate, from about six months of age, and the energy and fluid content of the feed reduced, the deficit energy and fluid being given as solids and fruit juices or other suitable drinks. Gradually a variety of suitable items are introduced using an exchange 'unit' system for protein (Table 8.2b) or the specific amino acid (*see* later, Tables 10.14, 10.17, 10.18) for cereal, potato and baby foods. By one year of age as full a diet as possible, within the scope of the diet prescription, with as much variety as possible should be given. The low-protein recipes given in Chapters 8 and 9 can be adapted for use in these diets.

PATIENT MANAGEMENT

The dietary treatment of amino acid disorders is highly complex and potentially hazardous. For good results these children should be treated in centres with appropriate expertise including biochemical and dietetic facilities. A team approach is essential. Initial contact between the parents, the paediatrician and the dietitian is important, and may determine long-term success or failure of treatment (Smith & Francis 1982). Anxiety and feeding problems related to treatment are similar to those experienced in the management of phenylketonuria (Chapter 9), but are exacerbated by the uncertain long-term prognosis, the child's poor appetite in many cases, and the need for emergency regimen during illness. Parents need a full explanation of the disorder, its treatment and its inheritance, and continual support and regular contact with the treatment team. Specific instructions regarding illness regimen should be taught to parents and junior medical staff at the hospital and the general practitioner should be informed.

Diets inevitably cause upheaval in the family, and there is an increased risk of feeding problems and malnutrition. The clinical consequences of energy deficit, poor control and undernutrition may necessitate hospitalization and/or an enteral feeding regimen of an appropriate formula or supplement to prevent the child coming to harm.

Early diagnosis and treatment is the single most important factor in determining the intellectual outcome of patients with maple syrup urine disease (Naughten *et al.* 1982). This is probably true for many of the other amino acid disorders (Brusilow 1985). Even patients who survive their initial illness may die later as a result of intercurrent infections accompanied by acute metabolic relapse and clinical deterioration. Although dietetic control is frequently easier as the child gets older, intercurrent infections can still cause acute deterioration and death at least into late adolescence. The present mode of dietary treatment, at least in patients with the classical forms of the amino acid disorders, necessitates lifelong treatment.

Liver transplants and new modes of treatment may alter the outcome of treated patients in the future.

Prenatal diagnosis, in affected families, is already possible for a number of the amino acid disorders, and genetic engineering may alter the course of events in the future (Lloyd & Scriver 1985).

Experience in maternal phenylketonuria (*see* Chapter 9) suggests that exposure of the fetus to chemical abnormalities from implantation onwards may cause damage *in utero*. There is some suggestive evidence that similar though less severe effects occur in the hereditary hyperammonaemias (Palmer *et al.* 1974, Brusilow 1985) and homocystinuria (Van Sprang & Wadman 1971) and other amino acidopathies; further experience will be acquired as treated patients reach adulthood (Levy 1985, Lloyd & Scriver 1985, Stacey 1985).

INDIVIDUAL AMINO ACID DISORDERS

The disorders discussed are those in which dietary treatment has been established or is of nutritional importance. New disorders or variants of old ones are continually being added so the list discussed is far from complete. The dietary regimens included are only a guide to management, as each patient diagnosed is different and information in this field is continually growing. Further amino acid disorders are mentioned by Smith and Francis (1982), Stanbury *et al.* (1983), Leonard *et al.* (1984), Collins and Leonard (1985), and Lloyd and Scriver (1985).

Maple syrup urine disease (MSUD)

This abnormality, so called because of the odour of the urine, is an inborn error of the metabolism of the branched chain amino acids leucine, isoleucine and valine, which are degraded by three separate but related pathways (Fig. 10.2). The underlying biochemical defect in the classical form of MSUD is the failure of oxidative decarboxylation of the α-ketoacids

derived from the branched chain amino acids. As a result these amino acids and their corresponding ketoacids are greatly increased in blood, erythrocytes, cerebrospinal fluids and urine (Snyderman 1976). Thus intake of the branched chain amino acids

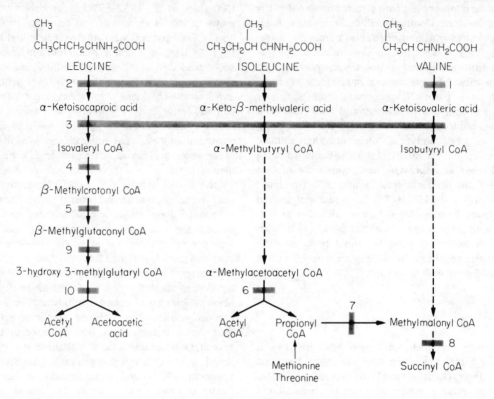

Group		Disorders
Plasma amino acids raised	1	Hypervalinaemia
	2	Hyperleucine isoleucinaemia
	3	Maple syrup urine disease
		classical
		mild
		intermittent
Organic acidaemias	4	Isovaleric acidaemia
leading to:		('sweaty feet syndrome')
vomiting	5	β-methylcrotonylglycinuria
ataxia		('cat's urine syndrome')
hypotonia	6	α-methylacetoacetic aciduria
ketosis	7	Propionic acidaemia
acidosis	8	Methylmalonic acidaemia
hypoglycaemia	9	β-methylglutaconic aciduria
convulsions	10	β-hydroxy-β-methylglutaric aciduria
mental retardatio		
coma		
death		

Fig. 10.2 Degradation of the branched chain amino acids. Adapted from Smith & Francis (1982).

can be titrated against plasma levels. Allo-isoleucine is elevated in blood when isoleucine levels are raised.

In the classical form of the disease, there is acute neurological deterioration in the neonatal period, accompanying organic acidaemia with varying degrees of metabolic acidosis. Affected patients appear normal at birth, but soon develop feeding difficulties, vomiting, lethargy, respiratory irregularity, and severe neurological signs such as convulsions, coma, apnoeic spells, and, if untreated, early death or severe brain damage results (Snyderman 1972, Hammersen *et al.* 1978, Di George *et al.* 1982). Adequate and immediate therapy during this acute phase of MSUD is essential for survival and normal development. Naughten *et al.* (1982) reported the outcome of 12 patients with classical MSUD presenting in the neonatal period and suggested the single most important factor in determining the outcome appeared to be the interval between the first symptoms and making the diagnosis. Dietary treatment must be instigated as soon as possible after symptoms occur, even a delay of a few days may affect the outcome. A delay of more than 14 days was invariably associated with mental retardation and cerebral palsy. Prompt and adequate dietary treatment allows survival and is also important to the intellectual development: normal, or near-normal, development has been reported (Snyderman 1972, Clow *et al.* 1981, Di George *et al.* 1982, Naughten *et al.* 1982), provided that treatment is started early enough, and the child survives the hazards of intercurrent infections (Naughten *et al.* 1982).

Two patients with MSUD, both of whom died at four months, were compared by Hammersen *et al.* (1978). The one who was treated from early infancy but died during a metabolic crisis had almost normal myelination of the brain; the other, who had not been treated, showed myelin deficiency, thus documenting the effect of treatment on brain myelination.

Several variant forms of MSUD with varying degrees of enzyme activity have been described (Zaleski *et al.* 1973); one form runs an intermittent course (Gompertz 1972), another variant described by Scriver (1973) responds to the cofactor thiamine and requires no dietary restrictions. In many of the variant forms of MSUD mental development is normal.

In patients with MSUD, including those with the variant forms, intercurrent infections and other causes of catabolism precipitate biochemical and clinical deterioration, which can be life-threatening (Gretter *et al.* 1972) and require emergency treatment as described above.

TREATMENT OF MSUD

Treatment was first described in 1963 by Westall using a synthetic diet low in leucine, isoleucine and valine, which continues to be the basis of treatment. Classical MSUD requires:

1 Emergency treatment (discussed above) of the acute intoxication syndrome which develops in the first days of life, and during relapse induced by infections or catabolism.
2 Dietary treatment limiting the intake of leucine, isoleucine, and valine to that required for growth, thus maintaining plasma levels within a safe range (between 100 and 700 μmol/l for leucine and 100 and 400 μmol/l for isoleucine and valine), as ascertained by regular biochemical monitoring.

The amount of leucine tolerated requires severe limitation of dietary protein, necessitating supplementation with a leucine-, isoleucine- and valine-free amino acid mixture. MSUD Aid (Table 10.6) has been used successfully for many years as the protein substitute. Recently the Milupa products MSUD 1 and 2 have become available, and a new product, Maxamaid MSUD, by Scientific Hospital Supplies is currently being assessed. A supplement of 2 to 3 g amino acids/kg per day provides the major intake of nitrogen in the diet. Appropriate vitamin and mineral supplements must be added, and adequate total nitrogen, essential fatty acids and energy intake are necessary.

Leucine, isoleucine and valine are essential amino acids and must be provided in the diet. During initial treatment, as soon as one of the amino acid plasma levels falls to below 700 μmol/l, a small supplement, initially in the range of $\frac{1}{4}$ of the theoretical requirement, i.e. 25 to 30 mg/kg per day, of that amino acid, is added to the feed as the synthetic L-amino acid. As a second blood level falls to below 700 μmol/l, a supplement of that L-amino acid is added, and similarly with the third amino acid. Leucine is usually the slowest to fall to the safe range (Snyderman 1976). The intake of the branched chain amino acids is then incrementally increased according to tolerance monitoring by initially daily measurement of plasma amino acid levels, titrating the intake of each amino acid separately against the blood level of that amino acid. Once some stability has been achieved, but without undue delay, the synthetic branched chain amino acids are replaced by small measured quantities of conventional protein, in the infant as an appropriate 'milk', e.g. human milk or modified whey-based milk such as Aptamil, Gold Cap SMA, Osterfeed or Premium (Table 10.5), and as 50 mg leucine exchanges (Table 10.10) in the older patient. Any deficit of isoleucine or valine continues to be given as a small, accurate supplement of the synthetic L-amino acid. The introduction of natural

food as soon as possible is important, to avoid deficiency of unknown nutrients (Snyderman 1976).

The theoretical requirement for branched chain amino acids compared with the actual intake tolerated by patients with MSUD reported by different workers is summarized in Table 10.11. The theoret-

Table 10.10　Quantity of food containing 50 mg leucine in the weight specified: leucine exchanges and their contribution of the branched chain amino acids.

	Weight of food (to nearest 5 g)	Leucine (mg)	Isoleucine (mg)	Valine (mg)
Milk				
15 ml cow's milk		50	27	36
30 ml double cream		46	25	34
20 ml single cream		48	27	36
Cereals				
5 g All bran		49	25	37
5 g Cornflakes		54	16	21
7 g Grapenuts		55	28	41
5 g Puffed Wheat		52	26	34
12 g Sugar Puffs		50	25	34
5 g muesli		50	27	36
5 g oatmeal—raw		48	26	34
5 g Ready Brek		48	25	34
10 g Rice Krispies		51	24	36
7 g Shredded Wheat and Spoon Size Shredded Wheat		53	27	36
7 g Weetabix		57	29	39
10 g Rice—raw		56	26	39
25 g Rice—boiled		48	22	33
Potatoes				
55 g boiled and milk-free mashed		48	33	41
30 g baked in skin, flesh only		48	33	39
40 g baked in skin, weighed with skin		52	34	44
30 g roast		51	36	42
20 g chips—fried		46	32	40
25 g frozen fried chips		45	33	38
55 g new—boiled		52	38	44
70 g new—canned		50	34	43
15 g crisps, plain or salted		57	39	48
10 g instant potato powder		55	38	46
40 g instant potato powder—made up according to manufacturer's instructions		48	33	40
40 g potato—raw		52	35	44
100 g sweet potato—boiled		58	39	48
Vegetables				
35 g brussels sprouts—boiled		53	42	49
30 g broccoli tops—boiled		48	36	45
15 g baked beans—canned		59	32	36
15 g peas—boiled fresh or frozen		53	35	36
15 g peas canned garden (drained)		48	30	33
10 g peas canned processed		43	27	29
45 g cauliflower—boiled		50	32	42

See also Table 10.5 for the composition of various modified milks.

Table 10.11 Branched chain amino acid intakes in MSUD (mg/kg per day).

	Normal infant requirement (i)	Maple syrup urine disease					
		3 months (i)	3 months (ii)	1 year (iii)	2 years (ii)	Infants (iv)	2 years (v)
Leucine	76 to 229	120	80 to 125	75	45	<140	205 to 615 mg/day (average 461 mg/day)
Isoleucine	102 to 119	60	50 to 75	40	25	<120	
Valine	80 to 105	90	60 to 90	60	35	<100	

(i) Holt (1967) (only one infant had a leucine requirement in excess of 150 mg/kg per day).
(ii) Snyderman (1976).
(iii) Dickinson *et al.* (1969).
(iv) Goodman *et al.* (1969). (The paper reported two patients with a tolerance level of leucine greater than 250 mg/kg per day during the second and third month of life, one tolerating 360 mg/kg per day at one point, and then an abrupt change to 140 mg/kg per day.
(v) Naughten *et al.* (1982). Actual intake leucine/day for 12 patients at age two years.
Close biochemical monitoring is essential, as individual tolerance varies.

ical requirement in normal children at different ages is given in Table 10.4. Tolerance varies from child to child due to the degree of residual enzyme activity (Saudubray *et al.* 1982), fluctuating growth rate, and metabolic relapse with infections from time to time in the same child. Blood amino acid levels in the child must therefore be monitored biochemically: initially daily, then twice weekly and, later, weekly to monthly as some stability in control is achieved. The requirement, in general, decreases on a weight basis with age, but fluctuates with growth spurts. A dietary regimen devised to restrict the intake of the branched chain amino acids, with the aim of keeping blood levels in the range quoted above, has been found satisfactory for growth, and normal development is possible if treatment is started early enough (Naughten *et al.* 1982). The conventional protein intake should be measured accurately and the prescription adjusted according to blood level monitoring.

Infant and weaning diet
As soon as the infant is feeding well and is over the acute presenting illness, the following feeding schedule is appropriate. Normally the branched chain amino acids, as the milk formula feed, are given separately before the feed containing the MSUD Aid, minerals and energy supplement, which can be flavoured and fed to appetite provided the infant takes adequate for growth needs (*see* example Table 10.12). The prescription of the MSUD Aid feed is adjusted for age, weight and contribution of the conventional protein intake. Vitamins are given medicinally.

The breast-feeding regimen used for the infant with phenylketonuria (p. 239) could be adapted for the patient with MSUD, suppressing maternal lactation appropriately by a prescribed intake of an MSUD Aid feed made to a similar recipe to the example in Table 10.12 (ii), given before demand breast-feeds. This has been successful in an infant with a variant form of MSUD, but whether adequate biochemical control would be possible in the classical disease is doubtful (personal observation).

The parents are counselled about the condition and its management and taught the feeding regimen and how to make up the actual feeds, so that the child can be discharged as soon as well enough.

Even when the infant is relatively well, long overnight fasts should be avoided, as they can lead to poor biochemical control, since the branched chain amino acids rise with fasting. In the young infant, six feeds three- to four-hourly is an appropriate schedule with a change to five feeds once the infant is well controlled. The late-night feed should be continued until about a year old, when it can be replaced with a bedtime high-carbohydrate drink which is repeated early in the morning.

Weaning solids should be introduced from about four months, provided the infant is well enough. A similar regimen to that suggested in Chapter 9 for the infant with phenylketonuria can be adapted. The low-leucine low-protein fruit and vegetables (Table 10.13) are usually permitted without measurement in the diet as well as a range of negligible-protein foods and special products suitable for age (*see* Tables 9.2a and 9.9). Gradually the energy content and volume of the MSUD Aid feed is proportionally reduced and the quantity of amino acids increased as solids increase, thus maintaining adequate total intake of

Table 10.12   Example of a feeding regimen for an infant (weight 3 kg) with MSUD.

		Leucine (mg)	Isoleucine (mg)	Valine (mg)	Protein plus amino acids	Energy kJ	Energy kcal	Carbo-hydrate (g)	Fat (g)
(i) Conventional protein feed									
200 ml Aptamil, reconstituted (26 g Aptamil powder)	Eight × 25 ml feeds	312	130	156	3·0	546	130	14·2	7·2
+ 50 mg synthetic L-isoleucine			50						
+ 100 mg synthetic L-valine				100					
(ii) MSUD feed									
8 g MSUD Aid		Nil	Nil	Nil	7·8	123	31	Nil	Nil
4·0 g Metabolic Mineral Mixture*	Eight × 50 ml feeds	Nil	Nil	Nil	Nil	Nil	Nil	Nil	Nil
30 g Maxijul LE†		Nil	Nil	Nil	Nil	480	120	30	Nil
30 ml Calogen‡		Nil	Nil	Nil	Nil	555	135	Nil	15
Water to 400 ml									
(iii) 3 Ketovite Tablets	Given medicinally								
5 ml Ketovite Liquid									
Fluoride drops									
Total		312	150	256	10·8	1704	416	42·2	22·2
This provides (per kg per day)		104	50	85·3	3·6	568	129		
Theoretical recommended intake (per kg per day)		*See* Table 10.11			3 to 4	550	130		

(i) Other modified milks can be substituted (*see* Table 10.5).

(ii) Each 100 ml feed contains 2·0 g amino acids, 7·5 g carbohydrate, 3·75 g fat, 72·5 kcal, 294 kJ, 1·7 mmol sodium, 2·1 mmol potassium, 2 mmol calcium, 1·9 mmol phosphorus and a range of trace minerals.

* The mineral content of the feed must be adjusted according to total intake; normally not more than 1 g minerals per 100 ml feed should be added in infancy because of the osmolar and renal solute load. In older children a full dose of 8 g Metabolic Mineral Mixture per day is recommended. Aminogran Mineral Mixture can replace Metabolic Mineral Mixture. Sodium bicarbonate and/or potassium chloride, as indicated according to blood electrolytes, can be added.

† Fruit juice concentrate can replace part of the added carbohydrate to improve palatability. Other glucose polymers can replace the Maxijul LE.

‡ 50% oil emulsion contains essential fatty acids. Other brands of protein-free fat emulsion containing essential fatty acids, e.g. Prosparol, can replace Calogen.

protein substitute (MSUD Aid), dietary energy, minerals and vitamins. Appropriate finger foods should be offered to encourage chewing from about eight months.

The branched chain amino acid intake is adjusted according to tolerance, and should be divided between meals or feeds.

There are many nutritional advantages and greater accuracy of dietary intake when the branched chain amino acids are given as a modified milk throughout infancy, but this must be balanced with the importance of introducing solids and more variety in the diet. An exchange system giving the quantity of food containing 50 mg leucine with the corresponding isoleucine and valine contribution is given in Table 10.10. The priority order in which items are offered at each meal is important but alters when the child is unwell and parents should be instructed accordingly. The prescribed regimen should permit the child to self-feed and eat according to his/her appetite. Force-feeding should be avoided, though praise and reward schemes are appropriate, or a nasogastric tube feeding regimen during periods of metabolic relapse.

Toddler and older child's diet

The guidelines given for the dietary management of patients with phenylketonuria (Chapter 9) can be adapted when the child with MSUD is well. High

Table 10.13 Low-leucine, low-protein fruit and vegetables: permitted without measurement in diets for patients with MSUD.

(a) *Fruit*	Less than 50 mg leucine and/or less than 0·6 g protein/100 g. Fresh, frozen, canned unless otherwise stated.
	Apple, apricot, bilberry, cherry, cranberries, currants (dried), damsons, fruit pie filling, fruit salad, grapes, grapefruit, guavas, lemons, lychees (canned), mandarin, melon (honeydew and water melon), medlars, nectarines, oranges, paw paw, peaches, pears, pineapple, plums, pomegranate, quince, raisins, raspberries, rhubarb, strawberries, sultanas, tangerine.
	Banana is only permitted in limited quantity because of its higher protein/leucine content, e.g. $< \frac{1}{2}$ per day in under-two-year-olds. < 1 per day in over-two-year-olds.
(b) *Vegetables*	Less than 100 mg leucine or less than 1 g protein/100 g. Fresh, frozen or canned in salt brine unless otherwise stated.
	Asparagus (boiled), artichoke (globe, boiled*), aubergine, beans (French), beetroot, cabbage (boiled and raw white), carrots*, celery (boiled* or raw), chicory, cucumber*, lettuce*, marrow (boiled*), onion (raw*, boiled* or fried), peppers (green and red), pumpkin, spring greens, swede (boiled), tomato*, turnip*.

* These vegetables are lower in leucine (less than 50 mg) and/or protein (less than 0·6 g)/100 g.

levels of leucine, more than 1000 μmol/l, however, are potentially 'toxic', and the emergency regimen, modified as clinically indicated, may be temporarily necessary. Diet is needed indefinitely.

Infections and emergency regimen
Catabolism resulting from infections and trauma is a great hazard, requiring immediate intervention, as already discussed. An emergency regimen, devised from Table 10.9, should be given with temporary withdrawal, or reduction to <25%, of the usual prescription of the branched chain amino acid (leucine exchanges). This should be instigated at the first sign of infection(s). Blood for amino acid levels should be

obtained and accompanying metabolic acidosis or hypoglycaemia must be dealt with promptly. Parents should be taught a simple practical regimen to use; with support and daily telephone consultation many of them can manage minor infections at home. The protein substitute and minerals can be temporarily omitted if refused, but if tolerated help to maintain the amino acid balance in plasma. Vomiting and/or diarrhoea, neurological deterioration, and/or severe acidosis necessitate hospitalization and immediate treatment. Restabilization and biochemical monitoring are essential during the regrading onto the usual diet prescription as clinically tolerated. Catch-up growth subsequently may require a temporary increase in the branched chain amino acid prescription. Long periods of protein withdrawal and inadequate regimen should be avoided, as nutritional deficiencies and growth failure can result.

Classical homocystinuria: cystathionine β-synthetase deficiency

Homocystinuria is found in several inborn errors of metabolism. The most important is classical homocystinuria due to cystathionine β-synthetase deficiency which causes a partial or complete block in the conversion of homocysteine to cystathionine (Fig. 10.3) leading to the accumulation of homocystine, methionine and other sulphur-containing metabolites, but a low plasma cystine (Mudd & Levy 1983). Confirmation of the diagnosis can be made by measuring the enzyme activity.

Accumulation of plasma methionine is relatively slow, particularly in infants fed human or whey-based modified milk, and cases may be missed in newborn screening programmes aimed to detect raised methionine levels, especially if the test is taken on or before the sixth day of life (Wilcken & Turner 1978, Whiteman *et al.* 1979, Walker *et al.* 1981).

Transient neonatal hypermethioninaemia as a result of a high protein intake is probably benign, but it may be the first indication of underlying liver disease and should be investigated. Transient neonatal homocystinuria is also found.

There is another group of rare inborn errors of folate and B_{12} metabolism that cause homocystinuria with low methionine levels. These are diagnosed and managed differently: diet is not important but B_{12} and different folate species are used in their treatment (Scriver 1973, Mudd & Levy 1983).

The clinical manifestations of classical homocystinuria include mental retardation, which is usually mild, lens dislocation (ectopia lentis), skeletal abnor-

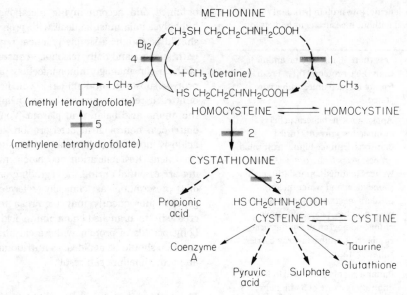

Fig. 10.3 Degradation of methionine and cystine. Key: (1) inherited tyrosinaemia with hypermethioninaemia, transient neonatal hypermethioninaemia; (2) cystathionine synthetase deficiency; (3) inherited cystathioninuria, neonatal cystathioninuria; (4) deficiency of adenosyl and methyl B_{12} leading to methylmalonic acidaemia, homocystinuria and hypomethioninaemia; (5) methyltetrahydrofolate reductase deficiency. From Smith & Francis (1982).

malities and a tendency to venous and arterial thrombosis which may be life-threatening (Thomas & Carson 1978, Carson 1982). Not all patients have the classical symptoms and some are asymptomatic, at least in childhood (Brenton *et al.* 1966, Carson 1982). The ectopia lentis is rare before the age of two years, but in untreated patients it develops in more than 90% of cases. Many patients are tall for age (Thomas & Carson 1978), have a fair complexion and malar flush. Although some patients do surprisingly well without treatment, most patients develop serious complications. There is a wide variation in the outcome of patients; those who are pyridoxine-responsive generally have a milder disease than those who do not (Collins & Leonard 1985).

Pyridoxine is a cofactor for the enzyme responsible for the conversion of homocysteine to cystathionine and the formation of cysteine. Approximately 40% of patients with classical homocystinuria respond to pyridoxine. A dose of pyridoxine of 100 to 500 mg/day, though occasionally of 1000 mg/day, may be necessary; with folic acid 10 to 20 mg/day is given with partial or complete biochemical remission (Brenton & Cusworth 1971, Wilcken & Turner 1978, Pullen 1980). If there is complete response to pyridoxine (plasma homocystine less than 10 μmol/l and plasma methionine less than 80 μmol/l on normal diet), dietary manipulation is unnecessary but pyridoxine and folic acid are continued indefinitely (Collins & Leon-

ard 1985). There is some evidence to suggest that pyridoxine is clinically beneficial to symptoms in the vitamin-responsive form of the disease and allows normal development of infants treated from the neonatal period (Carson 1982), but as complications may not arise until adult life it is still too early to be sure (Pullen 1980). Response to pyridoxine is consistent amongst siblings, suggesting it is genetically determined (Mudd & Levy 1983). All newly diagnosed patients with homocystinuria should have a trial of pyridoxine and the response measured by repeated biochemical testing (Collins & Leonard 1985).

Patients with homocystinuria have an increased requirement for folate. Supplements of folic acid are recommended in both the vitamin-responsive and the unresponsive classical forms of the disorder (Smith & Francis 1982).

Patients who have only a partial response to pyridoxine and folate therapy require a modified diet in addition.

Patients with a classical homocystinuria who do not respond to vitamin therapy are treated by a low-methionine, high-cystine diet (Coutts & Fowler 1967, Komrower & Sardharwalla 1971, Collins & Leonard 1985). This corrects the biochemical abnormality. Cysteine, which is normally synthesized from methionine via homocysteine, becomes an essential amino acid as a result of the metabolic block. Efficacy of dietary treatment is as yet unproven. There is some evidence that it is clinically beneficial; normal physical and mental development has been reported in patients treated from early infancy (Komrower & Sardharwalla 1971, Perry 1971), and affected individuals so treated seem to have less severe complications than their untreated siblings (Pullen 1980), but further evaluation is still needed as treated patients reach adulthood, because of the late onset of symptoms in many patients with this disease.

Dietary methionine intake is titrated against plasma levels of methionine, cystine and homocystine. There is no general agreement on the 'safe' upper limit of methionine, but one should probably aim at plasma levels close to the normal range (30 to 80 μmol/l) for methionine, cystine levels (from a fresh sample of blood as cystine and homocystine are unstable) in the normal range of $67 \pm 20\ \mu$mol/l, and absence (less than 5 μmol/l) of homocystine in blood and urine (Collins & Leonard 1985).

Emergency treatment during catabolic episodes is not necessary. However, the diet will need to be continued indefinitely since the risk of developing complications is high and is not reduced with age (Carson 1982, Collins & Leonard 1985). For example, the hazard of platelet stickiness and thrombosis is likely to persist for life. Whether dietary treatment will prevent it occurring is unknown. Aspirin has been used to reduce this risk.

Prenatal diagnosis of homocystinuria is now possible (Børresen & Boman 1982).

The effect of maternal homocystinuria is not yet well documented, though five successive spontaneous abortions in a pyridoxine-responsive patient were reported by Van Sprang *et al.* (1971). Histological changes were found in the placenta. Pyridoxine treatment during a sixth pregnancy resulted in the birth of a normal infant.

DIETARY TREATMENT OF CLASSICAL HOMOCYSTINURIA

Dietary methionine is restricted to that required for growth, and supplementary amino acids are given as a low-methionine protein substitute (Table 10.6) if the protein intake has to be reduced to such an extent that growth may be impaired. Since cystine cannot be synthesized normally it becomes an essential amino acid, and a supplement of 100 mg/kg per day in infants, and 1 to 2 g/day in children and adults, is recommended, unless provided by the protein substitute prescribed. Pyridoxine and folate supplements are recommended in addition to any vitamin and mineral supplements relevant to the dietary restrictions.

The basic principles of a low-methionine diet are similar to the low-phenylalanine dietary treatment of phenylketonuria (Chapter 9), but methionine is restricted instead of phenylalanine. However, pulses, soya, lentils and gelatine, which are relatively low in methionine (*see* Table 10.14), can be incorporated into the diet, thus reducing or eliminating the need for a protein substitute. The soya modified formulae suitable for infants are all supplemented with methionine; even so, Prosobee is slightly lower in methionine than most infant modified milks (Table 10.5). A convenient way of providing variety in the diet is by use of a 25 mg methionine exchange system (Table 10.15) to provide the dietary prescription of methionine required for individual tolerance.

Several low-methionine protein substitutes (Table 10.6) are available, but their nutritional contribution to the diet varies considerably, particularly regarding their vitamin and mineral content. All require sup-

Table 10.14 Protein, methionine and cystine content of different foods, per 100 g unless otherwise stated.

Foods	Protein (g)	Methionine (mg)	Cystine (mg)
Milk (cow's) } per	3·3	94	31
Prosobee } 100ml	2·0	33	20
Peas			
boiled, fresh or frozen (average)	5·2	50	58
canned garden	4·6	44	52
canned processed	6·2	59	69
dried raw and split, dried raw	21·8	210	240
dried boiled and split dried boiled	6·9/8·3	$\simeq$67	$\simeq$78
Chick-peas			
Bengal gram raw	20·2	260	290
cooked dahl	8	100	120
channa dahl	5·3	68	77
Red pigeon peas—raw	20	260	220
Butter beans			
raw	19·1	280	280
boiled	7·1	100	100
Haricot beans			
raw	21·4	240	170
boiled	6·6	74	53
Baked beans—canned	5·1	57	41
Lentils			
raw	23·8	190	230
split raw	7·6	61	73
masur dahl cooked	4·9	39	47
Soya flour			
full-fat	36·8	520	650
low-fat	45·3	640	790
Gelatine	84·4	760	Nil

Table 10.15 Quantity of food containing 25 mg methionine in the weight specified: methionine exchanges.

	Weight of food (to nearest 5 g)
Prosobee (Mead Johnson), normal reconstitution	75 ml
Milk, ordinary red or silver top	25 ml
Milk pudding and custard with ordinary milk	25 ml
Cream	
double	70
single	45
Potato	
raw (cook *after* weighing)	80
boiled	100
mashed (no milk added)	100
'new' boiled potatoes	100
chips	40
frozen chips, fried	50
roast	50
baked or jacket without skin	60
instant potato made up with water	80
crisps, plain or salt and vinegar	25
Cereals	
Weetabix	15
Shredded Wheat	15
Puffed Wheat	10
Sugar Puffs	25
Cornflakes	20
Rice Krispies	20
oatmeal, raw (cook after weighing)	10
porridge, cooked with water	100
macaroni	35
spaghetti	
dry weight	10
tinned in tomato sauce (no cheese)	85
rice	
raw (cook after weighing)	20
boiled and drained	50
semolina (dry weight)	15
lentils	
raw (cook after weighing)	15
boiled and drained	45
soup, canned lentil	50
Vegetables	
Peas	
boiled fresh, frozen	50
processed	45
dry (cook after weighing)	12
dry type, boiled and drained	40

Table 10.15 *continued*

	Weight of food (to nearest 5 g)
Vegetables continued	
beans	
broad beans	100
dry beans after cooking, e.g.	
butter, haricot, red kidney	25
baked beans in tomato sauce	50
spring greens	80
spinach, boiled	15
sweetcorn	
kernels	25
on cob	50
broccoli tops	55
sprouts	100
cauliflower	80
mushrooms, fried	30
Nuts	
peanuts—ground nuts, roasted/ salted	10
peanut butter	10
cashew	10
desiccated coconut	20
almonds	10
Fruit	
avocado pear	40
currants, dried	50
dates, dried	100
sultanas, dried	50
raisins, dried	80
Desserts	
yoghurt, fruit type and plain	25
ice-cream, dairy, non-dairy types	25
jelly, ordinary (a small serve is allowed freely)	200
Flour, bread and biscuits	
flour, white, plain or self-raising	15
bread	
brown, Hovis, wholemeal	15
white	20
crispbread (not starch-reduced type)	15
biscuits	
semi-sweet, shortbread	20
ginger nuts, sandwich type	25

Table 10.16 100–ml recipes for infant feeds low in methionine/histidine.

		Amino acid (g)	Protein equivalent (g)	Energy kJ	Energy kcal	Carbo-hydrate (g)	Fat (g)
(i) 5 g Albumaid Methionine Low *or* Albumaid Histidine Low	Select as appropriate	2	1·7	75	18	2·5	Nil
5 g Caloreen*		Nil	Nil	80	20	5·0	Nil
8 ml Prosparol†		Nil	Nil	148	36	Nil	4·0
Water to 100 ml							
	Each 100 ml	2	1·7	303	74	7·5	4·0
(ii) 4 g HOM I *or* HIST I	Select as appropriate	2·5	2·1	46	11	0·6	Nil
7 g Caloreen*		Nil	Nil	112	28	7·0	Nil
8 ml Prosparol†		Nil	Nil	148	36	Nil	4·0
Water to 100 ml							
	Each 100 ml	2·5	2·1	306	75	7·6	4·0

Conventional protein must provide essential methionine/histidine.

Both low-methionine feeds contain approximately 100 mg cystine/100 ml.

Each 100 ml feed (i) contains 1·6 mmol sodium, 1 mmol potassium, 0·9 mmol calcium, 2·4 mmol phosphorus, but very low levels of trace minerals. Supplements at least of iron, zinc and copper and vitamins as three Ketovite Tablets plus 5 ml Ketovite Liquid (Paines & Byrne) are essential in young children.

Each 100 ml feed (ii) contains 1·6 mmol sodium, 2 mmol potassium, 2·1 mmol calcium, 2·1 mmol phosphorus and a range of trace elements and most vitamins except vitamin D.

*Fruit juice concentrate can replace part of the carbohydrate to improve palatability. Other glucose polymers can replace Caloreen.

† 50% oil emulsion containing essential fatty acids. Other brands of protein-free oil emulsions high in essential fatty acids can replace Prosparol.

plements, and sources of essential fatty acids and energy must be provided in the diet.

Low-methionine infant feeds can be devised as in the example (Table 10.16); each contains 100 mg cystine in 100 ml. The essential methionine intake is supplied as human milk, Prosobee or a modified infant formula. The modified breast-feeding regimen suggested for infants with phenylketonuria could be adapted. An initial intake of 25 mg methionine per kg/day is prescribed in the bottle-fed infant and is adjusted according to plasma methionine and homocystine levels. Nutritional deficiencies should be avoided. Introduction of solids, finger foods and the older child's diet can follow the low-phenylalanine diet format.

Cystathionuria

This is due to an inherited defect of cystathionase which often responds to pyridoxine supplements (50 to 500 mg per day) (Stanbury *et al.* 1983). A transient defect occurs in newborns. Both conditions are probably harmless provided adequate cystine is provided in the diet. In the infant, breast-feeding, or a whey-based modified infant feed, because of their higher cystine content compared to other modified cow's milk-based feeds, is appropriate.

Cystinuria

Transport of the dibasic amino acids (ornithine, cystine, lysine and arginine) is affected in both the gut and kidneys (Stanbury *et al.* 1983), resulting in increased cystine in the urine with a tendency to cystine stone formation. The losses are not usually of nutritional importance unless protein intake is restricted. Lysine is an essential amino acid and arginine and cystine are essential at least in the young infant. A generous but not excessive dietary protein intake is appropriate to counteract urinary losses. A gross fluid intake is extremely important to prevent renal stone formation: in adults three litres of fluid per day is recommended.

Histidinaemia

This is due to an inherited defect of histidine metabolism with accumulation of histidine and its metabolites, including imadazole derivatives, due to a deficiency of histidase. Variant disorders have been reported.

There is disagreement regarding the necessity for dietary treatment of this disorder, since the biochemical findings of histidinaemia may be associated with complete normality, and clinical abnormalities and mental retardation are by no means inevitable in untreated patients (Neville & Lilly 1973, Popkin *et al.* 1974, Scriver & Levy 1983, Rosenmann *et al.* 1983, Coulombe *et al.* 1983).

Long-term follow-up of untreated patients and assessment of IQ and school progress reports will eventually determine whether screening and treatment of asymptomatic infants is justified, especially as the dietary treatment carries all the hazards associated with a synthetic diet.

Treatment, when given, consists of a low-histidine diet (Griffiths 1973, Snyderman *et al.* 1979a, Tada *et al.* 1980, Dyme *et al.* 1983). Some workers have only used dietary treatment during infancy or during the first two years, others have only treated symptomatic patients.

Table 10.17 Quantity of food containing 50 mg histidine in the weight specified: histidine exchanges.

	Weight of food (to nearest 5 g)
Milk	
50 ml	milk
70 ml	single cream
100 ml	double cream
35 g	yoghurt (natural or fruit-type)
15 g	whole egg
Cereals	
20 g	Cornflakes
35 g	Rice Krispies
20 g	Weetabix
20 g	oatmeal (raw)
20 g	Ready Brek
30 g	rice (raw)
90 g	rice (boiled)
25 g	bread (wholemeal)
30 g	bread (white)
Potato	
180 g	boiled or mashed
100 g	roast
70 g	chips
40 g	crisps (plain or salted)
100 g	baked (weighed without skin)
125 g	baked (weighed with skin)
45 g	peas—fresh or frozen
45 g	baked beans canned in tomato sauce

The principles of diet are similar to those used in the treatment of phenylketonuria with restriction of histidine instead of phenylalanine. Low-histidine protein substitutes are available (Table 10.6), and infant feeds can be devised as in the example (Table 10.16).

Histidine is an essential amino acid (Table 10.4), at least in infants and children (Holt 1967), and possibly in adults on prolonged synthetic diets (*Nutrition Reviews* 1970). The histidine requirement is supplied by either breast-feeding, human milk or a modified infant feed in the infant, and as a variety of foods (*see* 50-mg histidine exchanges, Table 10.17) in the older child. The intake is titrated to plasma histidine levels. Deficiency should be avoided. Raised levels are not clinically 'toxic' and therefore emergency regimens are not indicated during intercurrent infections.

Tyrosinaemias

Hereditary tyrosinaemia (also known as tyrosinosis and tyrosinaemia type I)

This is a rare metabolic disorder causing severe impairment of the liver and renal tubular dysfunction (Cohen *et al.* 1978, Hostetter *et al.* 1983, Gagné 1983). The primary defect is a deficiency of the enzyme fumarylacetoacetate lyase, which catalyses the final step of tyrosine degradation (Fig. 10.4). The diagnosis is made by measuring succinylacetone, which accumulates as a result of the metabolic block

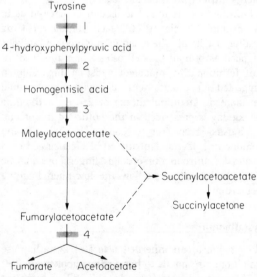

Fig. 10.4 Degradation of tyrosine. Key to inherited disorders of tyrosine metabolism: (1) tyrosine aminotransferase deficiency; (2) Hawkinsinuria; (3) alcaptonuria; (4) hereditary tyrosinaemia type I.

(Collins & Leonard 1985). Succinylacetoacetate also accumulates. The liver disease may begin prenatally and may already be advanced at birth (Hostetter *et al.* 1983).

An acute infantile form appears in the first weeks of life with progressive liver failure. Alpha-fetoprotein concentration is also increased (Hostetter *et al.* 1983). High levels of tyrosine, methionine and occasionally phenylalanine are found in blood, and tyrosyluria occurs. Despite dietary treatment the liver disease still progresses and it is usually fatal in the first year of life. Patients may be sensitive to even small increases in dietary protein intake, showing a marked deterioration in liver function with only a small rise in plasma tyrosine. It is thought the degradation of tyrosine continues in the liver despite the treatment, with the production of toxic metabolites such as succinylacetoacetate. Therapy aimed at reduction of the elevated tyrosine level is unlikely to be of fundamental value (Hostetter *et al.* 1983) in altering the course of the disease.

A chronic form of hereditary tyrosinaemia (type I) presents later with failure to thrive, gastrointestinal upset, cirrhosis of the liver, and renal tubular dysfunction, with secondary rickets and the Fanconi syndrome. High levels of tyrosine and methionine in blood are found. Mental retardation is not usually a feature (Halvorsen & Gjessing 1971).

A diet with restriction of tyrosine, phenylalanine and methionine has been used to correct the biochemical abnormality of amino acids, particularly in those with the chronic form of the disease (Fairney *et al.* 1968). Improvement has been noted even in those in whom the diet was started as late as one year, although some residual liver damage may remain. The patient of Fairney *et al.* (1968), who was treated from the age of 10 months, at 11 years old had an IQ of 97, had liver disease, was on the 50th percentile for height and weight and died of malignant hepatoma at 14 years.

Even with rigorous dietary treatment death usually ensues within the first decade of life (Cohen *et al.* 1978), due to either liver failure or hepatomata (Collins & Leonard 1985). Liver transplantation provides some hope for these children in the future, and prenatal diagnosis in affected families, with the possibility of a medical abortion, is now possible.

Other inherited disorders of tyrosine metabolism

Tyrosine aminotransferase deficiency, Richner–Hahnart syndrome or tyrosinaemia Oregan type, in which there is marked accumulation of tyrosine (Fig. 10.4) (Kennaway *et al.* 1971). The main features are skin lesions of hands and feet, a severe eye keratoconjunctivitis and sometimes mental retardation. Dietary treatment, low in both phenylalanine and tyrosine, corrects the biochemical abnormality and relieves both skin and eye symptoms.

Hawkinsinuria (Fig. 10.4) is a dominantly inherited defect of tyrosine metabolism with severe effects in infancy (Wilcken *et al.* 1981). This has been treated with high doses of vitamin C in pharmacological doses (1 g per day).

Transient neonatal tyrosinaemia

This occurs in newborn infants, particularly in those born prematurely, and is aggravated by high protein intakes. Walker *et al.* (1981) reported a reduction in the incidence of the transient neonatal amino acidaemias since the widespread use of lower protein modified milk for infant feeding. Transient neonatal tyrosinaemia is due to a block at the site of 4-hydroxyphenylpyruvic acid due to a deficiency of *p*-hydroxyphenylpyruvate oxidase (Fig. 10.4). Secondary hyperphenylalaninaemia occurs. Vitamin C is the cofactor for the enzyme and 50 to 100 mg per day usually corrects the defect. An appropriate protein intake, such as breast-feeding or use of a whey-based modified infant milk, largely prevents and corrects the biochemical abnormality. Liver disease is not present even when the biochemical abnormality persists for some time (Hostetter *et al.* 1983).

Raised tyrosine, phenylalanine and methionine also occur as a secondary effect of liver disease (Harries *et al.* 1969, Yu *et al.* 1971) and may simulate the hereditary disorders. Improvement in the liver condition results in remission of the biochemical abnormalities without specific therapy.

DIETARY TREATMENT OF HEREDITARY TYROSINAEMIA AND TYROSINE AMINOTRANSFERASE DEFICIENCY

The dietary regimen is based on the low-phenylalanine diet (Chapter 9), except that a protein substitute free of tyrosine and phenylalanine with or without methionine, is required (Table 10.6). The total intake of protein/nitrogen should not be higher than normal requirements and must be adjusted for the clinical condition, including the liver function. Supplementary individual amino acids may be necessary to correct the plasma amino acid profile, e.g. increased proportions of branched chain amino acids, cyst(e)ine and arginine may be needed due to the liver disease.

The protein substitute of choice is the Albumaid Phenylalanine/Tyrosine/Methionine Low (Table 10.6) as it ensures that an overload of methionine is avoided, the importance of which has been stressed by Michals et al. (1978). A feed for infants can be devised as described for the similar low-methionine product (Table 10.16i).

The essential intake of phenylalanine and methionine is provided by small quantities of conventional protein, aimed at keeping the plasma tyrosine within the normal range ± 1 SD (Gagné 1983). This may result in low plasma phenylalanine levels. However, in this condition the limit between deficiency and toxicity is narrow. Frequent biochemical monitoring of plasma amino acids is necessary, and caution should be exercised when increasing dietary protein intake. A modified whey-based milk in infants, and a variety of foods for the older child, provide the natural protein intake. The 50 mg phenylalalanine exchanges (Table 9.2) can be used, the tyrosine and methionine content being calculated as necessary. The methionine intake can be adjusted with supplements of the synthetic L-amino acid or combined use of the Albumaid Phenylalanine/Tyrosine Free product, which contains 600 mg methionine per 100 g, and Albumaid Phenylalanine/Tyrosine/Methionine Low. Both have a similar composition in other respects.

Appropriate mineral and vitamin supplements are essential. As a result of the liver disease additional vitamin D to correct the phosphataemic rickets and vitamin K to correct the hypoprothrombinaemia are frequently required, and vitamin A and E supplements may be desirable.

Although intercurrent infections do not cause the acute clinical deterioration seen in MSUD, a sudden increase in protein or plasma tyrosine is undesirable, and has been known to cause clinical deterioration, and therefore a high energy with reduced protein intake is advisable during periods of catabolism, as a temporary measure.

Organic acidaemias

A large number of defects in the degradation of the branched chain amino acids, threonine and methionine (Fig. 10.2 & Table 10.1), have been described; the commonest are methylmalonic acidaemia and propionic acidaemia apart from MSUD (see above). Recent helpful reviews have been given by Silken et al. (1981), Chalmers and Lawson (1982), Stanbury et al. (1983), Leonard et al. (1984), and Collins and Leonard (1985). Several of the defects may have a secondary raised glycine, e.g. propionic acidaemia

and methylmalonic acidaemia, and were previously known collectively as the ketotic hyperglycinaemias. Each of the disorders is characterized by the accumulation of organic acids, which vary with the site of the defect and give the disorders their names. Except in MSUD the plasma amino acid pattern is not diagnostic, as the amino acids involved in the metabolic block are broken down to organic acids and do not accumulate. It is necessary to examine the organic acids in plasma and urine to establish the diagnosis and understand the biochemical abnormality in order to devise appropriate treatment. A number of the enzymes concerned require specific vitamin cofactors. Several variants of each defect have been described, some of which respond to vitamin therapy (Table 10.3) as discussed earlier. The use of alternative pathways for removal of the toxic metabolite is possible in some disorders, e.g. glycine is given to detoxify isovaleric acid which is excreted as isovalerylglycine in isovaleric acidaemia (Kriegler & Tanaka 1976, Velazquez & Prieto 1980).

The more severe disorders in their classical form lead to ketosis, metabolic acidosis, vomiting, and neurological and other abnormalities in the neonatal period, and subsequent mental retardation commonly occurs if indeed the child survives (Table 10.1). Alternatively, the child may present with recurring episodes of ketoacidosis, which are often precipitated by infections or a sudden increase in dietary protein, and/or neurological problems, failure to thrive or mental retardation. The mildest forms may present with isolated episodes of ketoacidosis during intercurrent infections and the patient may appear normal in other ways (Stern & Toothill 1972). In contrast, other patients present with the clinical features of Reye's syndrome (Faull et al. 1976, Leonard et al. 1979).

The outcome of patients with these conditions depends on several factors: the precise nature of the inborn error; residual enzyme activity (Leonard et al. 1984, Rousson & Guibaud 1984); response to cofactor; the age at which symptoms present; age of diagnosis; and the neurodevelopmental status at the time of diagnosis. Although excellent results have been obtained in the vitamin-responsive disorders, and in others when the diagnosis is made early, provided the hazards of intercurrent infections are overcome and careful dietary control is maintained, patients, particularly with propionic acidaemia, presenting in the neonatal period do badly even when the diagnosis is made early and the patient is treated rigorously (Leonard et al. 1984). The outcome in the different variants of methylmalonic acidaemia has been reported in a large series (Matsui *et al.* 1983). Of those patients with no residual enzyme activity 60% died and all the others were handicapped. Those who were responsive to vitamin B$_{12}$ had a better outlook. The outcome of the other organic acidaemias is less well documented and reports are generally limited to only a few cases. Children with these disorders who survive the neonatal period and remain well with treatment may still deteriorate rapidly and even succumb during metabolic relapse associated with trauma or infections (Collins & Leonard 1985).

DIETARY TREATMENT OF PROPIONIC ACIDAEMIA, METHYLMALONIC ACIDAEMIA AND SIMILAR ORGANIC ACIDAEMIAS

The dramatic response to large doses of vitamin cofactors in some patients with organic acidaemias and their safe administration is in contrast to the difficult, often ineffective, low-protein diet therapy needed for the non-responsive disorders. Vitamin therapy (Table 10.3), appropriate to the metabolites found, should always be tried (*see* p. 270).

Protein-restricted diets are required in those patients who do not respond to cofactor vitamin therapy, or only partially do so. Sufficient protein for normal growth is required, and yet accumulation of metabolites should be prevented. As the responsible amino acids are not raised in blood, an arbitrary quantity of dietary protein, usually about 0·75 to 1·5 g protein/kg per day in reverse proportion to age and dependent on the growth rate, metabolic block and residual enzyme activity, together with a generous intake of dietary energy, is prescribed (Collins & Leonard 1985). At least the minimal quantity of protein to supply essential amino acids and nitrogen for growth needs (Table 8.2) should normally be given, except during episodes of intercurrent infections. During periods of catch-up growth higher protein intakes are often tolerated temporarily and if not supplied will inhibit such growth occurring.

The dietary protein intake can be provided in various concentrations of infant feeds (Table 10.18) to meet the dietary prescription, or as a variety of foods in the older child's diet (*see* Chapter 8). The intake should be monitored clinically and by blood amino acid profiles to ensure protein deficiency does not occur, and ideally the concentration of the abnormal blood and urine metabolite(s) should be assessed, and kept within minimum or safe levels. Generally the biochemical status is less satisfactory than in those disorders in which the protein intake can be more precisely regulated (Collins & Leonard 1985), as some protein is always degraded to form the metabolites.

During episodes of ketoacidosis, at the time of diagnosis or with metabolic relapse and during intercurrent illness, the temporary emergency regimen described on p. 282 with high-energy protein-free fluids (Table 10.9) is required.

Frequently these children self-select a low-protein intake, and are poor eaters, and feeding difficulties are common. Growth failure may result. Enteral feeding by nasogastric tube may be appropriate, using an appropriately devised feed. Any trend towards overweight, provided linear growth is normal, must be corrected by cautiously reducing the intake of both protein and energy, so that the weight velocity is reduced; weight loss should be avoided, as biochemical control will be lost. Individual assessment and supervision is necessary. Poor linear growth with overweight requires investigation of the cause of growth failure, including nutritional factors, but it is not always possible to achieve a normal growth rate even when nutritional deficiencies are corrected. Adequate energy must be provided from low-protein food, drinks and energy supplements. Vitamin and mineral supplements should be selected according to the contribution of the natural food intake, and essential fatty acids must be provided.

Supplementary amino acids appropriate for the metabolic block (Table 10.6) can be added to the diet if the protein intake is sufficiently low to possibly inhibit growth. The long-term benefit of this remains uncertain (Satoh *et al.* 1981, Leonard *et al.* 1984). They can be administered in a similar way to MSUD Aid in MSUD. Amino acids free of methionine, threonine, valine and isoleucine (SHS or Milupa) are available for use in propionic acidaemia and methylmalonic acidaemia.

Alternatively, where whole-protein intake has to be restricted, supplements of essential amino acids, e.g. Dialamine (Table 10.6), in conjunction with a low-protein high-energy diet may improve growth.

Acidosis should be corrected, and methylmalonate excretion is increased if the urine is kept alkaline. Sodium overload, particularly in the young infant, must be avoided by careful selection of any mineral supplement needed nutritionally.

Hypoglycaemia is a feature of some conditions and requires frequent carbohydrate feeding and avoidance of fasts.

Administration of glycine (250 mg/kg per day) has been used to reduce the accumulation of some organic acids, e.g. isovaleric acid, which is then excreted as a glycine conjugate (Krieger & Tanaka 1976, Velazquez & Prieto 1980).

Table 10.18   Examples of low-protein infant feeds.

	Low-protein feeds*†						Full-strength Gold Cap SMA‡	Human milk§ (100 ml)
Ingredients/100 ml feed								
†Gold Cap SMA								
Powder (g)	1·5	2·5	5	7·5	10	13	13	—
Glucose polymer (g)	15	14	12	10	10	8	Nil	—
50% oil emulsion (ml)	8	7	6	4	Nil	Nil	Nil	—
Water (ml)	100	100	100	100	100	100	100	—
Composition/100 ml								
Protein (g)	0·18	0·3	0·6	0·9	1·2	1·5	1·5	1·3
Carbohydrate (g)	15·8	14·4	14·8	14·8	15·6	15·2	7·2	7·4
Fat (g)	4·4	4·2	4·4	4·1	2·8	3·6	3·6	4·2
*Sodium (mmol)	0·08	0.13	0·26	0·38	0·5	0·65	0·65	0·65
*Potassium (mmol)	0·17	0·28	0·55	0·85	1·1	1·45	1·45	1·5
*Calcium (mmol)	0·13	0·22	0·44	0·66	0·88	1·1	1·1	0·88
Energy (kJ)	435	418	418	402	380	405	275	296
(kcal)	104	100	100	96	91	97	65	70
% energy from protein	0·7	1·2	2·4	3·8	5·3	6·2	9·2	7·4
150 ml/kg body weight provides								
Protein (g/kg)	0·27	0·45	0·9	1·35	1·8	2·25	2·25	1·95
Energy (kJ/kg)	650	628	628	600	570	608	408	440
(kcal/kg)	156	150	150	144	136	145	98	105

* Supplementary macro and micro minerals, electrolytes and bicarbonate may be indicated in conjunction with the low-protein feeds.

† Comprehensive vitamins, e.g. three Ketovite Tablets and 5 ml Ketovite Liquid, are recommended with these low-protein feeds.

‡ Other brands of whey-based low-protein infant modified milks may be calculated and used as an alternative.

§ *The Composition of Mature Human Milk* (DHSS 1977).

In the organic acidaemias in which there is accumulation of propionyl CoA, carnitine has been used as an effective strategy for the elimination of the propionyl groups (Bohan & Roe 1982, Roe *et al.* 1982, Roe *et al.* 1983). Carnitine acts by detoxifying the propionyl groups, thereby releasing CoA and restoring ATP biosynthesis and concentration toward normal; thus it may be used to maintain mitochondrial and cellular homeostasis in methylmalonic and propionic acidaemias. A dose of 100 mg/kg per day of carnitine with 150 mg/kg per day of glycine given in divided doses in conjunction with the appropriate low-protein diet, has been suggested in propionic acidaemia by Bohan and Roe (1982). The long-term effectiveness of such a regimen awaits further evaluation.

Although sodium benzoate is effective in reducing the hyperammonaemia of the urea cycle disorders (*see* later), it is contraindicated in the secondary hyperammonaemias associated with the organic acidaemias, particularly when there is propionyl CoA accumulation, due to the risk of benzoate accumulation in the mitochondria as a result of an inadequate supply of CoA and ATP (Bohan & Roe 1982, Collins & Leonard 1985).

Disorders of fat oxidation

A group of disorders of the breakdown of β-oxidation of fatty acids occur, and include long-, medium-, and short-chain acyl CoA dehydrogenase deficiency, systemic carnitine deficiency, hepatic carnitine palmitoyl transferase deficiency and multiple acyl CoA dehydrogenase deficiency (glutaric aciduria type II) (Duran *et al.* 1984). Patients present with hypoglycaemia and low ketone body concentrations and are often initially diagnosed as having Reye's syndrome (Leonard *et al.* 1979). Dicarboxylic aciduria occurs (Durnan *et al.* 1984). Great care is needed to identify the metabolic block correctly and to devise the correct treatment (Collins & Leonard 1985). Some of the disorders are cofactor-responsive.

Fasts must be avoided. During illness, trauma and metabolic relapse it is essential to give frequent carbohydrate-containing fat-free fluids, e.g. two to three-hourly drinks of 15 to 20% solution of carbohydrate(s), glucose polymer, sweetened fruit juice, Lucozade, etc, to provide approximately 20 g carbohydrate/kg per day as a temporary emergency regimen. Fat is poorly tolerated for obvious reasons, especially during metabolic relapse, and protein restriction may also be necessary; thus the patient is dependent on carbohydrate intake during such episodes. When well a diet with a moderate reduction of fat and protein intake with extra between-meal carbohydrate-containing drinks and/or snacks is recommended. Fasts, even overnight, should be avoided by giving a late-night and early-morning carbohydrate-containing drink or snack, which should also be given if the child refuses to eat at meal times.

Carnitine is essential for fatty acid transport into the mitochondria prior to oxidation. Deficiency of carnitine may occur as either a primary or more commonly a secondary disorder. Carnitine supplements are helpful if there are low plasma and urine levels of carnitine (Durnan *et al.* 1984, Leonard *et al.* 1984).

Carnitine may be an essential nutrient in the newborn infant. Deficiency has been reported (Slonim *et al.* 1981) as a cause of non-ketotic hypoglycaemia in an infant fed on a soya formula which was carnitine-free. Clinical improvement occurred with carnitine treatment.

Pyruvate dehydrogenase deficiency

In contrast to the above disorders this condition requires treatment with a high-fat, ketogenic diet, as carbohydrate and metabolic relapse increase plasma alanine, pyruvate and lactate (Falk *et al.* 1976).

Urea cycle disorders: hyperammonaemias

Disorders of the urea cycle are the result of enzyme deficiencies, leading to ammonia intoxication with high levels in blood and cerebrospinal fluid, which may exceed those found in hepatic failure. Although rare conditions, they have been diagnosed with increasing frequency during the last few years (Brusilow 1985). Between 50 and 90% of waste nitrogen is excreted as urea. Ammonia is produced from amino acid degradation in the tissues and bowel

lumen and enters the urea cycle in the liver (Fig. 10.5). Distinct disorders have been described due to each of the specific enzyme deficiencies (Table 10.1) (Walser 1983, Brusilow 1985). Arginase deficiency (argininaemia) is distinct from the other disorders in many respects and is discussed separately (*see* p. 304).

Ornithine carbamyltransferase (OCT) deficiency is the commonest of the urea cycle disorders. It is unusual in that it is inherited as a sex-linked dominant (Palmer *et al.* 1974). The defect in the severely affected 'hemizygous' male is almost always lethal, but mildly affected boys are not uncommon. Because of Lyonization of one X chromosome, the disease has a variable clinical expression in the heterozygous female. Fetal damage occurs, probably due to both maternal and fetal disorders, and spontaneous abortion is common (Palmer *et al.* 1974).

The urea cycle disorders vary widely in their severity and may present at almost any age in childhood, but most commonly present in the neonatal period. All patients, including those with milder disease, may have episodes of acute illness. Ammonia accumulation is toxic, particularly to the neurological system, and causes vomiting, convulsions, focal neurological signs and cerebral oedema, which may lead to coma and death (Collins & Leonard 1985). This may occur in the neonatal period or during episodes of catabolism (Mantagos *et al.* 1978). Symptoms may be episodic and are aggravated by dietary protein, infections and starvation. Early symptoms are headache, irritability, ataxia, confusion, abnormalities of behaviour, and vomiting. Chronic ammonia accumulation is characterized by periodic episodes as mentioned above, mental retardation and neurological abnormalities. Particularly in those who present in the neonatal period, outcome is poor (Msall *et al.* 1984). Patients with milder disease can grow and develop normally if the treatment is started early and if the child survives episodes of catabolism. Anorexia, feeding difficulties, and failure to thrive are common.

Plasma ammonia levels in the urea cycle disorders are usually grossly elevated, more than 400μmol/l* in those who present in the neonatal period, and may continue to rise rapidly. The normal plasma ammonia level in children is less than 40μmol/l* with slight elevation in individuals taking a high-protein diet. During episodes of acute encephalopathy in older children plasma ammonia usually exceeds $250\ \mu$mol/l* (Collins & Leonard 1985). A rise in ammonia may only be detected after protein-loading in

---

* Ammonia conversion factor: μmol/l $\div 0\cdot714 = \mu$g/100 ml.

some defects and the milder variants. Between episodes they may be normal, particularly if the protein
intake is low. Plasma glutamine and alanine are
raised, and arginine reduced, in all but arginase deficiency. Characteristic amino acids are elevated in
citrullinaemia, arginase deficiency and arginosuccinic aciduria. In all but the carbamyl phosphate
synthetase defect orotic acid is raised, which is diag-
nostically helpful. Specific biochemical abnormalities
accompany each disorder (Walser 1983). Diagnosis
is made by measuring plasma ammonia and amino
acids. Confirmation of the diagnosis can be made by
measuring the activity of the appropriate enzymes in
suitable tissue (Walser 1983).

Hyperammonaemia also occurs in familial protein
intolerance (Kekomakie *et al.* 1967), the organicacidaemias, e.g. methylmalonic acidaemia (Cathelinaeu
et al. 1981, Bohan & Roe 1982), Reye's syndrome,
and most commonly as a result of hepatic failure.
Transient neonatal hyperammonaemia also occurs
and responds to supplements of arginine.

TREATMENT

The aim of treatment is to keep the plasma ammonia
level in a safe range by diet and supplements of arginine, sodium benzoate, phenylacetate and/or citrulline (Brusilow 1985). The dietary total protein
intake is limited, but must provide for growth needs.
This usually means a protein intake of 0·5 to
1·5 g/kg per day, depending on the child's age and
severity of the defect, to minimize ammonia accumulation. Normal ammonia levels are rarely achieved
but treatment should be aimed to keep them below
80 μmol/l.

The dietary protein is given, as suggested earlier,
as frequent small feeds or meals with a high energy
intake and arginine supplements (*see* below). Many
patients self-select a low-protein diet and have a poor
appetite. Supplements of appropriate vitamin and minerals (Table 10.8) are given to ensure the nutritional adequacy of the diet.

During periods of acute ammonia intoxication—at
diagnosis, and during infections or other catabolic
episodes—an emergency high-energy protein-free regimen, as already described (p. 282, Table 10.9), is
required temporarily. Ammonia can be removed by
dialysis when clinically indicated (Hopkins *et al.*
1969, Brusilow 1985).

Arginine deficiency probably contributes to the associated growth failure and hair changes which are
features of these disorders.

Arginine is normally synthesized in the urea cycle
(Fig. 10.5), but because of the metabolic block in the
hereditary hyperammonaemias synthesis is reduced
and arginine becomes an essential or semi-essential
amino acid (Kline *et al.* 1981, Smith & Francis 1982).
Arginine supplements, except in arginase deficiency,
are thus required in the urea cycle disorders in a
dose of 100 mg/kg per day. Alternatively, citrulline,
170 mg/kg per day, can be used to provide the essential arginine, and has advantages over arginine itself
because citrulline contains one less nitrogen atom
than arginine, and even in infants with either carbamyl phosphate synthetase or ornithine carbamyltransferase deficiency it is rapidly converted to arginine via the intact part of the urea cycle (Fig. 10.5)
(Brusilow 1985).

Arginine is also useful in reducing hyperammonaemia (Brusilow 1984, 1985). In citrullinaemia and
arginosuccinic aciduria large doses of arginine as free
base (up to 700 mg/kg per day) can replenish ornithine synthesis and thus reduce ammonia accumulation significantly. The resultant increased citrulline
is less toxic than ammonia and is readily excreted
in urine (Brusilow & Batshaw 1979, Batshaw *et al.*
1981, Brusilow 1985).

Severely affected patients tolerate very little
protein, and progressive ammonia accumulation
occurs. Replacement of a proportion of the dietary
protein prescription with a small supplement of essential amino acids (Table 10.6) is useful in reducing
total nitrogen intake, and yet provides for growth
needs (Snyderman *et al.* 1977, Collins & Leonard
1985). Keto analogues provide carbon skeletons of
the essential amino acids without the NH_2 groups
(Batshaw *et al.* 1976, Brusilow *et al.* 1979) and theoretically could be transaminated to form their essential amino acids, thus utilizing available nitrogen.
However, apart from the disadvantage of the extremely bitter taste of the keto analogues, they are
not readily utilized and their contribution to dietary
therapy has been disappointing (personal observation).

Sodium benzoate has been used as another form of
therapy to remove ammonia and has made a dramatic difference to the management of these disorders.
This compound is conjugated in the liver with glycine
to form hippuric acid, which is rapidly excreted in
the urine by the kidney, thereby creating an alternative route for excretion of waste nitrogen which
can be highly effective in reducing plasma ammonia
(Batshaw & Brusilow 1980). It can be used both as
an adjunct to long-term dietary management and in
the treatment of acute hyperammonaemia episodes

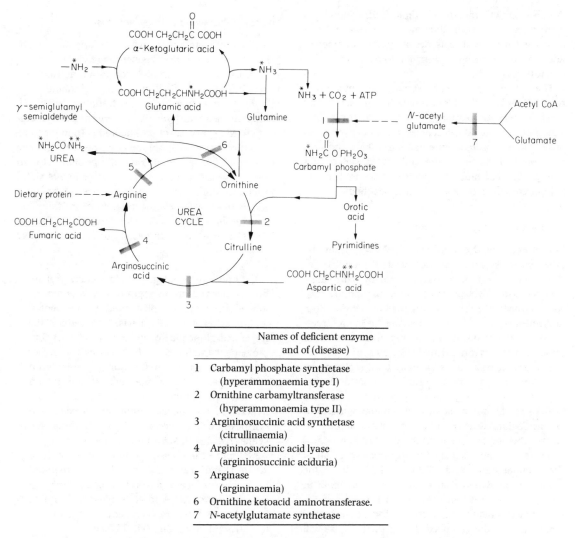

Fig. 10.5 Conversion of ammonia to urea. Amino groups (NH_2) enter the cycle either as carbamyl phosphate* or as aspartic acid**. Adapted from Smith & Francis (1982).

(Collins & Leonard 1985). Another alternative is the use of phenylacetic acid or sodium phenylacetate which conjugates with glutamine and can be excreted as phenylacetylglutamine, thus removing waste nitrogen (Brusilow 1985). This can be used in conjunction with sodium benzoate. Preliminary work on other alternatives, such as phenylbutyrate, to enhance removal of waste nitrogen are being explored currently by some units (Brusilow 1985). However, the safety and usefulness of sodium benzoate and/or phenylacetate in the neonatal period remains in doubt (Green 1981, Green *et al.* 1983, Brusilow 1985). There is a risk of both sodium over-

load and benzoate accumulation in mitochondria.

Lactulose is used in hepatic ammonia intoxication to reduce absorption of ammonia by the bowel lumen. This could be useful in acute episodes of hyperammonaemia in the urea cycle defects. However, it causes malabsorption and therefore is less suitable for long-term use in the treatment of chronic hyperammonaemia.

Many reports emphasize the poor growth of patients with urea cycle disorders. Selected or prescribed low-protein diets, arginine and energy deficiency all probably play a part. These patients are frequently poor eaters and have periodic food refusal.

A slower growth rate than optimal for the individual further impairs protein tolerance. The aim of treatment must be to avoid episodes of hyperammonaemia and yet provide adequate nutrition to maintain a normal rate of growth.

The child's treatment should be monitored regularly—clinically for growth parameters, and biochemically for plasma ammonia and the amino acid profile, to avoid deficiencies and under- or over-prescription of protein. Parents require help and support, particularly when the child is unwell or not eating. The diet must be continually revised in the light of growth, clinical and biochemical findings.

Arginase deficiency (argininaemia)

This disorder of the urea cycle is distinct from the other disorders and may not present until two or three years of age. It is characterized by neurodegeneration with developmental regression and progressive spasticity (Walser 1983, Brusilow 1985). Both arginine and total dietary protein are toxic, and treatment is therefore distinct to that required in the other urea cycle defects (Snyderman et al. 1979b).

The treatment requires virtually total replacement of dietary protein with an essential amino acid mixture free of arginine, given in an appropriate dose for growth needs, but avoidance of ammonia accumulation. Sodium benzoate is an important adjunct to dietary therapy to remove ammonia. The amino acid supplement should supply the requirement of all of the essential amino acids (Table 10.4), ideally in the proportion in which they occur in human milk, in the infant, and reference protein in the older child. Just sufficient additional nitrogen for non-essential amino acid synthesis is needed, or growth failure will occur. Dialamine (Table 10.6) has been used as the source of essential amino acids in the older child treated with this disorder. A virtually synthetic diet is necessary, as even traces of dietary protein can be significant. The diet must be supplemented with adequate energy, essential fatty acids, all vitamins and minerals to maintain weight and provide for growth needs. An extremely limited range of negligible-protein foods is permitted: even the protein content of special low-protein bread, biscuits, pasta, fruit and vegetables, etc. must be taken into account in the diet prescription. A high-energy protein-free regimen is essential during episodes of metabolic relapse, and even when well energy deficit must be avoided. Nasogastric tube feeding may be necessary to maintain optimal nutrient intake.

Hyperornithinaemia with gyrate atrophy

Hyperornithinaemia with gyrate atrophy of the choroid and retina is a rare degenerative retinopathy due to a deficiency of ornithine ketoacid aminotransaminase. Ornithine is raised and lysine, glutamine and glutamate are reduced in concentration in the blood. Glutamate semialdehyde is an intermediate metabolite in the synthesis of proline and is thought to be the major pathway for proline synthesis in the eye (Tada et al. 1984). Patients usually present between 5 and 10 years of age with progressive loss of sight, particularly night vision. There is uncertainty about whether the eye defects are related to ornithine excess or proline deficiency (Valle et al. 1980, Tada et al. 1984); thus two approaches to treatment have been reported.

(a) Ornithine is not present in dietary protein, but is derived from arginine. A low-protein low-arginine diet supplemented with essential amino acids has been devised to reduce the hyperornithinaemia by Valle et al. (1980). Improvement (McInnes et al. 1981) or no further deterioration in visual function in patients on such a diet have been reported. Over restriction of arginine resulted in clinically significant hyperammonaemia as a result of reduced protein synthesis during a period of hypo-ornithinaemia (Valle et al. 1980, McInnes et al. 1981).

McInnes et al. (1981) found that a range of 12 to 18 mg arginine/kg per day was required in teenagers given a total protein intake of 0·8 g/kg per day, to maintain plasma ornithine levels in the arbitrary therapeutic range of 150 to 250 μmol/l (normal 30 to 120 μmol/l).

A diet could be devised using these principles and those given under 'Arginase deficiency', with small supplements as tolerated of dietary protein, for patients of different ages. Arginine and total protein intakes would be expected to be greater in the younger age groups in order to promote growth, and prevent deficiency and hyperammonaemia. The diet must be monitored to avoid deficiency. Blood ammonia, ornithine, arginine and the amino acid profile, as well as clinical parameters, must be monitored.

(b) By contrast, Tada et al. (1984) have proposed that proline deficiency is the important factor and they treat patients with proline supplements (3 g per day), apparently with equally good results.

Long-term continual ophthalmological follow-up will be required to determine if the chorio-retinal degeneration is halted, or indeed reversed, by these therapeutic approaches.

Hartnup disease

This is due to defective transport of the neutral amino acids, including tryptophan, into mucosal cells and renal tubular cells (Milne 1972, Wilcken *et al.* 1977). The amino acid losses are usually insignificant. A pellagra-like clinical picture with ataxia is a rare complication, occurring only in some patients, and is relieved by nicotinamide (niacin) administration (100 to 250 mg per day). Normally about one-third of the daily nicotinic acid requirement is derived from dietary tryptophan (Milne 1972).

Disorders of tryptophan

Several disorders related to tryptophan degradation have been described and cause 'pellagra'. One of them, xanthurenic aciduria, is responsive to pyridoxine, 10 to 100 mg per day (Scriver & Rosenburg 1973).

Tryptophanuria ('blue diaper syndrome') is a specific defect of the tryptophan transport system (Stanbury *et al.* 1983). Pellagra is not a feature of this condition.

Abnormalities of purine metabolism

Hyperuricacidaemia results from abnormal purine metabolism. This occurs in gout, which is reviewed in Davidson *et al.* (1979). It can also be secondary to renal and various metabolic disorders, e.g. glycogen storage disease type I.

A rare genetic deficiency of the enzymes associated with uric acid, adenine and purine metabolism has been reported (Seegmiller 1976, Simmonds *et al.* 1980, Simmonds *et al.* 1981, Stanbury *et al.* 1983). Correct diagnosis is essential in order to devise appropriate treatment.

About 80% of dietary purines are absorbed and metabolized to uric acid. However, diet only accounts for approximately 50% of uric acid in the blood of normal individuals, the remainder being formed as a result of endogenous production. Most of the uric acid so formed is lost from the body urine. Uric acid is less soluble in very acid solutions and precipitates as uric acid renal stones in some patients with gout and other conditions with hyperuricacidaemia in whom a high fluid intake is recommended.

A low-purine diet does reduce blood urate levels, and although alternative treatment is available for most patients with gout, avoidance of excess purine intake is logical. Such patients are advised to avoid liver, kidneys, sweetbreads, sardines, anchovies, fish roes, pulses, legumes (including soya), and meat and yeast extracts. Feasts, fasts and alcohol are also inadvisable (Davidson *et al.* 1979).

Patients with the inherited enzyme defects associated with purine, adenine and uric acid metabolism may need a more formalized diet reducing purine intake (Table 10.19). The purine content of foods is now available in Clifford and Story (1976) and *Geigy Scientific Tables* (1981). Many of the older tables, due to inadequate analytical methods employed, are unreliable. Adequate intake of fluids and specific treatment appropriate for the metabolic defect concerned are recommended, e.g. allopurinol or avoidance of excess urine acidity (Simmonds *et al.* 1980, 1981). The diet must be nutritionally adequate for growth. During intercurrent infections, a high fluid intake and adequate energy from carbohydrates is advised.

Severe renal damage can develop in both uric acid and 2,8-DHA stone-formers prior to correct diagnosis and treatment. Whether modern treatment will prevent this requires further evaluation.

Caffeine is not metabolized to uric acid and therefore is not restricted during treatment with a low-purine diet. However, caffeine only differs from uric acid in having three extra methyl groups on the purine ring. Caffeine should therefore be avoided temporarily during studies of purine and uric acid metabolism as it can interfere with laboratory analysis (Simmons *et al.* 1981). Caffeine is present in tea, coffee, cocoa, chocolate, cola and Lucozade.

CONCLUSION

The amino acid disorders are demanding for all involved in treatment, including the clinical team, parents and patient. The diet must be modified for age and growth and requires clinical and biochemical monitoring. Parents need encouragement and support, particularly when the child is unwell or not eating for any reason. They demand, perhaps more than in any other situation, the science and practical application of dietetics.

Table 10.19 Low-purine diet*.

(a) Allowed and forbidden foods.

Foods permitted freely or in restricted quantity	Foods not permitted
Milk and modified infant milks. Milk products. Yoghurt, ice-cream.	Soya formula
Egg, cheese. Butter, margarine, fats and oils in moderation (avoid fried foods).	
Meat: lamb, beef, chicken, pork, ham, bacon, minced beef. ⎫ ⎬ One serve only per day White fish, cod, plaice, haddock, fish fingers ⎭	Liver, kidney, heart, brains, sweetbreads. Game: venison, pheasant, partridge, grouse. All meat extracts: Oxo, Bovril. etc. All yeast extracts: Marmite†, Vegemite†, Barmene†, etc. Soups and gravies containing meat and yeast extracts, stock cubes, gravy made with meat juices. Textured vegetable proteins based on soya. Meat pastes and paté. Meat casseroles. Made-up dishes containing soya proteins, meat extracts, e.g. beefburgers.
	Fish roes, herring, kippers, sardines, smelts, sprats, anchovies, salmon, trout, mackerel, tuna and other fatty fish. Scallops, mussels, shrimps, clams, squid, oysters. Fish paste.
Cereals: Rice Krispies, Ricicles, Cornflakes, Frosties, Farley's Original Rusk, Baby Rice. White flour, semolina, rice, sago, custard powder, etc. Pasta. Bread/rolls—white only. Plain cakes, e.g. Swiss roll and sponge type. Plain biscuits, e.g. Marie, Osborne, rich tea.	Oats: porridge, muesli and Swiss-style cereals. Cereals: Weetabix, Shredded Wheat, Puffed Wheat, Bemax, All Bran, bran and bran products. Rye and rye products, e.g. pumpernickel. Wholemeal, brown and wholegrain breads. Digestive biscuits, Crackerwheat, etc. Ryvita and similar crispbreads. Rich cakes, e.g. cream cakes, Madeira, Christmas type. Wholemeal rusks, e.g. Farley's.
All fruits, nuts (whole nuts only after four years old).	
Vegetables including carrots, runner and French beans, cabbage, salad vegetables. Potatoes, chips and crisps—plain, salted.	Pulses and legumes: peas, beans including baked beans, lentils. Spinach, asparagus, mushrooms. Soya. Crisps flavoured with meat and/or yeast extracts, etc.
Sugar, peanut butter, jam, marmalade, honey. Boiled sweets, jelly. Tomato ketchup, salad cream.	

Table 10.19(a) *continued*

Foods permitted freely or in restricted quantity	Foods not permitted
‡Chocolate and ‡chocolate-containing products, e.g. ‡chocolate biscuits, ‡chocolate ice-cream.	
Water, fruit juice, squashes, lemonade and fruit-flavoured fizzy drinks.	Alcohol
Decaffeinated coffee.	
‡Tea, ‡coffee, ‡cocoa, ‡chocolate, ‡Horlicks, ‡Bournvita, ‡Lucozade, ‡Coca Cola, ‡Pepsi, ‡Tab, ‡cola, etc.	

* Adapted from information from the Purine Metabolism Unit, Guy's Hospital, London. Clifford and Story (1976) and *Geigy Scientific Tables* (1981) provide details of the purine content of foods.

† Particularly high in adenine.

‡ Contain caffeine and should be avoided during purine metabolism studies (*see* text).

(b) Example of low-purine diet menu.

Breakfast	Cornflakes, Rice Krispies, Farley's Original Rusk
	Milk, sugar
	White bread or toast
	Scraping butter/margarine
	Marmalade, jam, honey
	Egg optional
	Milk or fruit juice*
Snacks	Fruit juice, fruit, water*
Lunch/supper	Average serve meat/fish from permitted list *once* daily, e.g. minced beef, chicken, fish fingers, lamb, beef, pork
	Avoid gravy
	Potato, rice, spaghetti
	Permitted vegetables, carrot, cabbage, French/runner beans, salad
	Tomato ketchup or salad cream
	Fruit and custard or milk pudding or jelly and ice-cream or yoghurt
	Water to drink*
Lunch/tea	White bread or rolls
(may be adapted	Scraping butter/margarine
to a packed	Egg or cheese dish, e.g. boiled egg, omelette, macaroni cheese
sandwich	Peanut butter, jam, honey
school lunch)	Salad and/or permitted vegetables, e.g. tomato
	Chips or crisps (plain or salted)
	Fruit, fresh, dried. Nuts in older children
	Water, fruit juice, milk*

* A high fluid intake is recommended. Tea and coffee are permitted except during purine metabolic studies.

REFERENCES

ACOSTA P.B. (1982) Construction of an amino acid-restricted diet. In *Practice of Pediatrics* (ed. Kelley V. C.), Chapter 69. New York: Harper & Row.

ACOSTA P.B. (1985) The contribution of therapy of inherited amino acid disorders to knowledge of amino acid requirements. In *Congenital Metabolic Disease. Diagnosis and Treatment* (ed. Wapnir R.). New York: Marcel Dekker Inc.

AGGETT P.J. & DAVIES N.T. (1983) Some nutritional aspects of trace metals. *J. Inherited Metabolic Disease* 6, Suppl. 1, 22–30.

ALEXANDER F.W., CLAYTON B.E. & DELVES H.T. (1974) Mineral and trace-metal balances in children receiving normal and synthetic diets. *Quart. J. Med.* NS 43, 89.

BATSHAW M.L. & BRUSILOW S.W. (1980) Treatment of hyperammonaemic coma caused by inborn errors of urea synthesis. *J. Pediat.* 97, 893–900.

BATSHAW M.L., BRUSILOW S. & WALSER M. (1976) Long term management of a case of carbamyl phosphate synthetase deficiency using ketoanalogues and hydroxyanalogues of essential amino acids. *Pediatrics* 58, 227.

BATSHAW M.L., THOMAS G.H. & BRUSILOW S.W. (1981) New approaches to the diagnosis and treatment of inborn errors of urea synthesis. *Pediatrics* 68, 290–7.

BESSMAN S.P. (1979) The justification theory: the essential nature of the non essential amino acids. *Nutr. Rev.* 37, 209.

BICKEL H., GUTHRIE R. & HAMMERSEN G. (eds.) (1980) *Neonatal Screening for Inborn Errors of Metabolism.* Berlin: Springer–Verlag.

BOHAN T.P. & ROE C.R. (1982) Treatment of inborn errors of urea synthesis (letter). *New Engl. J. Med.* 307, 1212.

BØRRESEN A.L. & BOMAN N. (1982) Prenatal diagnosis. *Lancet* Oct. 16, p. 875.

BRENTON D.P. & CUSWORTH D.C. (1971) The response of patients with cystathionine synthetase deficiency to pyridoxine. In *Inherited Disorders of Sulphur Metabolism, Proceedings of the 8th Symposium of the Society for the Study of Inborn Errors of Metabolism* (eds. Carson N.A.J. & Raine D.N.), p. 264. Edinburgh: Churchill Livingstone.

BRENTON D.P., CUSWORTH D.C. & DENT C.E. (1966) Homocystinuria. Clinical and dietary studies. *Quart. J. Med.* NS 35, 325.

BRUSILOW S.W. (1984) Arginine, an indispensible amino acid for patients with inborn errors of urea synthesis. *J. Clinical Investigations* 74, 2144–8.

BRUSILOW S.W. (1985) Inborn errors of urea synthesis. In *Genetic and Metabolic Disease in Paediatrics* (eds. Lloyd J. & Scriver C.), pp. 140–65. London: Butterworth.

BRUSILOW S.W. & BATSHAW M.L. (1979) Arginine therapy of ariginosuccinase deficiency. *Lancet* i, 124.

BRUSILOW S.W., VALLE D.L. & BATSHAW M.L. (1979) New pathways of nitrogen excretion in inborn errors of urea synthesis. *Lancet* ii, 452.

BUIST N.R.M. & JHAVERI B.M. (1973) A guide to screening newborn infants for inborn errors of metabolism. *J. Pediat.* 82, (No. 3), 511–22.

CARSON N.A.J. (1982) Homocystinuria: clinical and biochemical heterogenicity. In *Inborn Errors of Metabolism in Humans* (eds. Cockburn F. & Gitzelman R.), pp. 53–67. Lancaster: MTP Press.

CATHELINAEU L., BRIAND L. & OGIER H. (1981) Occurrence of hyperammonia in the course of 17 cases of methylmalonic acidaemia. *J. Pediat.* 99, (No. 2), 279–80.

CHALMERS R.A. & LAWSON A.M. (1982) *Organic Acids in Man.* London: Chapman & Hall.

CLAYTON B.E. (1975) The principles of treatment by dietary restriction as illustrated by phenylketonuria. In *Treatment of Inherited Metabolic Disease* (ed. Raine D.N.) pp. 1–32. Lancaster: MTP Press.

CLAYTON B.E., JENKINS P. & ROUND J.M. (1980) *Paediatric Chemical Pathology: Clinical Tests and Reference Ranges*, Oxford: Blackwell Scientific Publications.

CLIFFORD A.J. & STORY D.L. (1976) Levels of purines in foods and their metabolic effects in rats. *J. Nutr.* 106, 435–42.

CLOSE J.H. (1974) The use of amino acid precursors in nitrogen accumulation diseases. *New Engl. J. Med.* 290, 663.

CLOW C.L., READE T.M. & SCRIVER C.R. (1981) Outcome of early and long term management of classical MSUD. *Pediatrics* 68, 856–62.

COHEN B.E., KEREN G. & CRISPIN M. (1978) Congenital tyrosinaemia. *Monogr. hum. Genet.* vol. 9, 118–22. Basle: Karger.

COLLINS F.S., SUMMER G.K., SCHWARTZ R.P. & PARKE J.C. JR. (1980) Neonatal arginosuccinicaciduria—survival after early diagnosis and dietary management. *J. Pediat.* 96, 429–31.

COLLINS J.E. & LEONARD J.V. (1985) The dietary management of inborn errors of metabolism. *Hum. Nutr.: Appl. Nutr.* 39A, 255–72.

COOPER A., BETTS J.M., PEREIRA G.R. & ZIEGLER M.M. (1984) Taurine deficiency in the severe hepatic dysfunction complicating total parenteral nutrition. *J. pediat. Surg.* Vol. 19, No. 4, 462–5.

COULOMBE J.T., KAMMERER B.L., LEVY H.L., HIRSCH B.Z. & SCRIVER C.R. (1983) Histidinaemia, part III: Impact—a prospective study. *J. Inherited Metabolic Disease* 6, 58–61.

COUTTS J.M.J. & FOWLER B. (1967) Low methionine diet for homocystinuria with reference to 2 cases. *Nutrition* 21, 1, 35–42.

DAVIDSON SIR S., PASSMORE R. & BROCK J.F. (1979) *Human Nutrition and Dietetics*, 7th Edition, p. 364. Edinburgh: Churchill Livingstone.

DHSS (1977) *The Composition of Mature Human Milk.* London: HMSO.

DICKINSON J.P., HOLTEN J.B., LEWIS G.M., LILLEWOOD J.M. & STEEL A.E. (1969) MSUD. Four years experience with dietary treatment of a case. *Acta paediat. scand.* 58, 341–51.

DI GEORGE A.M., REZVANI I., GARIBALDI L.R. & SCHWARTZ M. (1982) Prospective study of MSUD for the first four days of life. *New Engl. J. Med.* Vol. 307, No. 24, 1492–5.

DURAN M., DeKLERK J.B.C., WADMAN S.K., BRUINVIS L. & KETTING D. (1984) The differential diagnosis of dicarboxylic aciduria. *J. Inherited Metabolic Disease* 7, 48–51.

DYME I.Z., HORWITZ S.J., BACCHUS B. & KERR D.S. (1983)

Histidinemia. A case with resolution of myoclonic seizures after treatment with a low histidine diet. *Amer. J. Dis. Child.* **137**, 256–8.

EFRON M.L. (1967) Diet therapy for inborn errors of amino acid metabolism. *J. Amer. diet. Ass.* **51**, 40.

FAIRNEY A., FRANCIS D. & ERSSER R.S. (1968) Diagnosis and treatment of tyrosinosis. *Arch. Dis. Childh.* **43**, 540.

FALK R.E., CEDERBONIM S.D., BLASS J.P., GIBSON G.E., KARK R.A. & CARREL R.E. (1976) Ketotic diet in the management of pyruvate dehydrogenase deficiency. *Pediatrics* **58**, 713–21.

FAO/WHO (1973) *Energy and Protein Requirements.* Report of a joint FAO/WHO *ad hoc* expert committee (WHO Technical Report Series No 522 and FAO Nutrition Meeting Report Series No 52). Geneva: WHO/FAO.

FAULL K., BOLTON P., HALPERN B., HAMMOND J., DANKS D.M., HÄHNEL R., WILKINSON S.P., WYSOCKI S.J. & MASTERS P.L. (1976) Patient with defect in leucine metabolism. *New Engl. J. Med.* **294**, 1013.

FORSUM E.F. & HAMBRAEUS L. (1972) Biological evaluation of a whey protein fraction with special reference to its use as a phenylalanine-low source in the dietary treatment of phenylketonuria. *Nutrition and Metabolism* **14**, 48.

FRANCIS D.E.M. (1986) *Nutrition for Children.* Oxford: Blackwell Scientific Publications.

GAGNÉ R. (1983)—Liver disease in hereditary tyrosinaemia (letter). *New Engl. J. Med.* **309**, 17, 1063.

GAULL G.E., RASSIN D.K. & RÄIHÄ N.C.R. (1977) Milk protein quantity and quality in low birthweight infants. III Effects of sulphur amino acids in plasma and urine. *J. Pediat.* **90**, 348.

GEGGEL M.D., AMENT M.E., HECKENLIVELY J.R., MARTIN D.A. & KOPPLE J.D. (1985) Nutritional requirement for taurine in patients receiving long-term parenteral nutrition. *New Engl. J. Med.* **312**, 142–6.

GEIGY SCIENTIFIC TABLES (1981) Vol. 1 *Units of Measurement, Body Fluids, Composition of the Body, Nutrition*, 8th Revised Edition (ed. Lentner C.). Basle: Ciba–Geigy.

GOLDMAN H.I., GOLDMAN S. & KAUFMAN I.R. (1974) Late effects of early dietary protein intake on low birth weight infants. *J. Pediat.* **85**, 764.

GOMPERTZ D. (1972) Organicacidaemias. In *Proceedings of Society for the Study of Inborn Errors of Metabolism, No. 9* (eds. Stern J. & Toothill C.). Edinburgh: Churchill Livingstone.

GREEN T.P. (1981) Sodium benzoate in treatment of hyperammonaemia in new-borns (Abstract). *Pediat. Res.* **15**, 630.

GREEN T.P., MARCHESSAULT R.P. & FREESE D.K. (1983) Disposition of sodium benzoate in newborn infants with hyperammonaemia. *J. Pediat.* **102**, 785–90.

GRETTER T.E., LONSDALE D. & SHAMBERGER R.J. (1972) Maple syrup urine disease variant. *Cleveland Clinic Quarterly* **39**, (No. 3), 129–33.

GRIFFITHS M. (1973) Clinical aspects of the dietary treatment of histidinaemia. A report of 4 cases. In *Treatment of Inborn Errors of Metabolism, proceedings of the 10th Symposium of the Society for the Study of Inborn Errors of Meta-*

bolism (eds., Seakins J.W.T., Saunders R.A. & Toothill C.) p. 87. Edinburgh: Churchill Livingstone.

HALVORSEN S. & GJESSING L.R. (1971) Tyrosinosis. In *Phenylketonuria and Some Other Inborn Errors of Amino Acid Metabolism* (eds. Bickel H., Hudson F.P. & Woolf L.I.), p. 301. Stuttgart: Georg Thieme.

HAMMERSEN G., WILLE L. & SCHMIDT H. (1978) Maple syrup urine disease: emergency treatment of the neonate. *Monogr. hum. Genet.* **9**, 84–9. Basle: Karger.

HANSEN A.E., STEWART R., HUGHES G. & SÖDERHJELM LARS (1962) The relation of linoleic acid to infant feeding. A review. *Acta paediat. scand.* Suppl. **137**, 721–6.

HARRIES J.T., SEAKINS J.W.T. & ERSSER R.S. (1969) Recovery after dietary treatment of an infant with features of tyrosinosis. *Arch. Dis. Childh.* **44**, 258–67.

HARRIES J.T., PIESOWICZ A.T., SEAKINS J.W.T., FRANCIS D.E.M. & WOLFF O.H. (1971) Low proline diet in type I Hyperprolinaemia. *Arch. Dis. Childh.* **46**, 72–81.

HARRIS R.J. (1971) Infection in maple syrup urine disease (letter). *Lancet* **ii**, 813–4.

HOBBS J.R. (1981) Bone marrow transplantation for inborn errors of metabolism. *Lancet* Oct. 3, 735.

HOLT L.E. JR. (1967) Protein and amino acid requirements. Suppl. *Curr. ther. Res.* **9**, 3, 149.

HOLT L.E. JR. & SNYDERMAN S.E. (1965) Protein and amino acid requirements of infants and children. *Nutrition Abstract Review* **35**, 1–13.

HOPKINS I.J., CONNELLY J.F., DAWSON A.G., HIRD F.J. & MADDISON T.G. (1969) Hyperammonaemia due to ornithine transcarbamylase deficiency. *Arch. Dis. Childh.* **44**, 143–8.

HOSTETTER M.K., LEVY H.L., WINTER H.S., KNIGHT G.J. & HADDOW J.E. (1983) Evidence for liver disease preceding amino acid abnormalities in hereditary tyrosinemia. *New Engl. J. Med.* **308**, 1265–7.

KEKOMAKI M., VISAKORPI J.K. & PERHEENTUPA J. (1967) Familial protein intolerance with deficient transport of basic amino acids. An analysis of ten patients. *Acta paediat. scand.* **56**, 617.

KENNAWAY N.G. & BUIST N.R.M. (1971) Metabolic studies in a patient with hepatic cytosol tyrosine aminotransferase deficiency. *Pediat. Res.* **5**, 287.

KLINE J.J., HUG G., SCHUBERT W.K. & BERRY H. (1981) Arginine deficiency syndrome. Its occurrence in carbamyl phosphate synthetase deficiency. *Amer. J. Dis. Childh.* **135**, 437–42.

KOMROWER G.M. & SARDHARWALLA I.B. (1971) The dietary treatment of homocystinuria. In *Inherited Disorders of Sulphur Metabolism, Proceedings of the 8th Symposium of the Society for the Study of Inborn Errors of Metabolism* (eds. Carson N.A.J. & Raine D.N.), p. 254. Edinburgh: Churchill Livingstone.

KON S.K. & COWIE A.T. (1961) *Milk: The Mammary Gland and its Secretion*, Vol. II. London: Academic Press.

KRIEGER I & TANAKA K. (1976) Therapeutic effects of glycine in isolvaleric acidaemia. *Pediat. Res.* **10**, 25.

LAWSON M.S., CLAYTON B.E., DELVES H.T. & MITCHELL J.D. (1977) Evaluation of a new mineral and trace metal supplement for use with synthetic diets. *Arch. Dis. Childh.* **52**, 62–7.

LEONARD J.V. & DAISH P.D. (1985) Evaluation of cofactor effectiveness. *J. Inherited Metabolic Disease* **8** Suppl. I, 17–19.

LEONARD J.V., SEAKINS J.W.T. & GRIFFIN N.K. (1979) β-Hydroxy-β-methylglutaricaciduria presenting as Reye's syndrome. *Lancet* (March 24), 680.

LEONARD J.V., DAISH P.D., NAUGHTEN E.R. & BARTLETT K. (1984) The management and long term outcome of organic acidaemias. *J. Inherited Metabolic Disease* **7**, 13–17.

LEVY H. (1985) Effect of mutation on maternal–fetal metabolic homeostasis: maternal aminoacidopathies. In *Genetic and Metabolic Disease in Paediatrics* (eds. Lloyd J. & Scriver C.), pp. 250–267. London: Butterworth.

LINDBLAD B.S. (1976) Protein and amino acid metabolism during development. In *The Fetus: Physiology and Medicine* (eds. Beard R.W. & Nathanielsz P.W.), p. 80. Philadelphia: Saunders.

LLOYD J. & SCRIVER C. (eds.) (1985) *Genetic and Metabolic Disease in Paediatrics*. London: Butterworth.

LOMBECK I., KASPEREK K., FEINENDEGEN L.E. & BREMER H.J. (1978) Trace element disurbance in dietetically treated patients with phenylketonuria and maple syrup urine disease. *Monogr. hum. Genet.* **9**, 114–19.

LOMBECK I., EBERT K., KASPEREK K., FEINENDEGEN L.E. & BREMER H.J. (1984) Selenium intake of infants and young children, healthy children and dietetically treated patients with phenylketonuria. *European J. pediat.* **143**, 99–102.

LOZY M. & HEGSTED D.M. (1975) Calculation of the amino acid requirement of children at different ages by the fractorial method. *Amer. J. clin. Nutr.* **28**, 1052.

MCINNES R.R., ARSHINOFF S.A., BELL L. & MCCULLOCK J.C. (1981) Hyperornithinaemia and gyrate atropy of the retina; improvement of vision during treatment with a low-arginine diet. *Lancet* (March 7), 513–17.

MAMUMES P., PRINCE P.E. & THORNTON N. (1976) Intellectual deficits after transient tyrosinaemia in the term neonate. *Pediatrics* **57**, 675.

MANN T.P., WILSON K.M. & CLAYTON B.E. (1965) A deficiency state arising in infants on synthetic foods. *Arch. Dis. Childh.* **40**, 364.

MANTAGOS S., TSAGARAKI E. & BURGESS A. (1978) Neonatal hyperammonaemia with complete absence of liver carbamyl phosphate synthetase activity. *Arch. Dis. Childh.* **53**, 230–4.

MATSUI S., MAHONEY M.J. & ROSENBERG L.E. (1983) The natural history of the inherited methylmalonic acidaemias. *New Engl. J. Med.* **308**, 15, 857–61.

MENKES J.H., WELCHER D.W. & LEVI H.S. (1972) Relationship of elevated blood tyrosine to the ultimate intellectual performance of premature infants. *Pediatrics* **49**, 218.

MICHALS K., MATALON R. & WONG P.W.K. (1978) Dietary treatment of tyrosinaemia type I (research). *J. Amer. diet. Ass.* **73**, 507–14.

MILNE M.D. (1972) Renal tubular dysfunction. In *Disease of the Kidney*, 2nd Edition (eds. Strauss M.B. & Welt L.G.), p. 1071. Boston: Little, Brown & Co.

MOCK D.M., DE LORIMER A.A., LIEBMAN W.M., SWEETMAN L. & BAKER H. (1981) Biotin deficiency—an unusual complication of parenteral alimentation. *New Engl. J. Med.* April 2, **304**, (14) 820–3.

MSALL M., BATSHAW M., SUSS R., BRUSILOW S.W. & MELLITIS E.D. (1984) Neurologic outcome in children with inborn errors of urea synthesis. *New Engl. J. Med.* **310**, 1500–5.

MUDD S.H. & LEVY H.L. (1983) Disorders of transsulfuration. In *The Metabolic Basis of Inherited Disease*, 5th Edition (eds. Stanbury J.C., Wyngaarden J.B., Fredrickson O.S., Goldstein J.L. & Brown M.S.) pp. 522–59. New York: McGraw-Hill.

MUNRO H.N. (1970) Free amino acid pools and their role in regulation. In *Mammalian Protein Metabolism* (ed. Munro H.N.), p. 299. New York: Academic Press.

NAKAGAWA I. *et al.* (1971) A conspectus of research on amino acid requirements of man, In *Journal of Nutrition* (Irwin I. & Hegsted D.M.) **101**, 553.

NAUGHTEN E.R., JENKINS J., FRANCIS D.E.M. & LEONARD J.V. (1982) Outcome of maple syrup urine disease. *Arch. Dis. Childh.* **57**, 918–21.

NAYLOR E.W. (1981) Screening for urea cycle disorders. *Pediatrics* **68**, 453–7.

NEVILLE B.G.R. & LILLY P.M. (1973) Histidinaemia: its significance in neonatal screening. *Arch. Dis. Childh.* **48**, 325.

Nutrition Review (1970) Evidence of liver damage in subjects fed amino acid diets lacking arginine and histidine **28**, 9, 229–32.

NYHAN W.L., FAWCETT N., ANDO T., RENNERT O.M. & JULIUS R.L. (1973) Response to dietary therapy in B$_{12}$ unresponsive methylmalonic acidemia. *Pediatrics* **51**, 539–48.

NYMAN R. *et al.* (1979) Observations on the composition of milk substitute products for treatment of inborn errors of amino acid metabolism. Comparisons with human milk. A proposal to rationalise nutrient content of treatment products. *Amer. J. clin. Nutr.* **32**, 1279.

PALMER T., OBERHOLZER V.G. & BURGESS E.A. (1974) Hyperammonaemia in 20 families. Biochemical and genetical survey including investigations in three new families. *Arch. Dis. Childh.* **49**, 443.

PAUL A.A., SOUTHGATE D.A.T. & RUSSELL J. (1980) *First Amino Acid Supplement to the Composition of Foods* (McCance & Widdowson). London: HMSO.

PERRY T.L. (1971) Treatment of homocystinuria with a low. methionine diet and supplemental L-cystine. In *Inherited Disorders of Sulphur Metabolism, Proceedings of the 8th Symposium of the Society for the Study of Inborn Errors of Metabolism* (eds. Carson N.A.J. & Raine D.N.), p. 245. Edinburgh: Churchill Livingstone.

POHLANDT F. (1974) Cystine: a semi-essential amino acid in the newborn infant. *Acta paediat. scand.* **63**, 801.

POHLANDT F. (1978) Plasma amino acid concentrations in newborn infants breast fed *ad libitum*. *J. Pediat.* **92**, 614.

POPKIN J.S., CLOW C.L. & SCRIVER C.R. (1974) Is hereditary histidinaemia harmful? *Lancet* **i**, 721.

PULLON D.H.H. (1980) Homocystinuria and other methioninaemias. In *Neonatal Screening for Inborn Errors of Meta-*

bolism (eds. Bickel H., Guthrie R. & Hammersen G.), p. 29. Berlin: Springer–Verlag.

ROE C. & BOHAN T. (1982) L-Carnitine therapy in propionicacidaemia. *Lancet* June 19, 1411–12.

ROE C.R., HOPPEL C.L., STACEY T.E., MILLINGTON D.S., CHALMERS R.A. & TRACEY B.M. (1983) Metabolic response to carnitine in methylmalonic acidaemia—an effective strategy for elimination of propionyl groups. *Arch. Dis. Childh.* **58**, 916–20.

ROSENMANN A., SCRIVER C.R., CLOW C.L. & LEVY H.L. (1983) Histidinaemia. Part II: Impact; a retrospective study. *J. Inherited Metabolic Disease* **6**, 54–7.

ROUSSON R. & GUIBAUD P. (1984) Long term outcome of organic acidurias: survey of 105 French cases. *J. Inherited Metabolic Disease* **7**, 10–12.

ROYSTON N.J.W. & PARRY T.E. (1962) Megaloblastic anaemia complicating dietary treatment of phenylketonuria in infancy. *Arch. Dis. Childh.* **37**, 430.

SALLAN S. & COTTOM D. (1969) Peritoneal dialysis in maple syrup urine disease. *Lancet* **ii**, 1423–4.

SATOH T., NARISAWA K., IGARASHI Y., SAITOH T. *et al.* (1981) Dietary therapy in 2 patients with vitamin B_{12} unresponsive methylmalonic acidaemia. *Europ. J. Pediat.* **135**, 305–12.

SAUDUBRAY J.M., AMÉDÉ E.O., MUNNICH A., OGIER H., DEPONDT E., CHARPENTIER C., COUDÈ F., REY F. & FRÉZAL J. (1982) Hétérogénéité de la leucinose: heterogenicity of MSUD—correlation between clinical aspects, protein tolerance and enzyme defect. *Archives Francaise de Pediatrie* **39**, Suppl. 2, 735–44.

SCRIVER C.R. (1973) Hereditary vitamin dependencies. In *Treatment of Inborn Errors of Metabolism, Proceedings of the 10th Symposium of the Society for the Study of Inborn Errors of Metabolism* (eds. Seakins J.W.T., Saunders R.A. & Toothill C.), p. 127. Edinburgh: Churchill Livingstone.

SCRIVER C.R. & LEVY H.L. (1983) Histidinaemia. Part I: Reconciling retrospective and prospective findings. *J. Inherited Metabolic Disease* **6**, 51–3.

SCRIVER C.R. & ROSENBERG L.E. (1973) *Amino Acid Metabolism and its Disorders: Major Problems Clinical Pediatrics*, pp. 1–478. Philadelphia: Saunders.

SEEGMILLER J.E. (1976) Genetic defects in human purine metabolism leading to urolithiasis. In *Urolithiasis Research* (eds. Fleisch H., Robertson W.G., Smith D.H. & Vahlensieck W.), pp. 147–55. New York: Plenum Press.

SIMMONDS H.A., WARREN D.J., CAMERON J.S., POTTER C.F. & FAREBROTHER D.A. (1980) Familial gout and renal failure in young women. *Clinical Nephrology* Vol. **14**, No. 4, 176–82.

SIMMONDS H.A., CAMERON J.S., DILLON M.J., BARRATT T.M. & VAN ACKER K.J. (1981) 'Uric acid' stones in children: problems of diagnosis and treatment in a new defect—adenine phosphoribosyltransferase deficiency. *Fortschr. Urol. Nephrol.* **16**, 52–7.

SLONIM A.E., BORUM P.E., TANKA K. *et al.* (1981) Dietary dependent carnitine deficiency as a cause of non-ketotic hypoglycaemia in an infant. *J. Pediat.* **99**, 551–5.

SMITH I. (1985) The hyperphenylalaninaemias. In *Genetic*

and Metabolic Disease in Paediatrics (eds. Lloyd J. & Scriver C.), pp. 166–210. London: Butterworth.

SMITH I. & FRANCIS D.E.M. (1982) Disorders of amino acid metabolism. In *Textbook of Paediatric Nutrition*, 2nd Edition (eds. McLaren D.S. & Burman D.), pp. 295–323. Edinburgh: Churchill Livingstone.

SNYDERMAN S.E. (1972) *Organic Acidurius, Proceedings of the 9th Symposium of the Society for Study of Inborn Errors of Metabolism* (eds. Stern J. & Toothill C.). Edinburgh: Churchill Livingstone.

SNYDERMAN S.E. (1975) Maple syrup urine disease. In *Treatment of Inherited Metabolic Disease* (ed. Raine D.N.), pp. 71–90. Lancaster: MTP Press.

SNYDERMAN S.E. (1976) Branched chain ketoaciduria (maple syrup urine disease). *Clinics in Perinatology* **3**, 1, 41–52.

SNYDERMAN S.E., HOLT L.E. & NORTON P.M. (1968) The plasma aminogram. I. Influence of the level of protein intake and a comparison of whole protein and amino acid diets. *Pediat. Res.* **2**, 131.

SNYDERMAN S.E., SANSARICQ C., CHEN W.J., NORTON P.M. & PHANSALKER S.V. (1977) Arginemia. *J. Pediat.* **90**, 563–8.

SNYDERMAN S.E., SANSARICQ C., NORTON P.M. & MANKA M. (1979a) The nutritional therapy of histidinaemia. *J. Pediat.* **95**, 712–15.

SNYDERMAN S.E., SANSERICQ C., NORTON P.M. & GOLDSTEIN F. (1979b) Arginemia treated from birth. *J. Pediat.* **95**, 61–3.

STACEY T.E. (1985) Effect of mutation on maternal-fetal metabolic homeostasis: general concepts. In *Genetic and Metabolic Disease in Paediatrics* (eds. Lloyd J. & Scriver C.), pp. 234–49. London: Butterworths.

STANBURY J.B., WYNGAARDEN J.B., FREDRICKSON D.S., GOLDSTEIN J.L. & BROWN M.S. (eds.) (1983) *The Metabolic Basis of Inherited Disease*, 5th Edition. New York: McGraw-Hill.

STERN J. & TOOTHILL C. (eds.) (1972) *Organic Acidurias, Proceedings of the 9th Symposium of the Society for the Study of Inborn Errors of Metabolism*. Edinburgh: Churchill Livingstone.

TADA K. (1980) A revised recommendation in nutritional treatment of histidinaemia. *Acta paediat. jap.* **84**, 559.

TADA K., SAITO T., HAYASAKA S. & MIZUNO K. (1984) Hyperornithinaemia with gyrate atrophy: pathophysiology and treatment. *J. Inherited Metabolic Disease* **6**, suppl. 2, 105–6.

THOMAS P.S. & CARSON N.A.J. (1978) Homocystinuria. The evolution of skeletal changes in relation to treatment. *Annales de Radiologie* **21**, 95–104.

VAN SPRANG F.J. & WADMAN S.K. (1971) Treatment of homocystinuria. In *Inherited Disorders of Sulphur Metabolism, Proceedings of the 8th Symposium of the Society for the Study of Inborn Errors of Metabolism* (eds. Carson N.A.J. & Raine D.N.) p. 275. Edinburgh: Churchill Livingstone.

VALLE D., WALSER M., BRUSILOW S.W. & KAISER-KUPFER M. (1980) Gyrate atrophy of the choroid and retina. *J. clin. Invest.* **65**, 271–377.

VELAZQUEZ A. & PRIETO E.C. (1980) Glycine in the acute management of isovalericacidaemia. *Lancet*, Feb. 9, 313.

WALKER V., CLAYTON B.E., ERSSER R.S., FRANCIS D.E.M., LILLY

P., SEAKINS J.W., SMITH I. & WHITEMAN P.D. (1981) Hyperphenylalininaemia of various types among three quarters of a million neonates tested in a screening programme. *Arch. Dis. Childh.* **56**, 10, 759–64.

WALSER M. (1983) Urea cycle disorders and other heredary hyper-ammonemic syndromes. In *The Metabolic Basis of Inherited Disease*, 5th Edition (eds. Stanbury J.C., Wyngaarden J.B., Fredrickson D.S., Goldstein S.L. & Brown M.S.), pp. 402–38. New York: McGraw-Hill.

WESTALL R.G. (1963) Dietary treatment of a child with maple syrup urine disease (branched-chain ketoaciduria). *Arch. Dis. Childh.* **38**, 485–91.

WHITEMAN P. (1983) Inborn lysosomal storage disorders affecting the nervous system. In *Clinical Neuropathology* (eds. Weller R.O., Swash M. & McLellan D.L.), p. 227. Berlin: Springer-Verlag.

WHITEMAN P.D., CLAYTON B.E., ERSSER R.S., LILLY P. & SEAKINS J.W.T. (1979) Changing incidence of neonatal hypermethioninaemia: implications for the detection of homocystinaemia. *Arch. Dis. Childh.* **54**, 593–8.

WILCKEN B. & TURNER G. (1978) Homocystinuria in New South Wales. *Arch. Dis. Childh.* **53**, 242–5.

WILCKEN B., YU J.S. & BROWN D.A. (1977) Natural history of Hartnup disease. *Arch. Dis. Childh.* **52**, 38–40.

WILCHEN B., HAMMOND J., HOWARD N., BOHANE T., HOCART C. & HALPERN B. (1981) Hawkinsinuria. A dominantly inherited defect of tyrosine metabolism. *New Engl. J. Med.* **305**, 15, 865–9.

YU J.S., WALKER–SMITH J.A. & BURNARD E.D. (1971) Neonatal hepatitis in premature infants simulating hereditary tyrosinosis. *Arch. Dis. Childh.* **46**, 306–9.

ZALESKI L.A., DANCIS J. & COX R.P. (1973) Variant maple syrup urine disease in mother and daughter. *CMA Journal* (Aug. 18) **109**, 299–304.

CHAPTER 11

Ketogenic diets in the treatment of childhood epilepsy

A ketogenic diet has been tried in most forms of childhood epilepsy with varying degrees of success. However, although some patients with tonic–clonic fits may respond favourably, it is more successful in children who have myoclonic epilepsy (Bower *et al.* 1982) which tends to be particularly resistant to conventional anticonvulsants.

Various dietary regimes have been proposed as a treatment of epilepsy (Livingston 1972). The use of a ketogenic diet was initiated by Wilder (1921) following observations that starvation resulted in control of seizures but the beneficial effect was lost when food was reintroduced. He aimed to simulate the ketosis–acidosis associated with starvation by means of high-fat, low-carbohydrate diets. Although beneficial effects were reported with such a diet, due to its complexity it has been used only spasmodically except in a few centres. Keith (1963) and Livingston (1972) have extensive experience with the 'traditional' ketogenic regimen over more than 50 years. Interest has escalated since medium-chain triglycerides (MCT) were found to produce ketosis more readily than other dietary fat, and an MCT-based ketogenic diet was shown to be effective by Huttenlocher *et al.* (1971). Also, despite improvement in anticonvulsant therapy, not all children respond to drug therapy, and concern has been expressed about the long-term effects, especially of high doses.

Little is known about the mode of action of the ketogenic diet in the control of seizures, or of the metabolic effects. Many theories have been suggested (Livingston 1972, Schwartz *et al.* 1980, Bower *et al.* 1982): the ketone bodies may be utilized by the brain for oxidative metabolism in place of glucose; the lipid in the cell membrane may be affected; or the amino acid changes (e.g. decreased alanine) may affect cerebral neurotransmitter formation.

Because of the complexity of the dietary regimen most workers only recommend it in patients who fail to respond to anticonvulsant therapy (Dodson *et al.* 1976). Only some children respond to the diet and certain factors influence its effectiveness:

(a) *Type of epilepsy.* The best response has been found in controlling the seizures of childhood myoclonic epilepsy (Bower *et al.* 1982). Just over 50% of patients respond and a further 25% show some improvement (Livingston 1972, Dodson *et al.* 1976, Schwartz *et al.* 1980). Those with tonic–clonic (grand mal) epilepsy may be helped, but the diet is essentially ineffective in most patients with other types of epilepsy (Huttenlocher *et al.* 1971, Livingston 1972).

(b) *Age of patient.* The diet is most effective in two- to five-year-olds. Such children become ketotic quickly and maintain an adequate level of ketosis with the diet. The diet becomes progressively less effective with each additional year of age and from teenage is rarely successful (Huttenlocher 1971, Livingston 1972). The very young child, especially under one year of age, rarely produces a significant degree of ketosis (Schwartz *et al.* 1980, Livingston 1972). Urine ketones may be negative, despite increased plasma β-hydroxybutyrate (BHB) levels, due to the relatively large fluid intake and dilute urine passed by infants (Clark & House 1978). However, Bower *et al.* (1982) report details of a child in whom seizures were controlled on a MCT ketogenic diet started at eight months of age. The diet was maintained for one year and the child remained seizure-free, though severely subnormal, subsequently.

Infants are at greatest risk from nutritional inadequacies of the dietary regimen and therefore the regimen is not recommended for this age group.

(c) *Motivation of patient.* A great deal of motivation and co-operation is required between parents and patients, and dietetic and medical teams in carrying out the diet. It must be rigidly adhered to, otherwise ketosis disappears and the entire beneficial effect can be lost, e.g. fitting may return within hours of indulgence in concentrated carbohydrate, whether by pilfering or accidentally, for example in medicines (Dodson *et al.* 1976).

Three basic ketogenic dietary regimen have been used, though several variations of each have been described by different workers:

(i)   Traditional ketogenic diet in which 87 to 90% of energy is given as dietary fat.

(ii)   MCT ketogenic diet in which MCT provides 60% energy intake and dietary fat a further 10 to 12% energy.

(iii)   Combined fat ketogenic diet in which MCT provides 30% energy and dietary fat at least 40% energy.

Schwartz *et al.* (1980) have published data comparing regimens (i) and (ii).

1   The traditional regimen gave a higher degree of plasma ketones and is probably more effective than the MCT regimen, but these workers failed to show conclusively that one diet was better than the other, thus confirming the earlier observations of Huttenlocher *et al.* (1971). In many cases the total ketones reached levels seen in diabetic pre-coma. The ketone levels in the evening were higher than on fasting in patients on the ketogenic diet, in contrast to normal subjects who show higher ketone levels in the morning following the overnight fast.

2   Blood glucose levels were lower on the ketogenic diet, especially after lunch and supper, compared with normal subjects. No severe hypoglycaemia was reported by Schwartz and co-workers (1980), but this has been reported by others using the traditional ketogenic diet (Livingston 1972, Dobson *et al.* 1976).

3   The blood alanine levels were significantly lower on the traditional diet than the MCT diet (Schwartz *et al.* 1980). Data on other amino acids were not reported in detail, but branched-chain amino acids and phenylalanine were said to be increased.

4   Cholesterol levels were not changed by the diets used in the study by Schwartz *et al.* (1980) but have been said by others to be raised, together with lipaemia.

The three dietary regimens contain different proportions of nutrients (Table 11.1). A more varied diet with a higher intake of natural food is possible with the MCT regimen. Up to twice as much protein and three times the carbohydrate intake is permitted,

Table 11.1   Energy distribution in various ketogenic diets per 4200 kJ/1000 kcal.

Type of ketogenic diet	Fat		Protein* (g) (% energy)	Carbohydrate (g) (% energy)
	Dietary fat (g) (% energy)	MCT (g) (% energy)		
(i) Traditional 3:1 ratio, i.e. 3 g fat:1 g protein plus carbohydrate	97 (87)	Nil	15	18
			Total 33 g (13)	
Traditional 4:1 ratio i.e. 4 g fat:1 g protein plus carbohydrate	100 (90)	Nil	15	10
			Total 25 g (10)	
(ii) MCT = 60% energy plus coincidental dietary fat	12 (11)	72† (60)	25 (10)	50 (20)
	(*Total* 71)		*Total* 1250 kJ/300 kcal	
(iii) Combined fat plus MCT. 30% energy as MCT plus 40% dietary fat energy	45 (40)	35 (30)	25 (10)	50 (20)
	(*Total* 70)		*Total* 1250 kJ/300 kcal	

* At least 1 g protein/kg per day must be provided in the diet to ensure adequate for growth.

† 72 g MCT oil is contained in approximately 140 ml Liquigen MCT emulsion.

there is less risk of nutritional deficiency, and it is easier to prepare from the family's meals. However, fewer ketones are produced with such a diet, and gastrointestinal symptoms, including abdominal pain, vomiting and diarrhoea, may occur due to the large doses of MCT. The large volume of MCT is difficult to incorporate in the diet and the MCT drinks can cause feeding problems.

The traditional diet has the disadvantage of being very dependent on the dietitian providing an individualized regimen, as each meal should contain the correct proportions of fat, carbohydrate and protein. Growth failure, alopecia, hyperlipidaemia, hypercholesterolaemia, hyperuricacidaemia and renal calculi due to hypercalciuria have all been reported as complications of the traditional ketogenic diet (Livingston 1972, Dodson *et al.* 1976).

Recently combined-fat regimens [Table 11.1(iii)] have been devised by the Dietetic Department, John Radcliffe Hospital, Oxford, and at the author's clinic. These have the advantages of both regimens, giving more flexibility and variety than the traditional diet (i) and fewer gastrointestinal symptoms than the full MCT diet (ii). It is now the author's preferred regimen.

Before the final decision to embark on a ketogenic diet is taken, the parents should be seen by the dietitian and fully informed about the regimen, the necessity to weigh the diet, and need for full compliance. A diet history should be taken and the child's food preferences considered. The financial implications of the diet must be discussed. The child should have the opportunity to taste the special foods used in the ketogenic regimen.

Anticonvulsant drug therapy is continued unchanged for the first six weeks or more of treatment with the diet, thereafter the dose may be gradually reduced or omitted in some responsive patients. Acetazolamide is contraindicated in some patients on a ketogenic diet as it can lead to severe metabolic acidosis (Dobson *et al.* 1976). An alternative should normally replace acetazolamide before starting the dietary regimen. Medicines should ideally be in a carbohydrate-free base.

Anticonvulsants disturb calcium and vitamin D metabolism, and rickets can occur. This may be resistant to calciferol but is responsive to 25-hydroxycholecalciferol. Phophylactic vitamin D and calcium are recommended. Folate deficiency with megaloblastic anaemia also occurs with anticonvulsants, and therefore folic acid supplements are important. In addition, comprehensive vitamin–mineral supplements (Table 11.2) are necessary to ensure the nutritional adequacy of ketogenic diets.

Table 11.2 Examples of vitamin–mineral supplements for ketogenic diets.

Daily either:
   (a) 4 to 8 g Aminogran Mineral Mixture*/Metabolic
        Mineral Mixture†
        + 3 Ketovite Tablets ⎫‡
        + 5 ml Ketovite Liquid ⎭

   (b) 1 Forceval capsule‡
        + 1 SandoCal tablet§

   (c) 12 Cow & Gate Supplementary Vitamin Tablets‡
        + 1 SandoCal tablet§
        + 0·6 ml Abidec‡

* Aminogran Food Supplement is contraindicated.
† Comprehensive mineral mixtures.   ⎫ *See* Francis 1986.
‡ Comprehensive vitamin supplements ⎭
§ Contains some carbohydrate but is more palatable than other calcium supplements. One tablet contains $\simeq 400$ mg elemental calcium.

INTRODUCTION OF DIET

The diet should be introduced in hospital, after ensuring that the child is not prone to ketotic hypoglycaemia, which contraindicates a ketogenic diet.

Opinions vary regarding the necessity to fast the child, for varying lengths of time, before starting the diet. Livingston (1972) suggested a 3 to 5 days' fast with only water; Dodson *et al.* (1976) suggested 48 hours. But Gordon (1977) suggested it was not necessary to starve the child before starting the dietary regimen, and recommended that the diet be introduced slowly, especially the MCT, and therefore during the first few days there is an energy deficit. Although starvation may induce ketosis more quickly, the author has found that gradual introduction of the diet over 4 to 10 days after an initial 12 to 16 hour overnight fast is appropriate for the majority of children. This is particularly important with the MCT regimen, as it helps avoid many of the gastrointestinal side-effects associated with large doses of MCT. It also allows the child and parents to get used to the new foods gradually.

ENERGY INTAKE

Livingston (1972) suggested 60 to 80 kcal/kg per day (250 to 335 kJ/kg per day) for two- to five-year-olds. Dodson *et al.* (1976) and Bower *et al.* (1982) suggested 75 kcal/kg per day (314 kJ/kg per day) as an initial energy intake. However, the energy intake for any individual patient varies and must be assessed carefully, taking into account the child's age, weight, previous dietary intake, energy expenditure, and relevant clinical condition (mobility, obesity, severity of seizures). The energy intake of the proposed diet at any time must be precise, as the exact intake has to be consumed each day; overestimation leads to diet refusal and possibly loss of ketosis, or to obesity. Inadequate energy prescription can be equally a problem, causing hunger, weight loss, poor growth, or pilfering by the child, with loss of ketosis. The energy intake should therefore only be adjusted once the full diet plus fat or MCT intake is being taken, but will need to be adjusted from time to time to meet the individual's needs, taking care not to overprescribe when increased dietary bulk is more appropriate and can be met by increasing the free foods intake.

Ketogenic diet construction

During metabolism ketones are formed from 90% of fat and 42% protein, but none is produced from carbohydrate.

To produce ketones it is essential to increase the ketogenic content of the diet, i.e. an increased proportion of energy from fat with a reduced protein and carbohydrate intake.

(i)   Traditional ketogenic diet

This ketogenic diet is based on dietary fat contributing 87 to 90% of the energy intake. The diet is frequently expressed as a ratio of gram of fat to gram of carbohydrate plus protein. A ratio of 3:1 is equivalent to 87% energy from fat; a ratio of 4:1 is equivalent to 90% energy from fat.

Dodson et al. (1976) suggested that a 3:1 ratio be used for children under five years old, and a 4:1 ratio be used for children of five years old or more, whereas Livingston (1972) and Schwartz et al. (1980) used traditional diets with a 4:1 ratio. There is, however, a degree of individual response in the amount of fat needed to produce ketone levels in the treatment range of ≥ 2 mmol/l plasma BHB (Bower et al. 1982). It is essential the diet contains adequate protein for growth: at least 1 g/kg per day. The remainder of the dietary energy is given as carbohydrate.

The traditional ketogenic diet is calculated as follows:

The energy requirement is assessed.

The daily protein, fat and carbohydrate is calculated from the distribution of energy from Table 11.1(i) for the fat ratio initially required.

Table 11.3   Suggested 'milk-shakes' for ketogenic diet.

		Carbohydrate (g)	Protein (g)	Fat (g)	kJ	kcal
(a)	15 g skimmed milk powder* Essence or coffee flavouring	7·9	5·5	Trace	227	53

	30 ml Prosparol, Calogen or
	  Liquigen or
	  double cream or
	60 ml single cream
	Water to 75 to 150 ml
		Nil	Nil or 0·5
			from cream
				15	555	135

	Total	7·9	5·5 or 6	15	782	188
(b)	30 ml 'diabetic'/low-calorie squash or	Trace	Trace	Nil	Trace	Trace
	1 to 2 drops vanilla essence or 1 tsp coffee powder or unsweetened cocoa powder 2 drops saccharin solution or 1 tablet saccharin	Nil to trace	Nil	Nil	Nil	Nil

	30 ml Calogen, Prosparol or
	  Liquigen or
	  double cream or
	60 ml single cream
	Water to 75 to 300 ml
		Nil	Nil or 0·5
			from cream
				15	555	135

	Total	Trace	Nil or 0·5	15	555	135

* The protein plus carbohydrate content must be taken into account in the diet calculations.

Each meal should contain the same ratio of nutrients and must be calculated individually. It will be noted that a 4:1 ratio diet has one-tenth of the kcal daily requirement as gram of fat.

Provided the minimum protein requirement is met, then for practical purposes, protein and carbohydrates are interchangeable. Refined carbohydrates should be avoided in all ketogenic diets, but this is particularly important in traditional ketogenic diets in order to provide a balanced diet and adequate bulk within the limitations of the diet.

The fat is given as butter, margarine, oils, mayonnaise or 50% arachis oil emulsions, Prosparol or Calogen. A home-made oil emulsion can be made with an edible gum or egg-yolk (*see* Recipes). Double cream is palatable and can be used, but is expensive and increases the protein intake slightly. Some of the fat can be incorporated into 'milk-shakes' (Table 11.3).

Imagination is needed in preparing the diet so as to introduce variety and find ways in which to utilize the large amount of fat. Cream or butter can be added to vegetables and soups. Cream can be diluted and used to replace milk in tea or coffee, or used with cereal. Or it can be made into egg custard or junket, or added to carbohydrate-free jelly and/or frozen as an 'ice-cream', and served with fruit (unsweetened) from the meal allowance. Or it can be whipped and served as a mousse, flavoured with essences such as vanilla or almond, or sprinkled with spices such as cinnamon. Oil can be incorporated into salad dressing or mayonnaise with egg-yolk and vinegar, or used for frying, provided all the oil is served and eaten. Butter can be added to scrambled egg or savoury egg custard, and some children will eat it by itself or flavoured with Bovril or Marmite. Fat used in cooking may be given as an extra.

A limited list of very low-energy foods (Table 11.4) can be incorporated in the diet. In the traditional ketogenic diets, the low-carbohydrate vegetables must be limited to small serves 2 to 3 times daily, as even these contribute a small but significant protein and carbohydrate intake. Low-calorie fruit drinks/squash often contain some carbohydrate or sorbitol and are therefore not suitable; a sugar- and carbohydrate-free brand, e.g. Rose's or Boots 'diabetic'/low-calorie squash, should be selected. A number of sugar-free carbonated beverages are suitable. Use of these items should be made to give variety and bulk to the diet. For example, ice-lollies can be made from frozen sugar-free drinks. Low-calorie clear soups

Table 11.4 Free foods for use with ketogenic diets.

Salt, pepper, herbs, spices, Bovril, Marmite, stock cubes and Oxo, food essences, food colourings

Clear soups made from meat stock, stock cubes or Bovril and permitted vegetables

Vinegar, oil and vinegar dressing

Sugar-free drinks, e.g. Rose's and Boots 'Diabetic' Squash, Tab, Diet Pepsi, OneCal, Slimline drinks

'Diabetic' jelly (sugar-free)

Sugar-free pastilles in limited quantity (3 to 4/day)

Saccharin, aspartame or Acesulfame K, e.g. Sweetex, Hermesetas (not sorbitol or powdered sweeteners)

Ice-lollies made from diluted 'diabetic' sugar-free squash

Black tea and coffee (cream and artificial sweetener may be added). Consommé

Vegetables
In small quantity in traditional ketogenic diets.
Unlimited in MCT ketogenic diets.
Fresh, frozen or tinned in brine and no added sugar.

Aubergine, asparagus, bean sprouts, broccoli, Brussels sprouts, cabbage, cauliflower, celery, chicory, Chinese leaves, cress, courgette, cucumber, endive, green beans (French and runners), green and red peppers, kale, leek, lettuce, marrow, mushroom, mustard and cress, okra, olives, onion, radish, rhubarb, sauerkraut, spinach, spring greens, Swiss chard, tomatoes and unsweetened tomato juice, zucchini. Fresh mint, parsley and herbs. Pickled onions.

Nuts
One of the following can be included (shelled weight/day).
Barcelona nuts, 30 g (1 oz)
Brazil nuts, 30 g (1 oz)
Walnuts, 15 g ($\frac{1}{2}$ oz)

Additional items permitted in MCT ketogenic diets
1 to 2 teaspoons cocoa powder (unsweetened)
Small serve carrot, turnip and beetroot
Small serve unsweetened grapefruit, lemon, melon, stewed gooseberries, blackberries, loganberries, fresh blackcurrants, whitecurrants, redcurrants
Up to 15 g ($\frac{1}{2}$ oz) almonds
Bran up to 10 g/day adds bulk to the diet. Soya bran is preferable to wheat or rice bran.

Table 11.5   Examples of traditional ketogenic diet meals.

Each approximately equals 2100 kJ, 500 kcal, 50 g fat, 7 to 8 g protein, 7 g carbohydrate, i.e. approximately 4:1 ratio of fat: carbohydrate plus protein. Cooked weight of foods.

			Protein (g)	Fat (g)	Carbohydrate (g)
(i)	50 g egg, e.g. scrambled, poached, boiled		6·1	5·5	Nil
	20 g butter		Nil	15·0	Nil
	15 g wholemeal bread		1·4	0·4	6·3
	60 ml Prosparol/Calogen or double cream (Table 11.3)		Nil to 1·0	30	Nil to 1·2
		Total	7·5 to 8·5	50·9	6·3 to 7·5
(ii)	10 g muesli		1·3	0·8	6·6
	50 g egg, scrambled with butter		6·1	5·5	Nil
	20 g butter		Nil	15·0	Nil
	60 ml Calogen/Prosparol or double cream (Table 11.3)		Nil to 1·0	30	0 to 1·2
		Total	7·4 to 8·4	51·3	6·6 to 7·8
(iii)	20 g beef or lamb—lean only, cooked weight		5·0	2·2	Nil
	20 g chips		0·8	2·2	7·5
	Vegetables/salad from Table 11.4		Trace	Nil	Trace
	15 ml oil or 20 g butter for vegetables		Nil	15·0	Nil
	60 ml Prosparol/Calogen or double cream (Table 11.3)		0 to 1·0	30	0 to 1·2
		Total	5·8 to 6·8	49·4	7·5 to 8·7
(iv)	50 g egg, e.g. hard-boiled		6·1	5·5	Nil
	15 g crisps		0·9	5·4	7·4
	Tomato and/or celery		Trace	Nil	Trace
	80 ml Calogen/Prosparol or double cream (Table 11.3)		0 to 1·2	40	0 to 1·6
		Total	7·0 to 8·2	50·9	7·4 to 9·0
(v)	Clear soup with permitted vegetables (Table 11.4)		Trace	Nil	Trace
	25 g cheddar cheese		6·5	8·4	Nil
	75 g orange		0·6	Nil	6·4
	80 ml Prosparol/Calogen or double cream (Table 11.3)		0 to 1·2	40	0 to 1·6
		Total	7·1 to 8·3	48·4	6·4 to 8
(vi)	20 g roast chicken, cooked weight		5·0	1·1	Nil
	15 g chips		1·7	0·6	5·6
	Vegetables from Table 11.4		Trace	Nil	Trace
	100 ml double cream, e.g. whipped and flavoured with cinnamon		1·5	50	2·0
		Total	8·2	51·7	7·6
(vii)	25 g cheddar cheese		6·5	8·4	Nil
	15 g bread		1·4	0·4	6·3
	40 g butter (and Marmite/Bovril)		Nil	30·0	Nil
	Salad vegetables (Table 11.4)		Trace	Nil	Trace
	1 walnut		Trace	Trace	Trace
	10 ml oil for oil and vinegar dressing		Nil	10	Nil
		Total	7·9	48·4	6·3

Table 11.5 *continued*

		Protein (g)	Fat (g)	Carbohydrate (g)
(viii)	25 g tuna fish or sardines	5·8	1·1	Nil
	Salad vegetables (Table 11.4)	Trace	Nil	Trace
	75 g stewed apple (no sugar)	Trace	Nil	6·0
	100 ml double cream, whipped and added to sugar-free jelly	1·5	50	2·0
	Total	7·3	51·1	8·0
(ix)	30 g grilled or poached cod, haddock, plaice	6·3	0·3	Nil
	30 g butter	Nil	22·5	Nil
	Vegetables (Table 11.4)	Trace	Nil	Trace
	100 g dessert pear	0·2	Nil	7·6
	60 ml Calogen/Prosparol or double cream (Table 11.3)	0 to 1·0	30	0 to 1·2
	Total	6·5 to 7·5	52·8	7·6 to 8·8
(x)	8 g Cornflakes	0·7	0·1	6·8
	25 g bacon, fried back bacon, lean and fat	6·2	10·0	Nil
	Fried tomatoes and mushrooms using 20 ml oil	Trace	20	Trace
	40 ml Prosparol/Calogen or double cream (Table 11.3)	0 to 0·6	20	0 to 0·8
	Total	6·9 to 7·5	50·1	6·8 to 7·6
Fluid diet alternative				
(xi)	100 ml milk	3·3	3·8	4·7
	20 g egg-yolk (one)	3·2	6·0	Nil
	80 ml Calogen/Prosparol or double cream	0 to 1·2	40	0 to 1·6
	Saccharin and vanilla essence	Nil	Nil	Nil
	Water to >200 ml			
	Total	6·5 to 7·7	49·8	4·7 to 6·3

can be made with stock cubes or Bovril and permitted vegetables to which cream or oil can be added.

Other diabetic products are not suitable or must be incorporated into the diet calculations, e.g. small quantities of plain diabetic chocolate can be given as a treat occasionally, e.g. at Easter, birthdays and Christmas. Fruit canned in water must be used as a carbohydrate or energy exchange in the diet.

Various diets can be devised from the examples of meals (Table 11.5) which contain approximately a 4 : 1 ratio, 2100 kJ, 500 kcal, 50 g fat, 7 to 8 g protein and 7 g carbohydrate. Multiples of these meals can be used to devise diets of the required energy intake.

The vitamin and mineral supplements suggested in Table 11.2(a) are essential with this limited diet.

(ii) *MCT ketogenic diets containing 60% energy as MCT*

Medium-chain triglycerides (MCT) are more ketogenic than ordinary fat and therefore a lower proportion of total fat can be incorporated into this diet. Huttenlocher *et al.* (1971) suggested that a diet containing 60% energy as MCT was at least as effective as a 3 : 1 ratio ketogenic traditional diet. However, as much as 70% energy as MCT may be needed in some patients to produce adequate ketones. A further 10 to 15% energy is provided by dietary fat from conventional foods, which provide the remaining energy, together with protein and carbohydrate. As the diet contains less fat a higher protein intake is possible [Table 11.1(ii)] and the diet in general is less rigid and more acceptable. The MCT is given largely as Liquigen which contains a 52% MCT emulsion in water, or as MCT oil incorporated into food and drinks or as a home-made emulsion (*see* Recipes).

The energy requirement is assessed and the minimum protein intake calculated (1 g protein/kg per day). The prescription of MCT and Liquigen is calculated from Table 11.1(ii). Liquigen should be diluted to at least 1½ times the volume with extra water or fluid, or can be given as 'milk-shakes'; examples are given in Table 11.3. The skimmed milk powder in recipe (a) must be calculated into the protein and carbohydrate or energy allowances. The daily quantity of MCT or Liquigen should be divided into 4 to 6 doses given throughout the day, including bedtime. The prescribed MCT and Liquigen should be introduced gradually over 4 to 10 days. To avoid the development of gastrointestinal symptoms, such as abdominal pain, diarrhoea and/or vomiting, the child should be taught to take the MCT-containing drink slowly and throughout the meal. Alternatively, Liquigen can be added to a cup of tea or coffee, incorporated in recipes such as sugar-free jelly, which can also be frozen to make an 'ice-cream' or 'mousse' substitute, made into custards or sauces, added to mashed potatoes and soups, and incorporated into sugar-free biscuits, cakes or pastry. The protein and carbohydrate or energy content of the ingredients used in the recipes must be calculated into the dietary allowances. A Liquigen recipe leaflet is available from Scientific Hospital Supplies, and some but not all of the recipes can be adapted for use in the ketogenic diet. Care must be taken to ensure MCT is not overheated, as a bitter taste is formed due to the low smoke point. However, the oil can with care (see Chapter 7) be used for frying, but it is important to ensure that the child consumes the full quantity. Liquigen can be heated gently but should only be kept at 100°C for short periods or the emulsion will break down. The emulsion is less stable in acid and therefore fruit or fruit flavourings, vinegar or lemon juice may cause curdling. Liquigen should be added slowly to hot drinks such as tea or coffee after they have been poured in order to prevent breaking the emulsion.

The rest of the dietary energy is made up from carbohydrate and protein [Table 11.1(ii)] using either:

(a)   The energy exchanges (Table 11.6), which should be distributed between meals and snacks as shown in the example (Table 11.7). Concentrated carbohydrates should be avoided and several energy exchanges of the protein foods such as meat should be incorporated to ensure an adequate protein intake in the diet.

(b)   Alternatively, the 10 g carbohydrate exchanges used in the diabetic diet (Table 5.2, p. 134) and 6 g protein exchanges used in low-protein diets (Table 8.4, p. 205) can be used to devise the diet prescription. Milk is counted as both a protein and carbohydrate exchange and

Table 11.6   Energy exchanges: quantity of food which when eaten in the stated quantity supplies 420 kJ, 100 kcal.

*	25 g Cheddar cheese or Parmesan or cream cheese
*	20 g Stilton Cheese
*	100 g cottage cheese
*	200 g natural yoghurt
*	80 g lean ham or very lean bacon
*	40 g meat (various) or fried meats or bacon
*	50 g chicken, turkey or very lean meat or veal, liver, kidney
*	25 g sausage, e.g. salami type
*	30 g English type or liver sausage; beef burger
*	100 g baked fish or steamed or poached, smoked and 'white' fish
*	50 g fish in batter—fried
*	50 g fatty fish, kippers, sardine, salmon
*	30 g Camembert cheese or Danish blue or processed
*	150 g milk
*	300 g skimmed milk
	200 g peas
	300 g apple, eating, weighed with core and skin
	400 g apricot, fresh, raw
	300 g orange, fresh only
	125 g banana (peeled)
	160 g grapes
	225 g pear, weighed with core and skin
	250 g pear, flesh only
	225 g pineapple, fresh
	225 g pomegranate
	250 g peach, flesh only
	300 g peach, weighed with stone
	45 g bread
	30 g cereals, unsweetened, e.g. Cornflakes, Rice Krispies
	25 g cream crackers and water biscuits
	30 g crispbread
	30 g flour (raw)
	30 g raw macaroni, spaghetti, rice, semolina
	80 g boiled rice
	24 g oatmeal, raw
	120 g potato, boiled
	80 g mashed potato with milk and butter
	150 g baked beans
	40 g chips
	65 g roast potato
	55 g fish fingers
	20 g crisps (plain or salt and vinegar)
†	125 g flavoured yoghurt
†	100 g fruit or nut yoghurt
†	60 g ice-cream
†	20 g biscuits, various plain type and digestive
†	20 g biscuits, chocolate, full-coated
†	30 g cakes and buns (no icing)
†	20 g fancy and fruit-type, rich, Madeira cake (no icing)

* High-protein exchanges.
† Contain concentrated, refined carbohydrate and therefore use sparingly e.g. for treats and not more than one item in any one day.

Table 11.7 Examples of a 5000 kJ/1200 kcal MCT ketogenic diet where MCT provides 60% energy. Suitable for a 2-year-old weighing 14 kg. Using energy exchanges.

Energy (5000 kJ/1200 kcal) { 60% as MCT = 86 g MCT oil or 165 ml Liquigen
40% as energy exchanges = 2000 kJ/480kcal or 4¾ energy exchanges*

Menu suggestion

165 ml Liquigen } Six × 70 ml Liquigen drinks†
Water to 420 ml

		Energy exchanges (kJ/kcal)
Breakfast	70 ml Liquigen drink	
	15 g Cornflakes (unsweetened cereal)	½
	75 ml milk	½ } = 1½ exchanges
	22 g bread (may be toasted) (plus butter)	½
	Mushroom and tomatoes (Table 11.4)	
Mid-morning	70 ml Liquigen drink	
Lunch	70 ml Liquigen drink	
	40 g ham	½
	22 g bread (plus butter)	½ } = 1¼ exchanges
	Salad vegetables (Table 11.4)	
	75 g apple (weighed with core and skin)	¼
Mid-afternoon	70 ml Liquigen drink	
	15 g crispbread (plus butter)	½ } = ½ exchange
	Pickled onions and olives (Table 11.4)	
Evening meal	70 ml Liquigen drink	
	Clear soup (Table 11.4)	
	30 g sausages—English-type, cooked weight	1
	20 g chips	½ } = 1½ exchanges
	Vegetables (Table 11.4)	
	Unsweetened stewed blackcurrants (Table 11.4)	
Bedtime	70 ml Liquigen drink	

Vitamin–mineral supplement, e.g. one Forceval capsule plus one SandoCal tablet.

* *See* energy exchanges, Table 11.6.
† May be flavoured, used in cooking or mixed with food.

the other carbohydrate exchanges will provide some additional protein. The MCT and exchanges should be distributed throughout the meals similarly to the examples given in Table 11.8. Some MCT should be included at bedtime in order to maintain overnight ketosis.

Carbohydrate Countdown by the British Diabetic Association gives both carbohydrate and energy values of a number of foods and can be used to increased variety in the diet.

Minor differences between the two regimens exist

and, in general, the energy exchange system (a), first described by Clarke and House (1978), has been found easier for parents to use and adequately achieves ketosis, so long as the prescription is adjusted for the individual according to the results of monitoring for ketones and the energy needs of the child.

(iii) Combined fat and MCT ketogenic diet containing 30% energy as MCT, and 40% energy as dietary fats (30% as prescribed fat exchanges and 10% from natural foods)

This combined diet overcomes the necessity for large

Table 11.8 Example of a 5000 kJ/1200 kcal MCT ketogenic diet where MCT provides 60% energy. Suitable for a 2-year-old weighing 14 kg. Using protein and carbohydrate exchanges.

Energy (5000 kJ/1200 kcal)
- 60% as MCT = 86 g MCT oil or 165 ml Liquigen
- 10% as protein = 30 g protein or five × 6 g protein exchanges*
- 20% as carbohydrate = 60 g carbohydrate or six × 10 g carbohydrate exchanges†
- 10% (approx.) as ordinary dietary fat is provided by the foods used in protein/carbohydrate exchanges.

Menu suggestion

165 ml Liquigen
Water to 420 ml } Six × 70 ml Liquigen drinks‡

Breakfast	70 ml Liquigen drink	
	Cereal (unsweetened), e.g. 1 Weetabix	= 1 carbohydrate exchange
	200 ml milk	= 1 carbohydrate exchange plus 2 protein exchanges
	Free foods, e.g. mushrooms and tomato (Table 11.4), fried	
Mid-morning	70 ml Liquigen drink	
Lunch	70 ml Liquigen drink	
	1 egg plus 25 g Cheddar cheese	= 2 protein exchanges
	20 g bread	= 1 carbohydrate exchange
	Butter	
	Salad vegetables, Table 11.4	
	1 fruit, e.g. 1 apple/orange	= 1 carbohydrate exchange
Mid-afternoon	70 ml Liquigen drink	
	< 15 g almonds or walnuts	
	Pickled onions, olives	
Evening meal	70 ml Liquigen drink	
	Clear soup (Table 11.4)	
	40 g meat	= 2 protein exchanges
	Thin gravy	
	Free vegetables from Table 11.4	
	30 g chips or 50 g boiled potato	= 1 carbohydrate exchange
	2 cream cracker biscuits and butter	= 1 carbohydrate exchange
Bedtime	70 ml Liquigen drink	

Vitamin–mineral supplement, e.g. 1 Forceval capsule plus 1 SandoCal tablet.

* 6 g protein exchanges (*see* Table 8.4).
† 10 g carbohydrate exchanges (*see* Table 5.2).
‡ May be flavoured, used in cooking or mixed with food.

quantities of MCT and carries some of the advantages of both the other types of ketogenic diets.

The assessed energy requirement is distributed between nutrients [Table 11.1(iii)] as follows:

(a)   30% energy from MCT/Liquigen.

(b)   30% energy from fat exchanges (Table 11.9).

(c)   40% energy from natural foods which will provide protein, carbohydrate and additional dietary fat, given as energy exchanges (Table

Table 11.9 Fat exchanges containing 15 g fat.

20 g butter or ordinary margarine
15 ml oil (MCT or vegetable oil)
15 ml oil plus 15 ml vinegar or lemon juice as dressing
30 ml double cream, Prosparol, Calogen, Liquigen
2 egg-yolks or 2 standard eggs
60 ml single cream
20 ml mayonnaise (recipe, *see* p. 327).

11.6); *or* from 10 g carbohydrate and 6 g protein exchanges as described above.

The diet prescription is distributed between meals (Table 11.10) and adjusted for the individual's needs.

The parents need detailed, careful instruction regarding menu planning and food preparation before the child's discharge. A suggested out-patient diet plan is given in Table 11.11.

Table 11.10 Example of a 5000 kJ/1200 kcal ketogenic diet using combined fats. Suitable for a 2-year-old weighing 14 kg.

Energy (5000 kJ/ 1200 kcal)
- 30% as MCT = 43 g MCT oil = 85 ml Liquigen
- 30% as fat exchanges = 40 g fat = $2\frac{2}{3}$ × 15 g fat exchanges*
- 40% as energy exchanges = 2000 kJ/480 kcal or $4\frac{3}{4}$ energy exchanges†

Menu suggestion

85 ml Liquigen
Water to 210 ml } Six × 35 ml Liquigen drinks‡

		Fat exchanges	Energy exchanges (kJ/kcal)
Breakfast	35 ml Liquigen drink		
	62 g banana		$\frac{1}{2}$
	75 baked beans		$\frac{1}{2}$
	22 g bread (may be toasted)		$\frac{1}{2}$ } = $1\frac{1}{2}$ energy exchanges plus 1 fat exchange
	20 g butter	1	
Mid-morning	35 ml Liquigen drink		
Lunch	35 ml Liquigen drink		
	25 g Cheddar cheese		1
	15 g crispbread		$\frac{1}{2}$
	20 g butter	1	} = $1\frac{1}{2}$ energy exchanges plus 1 fat exchange
	Salad vegetables, Table 11.4		
	Melon or $\frac{1}{2}$ grapefruit, Table 11.4		
Mid-afternoon	35 ml Liquigen		
	<15 g walnuts or almonds or 30 g Brazil nuts		
Evening meal	35 ml Liquigen drink		
	25 g chicken, cooked weight		$\frac{1}{2}$
	60 g boiled potato		$\frac{1}{2}$
	Thin gravy		} = $1\frac{3}{4}$ energy exchanges plus $\frac{2}{3}$ fat exchange
	Vegetables, Table 11.4		
	100 g natural yoghurt		$\frac{1}{2}$
	100 g fresh apricots		$\frac{1}{4}$
	20 ml double cream	$\frac{2}{3}$	
Bedtime	35 ml Liquigen drink		

Vitamin–mineral supplement, e.g. 1 Forceval capsule plus 1 SandoCal tablet.

*Table 11.9.
†Table 11.6.
‡May be flavoured, used in cooking or mixed with food.

Table 11.11 Out-patient menu plan—daily prescription for a child on a ketogenic MCT diet or combined fat diet.

1 ...ml Liquigen ⎱ Divide into six drinks.
  ...water ⎰ Give with meals and snacks.

Flavouring can be added, such as saccharin, coffee, tea, 'diabetic' squash, vanilla essence, peppermint essence, consommé, Worcester sauce, spices, e.g. cinnamon.

2 ... 15 g fat exchanges (Table 11.9).

3 Normal food must be restricted to a total of ... kJ/kcal per day. Energy exchanges are given in Table 11.6.
  Include two or three energy exchanges of protein foods marked *(as below for †) in Table 11.6.

Use refined carbohydrate foods very sparingly, marked * in Table 11.6.

Daily ... kJ/kcal = ... energy exchanges.

Divide into meals:
Breakfast ...   kJ/kcal and ... 15 g fat exchanges.
Mid-morning ...   kJ/kcal and ... 15 g fat exchanges.
Lunch ...   kJ/kcal and ... 15 g fat exchanges.
Snack ...   kJ/kcal and ... 15 g fat exchanges.
Evening meal ...   kJ/kcal and ... 15 g fat exchanges.
Bedtime ...   kJ/kcal and ... 15 g fat exchanges.

4 Give appropriate vitamin and mineral supplements daily, e.g. 1 Forceval capsule and 1 SandoCal tablet.

Menu suggestion

Breakfast   ...ml Liquigen drink
                     ... energy exchange cereal ⎱ Table 11.6
                     ... energy exchange bread ⎰
                     ... fat exchanges butter ⎱ Table 11.9
                     ... fat exchanges egg ⎰
                     Tea/coffee/'diabetic' squash

Mid-morning   ...ml Liquigen drink
                     ... energy exchange, Table 11.6

Lunch   ...ml Liquigen drink
                     ... energy exchange meat/fish, Table 11.6
                     Vegetables from free list, Table 11.4
                     1 tablespoon thin gravy
                     ... energy exchange potato/chips ⎱ Table 11.6
                     ... energy exchange fruit ⎰
                     ... fat exchanges butter/oil, etc., Table 11.9
                     Tea/coffee/'diabetic' squash

Snack   ...ml Liquigen drink
                     Free foods from Table 11.4
                     ... energy exchange, Table 11.6

Supper   ...ml Liquigen drink
                     Clear soup from free list, Table 11.4
                     ... energy exchange meat/fish, Table 11.6
                     Vegetables from free list, Table 11.4
                     ... energy exchange bread/potato, Table 11.6
                     ... fat exchanges butter/oil, etc., Table 11.9
                     ... energy exchange fruit, Table 11.6
                     Tea/coffee/'diabetic' squash

Bedtime   ...ml Liquigen drink

Vitamins and minerals   1 Forceval capsule plus 1 Sandocal tablet

MONITORING OF THE KETOGENIC DIET

The diet is monitored by testing for urinary ketones twice daily with Ketostix or Acetest tablets. The tests are usually made before breakfast and the evening meal, ideally aiming at moderate to high ketones (3·9 to 15·7 mmol/l urine). Characteristically, the morning test shows fewer ketones than later in the day. Schwartz *et al.* (1980) have reported that some children maintained on the diet continued to have pre-breakfast seizures. An increase in the fat content of a late evening or bedtime drink helps rectify this tendency.

Urinary ketones may not appear for a week or more after initiating the diet, particularly if the child is not fasted initially, and/or the diet is introduced slowly. Urinary ketones are affected by excess fluid intake and are particularly unreliable in infants. The urinary test for ketones is only semi-quantitative and does not accurately reflect the actual concentration of ketones in blood.

To obtain reliable results the 'Ketostix' strips must be kept cool and dry. The strip is dipped into a fresh specimen of urine or passed through the urine stream and the colour is read after 15 seconds and compared with the standard chart to get a semi-quantitative result.

Blood monitoring of β-hydroxybutyrate (BHB) is recommended during stabilization and then monthly, aiming at more than 2 mmol/l once the diet is established. Maximum concentration may not be reached for approximately one month after starting treatment. It has also been noted that clinical response to the diet may be delayed by 10 to 20 days after the diet is established (Dodson *et al.* 1976). A dietary trial of 6 to 8 weeks is therefore necessary before lack of response to the diet is definite. Even then, the diet should be discontinued slowly.

Clinical and EEG response have been positively correlated with plasma ketones (BHB) by Stephenson *et al.* (1977) in patients who had been on the diet for over two months; Bower *et al.* (1982) found the level of ketones correlated with a good clinical response, but only in some children.

The child's clinical progress and growth should be checked regularly, and parental support in maintaining the diet is essential. Growth failure has frequently been reported with ketogenic dietary regimens (Livingston 1972, Dodson *et al.* 1976). This may be due to dietary deficiencies or a specific effect of the ketogenic diet. Livingston (1972) reported that catch-up growth subsequently occurred when the diet was discontinued.

LOSS OF KETONES

A sudden interruption of diet, with loss of ketones, especially during infection, can precipitate fits.

Causes of ketone loss include inaccuracies in the dietary measurements; rejection of part of the fat/MCT intake; inappropriate timing of the fat supplements; use of concentrated carbohydrates in the diet, even when used as part of the dietary prescription or given inadvertently in medicines; a large fluid intake (more than 1000 ml/day) which is diluting the urinary ketones; diarrhoea (or vomiting) causing a reduction of actual intake of fat.

Different children respond to ketones differently and require individual assessment. Some are better with moderate levels rather than higher levels of ketones (Schwartz *et al.* 1980), though usually the reverse is true.

Loss of urinary ketones necessitates full dietary and clinical investigation. Plasma β-hydroxybutyrate (BHB) should be checked if possible, especially if no obvious cause can be found for the loss of urinary ketones. If none of the above appears to be responsible for the loss of ketones, and they do not return within a few days, the dietary carbohydrate intake should be slightly reduced, e.g. by 200 kJ (50 kcal) and/or the fat/MCT intake increased, e.g. by 10 ml Liquigen or 5 g fat per day.

ILLNESS

Medicines should ideally be carbohydrate-free, so it is essential to alert both the general practitioner and pharmacist in order that prescribed medications are correctly selected. The parents should be advised to use only prescribed medicines. Clearly, a medical adviser must have discretion in prescribing medications appropriately. Examples of carbohydrate-free medicines include Panadol Tablets, Pholcomed Diabetic cough mixture, capsule and parenteral preparations.

Frequently ketosis is lost, and anorexia is common, with intercurrent infections, and fitting can occur. The full diet can be temporarily stopped and replaced with frequent drinks of low-carbohydrate fluids; starvation will maintain the ketosis. Alternatively, the diet quantities may be reduced, but the ratio of fat should be maintained if possible. Once the above are tolerated, the diet should be proportionally reintroduced over 3 to 7 days to the full intake, taking care to introduce the fat/MCT to a full quantity before the full conventional food intake is included.

Diarrhoea can occur or be aggravated by MCT. A temporary reduction of the MCT prescription is appropriate with small daily increments to the full dose as tolerated. Some children do not tolerate the full 60% MCT diet (ii) in which case the combined 30% MCT and 40% dietary fat regimen (iii) is more appropriate and will often be tolerated.

Hospitalization is necessary in some cases of illness and if dehydration, electrolyte imbalance or metabolic acidosis occurs, as these require immediate correction. Discretion in the choice of parenteral fluid must lie with the attending medical officer: monitoring of blood sugar and urinary ketones is important and it is recommended that the lowest carbohydrate content possible be given, e.g. 4·3% glucose in $\frac{1}{5}$ normal saline = 69 kJ (17 kcal) and 3·1 mmol sodium per 100 ml, whereas $\frac{1}{5}$ normal saline in sterile water = nil energy and 3·1 mmol sodium per 100 ml.

Oral rehydration with carbohydrate-free electrolyte mixtures, which can be made by most pharmacists, is recommended in preference to the low-carbohydrate mixtures such as Dextrolyte, Dioralyte or Rehidrat. If the child cannot eat, fluids can be substituted or a home-made enteral feed containing the ketogenic proportions of carbohydrate, protein and fat, devised using milk, egg, cream, Calogen or Prosparol and/or Liquigen, plus vitamin and mineral supplements, can be given by nasogastric tube. Tables 11.5 and 11.12 give examples of suitable fluids.

Special occasions and school meals
The child should be encouraged to participate in social eating, but in the majority of situations the parents will need to supply a tuck box of appropriate food. The school should be informed of the necessity to adhere strictly to the diet. Treats of sweets or pilfering can be potentially harmful as they will cause loss of ketones and the possible return of seizures.

Celebrations such as birthdays and Christmas demand special foods. The permitted free food and dietary prescription foods should be used to the full and can be presented in various ways, for example:

A 'hedgehog' can hold diced 'free' vegetables on cocktail sticks; sugar-free drinks can be served in a fun glass or with a straw; sugar-free ice-lollies can be frozen in different shapes; mousse, ice-cream or jelly (sugar-free) can incorporate fat exchanges or cream.

Plain 'diabetic' Easter eggs and diabetic Christmas pennies can be given occasionally, e.g. 10 g once a week.

Trifle can be made with plain sponge (no sugar) and fruit from the dietary allowance with sugar-free diabetic jelly and double cream from fat exchanges.

'Sugar-free' gums, e.g. Dentine Gum and Orbit, should only be used for treats as they can contain some carbohydrate.

Choux pastry cases (*see* recipe) can be filled with lots of whipped double cream (no sugar) and used as an extra for treats and parties or even a visit to granny or friends. Use with candles for a birthday cake or make a sponge cake and use whipped cream with food colouring as decoration (no sugar) and add candles; the sponge cake should be used as part of the dietary allowance.

DIET DURATION AND DISCONTINUATION

Not all patients respond to a ketogenic diet. However, the beneficial effect of the diet may not be obvious initially, and a six- to eight-week trial is recommended before considering the possibility that the child has not responded. Even so, at whatever stage the diet is stopped it should be discontinued gradually over 10 to 14 days, as a sudden increase in carbohydrate can precipitate seizures. The normal food

Table 11.12   Example of a fluid or enteral feed for use as a substitute for a ketogenic diet*.

	Energy		Protein (g)	Fat (g)	Carbohydrate (g)
	kJ	kcal			
60 ml milk (full-fat)	172	40	2·0	2·3	2·8
15 ml Liquigen/Calogen/Prosparol and/or double cream	278	68	0 to trace	7·5	Nil
Flavouring (carbohydrate-free)	Nil	Nil	Nil	Nil	Nil
Water to >100 ml					
Total	450	108	2	9·8	2·8

* Contains 82% energy from fat plus MCT.
An appropriate volume for energy needs should be fed.
Vitamin and iron supplements are recommended if used for more than a few days.

intake is gradually increased and the fat decreased proportionally. Concentrated refined carbohydrates should be avoided even after the diet is discontinued.

Dietary indiscretion on repeated occasions or where the diet becomes a battle between parents and child may warrant diet discontinuation, particularly if it has not caused a marked clinical improvement. Parental support is essential during dietary treatment, but also when the diet is discontinued, because most parents of children with epilepsy are highly motivated and admission of their failure or the diet's failure can be very distressing for the family.

Children who respond to the diet may be able to have their anticonvulsants gradually reduced or stopped. This is the basic aim of the dietary regimen. There is no consensus of opinion regarding when to discontinue the diet in those who respond. Clarke and House (1978) reported success in a child in whom the diet was discontinued after 18 months and who remained fit-free. Livingston (1972) suggested two years on the traditional 4:1 regimen followed by six months on each of a 3:1 then 2:1 regimen before a normal diet was permitted, a total of three years on a ketogenic diet. To some patients the beneficial effect of the diet is only temporary, even when ketosis is maintained.

Growth failure has been reported; at what stage growth failure warrants discontinuation of the diet must be determined by the paediatrician.

The dietitian must ensure the nutritional adequacy of the regimen prescribed and the practical application of the prescribed diet in overcoming feeding difficulties and maintaining ketosis at the desired level.

REFERENCES

Bower B.D., Schwartz R.H., Eaton J. & Aynsley-Green A. (1982) The use of ketogenic diets in the treatment of epilepsy. In *Topics in Perinatal Medicine* (ed. Wharton B.), pp. 136–40. London: Pitman Medical.

Burman D., Perham T.G.M. & Clothier C. (1982) Nutrition in systemic disease. In *Textbook of Paediatric Nutrition*, 2nd Edition (eds. McLaren D.S. & Burman D.I.), p. 370. Edinburgh: Churchill Livingstone.

Clarke B.J. & House F.M. (1978) Medium chain triglyceride oil in ketogenic diets in the treatment of childhood epilepsy. *J. hum. Nutr.* **32**, 111–16.

Dodson W.E., Prensky A.L. & De Vivo D.C. (1976) Management of seizure disorders: selected aspects. *J. Pediat.* **9**(5), 695–703.

Francis D.E.M. (1986) *Nutrition for Children.* Oxford: Blackwell Scientific Publications.

Gordon N. (1977) Medium chain triglycerides in a ketogenic diet. *Develop. Med. Child Neurol.* **19**, 535–44.

Huttenlocher P.R., Wilbourn A.J. & Signore J.M. (1971) Medium chain triglycerides as a therapy for intractable childhood epilepsy. *Neurology* **21**, 1097–1103.

Keith H.M. (1963) *Convulsive Disorders in Children with Reference to Treatment with Ketogenic Diet.* Boston: Little, Brown & Co.

Livingston S. (1972) Dietary treatment of epilepsy. In *Comprehensive Management of Epilepsy in Infancy, Childhood and Adolescence*, pp. 378–405, Springfield, Illinois: Charles C. Thomas.

Schwartz R.H., Aynesley-Green A. & Bower B.D. (1980) Clinical and metabolic aspects of the ketogenic diets. *Research and Clinical Forums* **2** (2), 63–73.

Stephenson J.B.P., House F.M. & Stromberg P. (1977) Medium chain triglycerides in a ketogenic diet. *Develop. Med. Child Neurol.* **19**, 693–6.

Wilder R.M. (1921) The effect of ketonuria on the course of epilepsy. *Mayo Clinic Bulletin* **2**, 307.

Recipes

Mayonnaise (20 ml = 1 fat exchange)

2 egg-yolks
$\frac{1}{2}$ × 5 ml tsp mustard
125 ml salad oil
Salt, pepper
15 ml vinegar of your choice

Ensure ingredients are at room temperature.

Mix egg-yolks and seasonings in a bowl. *Slowly* whisk in oil to egg-yolks, drop by drop initially, to form an emulsion. If using an electric mixer, switch onto maximum speed and use the balloon whisk. Add the vinegar to thin down the mixture to the correct consistency. Season to taste. Add chopped parsley, capers or tarragon if desired.

Choux pastry cases

40 g butter or margarine
125 ml water
65 g flour (plain)
2 eggs, beaten

Place butter and water in a saucepan and bring to boil. Remove from heat, add the flour and beat well. Cook until paste comes away from the sides. Leave to cool, add eggs gradually, beating continuously. The mixture should be a soft piping consistency which will hold its shape. Place teaspoons or pipe in shapes onto a *well*-greased tin. Cook in a hot oven at 200°C (400°F, gas No. 6) for 30 to 40 minutes until well risen, crisp and golden-brown. Cool and store in an airtight tin until required. Split and serve filled with lots of whipped double cream (no sugar). Add food essence or food colouring to cream and sweeten with saccharin as desired. *Do not* add chocolate or icing, but 1 teaspoon cocoa (unsweetened) may be added to the cream.

CHAPTER 12

Low-calcium diets

Hypercalcaemia

Hypercalcaemia of infancy is characterized by irritability, failure to thrive, anorexia, vomiting, and constipation, and is often associated with thirst and polyuria. The serum and urinary calcium levels are raised due to increased intestinal absorption of calcium, and there may be calcium deposits in many tissues, with resultant renal damage and mental retardation (Forfar & Arneill 1984). The syndrome was first reported in 1952 by Fanconi et al.; also by Lightwood (1952) and Payne (1952). Since then large series of infants with hypercalcaemia have been reported (Ferguson & McGowan 1954, Fellers & Schwartz 1958, and recent review by Martin et al. 1984).

Two different forms of hypercalcaemia

Two different forms of hypercalcaemia occur (Burman & McLaren 1982):

(i) The mild form. This was common in Britain in the 1950s and appeared to be related to excess vitamin D intake. The vitamin D supplementation of infant foods was reduced and a subsequent survey suggested a reduced incidence of the condition (Oppe 1964).

This form responds well to a low-calcium diet ($\leqslant 3.7$ mmol, 150 mg per day) without dietary vitamin D. As soon as the hypercalcaemia is corrected a normal diet can be resumed.

As vitamin D intake was not always excessive a degree of hypersensitivity to the vitamin was suggested. The DHSS has recently reviewed calcium status in the United Kingdom in the report on osteomalacia and rickets (DHSS 1980). It recognized that vitamin D supplements aimed at prevention of these conditions will inevitably precipitate hypercalcaemia in a few susceptible individuals.

(ii) Fanconi-type idiopathic infantile hypercalcaemia and Williams–Beuren syndrome. The rare severe form is a syndrome including hypercalciuria, hypercalcae-

mia, nephrocalcinosis, osteosclerosis, elfin face, mental retardation and cardiac disease (Black & Bonham Carter 1963); hypercalcaemia is not an inevitable finding. The onset of symptoms is during the first six months of life in 80% of all reported cases (Oppe 1964, Martin et al. 1984), but the diagnosis may be delayed. An estimated incidence for the past 20 years has been approximately 18 cases per year in the U.K., 1 in 47 000 livebirths (Martin et al. 1984).

Although the aetiologies of Fanconi-type idiopathic infantile hypercalcaemia and Williams–Beuren syndrome are unknown, they are congenital anomalies, since the birth weight of the two groups studied by Martin and colleagues (1984) was significantly less than normal, and cardiac murmurs were often noted at birth. They are generally thought to be the same syndrome. Martin et al. (1984) compared the clinical features of 76 cases diagnosed with Fanconi-type hypercalcaemia and 41 with Williams–Beuren syndrome and showed there was a greater degree of feeding problems and failure to thrive in those with Fanconi-type idiopathic hypercalcaemia, who generally required treatment of the biochemical abnormality with a low-calcium diet. The symptoms of hypercalcaemia are non-specific, which may explain the delay in diagnosis from the onset of symptoms, and there was an even greater delay in the diagnosis of the majority classified as having Williams–Beuren syndrome without hypercalcaemia.

Metabolic balance studies have shown consistently that the infants with hypercalcaemia absorb calcium more avidly than matched controls (Martin et al. 1984). Clinical studies have usually failed to find evidence of excess vitamin D intake during infancy or increased maternal intake during pregnancy. Where hypercalcaemia is borderline, a calcium load test (Barr & Forfar 1969) and documentation of hypercalciuria are necessary to assess the need for dietary treatment. Short-term steroid treatment may be helpful in some patients.

Treatment of hypercalcaemia in children aims initially to reduce the calcium intake to $\leqslant 3.7$ mmol

(150 mg) calcium per day, and occasionally in infants a minimal intake of 1·2 to 1·5 mmol (50 to 60 mg) calcium per day is required. Added vitamin D is omitted, at least temporarily, from the diet. Dietary treatment improves the symptoms of vomiting and slow weight gain, but it does not necessarily improve the outcome, and feeding problems frequently persist with many patients continuing on a diet of fluids and purées for several years because of the chewing and swallowing difficulties.

Dietary calcium intake needs to be reassessed from time to time in the light of plasma calcium (normal 2·13 to 2·62 mmol/l) and urinary calcium (normal 0 to 0·1 mmol/kg weight per 24 h) levels (Martin *et al.* 1984). Prolonged or overtreatment can cause asymptomatic hypocalcaemia and can result in iatrogenic rickets in the growing long bones. This should be prevented because of the risks to childhood dentition (Martin *et al.* 1984), as well as the potential risk of symptomatic hypocalcaemia, though no case of the latter was reported in the study by Martin *et al.* (1984). Once the serum and urinary calcium levels are normal, after perhaps 6 to 12 months of treatment, a controlled calcium intake of $\simeq 7·5$ to 10 mmol (300 to 400 mg) in the light of clinical and biochemical findings will be needed long-term, with appropriate monitoring and review. The calcium load test and urinary calcium to creatinine ratio (normal range $0·4 \pm 0·17$) are helpful in assessing calcium tolerance (Ghazali & Barratt 1974). At this stage a normal intake of vitamin D, 7·5 to 10 μg (300 to 400 i.u.) daily, may be considered appropriate.

Even with treatment, prognosis is poor. A parents support group for these patients has been formed.

Other conditions requiring a low-calcium dietary regimen

A low-calcium diet with or without vitamin D supplements is used in a number of other conditions affecting calcium metabolism, such as temporarily in patients who have received excessive amounts of vitamin D. A reduced calcium intake to $\leqslant 20$ mmol (800 mg) and occasionally to 7·5 mmol (300 mg) is required permanently in patients with renal calculii due to idiopathic hypercalciuria (p. 202).

The rare inherited calcium disorder, osteopetrosis (Yu *et al.* 1971, Burman & McLaren 1982), also known as marble bone disease, causes an increased density of bone which encroaches on bone marrow and foramina in the skull; blindness, deafness, splenomegaly, anaemia, and thrombocytopenia can result.

Lifelong treatment, including a minimum calcium intake $\leqslant 3·7$ mmol (150 mg) per day, is required.

LOW-CALCIUM DIETS

The low-calcium milk substitute Locasol—new formula (Table 12.1)—is used as the basis of nutrition in infants and toddlers and can be used to replace milk in the diet of children and adults. A modified infant milk formula or human milk may be sufficiently low in calcium in some cases, or a module formula can be devised for specific patients (Table 12.1).

The low- and high-calcium foods are indicated in Table 12.2 and sample menus for a very-low calcium diet $\leqslant 3·7$ mmol (150 mg) per day are given in Table 12.3. Added vitamin D is usually omitted, at least temporarily.

The diet devised must be nutritionally adequate in other respects, except for calcium and vitamin D. However, protein intake should not be excessive and may need modification if the blood urea is raised and renal function impaired. A generous fluid intake should be encouraged.

The new formula Locasol is nutritionally complete except for calcium and vitamin D. If Locasol is not used as the basis of the diet the Cow & Gate Supplementary Vitamin Tablets (dose according to age of 6 to 12 tablets per day) are a suitable low-calcium form of trace minerals, water-soluble vitamins and fat-soluble vitamins, without vitamins A and D. Vitamin A (free of vitamin D) can be given as the precursor carotene, from natural foods such as apricots, carrots, yellow and green vegetables or fruit juices. Alternatively, three Ketovite Tablets plus vitamin B_{12} and a source of carotene provide a comprehensive range of vitamins. However, Ketovite Liquid, which contains 10 μg vitamin D in the standard 5 ml dose, may be contraindicated.

Hard water contains a considerable amount of calcium. Local water boards can give details of the calcium content of the water supply and type of hardness. Occasionally, hardness of water can be removed by boiling; alternatively, distilled or de-ionized water can be obtained from pharmacies. A home water softener unit is the most convenient way of obtaining low-calcium water, but the type of softener must be selected with care if the water is to be used for infants, due to the resultant high sodium content of the water produced by sodium-exchange resins. Some, but not all, bottled natural spring waters contain calcium (e.g. Evian contains 2 mmol/l calcium); some are not bacteriologically safe, especially for infant

Table 12.1 Examples of low-calcium milk substitute feeds for infants and children.

	Calcium (mg*)	Phos- phorus (mmol)	Potassium (mmol)	Sodium (mmol)	Energy kJ	Energy kcal	Carbo- hydrate (g)	Protein (g)	Fat (g)
(a) 13·1 g Locasol†	≤7·0	1·8	2·5	1·2	275	66	7·3	1·9	3·4
Water to 100 ml‡			Trace	Trace					
100 ml *total*	≤7·0	1·8	2·5	1·2	275	66	7·3	1·9	3·4
(b) 25 g Comminuted Chicken	2·3	0·4	0·3	0·1	62	15	Nil	1·9	0·8
8·5 g glucose polymer			Trace	Trace	137	32·6	8·2		
5 ml Prosparol				Trace	92·5	22·5			2·5
1 mmol potassium chloride			1·0						
0·2 g Calcium-free Mineral Mixture§	Nil	0·9	1·1	0·8					
Water to 100 ml‡			Trace	Trace					
100 ml *total*	2·3	1·3	2·4	0·9	304	70	8·2	1·9	3·3
(c) 2 g Maxipro HBV	6·0	0·3	0·2	0·2	30	7	Trace	1·8	Nil
7 g glucose polymer			Trace	Trace	112	28	7		
7 ml Prosparol				Trace	130	31·5			3·5
0·3 g calcium-free Mineral Mixture§	Nil	4	1·6	1·3					
Water to 100 ml‡			Trace	Trace					
100 ml *total*	6·0	1·7	1·8	1·5	272	66·5	7	1·8	3·5
(d) 50 ml Osterfeed‖	18	0·5	0·75	0·4	142	34	3·5	0·75	1·9
1 g Maxipro HBV	3	0·1	0·1	0·1	15	3·5	Trace	0·9	Nil
7 g glucose polymer			Trace	Trace	112	28	7·0		
Appropriate quantity of Calcium-free Mineral Mix- ture can be prescribed§									
Water to 100 ml‡			Trace	Trace					
100 ml *total*	21	0·6	0·85	0·5	269	65·5	10·5	1·65	1·9
(e) Comparison with human milk and a whey-based infant formula									
100 ml mature human milk	34	0·5	1·5	0·6	289	69	7·2	1·3	4·1
100 ml Osterfeed‖	36	1·0	1·5	0·8	284	68	7	1·5	3·8
(f) Social replacement of milk (low nutritional value; unsuitable for infants and young children)									
10 g Coffee-mate	1·3	1·2	2·3	0·6	224	54	5·8	0·3	3·4
Water to 100 ml‡			Trace	Trace					
100 ml *total*	1·3	1·2	2·3	0·6	224	54	5·8	0·3	3·4

Vitamin supplements are essential with feeds (b) to (d) as either:

6 to 12 Cow & Gate Supplementary Vitamin tablets plus a source of carotene.

Or Ketovite Tablets, and vitamin B₁₂, and a source of carotene (Ketovite Liquid contains vitamin D).

* Milligram of calcium are used because of the low values given in this table. To convert to millimole divide milligram value by 40.

† New complete formula 1985. Renal solute load 130 mmol/l.

‡ Calcium content of water varies; low-calcium water, or de-ionized or distilled water should be used.

§ The dose of Calcium-Free Mineral Mixture (*see* Francis 1986) is based on a maximum of 0·5 g/kg per day to 4 g/day. As this mineral mixture contains very little chloride the feed is lower than recommended unless potassium chloride supplements are prescribed.

‖ Other modified infant formulae may be selected as appropriate.

Table 12.2 Low-calcium diet.

Foods allowed	Foods forbidden or restricted
Water: low-calcium, distilled, de-ionized, softened or suitable bottled water.	Tap water, hard water containing calcium.
Milk substitute (*see* Table 12.1): Locasol	Milk, cheese, cream, ice-cream. Filled milks, Casilan, Complan, etc.
Flour: 100% wholemeal, stone-ground flour (Allinson's), unfortified flour, potato flour, cornflour, rice flour, arrowroot.	Flour fortified with calcium, white flour, bread and commercially baked goods.
Cakes, biscuits, and pastries made with appropriate unfortified low-calcium flour.	Pastries, cakes, biscuits made from fortified flour.
Low-calcium baking powder.	Baking powder unless known to be low-calcium.
Matzos	
Bread: Allinson's, stone-ground or 100% wholemeal, home-made from a suitable low-calcium flour.	Breads made with fortified flour.
Macaroni, rice, semolina, dry cereals, and spaghetti without cheese.	Baby cereals and rusks containing milk powder, calcium and/or vitamin D.
Custard powder, sago, tapioca, oats.	
Pasta, pulses.	
Porridge made without milk.	
Cornflakes, Rice Krispies, Weetabix, Puffed Wheat, Sugar Puffs, etc.	Special K, muesli containing milk powder.
All meats, poultry, ham, bacon.	
Egg—limit intake (*see* Table 12.4).	
Fish (except bones)	Fish bones, e.g. in sardines, Fish in batter, fish fingers.
Fruit, fruit juices and vegetables except those listed elsewhere. Oranges—limit to 2 to 3 oranges per week.	Spinach, broccoli, watercress, olives. Concentrated orange juices. Dried fruit such as figs, dates, currants, sultanas, raisins.
Sugar, brown, white, pure icing sugar.	Free-flowing icing sugars containing calcium.
Jam, honey, jelly, syrup, marmalade.	Lemon curd.
Plain boiled sweets, lollies, candies. Carbonated beverages such as Coke, lemonade, Lucozade.	Chocolate, fudge, toffee, fruit gums, ice-cream.
Table jellies.	Agar, Carrageen, Quick Jel.
Butter (restrict quantity if vitamin D limited). Lard, cooking fats and oils. Catering margarines without vitamins.	Margarines (contain high quantities of vitamin A and D)
Salt, pepper, herbs, spices.	
Tea, coffee—black or with milk substitute. Coffee-mate (Carnation) and coffee creamers low in calcium	Malted drinks and similar beverages.

Table 12.3 Sample menus for a low-calcium diet ⩽ 3·7 mmol, 150 mg calcium per day.

(a)	*Older child's diet*	
	Breakfast	Cornflakes, Rice Krispies, Weetabix
		Sugar
		Milk substitute low in calcium, Locasol
		Bacon or ham/egg (alternate days)—optional
		100% wholemeal bread and butter and jam or honey
		Tea/coffee and Coffee-mate
	Mid-morning	Fruit juice or squash made with low-calcium water
	Dinner	Meat or chicken or mince or fish (cooked without milk)
		Thin gravy, or gravy thickened with cornflour
		Milk-free mashed potatoes, or boiled, or roast, or chips
		Carrots and/or vegetables permitted
		Fruit, fresh, tinned or stewed
		Custard made with Locasol, or Coffee-mate and water
	Tea	Tea/coffee and Coffee-mate or fruit juice or Locasol
	Supper	Ham, meat or fish
		Crisps, or chips and/or 100% wholemeal bread and butter
		Salad or vegetables permitted
		Home-made biscuits using a suitable flour
		Fruit
	Bedtime	Tea/coffee and Coffee-mate or fruit juice or Locasol

(b)   *Weaning or toddler diet*

In addition to milk substitute, Locasol feeds

	a.*m.*	Weetabix or porridge
		Milk substitute, Locasol
	Midday	Minced meat or flaked fish ⎫
		Boiled potato ⎪
		Permitted vegetable ⎬ May be puréed
		Gravy ⎭
		Custard made from Locasol ⎫ Optional
		Mashed or purée fruit ⎭
		Fruit juice diluted with low-calcium water
	p.m.	Alternate days boiled egg and wholemeal bread and butter
		or meat and vegetables as midday
		or suitable commercial baby food low in calcium
		Locasol with cereal or as custard

feeds. The water selected should be low in sodium as well as calcium, and bacteriologically safe, especially if intended for infants.

Although plans were made to end the requirement that white flour and bread should be fortified with calcium and B vitamins, this decision has recently been reprieved. Flour and breads will continue to be fortified with calcium by law in the United Kingdom, unless 100% wholemeal (DHSS 1981). Fortified flour is used in commercial cakes, biscuits, pastries and breads. Patients on a low-calcium diet should use unfortified flour, or wholemeal flour, which are lower in calcium; the latter can be sieved to remove excess husk if a 'whiter' flour is required. However, the wholegrain flours contribute fibre to the diet, which is useful in overcoming the constipation which is a frequent feature in patients with hypercalcaemia. Cornflour and rice flour are also low in calcium. Unfortified flour can be obtained from some mills on the receipt of a medical certificate. Low-calcium baking powder should be used in baking and can be made from the recipe on p. 000.

All commercial baby cereals and rusks contain either skimmed milk powder, calcium and/or vitamin D and should be avoided or replaced with a suitable crushed adult-type of low-calcium cereal, e.g. Weetabix or porridge.

Table 12.4   Calcium content of various foods.

100 g	Calcium mg	Calcium mmol
Arrowroot	7	0·2
Cornflour	15	0·4
Rice flour	4	0·1
Oatmeal (raw)	55	1·4
Porridge	6	0·2
Flour		
Plain, fortified	150	3·4
Self-raising, fortified	350	8·8
100% wholemeal	35	0·9
Unfortified brown	20	0·5
Unfortified white	15	0·4
Bread		
White	100	2·5
Hovis	150	3·4
Brown	100	2·5
Wholemeal (unfortified)	23	0·6
Allinson's (small bakeries)	23	0·6
Allinson's (supermarkets)	75	1·9
Chapatis	63*	1·6*
Biscuits, various	100*	2·5*
Weetabix	33	0·8
Cornflakes	3	0·1
Rice Krispies	7	0·2
Matzo	32	0·8
Egg, *one only*, 50 g	52	1·3
Human milk—mature, 100 ml	34	0·9
Modified whey-based infant formulae	46*	1·2*
Cow's milk 100 ml	120	3·0
Double cream 100 ml	50	1·3
Coffee-mate (Carnation)	13	0·3
Orange juice	12	0·3
Distilled or de-ionized water	Trace	Trace

* Average values.

The calcium content of various foods is given in Table 12.4. The degree of calcium restriction required in the treatment of a condition varies with the clinical findings. A calcium intake of 3·7 to 20 mmol (150 to 800 mg) can be devised from the data in Tables 12.1 to 12.4.

REFERENCES

BARR D.G.D. & FORFAR J.O. (1969) Oral calcium load test in infancy, with particular reference to idiopathic hypercalcaemia. *Brit. med. J.* 1, 477–80.

BLACK J.A. & BONHAM CARTER R.E. (1963) Association between aortic stenosis and facies of severe infantile hypercalcaemia. *Lancet* 2, 745–9.

BURMAN D. & McLAREN D.S. (1982) Element deficiency and toxicity (hypercalcaemia). In *Textbook of Paediatric Nutrition*, 2nd Edition (eds. Burman D. & McLaren D.S.), pp. 173–4. Edinburgh: Churchill Livingstone.

DHSS (1980) Report on Health and Social Subjects—Rickets and Osteomalacia, Report No. 19. London: HMSO.

DHSS (1981) Nutritional Aspects of Bread and Flour, Report No. 23. London: HMSO.

FANCONI G., GIARDET P., SCHLESINGER B., BUTLER H. & BLACK J.S. (1952) Chronische Hypercalcaemie, Kombiniert mit Osteoklerose, Hyperazotamie, Minderwuchs und Kongenital Missbildungen. *Helv. paediat. Acta* 7, 314–34.

FELLERS F.X. & SCHWARTZ R. (1958) Etiology of the severe form of idiopathic hypercalcaemia of infancy. *New Engl. J. Med.* 259, 1050–8.

FERGUSON A.W. & McGOWAN G.K. (1954) Idiopathic hypercalcaemia in infants. *Lancet* 1, 1272–4.

FORFAR J.O. & ARNEILL G.C. (1984) *Textbook of Paediatrics*, 3rd Edition, pp. 1279–82. Edinburgh: Churchill Livingstone.

GHAZALI S. & BARRATT T.M. (1974) Urinary excretion of calcium and magnesium in children. *Arch. Dis. Childh.* 49, 97–101.

LIGHTWOOD R.C. (1952) Idiopathic hypercalcaemia in infants with failure to thrive. *Arch. Dis. Childh.* 27, 302–3.

MARTIN N.D.T., SNODGRASS G.J.A.I. & COHEN R.D. (1984) Idiopathic infantile hypercalcaemia—a continuing enigma. *Arch. Dis. Childh.* 59, 605–13.

OPPE T.E. (1964) Infantile hypercalcaemia, nutritional rickets and infantile scurvy in Great Britain, British Paediatric Association Report. *Brit. Med. J.* 1, 1659–61.

PAYNE W.W. (1952) The blood chemistry in idiopathic hypercalcaemia. *Arch. Dis. Childh.* 27, 302.

YU J.S., OATES R.K., WALSH, K.H. & STUCKEY S.J. (1971) Osteopetrosis. *Arch. Dis. Childh.* 46, 257–63.

Parents support group
Infantile Hypercalcaemia Foundation Ltd,
c/o Lady Cooper, Mulberry Cottage, Mulberry Green,
Old Harlow, Essex, CM17 0EY.

CHAPTER 13

Galactosaemia, fructosaemia and favism: dietary management

Inborn errors of metabolism were described first by Garrod in 1909 and are due to enzyme defects. Many such disorders have subsequently been identified (Stanbury et al. 1983) and in some enzyme replacement therapy is possible (Whiteman 1983). In others, such as galactosaemia and fructosaemia, diet is the only effective treatment (Clayton & Francis 1978). The appropriate dietary regimens are described in this chapter; full details of the metabolic, clinical and genetic aspects of the conditions are described in standard texts (Cornblath & Schwartz 1976a, Burman et al. 1980, Stanbury et al. 1983).

GALACTOSAEMIA

Two major disorders associated with galactose metabolism by erythrocyte enzymes, and responsive to dietary treatment, have been described: (i) deficiency of galactose-1-phosphate uridyltransferase required to metabolize galactose to glucose results in classical galactosaemia, and (ii) deficiency of galactokinase which catalyses the formation of galactose-1-phosphate from galactose. The metabolism of galactose and glucose are complex, but are summarized in Fig. 13.1. A number of modifications of the classical syndromes have been described (Gitzelmann & Hansen 1980, Stanbury et al. 1983) but are not relevant to a discussion of the dietary management.

Most dietary galactose is derived from lactose, the disaccharide of milk that is hydrolysed to galactose and glucose by the action of intestinal lactase, which shows normal activity in these patients.

Screening programmes of recent years suggest an incidence in Massachusetts, U.S.A., of 1 in 50 000 (Shih et al. 1971) and 1 in 40 000 for 1979 in Europe (Bickel et al. 1981). In the United Kingdom the diagnosis is usually made in a sick child, screening for galactosaemia in newborns being uncommon.

Classically, galactosaemia usually presents after the introduction of milk (human, cow's milk, modified milks) as failure to thrive, with vomiting, diarrhoea and impaired liver function with jaundice and hepatomegaly (Donnell et al. 1980). Severity and onset of symptoms vary widely, poor sucking may be noted within 48 hours of birth, or the condition may present as an acute fulminating disease with particular susceptibility to infection, such as by Escherichia coli. Without treatment the disease is usually rapidly fatal, but if the child survives without treatment he develops mental retardation, cirrhosis of the liver and cataracts. Early diagnosis and prompt treatment with a galactose-free diet can lead to excellent immediate results and a favourable long-term prognosis, though the outcome is not entirely certain, some patients having more or fewer problems in spite of good dietary care (Donnell et al. 1980).

Mass neonatal screening constitutes an essential first step in reducing mortality and morbidity among children with galactosaemia. Levy (1980) suggests that screening for galactosaemia is less well accepted because of the incorrect assumptions that it always presents in the neonatal period with at least jaundice and vomiting of milk and that this presentation will lead to appropriate investigation and correct diagnosis and treatment. However, this is not always the case, resulting in delayed or missed diagnosis. There is also concern over the ideal timing of a screening test programme, which would be ideal on cord blood but more practical if performed on the sample taken for the screening for phenylketonuria and hypothyroidism on the sixth to tenth day.

Biochemical findings include raised galactose-1-phosphate in erythrocytes, which is thought to be the toxic metabolite (Cornblath & Schwartz 1976a, Gitzelmann & Hansen 1980), proteinuria and amino aciduria, and raised serum galactose and urinary galactose with depressed blood glucose levels, providing the infant is obtaining dietary galactose. Cataracts may be present at birth or develop subsequently, and despite treatment remain permanent in some cases.

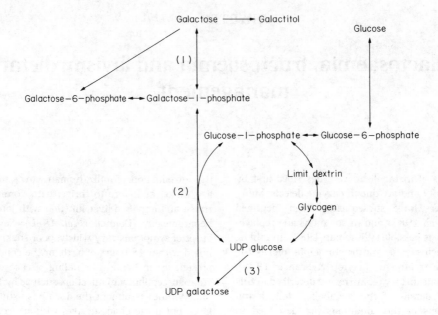

Enzymes involved :

    (I) Galactokinase
    (2) Galactose–I–phosphate uridyl transferase
    (3) Epimerase

Fig. 13.1 Schematic metabolism of galactose and glucose.

Diagnosis is confirmed by enzyme studies on erythrocytes. The enzyme test is relevant even when the infant is on a minimal galactose diet. In high-risk cases, such as siblings of children with galactosaemia, cord blood can be tested before lactose is ever given to the infant; a lactose-free feed, sugar or glucose water can be given in the meanwhile.

Dietary treatment

Dietary exclusion of galactose, and lactose from which it is derived, is necessary at least throughout childhood, and the major sources of lactose should probably be omitted for life (Brandt 1980). The diet must be nutritionally adequate to promote normal growth. Tables 13.1 to 13.4 give details of suggested diets. The lactose in milk (including human, cow, goat, ewe and the majority of infant formulae) is the major source of dietary galactose. However, lactose is used as a filler in medicines, especially tablets, and is also used in spices, such as retail monosodium glutamate powder, and artificial sweeteners such as Sweet 'n' Low and Canderel, which must also be omitted. Cow's milk proteins, provided they are lactose-free, are permitted, e.g. Coffee-mate, Casilan.

A nutritionally adequate galactose/lactose-free milk substitute (*see* Tables 1.4 & 1.5) should be selected and is essential during infancy and as a supplement to the diet, at least in pre-school age children. Thereafter a galactose/lactose-free social replacement of milk may be adequate (*see* Table 1.7) or calcium and vitamin supplements may suffice. Lactase-treated milks, such as Digestelact (Hunter Valley, Australia) or Lactalac (Co-operative Condensfabriek, Holland), which have merely split the lactose into galactose and glucose, are contraindicated in galactosaemia.

A number of plant foods contain raffinose, stachyose, and therefore galactosides, which together with nucleoproteins are potential sources of galactose (Table 13.1). However, because of the absence of human α-galactosidase, these are not digested by the intestinal mucosa to release galactose (Gitzelmann 1980). These oligosaccharides, when they reach the colon, are fermented by bacterial action and largely result in the release of various organic acids rather than galactose. Only a small amount of galactose is absorbed, except when the patient has diarrhoea, though no explanation is known for the latter (Gitzelman 1980). Traditionally, foods high in galactosides, i.e. pulses, spinach, cocoa, and whole soya (but not soy-isolate protein from which these oligosaccharides are removed during processing to remove the trypsin inhibitor), and those rich in nucleoproteins, i.e. liver, kidney, brain, sweetbread and egg have been limited or excluded from the diet during infancy and early childhood. It is probably unnecessary to exclude these foods, but opinions differ (Gitzelmann & Auricchio 1965, Gitzelman 1980, Donnell *et al.* 1980, Clothier & Davidson 1983). At present there are few documented studies correlating galactose-1-phosphate levels with different dietary components other than lactose. The inevitable differences from one patient to another make it difficult to give firm guidelines. Also, in early infancy high galactose-1-phosphate levels can be due to biosynthesis of galactose from UDP glucose (Fig. 13.1) and not necessarily due to dietary ingestion of lactose or galactose. This also occurs in pregnant women, even on a milk-free diet, and in normal infants. The essential requirement of galactose for brain cerebroside synthesis is provided in this way.

Apart from rigid dietary exclusion of galactose and lactose there is no way at present to prevent galactose-1-phosphate accumulation. Dietary lapse in

early infancy may result in immediate gastrointestinal symptoms, but there is some evidence that non-adherence to the diet is asymptomatic in the older child (Donnell *et al.* 1980, Kinmoth & Baum 1982). Ethanol inhibits hepatic galactose elimination and is best avoided (Brandt 1980).

It is important to chart serial measurements of height and weight in children with galactosaemia and recommended that the diet be monitored by erythrocyte galactose-1-phosphate estimations (Donnell *et al.* 1980), at least monthly in infants, two to three-monthly in children, and yearly thereafter, to ensure the diet is being adhered to adequately. The aim should be to maintain galactose-1-phosphate levels ideally in the normal range, i.e. below 0·57 μmol/g of haemoglobin (30 μg/ml of erythrocytes).

MINIMAL GALACTOSE/LACTOSE DIET

Infants. A nutritionally adequate galactose/lactose-free milk substitute, (full details are given in Tables 1.4 & 1.5) forms the basis of the diet. The formula should mimic the nutritional guidelines (except for lactose) given in *Artificial Feeds for the Young Infant* (DHSS 1980). The following are appropriate:

From birth	Pregestimil Pepdite 0–2	Hydrolysed protein lactose-free formalae with MCT
	S Formula Soya Prosobee Wysoy	Soy-isolate lactose-free formulae
From three months	Nutramigen	Hydrolysed casein formula
Children	Galactomin	Casein formula

The formulae containing MCT as partial replacement of fat are advised if the patient has steatorrhoea. Medicines and supplements must be lactose-free.

Weaning. Galactose/lactose-free solids are introduced as appropriate for age, excluding initially the foods rich in galactosides and nucleoprotein (Table 13.1). The introducing of egg is delayed till 6 to 8 months and is then given 2 to 4 times per week. Many commercial baby foods contain milk or other contraindicated ingredients and should be scrutinized with care. A sample weaning menu is given in Table 13.2.

Table 13.1 Foods containing galactosides or high in nucleoprotein.

| *Galactosides* | Most plant foods, especially pulses: peas, beans, lentils, dahl, legumes, chick-peas, gram. Spinach.
Soya (except soy-isolates)
Textured vegetable protein (TVP)
Cocoa and chocolate (NB many also contain milk/lactose)
Nuts |
| *Nucleoproteins* | Offal: liver, kidney, brain, sweetbread, liver sausage, and paté
Egg |

Table 13.2 Minimal galactose weaning diet menu. To
use in addition to galactose/lactose-free milk substitute
feeds, e.g. Nutramigen, Wysoy, Prosobee or S Formula.

8 to 10 a.m.	*Milk-free cereal, Robinson's Baby Rice, Farex Weaning Cereal, plain Ready Brek (Lyons), or Milupa Plain Rice Cereal
	Mix with milk substitute
	*Milk-free toast and Tomor margarine or milk-free low-fat spread
12 to 2 p.m.	Puréed or sieved meat or chicken (avoid offal)
	Milk-free mashed potato
	Gravy
	Puréed or sieved vegetables, e.g. tomato, carrot, cauliflower (avoid pulses)
Or	Suitable strained baby foods*
	*Custard made with milk substitute and/or jelly and/or purée fruit
Snack	Diluted fruit juice
	Milk-free rusk*
5 to 6 p.m.	*Custard made with milk substitute
Or	Milk-free rusk, e.g. Farley's Original Rusk
	Fruit purée
	Savoury suitable strained baby foods*
	*Milk-free toast and Tomor margarine or milk-free low-fat spread

* The ingredients of all commercial products should be
scrutinized and omitted if they contain lactose, milk, whey,
cream, pulses, offal, etc.

Toddlers. Finger foods such as milk-free bread or
rusk should be introduced from about eight months
to encourage chewing, minced foods should replace
purées, and the child should be encouraged to drink
from a cup and gradually to feed himself.

Provided galactose-1-phosphate levels are adequately controlled the foods containing galactosides
and nucleoproteins (Table 13.1) are permitted. Galac-
tose-1-phosphate levels should be monitored after
each major dietary change.

Young children. A varied diet selected from Table
13.3 is used throughout childhood. Commercially
prepared foods and medicines must be continually
scrutinized, as product changes frequently occur. Vitamin and mineral supplements (lactose-free) may be
required to provide an adequate intake of calcium,
riboflavin, vitamins A, D, C, B_{12} and folic acid, if these
are not taken in the form of an appropriate milk

substitute. A comprehensive vitamin–mineral supplement can be provided by:

Calcium Sandoz Liquid
6 to 12 Cow & Gate Supplementary Vitamin Tablets
5 ml Ketovite Liquid

Older children may be permitted foods which contain
traces of lactose (Table 13.4) but visible milk, ice-
cream, custard and actual lactose should be avoided.
Alcohol (beverages, gripe water, etc.) is probably best
avoided.

Results of treatment in patients with galactosaemia

Dietary treatment can be life-saving and symptoms
and signs of the disease remit (Kinmoth & Baum
1982), though cataracts may persist in some patients
and ultimately require surgery. Even on a well-controlled diet eye changes may progress (Donnell *et al.*
1980); in others they completely resolve with treatment. Throughout childhood growth rate is usually
slightly below that of normal children of a similar age.
Even with good dietary treatment the long-term outcome (intellectual development) is not entirely certain
(Nadler *et al.* 1969, Komrower & Lee 1970, Yu 1972,
Editorial 1982, Komrower 1982). In the group reported by Donnel *et al.* (1980) many developed well,
but others had more or less severe problems. In
general, patients from higher IQ families had higher
IQs, which may be related to genetic and sociological
factors. Other determinant factors for outcome are
the age of the diagnosis and instigation of dietary
treatment, with a more favourable outcome when
the diet is started at an earlier age, before the fourth
month, and good dietary compliance, which tends to
lapse with increasing age even when diet relaxation
is not advised. Diet may be less well adhered to in
those from a lower social class. Unfavourable intrauterine exposure to galactose (or its metabolites) of
the galactosaemic homozygote has been posed as
another cause of the variable outcome of treatment
(Donnell *et al.* 1980). Even when the mothers were
on a restricted lactose intake throughout pregnancy,
galactose-1-phosphate in cord blood erythrocytes is
elevated, suggesting that the fetus is exposed to this
metabolite in intrauterine life. Although it is unknown if maternal lactose restriction during pregnancy is beneficial to the outcome in the fetus,
because of endogenous production of lactose and galactose from quite early in the pregnancy it is recommended that the major sources of dietary lactose are
omitted throughout pregnancy in known galactosaemic heterozygotes until it is determined if the fetus

Table 13.3   Minimal galactose and lactose diet for children with galactosaemia.

(a) Allowed and forbidden foods.

Foods allowed	Foods forbidden and which may contain lactose/galactose*
Milk substitute	Lactose and galactose
	Lactase-treated milks
Infants	Milk sugar
Pregestimil	Human, cow's, goat's milk
Prosobee	Evaporated and skimmed milks, non-fat milks, modified
S Formula Soya	baby milks and other milk substitutes containing
Wysoy	galactose/lactose, enteral feeds containing lactose.
Over three months *See* Tables 1.4	Complan, Build-Up
Nutramigen and 1.5	Filled milks such as Five Pints, Fast Pints
Children	
Galactomin	
Milk-free margarines, e.g. Tomor, Telma, Vitaquell	Cream, butter, cheese, margarines, Outline spread
Low-fat milk-free spreads*	All ice-cream, non-milk fat ice-cream, milk puddings and
All edible oils, lard, pure fats	desserts
Non-dairy imitation cream*	Yoghurt
Meat, poultry, fish, bacon, ham, shellfish, eggs	Sausages, burgers and fish fingers, fish cakes, battered fish,
	unless known to be milk-free
	Made-up dishes with milk/lactose-containing ingredients
	Ham and cured meats from brine containing whey protein
	or EM 40
	Tinned meat and fish products
Cereals	Milk puddings, e.g. custard, creamed rice
Wheat, rye, barley, oats, rice, corn, millet, semolina,	Non-milk fat products
sago (cooked without milk)	Instant custard mix
Flour	Egg noodles, macaroni cheese, tinned spaghetti with
Plain, self-raising, wholemeal	cheese, Italian-type spaghetti
Macaroni*, spaghetti	Instant Whip, Angel Delight
Custard powder*	
Breakfast cereals	
Weetabix, Cornflakes, Rice Krispies, Shreddies, bran, All	
Bran	
Baby cereals	Baby cereals fortified with milk solids, e.g. Farley's
Robinson's Baby Rice, Farex Weaning Cereal, Milupa	Breakfast Cereal, low-sugar baby rusks, some muesli,
Plain Rice Cereal, Farley's Original Rusk only, plain	Special K, etc.
Ready Brek	
Bread, e.g. wholemeal, Hovis, plain white milk-free, VitBe,	Milk bread, Procea, etc.
granary breads	
Cakes and biscuits known to be free of lactose and milk	Cakes and biscuits known containing milk, lactein, butter,
	etc.
Fruit—all varieties	Pies and made-up dishes containing lactose or milk, etc.
Fruit juices	Instant potato* containing milk and/or butter
Nuts	Mashed potato containing milk and/or butter
Vegetables without butter, milk products	Potato salad*, vegetable salad*, salad creams, mayonnaise
Potatoes, plain crisps*	Flavoured crisps*
Milk-free soups* and consommé	Cream soups
Soup cubes, Oxo, Bisto, gravy mix*, Marmite, Bovril	
Salt, pepper	

Table 13.3 (a)   *continued*

Foods allowed	Foods forbidden and which may contain lactose/galactose*
Fresh herbs and pure spices, mustard, yeast	Spices containing lactose filler, e.g. retail monosodium glutamate
Sugar, jam, honey, jelly, syrup Food essences and colourings	Sugar substitutes containing lactose, e.g. Sweet 'n' Low, Canderel
Table jellies	
Tea, coffee, instant coffee (without milk) Milk-shake fruit flavourings Fruit drinks and squashes Carbonated beverages, slimming drinks Coffee-mate, Pareve-mate (kosher) coffee creamer Casilan	
Boiled sweets, lollies, pastilles, gums, ice-lollies without milk	Fudge, toffee Sweets containing hydrolysed milk, whey and/or milk sugar
Cocoa, pulses and offal (Table 13.1) if permitted	Milk chocolate, diabetic chocolate horlicks, Ovaltine, Bournvita Milo, etc.
Most liquid and capsule medicines are suitable*	Most tablets containing lactose filler Alcohol in beverages, gripe water, etc. is not advisable

* The ingredients of commercial products should be continually scrutinized for suitability and omitted if they contain lactose, milk, whey, etc.

(b) Example menu for a child with galactosaemia.

Breakfast	Weetabix, Cornflakes, porridge or milk-free muesli and/or fruit Sugar (optional) Milk substitute, e.g. Wysoy or Galactomin Bacon and tomato or egg (optional) Milk-free bread or toast Tomor margarine or milk-free margarine Marmalade, jam, honey, Marmite, Bovril, peanut butter Milk substitute, flavoured with tea or coffee and/or fruit juice
Mid-morning	Fruit juice or milk substitute
Lunch/dinner	Meat, chicken, fish, egg Potato—roast, boiled, chips Vegetables permitted } Without milk or butter Gravy Fruit, jelly Custard made with milk substitute and suitable custard powder Crumbles, fruit pie, tart (made without milk, butter)
Tea	Fruit or milk-free sandwich, biscuit or cake Milk substitute or fruit juice

Table 13.3 (b) *continued*

Supper/lunch Meat, chicken, fish, egg or milk-free made-up dishes, e.g. home-made beefburgers ⎫
Salad or vegetables permitted
Chips or plain crisps or jacket potato, rice or milk-free pasta
Milk-free bread or rolls, crispbread ⎬ Can be adapted
Tomor margarine or milk-free margarine to a sandwich
Marmite, jam, honey, peanut butter school lunch
Milk-free biscuit or cake
Fruit, nuts, dried fruit ⎭

Bedtime Milk substitute
Fruit and/or milk-free sandwich for older children

Calcium and vitamin supplement as appropriate

Table 13.4 Foods containing traces of lactose which may be permitted in older children with galactosaemia.

Butter
All margarines
Hard cheeses, e.g. Edam, Gouda, Cheddar
Dark chocolate (non-dairy)

has galactosaemia. Prenatal diagnosis of galactosaemia is possible (Fensom *et al.* 1979, Holten & Raymont 1980). At birth the infant should be deprived of lactose until the diagnosis is eliminated.

It has been shown that the heterozygous fetus of a homozygous galactosaemic mother is not exposed to raised galactose-1-phosphate tissue concentrations and has a better chance of ultimate IQ than the well-treated mother (Sardharwalla *et al.* 1980).

In a number of patients with galactosaemia there are reports of a difference between measured IQ and function, many having learning difficulties and distractability, which may be either primary or environmental, due to parental anxiety and the rigid dietary regimen needed for treatment (Komrower & Lee 1970, Donnell *et al.* 1980, Brandt 1980). Galactosaemia has recently been reviewed in an Editorial (1982) encouraging multicentre liaison and closer follow-up of these patients in the future, in order to gain greater insight into the condition and its management.

Duration of dietary treatment

It is generally agreed that dietary treatment of galactosaemia should be very strict in the first few years of life. Some workers have suggested a relaxed attitude towards the diet when the patient is older (Komrower 1970, 1973, Donnell & Bergren 1975) but

others disagree (Brandt 1980). The enzyme defect persists for life, and galactose-1-phosphate is very toxic and is rapidly formed in the liver from galactose. Although the diet is relatively simple it is socially inconvenient, particularly for a convenience food-oriented society in which many manufactured foods contain lactose and/or milk; however, the diet is harmless and can support normal growth. Any easement of the diet after the first few years should be minimal and only to make the diet more socially acceptable. Dietary change should be monitored by galactose-1-phosphate levels, which should ideally be below $0.57\,\mu mol/g$ of haemoglobin ($30\,\mu g/ml$ of erythrocytes). This usually means the galactoside- and nucleoprotein-rich foods (Table 13.1) are permitted, and those containing only traces of lactose (Table 13.4) may be acceptable from school age onwards.

Although controlled study data on diet relaxation are not available, it is suggested that patients with classical galactosaemia should continue the lactose-free diet for life (Brandt 1980). Many patients have discomfort on lactose ingestion, though obvious symptoms may not always occur with dietary indiscretion. Patients with atypical galactosaemia may be able to have a less strict diet from two years of age (Brandt 1980). Parental support and encouragement with appropriate dietary advise is essential for all patients.

GALACTOKINASE DEFICIENCY

This is a much rarer disorder of galactose metabolism, in which galactokinase activity is deficient but galactose-1-phosphate uridyltransferase activity is normal (Fig. 13.1) (Nelson & Hsia 1967, Cook *et al.* 1971, Gitzelmann & Hansen 1980). The condition causes cateracts due to galactitol accumulation in the lens of the eye, but no hepatic disorder or mental retardation occurs (Gitzelmann & Hansen 1980). As the condition is asymptomatic in the newborn it is usually only diagnosed once cataracts are identified. Abnormal galactose tolerance results in a raised concentration of galactose and galactitol in blood and urine. Preliminary studies indicate that cataracts improve if treatment (with a low-galactose, low-lactose diet) is begun early in life, but less satisfactory results are obtained if the cataracts have become dense. Dietary treatment in the occasional case diagnosed in infancy results in normal progress. (Thalhammer *et al.* 1968, Gitzelmann & Hansen 1980) Dietary treatment must continue for life.

The mothers of children with cataracts in whom galactokinase and/or galactose-1-phosphate uridyltransferase in erythrocytes is reduced should be advised to avoid lactose and milk during subsequent pregnancies (Harley *et al.* 1974).

FRUCTOSE INTOLERANCE

Hereditary fructose intolerance is somewhat similar to galactosaemia in its manifestation, but in this case fructose is not metabolized normally (Cornblath & Schwartz 1976b, Baerlocher *et al.* 1980, Woods 1980). Fructose absorption and its formation from sucrose by intestinal sucrase is normal. Fructose is normally a major dietary component, accounting for approximately 30% carbohydrate intake after early infancy.

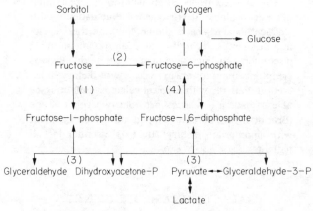

Enzymes involved:
  (1) Fructokinase
  (2) Hexokinase
  (3) Fructaldolase
  (4) Fructose-1,6-diphosphatase

Fig. 13.2 Schematic metabolism of fructose.

There are four enzymes involved in fructose metabolism (Fig. 13.2), i.e. hexokinase, fructokinase, fructaldolase and fructose-1, 6-diphosphatase. Deficiencies of the latter three have been described, however fructokinase deficiency, which gives rise to essential fructosuria, is a benign inborn error of metabolism which does *not* require dietary restriction although both fructosaemia and fructosuria occur. Many such patients are probably undetected in the community, and some are misdiagnosed as having diabetes mellitus.

Hereditary fructose intolerance

Hereditary fructose intolerance (HFI) is due to primary fructaldolase deficiency in which fructose-1-phosphate accumulates (Baerlocher *et al.* 1980). Symptoms occur with the ingestion of fructose (or sucrose), usually when foods such as fruit or sweetened cereals are introduced at weaning. Symptoms include sweating, trembling, nausea, vomiting, hypoglycaemia, unconsciousness and convulsions. The reaction is most severe in the young child and infant. Failure to thrive, poor feeding, diarrhoea, abdominal distension, jaundice and hepatomegaly occur, proceeding to liver failure and even death if fructose is not withdrawn. Self-selection of a fructose- and sucrose-free diet due to 'sweet' aversion is common. Fructosaemia, fructosuria and hypoglycaemia with symptoms of shock on ingestion of fructose are the most striking features. Diagnosis is by enzyme studies on a liver biopsy. The enzyme also occurs in the intestine and kidney (Baerlocher *et al.* 1980). A fructose load is dangerous and can even be fatal. Treatment must be started immediately and continued lifelong by total exclusion of fructose, sucrose, and possibly sorbitol, from the diet (*see later*, Table 13.5). Intravenous fructose is contraindicated. The dietary regimen causes almost immediate remission of symptoms, with the exception of the hepatomegaly which may take months to resolve (Baerlocher *et al.* 1980). Even small quantities of fructose in the diet can give chronic symptoms of failure to thrive, hypoglycaemia and liver disease.

Fructose-1, 6-diphosphatase deficiency

Fructose-1, 6-diphosphatase deficiency causes lactic acidosis (Baerlocher *et al.* 1980, Woods 1980). Symptoms include hypoglycaemia, hyperventilation, hepatomegaly, hypotomia, failure to thrive, vomiting and convulsions. Infants are most at risk and this diagnosis should be considered if lactic acidosis is present.

Patients with fructose-1, 6-diphosphatase deficiency do not appear to have the 'sweet' aversion commonly seen in patients with fructaldolase deficiency (HFI). Fasting, catabolism and infections, in fructose-1, 6-diphosphatase deficiency, cause hypoglycaemia and clinical deterioration, whereas in HFI fasting improves symptoms. Enzyme assay is possible. Glycogen is not metabolized normally and cannot be used to maintain glucose homeostasis. Treatment requires avoidance of fasts. During illness frequent glucose drinks with bicarbonate to correct acidosis should be administered, and fructose, sucrose, sorbitol and fat should be avoided.

Frequent carbohydrate intake is of primary importance to maintain normoglycaemia even when the child is well. A late night snack of starch-type carbohydrate (sucrose- and fructose-free) is advised, e.g. a cheese or ham sandwich with a glass of milk. However, adherence to a strict fructose-, sucrose-, sorbitol-free diet is unnecessary, though avoidance of *added* sugar, honey and fructose is recommended. Fruit is permitted in small quantities, as part of mixed meals, when the child is well. The total dietary carbohydrate should be high, possibly $\geqslant 65\%$ dietary energy, and fat intake slightly restricted to compensate.

Treatment is effective provided diagnosis is made early in life, although some irreversible damage may be present if the diagnosis is delayed (Cornblath & Schwartz 1976b, Baerlocher *et al.* 1980).

Patients with fructosaemia, probably largely due to dietary sucrose exclusion, have excellent teeth and few caries compared with their unaffected siblings (Cornblath & Schwartz 1976b).

Fructose-free diet

Fructose is the carbohydrate present in fruit and is sometimes referred to as fruit sugar or laevulose. It is present in invert sugar and is a component of sucrose, so this sugar in all its forms (cane, beet, brown, white, icing sugar and syrup) must be excluded from the diet as well as sources of fructose, including honey, all fruit, root vegetables, pulses and tomatoes. Sorbitol is also contraindicated.

Glucose sweets, liquid glucose and corn syrup solids may contain traces of sucrose; even some children's toothpastes contain sucrose. Dietetic and 'low-calorie' fruit squashes contain traces of fructose and sucrose from the natural fruit used in manufacture, and some diabetic products are sweetened with fructose or sorbitol, e.g. diabetic sweets and chocolate, fruit squashes.

Many manufactured products, including savoury foods such as sauces, soups, baby foods, salad creams and breakfast cereals, have added sugar as well as the obviously sweetened foods or those containing contraindicated ingredients, such as fruit, and therefore all such products must be continually scrutinized for suitability before use.

Bread, even unsweetened varieties, contains trace quantities of sugar used to start the yeast and may need to be limited or replaced with soda bread or bread made with a glucose starter. Potatoes contain traces of sucrose but this is reduced with storage.

All medicines in liquid form are likely to contain sucrose and/or sorbitol and must be replaced by alternatives; less commonly tablets may contain sucrose.

Glucose, glucose polymers, lactose, galactose, maltose, dextrin and starch are all suitable carbohydrates. Adequate carbohydrate intake is essential, especially in fructose-1, 6-diphosphatase deficiency, preferably as frequent glucose drinks, and/or starch-containing snacks.

A fructose-free diet is detailed in Table 13.5.

Sucrose-free ascorbic acid tablets (50 to 100 mg/day) are recommended, as this diet can be inadequate in this vitamin unless plenty of green vegetables are included.

GLUCOSE-6-PHOSPHATE DEHYDROGENASE DEFICIENCY: FAVISM

There is a wide spectrum of diseases associated with a deficiency of erythrocyte glucose-6-phosphate dehydrogenase (G-6-P-D). Favism occurs as a result of the deficiency of the B variant of the enzyme. An acute haemolytic anaemia is caused in susceptible individuals by eating *Vicia faba* beans (broad beans) or by inhaling their pollen. The patient becomes pale and may develop jaundice, haemoglobinuria and sometimes renal failure (Kattamis *et al.* 1976). Blood transfusions may be necessary, but recovery usually occurs.

It is well recognized throughout the Mediterranean area, particularly in southern Italy and Greece. It occurs in the relevant ethnic groups in the United Kingdom. The enzyme deficiency is a sex-linked gene and is fully expressed in males and in homozygous females. It is most commonly seen in children, and has even been reported in exclusively breast-fed infants whose mothers have eaten the 'fava' (broad) beans. The toxic agent in the beans is thought to be vicine or convicine, a pyrimidine glycoside (Mager *et al.* 1965). Oxidant drugs also precipitate haemolysis

Table 13.5 Fructose-free diet for treatment of hereditary fructose intolerance.

(a) Allowed and forbidden foods.

Foods allowed	Foods forbidden
Modified infant feeds without sugar/sucrose	Sweetened condensed milk
Milk, cheese, cream, butter, natural yoghurt	Infant feeds containing sucrose, e.g. Nutramigen, Wysoy
Unsweetened evaporated milk	and soya milks with sucrose
Coffee creamers, e.g. Coffee-mate	Sweetened milks and milk-shakes
Skimmed milks	Commercial ice-cream
Filled milks with non-milk fat	Fruit and flavoured yoghurts
Meat, fish, egg, offal, poultry, ham, bacon	Sugar brine tendersweet meats, e.g. ham
Tinned and frozen meat and fish provided only permitted	Meat and fish pastes
ingredients are included	Textured vegetable proteins
	Stews and casseroles containing ingredients such as
	carrots, peas, etc.
Cereals	Soya and soya flour
Wheat, rice, rye, barley, oats, sago, tapioca, flour,	Baby and breakfast cereals, e.g. Cornflakes, Rice Krispies,
semolina, pasta	muesli, Farley's and Liga low-sugar rusks
Baking powder	Sweetened custard and blancmange powders and pudding
Potato flour, cornflour, rice flour, custard powder	mixes
(unsweetened)	Baby foods unless ingredients are checked
Porridge oats, Ready Brek—plain (Lyons), Baby Rice	
(Robinsons or Milupa), Farex Weaning Cereal (Farley's),	
Aminex (Cow & Gate), Shredded Wheat	
Bread	Sweetened breads and buns
White, brown, wholemeal, unsweetened types, limit to 2	Cakes, biscuits and pastries
to 3 slices per day	
Cream and water cracker biscuits	
Crispbread, Ryvita, Vita-wheat	
Cakes and biscuits made with glucose replacing sucrose	
Glucose, glucose polymers, glucose drinks, e.g. Lucozade	Fructose, laevulose, fruit sugar, invert sugar, honey, sugar,
Lactose, galactose, starch, maltose and dextrins	syrup, jam, caramel, marmalade
Saccharin, aspartame, Nutrasweet, Canderel	Sorbitol, Sucron, sweetening agents containing sucrose
Sugar-free low-calorie fizzy drinks, e.g. Slimline, OneCal,	and/or sorbitol and/or fructose
Tab	Sweets, chocolate, nuts, candy, fizzy drinks, ice-lollies and
Tea, coffee, cocoa (unsweetened)	ice-cream unless home-made to suitable recipe
	Fruit juices and drinks, milk-shakes, chocolate beverages,
	lemon tea
	Diabetic and dietetic products including low-calorie
	squash, sweets, biscuits and fruits
	Glucose sweets
Potato—preferably stored for a week or two	All fruit
Chips, roast	Nuts
Crisps, plain or cheese flavouring	Root vegetables, tomato, pulses, e.g. peas, beans, lentils,
Asparagus, bamboo and bean shoots, courgettes,	sweetcorn and vegetables not listed as suitable
cauliflower, cabbage, celery, cress, chicory, French and	Tomato paste and purée
runner beans, broccoli, cucumber, lettuce, onion, spring	Baked beans
onion, green peppers, spring greens, marrow,	Tinned spaghetti and ravioli with tomato flavouring
mushroom, parsley, mint, sage, spinach, sprouts, pickled	
onions, garlic, radishes	

Table 13.5 (a) *continued*

Foods allowed	Foods forbidden
Butter, margarine, oils, lard, hard fats, suet	
Marmite, salt, pepper, herbs, mustard, chilli, pepper, curry powder	Bovril, Oxo, gravy browning, soups, sources, chutney, ketchup, soy sauce, salad creams, mayonnaise
Spices, essences, food colouring, oil and vinegar dressing	
Gelatine, rennet	Jelly
Tablet and capsule medicines known to be sucrose-free	Medicines sweetened with sucrose and/or sorbitol, i.e. all liquid medicines. Tablets containing sucrose are forbidden.
Processed, tinned and frozen foods containing only permitted ingredients. All products should be continually scrutinized for suitability.	Toothpaste containing sucrose
	Manufactured foods of unknown content or containing forbidden ingredients.

(b) Example of a minimal fructose diet.

All sugar should be avoided and unsweetened manufactured foods selected.

Breakfast	Porridge, plain Ready Brek, Shredded Wheat
	Milk (and glucose)
	Egg, bacon, ham, fish (optional)
	Bread/toast and butter, margarine
	Marmite
	Milk or tea, coffee, cocoa (no sugar)
Mid-morning	Milk, Lucozade, sugar-free drink
	Plain crisps
Lunch/supper	Meat, fish, liver, poultry, egg, cheese or meat dish containing only permitted ingredients, e.g. macaroni cheese, fish fingers
	Gravy or oil and vinegar dressing as appropriate
	Potatoes, chips, plain crisps, rice, pasta
	Permitted vegetables, e.g. cabbage/cauliflower/spinach
	Unsweetened milk pudding or natural yoghurt or sponge cake made with glucose and permitted ingredients
	Bread or crispbread/cream crackers and butter, margarine and cheese, Marmite
	Milk or tea, coffee, cocoa (no sugar)
Tea	Bread, crispbread, cream crackers and butter, margarine
	Cheese, Marmite, egg
	Plain crisps
	Home-made 'glucose biscuits'
	Milk and/or tea
Bedtime	Milk
	Cream crackers and cheese
Daily	50 to 100 mg ascorbic acid tablet (sucrose/fructose-free)

(Lunch/supper section note: Can be adapted to a packed sandwich lunch for school)

Footnote. Patients with fructose-1, 6-diphosphatase deficiency require frequent meals and glucose drinks and a less rigid fructose and sucrose exclusion (*see* text).

in these patients; more than 40 different drugs must be avoided, including analgesics, antipyretics, antimalarials and sulphonamides.

Treatment

The haemolysis is prevented by total exclusion of *Vicia faba* (broad) beans; both fresh and boiled dried beans should be omitted from the diet. Avoidance of the relevant drugs is also necessary.

In families with this trait the maternal diet during breast feeding should also exclude these items.

REFERENCES

BAERLOCHER K, GITZELMANN R & STEINMANN B (1980) In *Inherited disorders of Carbohydrate metabolism* (eds. Burman D., Holten J.B. & Pennock C.A.), pp. 163–90. Lancaster: MTP Press Ltd.

BICKEL H., BACHMANN C., BECKERS R., BRANDT N.J., CLAYTON B.E., CORRADO G. *et al.* (1981) Neonatal mass screening of metabolic disorders. *Europ. J. Paediat.* **137**, 133–9.

BRANDT N.J. (1980) How long should galactosaemia be treated? In *Inherited Disorders of Carbohydrate Metabolism* (eds. Burman D., Holten J.B. & Pennock C.A.), pp. 117–24. Lancaster: MTP Press Ltd.

BURMAN D., HOLTEN J.B. & PENNOCK C.A. (eds.) (1980) *Inherited Disorders of Carbohydrate Metabolism.* Monograph based upon proceedings of the 16th symposium of the Society for the Study of Inborn Errors of Metabolism. Lancaster: MTP Press Ltd.

CLAYTON B. & FRANCIS D.E.M. (1978) Inborn errors of metabolism in children. In *Nutrition in the Clinical Management of Disease* (eds. Dickerson J. & Lee H.), pp. 29–48. London: Edward Arnold.

CLOTHIER C.M. & DAVIDSON D.C. (1983) Galactosaemia workshop. *Hum. Nutr. appl. Nutr.* **37A**, 483–90.

COOK J.G.H., DON A. & MANN T.P. (1971) Hereditary galactokinase deficiency. *Arch. Dis. Childh.* **46**, 465–9.

CORNBLATH M. & SCHWARTZ R. (1976a) Hereditary galactose intolerance. In *Disorders of Carbohydrate Metabolism in Infancy* (Vol. III in the series *Major Problems in Clinical Paediatrics*), 2nd Edition (eds. Schaffer A. & Markowitz M.), pp. 294–321. Philadelphia: W.B. Saunders Co.

CORNBLATH M. & SCHWARTZ R. (1976b) Hereditary fructose intolerance. In *Disorders of Carbohydrate Metabolism in Infancy* (Vol. III in the series *Major Problems in Clinical Paediatrics*), 2nd Edition (eds Schaffer A. & Markowitz M.), pp. 322–42. Philadelphia: W.B. Saunders Co.

DHSS (1980) *Artificial Feeds for the Young Infant*, Report No. 18. London: HMSO.

DONNELL G.N. & BERGREN W.R. (1975) The galactosaemias. In *The Treatment of Inherited Metabolic Disease* (ed. Raine D.N.), pp. 91–114. Lancaster: MTP Press Ltd.

DONNELL G.N., KOCH R. & BERGREN W.R. (1969) Observations on results of management of galactosaemic patients.

In *Galactosaemia* (ed. Hsia D.Y.Y), p. 247. Springfield, Illinois: Thomas.

DONNELL G.N., KOCH R., FISHLER K. & NG W.G. (1980) Clinical aspects of galactosaemia. In *Inherited Disorders of Carbohydrate Metabolism* (eds. Burman D., Holten J.B. & Pennock C.A.), pp. 103–16. Lancaster: MTP Press Ltd.

EDITORIAL (1982) Clouds over galactosaemia. *Lancet* ii No. 8312, 1379.

FENSOM A.H., BENSON P.F., RODECK C.H., CAMPBELL S. & GOULD J.D.M. (1979) Prenatal diagnosis of a galactosaemia heterozygote by fetal blood enzyme assay. *Brit. med. J.* **i**, No. 6155, 21–2.

GARROD A.E. (1909) *Inborn Errors of Metabolism* (ed. Frowde H.). London: Hodder & Stoughton.

GITZELMANN R. (1980) Discussion. In *Inherited Disorders of Carbohydrate Metabolism* (eds. Burman D., Holten J.B. & Pennock C.A.), pp. 152–3. Lancaster: MTP Press: Ltd.

GITZELMANN R. & AURICCHIO S. (1965) The handling of soya or galactosides by a normal and galactosaemic child. *Pediatrics* **36**, 231.

GITZELMANN R. & HANSEN R.G. (1980) Galactose metabolism, hereditary defects and their clinical significance. In *Inherited Disorders of Carbohydrate Metabolism* (eds., Burman D., Holten J.B. & Pennock C.A.), pp. 61–102. Lancaster: MTP Press Ltd.

HARLEY J.D., MUTTON P., IRVING S. & GUPTA J.A. (1974) Maternal enzymes of galactose metabolism and the 'inexplicable' infantile cataract. *Lancet* **2**, 259.

HOLTEN J.B. & RAYMONT C.M. (1980) Prenatal diagnosis of classical galactosaemia. In *Inherited Disorders of Carbohydrate Metabolism* (eds Burman D., Holten J.B. & Pennock C.A.), pp. 141–8. Lancaster: MTP Press Ltd.

KATTAMIS C., KARAMBULA K., IOANNIDOU V. & HATZIKOO V. (1976) Jaundice and bilirubin levels in Greek children with favism. *Arch. Dis. Childh.* **51**, 233.

KINMOTH A.L. & BAUM J.D. (1982) Disorders of carbohydrate metabolism. In *Textbook of Paediatric Nutrition*, 2nd Edition (eds. McLaren D.S. & Burman D.), pp. 278–80. Edinburgh: Churchill Livingstone.

KOMROWER G.M. (1973) Treatment of galactosaemia. In *Treatment of Inborn Errors of Metabolism* (eds. Seakins J.W.T., Saunders R.A. & Toothill C.), pp. 113–20. Edinburgh: Churchill Livingstone.

KOMROWER G.M. (1982) Galactosaemia—thirty years on. The experience of a generation. F.P. Hudson memorial lecture. *J. inher. metab. Dis.* **5**, suppl. 2, 96–104.

KOMROWER G.M. & LEE D.H. (1970) Long term follow-up of galactosaemia. *Arch. Dis. Childh.* **45**, 241, 367–73.

LEVY H.L. (1980) Screening for galactosaemia. In *Inherited Disorders of Carbohydrate Metabolism* (eds. Burman D., Holten J.B. & Pennock C.A.), pp. 133–40. Lancaster: MTP Press Ltd.

MAGER J., GLASER G., RAZIN A., IZAK G., BIEN S. & HOAM M. (1965) Metabolic effects of pyrimidines derived from fava bean glycosides on human erthrocytes deficient in glucose-6-phosphate dehydrogenase. *Biochem. biophys. Res. Comm.* **20**, 235.

NADLER H.L., INOUYE T. & HSIA D.Y.Y. (1969) Clinical galactosaemia: a study of 55 cases. In *Galactosaemia* (ed. Hsia D.Y.Y.), p. 127. Springfield, Illinois: Thomas.

NELSON K. & HSIA D.Y.Y. (1967) Screening for galactosaemia and glucose-6-phosphate dehydrogenase deficiency in newborn infants. *J. Pediat.* **71**, No. 4, 582.

SALMAN TAJ EDIN (1971) Favism in breast fed infants. *Arch. Dis. Childh.* **46**, 121.

SARDHARWALLA I.B., KOMROWER G.M. & SCHWARTZ V. (1980) In *Inherited Disorders of Carbohydrate Metabolism* (eds. Burman D., Holten J.B. & Pennock C.A.), pp. 125–132. Lancaster: MTP Press Ltd.

SHIH V.E., LEVY H.L., KAROLKEWICZ V., HOUGHTON S., EFRON M.L., ISSELBACHER K.L., BEUTLER E. & MACCREADY R.A. (1971) Galactosaemia screening of newborns in Massachusetts. *New Engl. J. Med.* **284**, 753–7.

STANBURY J.B., WYNGAARDEN J.B., FREDRICKSON D.S., GOLDSTEIN J.L. & BROWN M.S. (eds.) (1983) *The metabolic Basis of Inherited Disease*, 5th Edition. New York: McGraw Hill.

THALHAMMER O., GITZELMANN R. & PANTLITSCHO M. (1968) Hypergalactosaemia and galactosuria due to galactokinase deficiency in a newborn. *Pediatrics* **42**, 441.

WHITEMAN P. (1983) Inborn lysosomal storage disorders affecting the nervous system. In *Clinical Neuropathology* (eds. Weller R.O., Swash M., McLellan D.L. & Schultz C.L.), p. 227. Berlin: Springer—Verlag.

WOODS H.F. (1980) In *Inherited disorders of carbohydrate metabolism* (eds. Burman D., Holten, J.B. & Pennock C.A.), pp. 191–204. Lancaster: MTP Press Ltd.

YU J.S. (1972) Screening tests for inborn errors of metabolism: special article. *Modern Medicine*, December, 753–8.

CHAPTER 14

Diets in various types of hypoglycaemia including glycogen storage disease, leucine-sensitive hypoglycaemia and ketotic hypoglycaemia

Hypoglycaemia is rare beyond the neonatal period, when it is particularly related to prematurity, low birth weight, and delayed feeding, and is also a feature of the infant who is born to a woman with diabetes mellitus. Early introduction of feeds, e.g. human milk soon after birth, usually prevents the problem. Other causes of dietetic interest include ketotic hypoglycaemia, leucine-sensitive hypoglycaemia, glycogen storage disease types I, III and VI (Cornblath & Schwartz, 1976, Hug 1980), galactosaemia and the fructosaemias (see Chapter 13), dumping syndrome following gastrectomy (Meyer et al, 1981), certain amino acid disorders and organic acidaemias related to branched-chain amino acid metabolism (see Chapter 10), in a rare systemic carnitine deficiency (Slonim et al. 1981), and hormone abnormalities such as Addison's disease and congenital adrenal hyperplasia and tumour of the pancreas. Secondary hypoglycaemia occurs in diabetes mellitus if inadequate carbohydrate is given to balance the administered insulin (see Chapter 5).

Hypoglycaemia can permanently damage the central nervous system, particularly in infants under six months, and therefore immediate steps must be taken to achieve normoglycaemia. The long-term growth failure associated with the hypoglycaemia of glycogen storage disease is largely overcome by continual carbohydrate administration aimed at maintaining normoglycaemia. Hypoglycaemia may be asymptomatic or associated with one or other of the following: listlessness, apathy, irritability, pallor, sweating, weakness, hunger, headache, visual disturbance, nausea, bizarre behaviour, mental confusion, convulsions and coma.

Frequent or continuous administration of carbohydrate intravenously or orally corrects hypoglycaemia. However, several secondary types of hypoglycaemia require specific dietary regimens, e.g. galactose-free diet in galactosaemia. Once hypoglycaemia is suspected and confirmed the cause should be sought, as the dietary regimens required to treat the primary condition vary considerably (Cornblath & Schwartz 1976, Burman et al. 1980).

Leucine-sensitive hypoglycaemia and amino acid disorders require a low-protein high-carbohydrate regime, avoiding 'fasts.'

In pancreatic tumour and type III glycogen storage disease, a high-protein diet to encourage gluconeogenesis is indicated.

Dumping syndrome requires a frequent feeding, low to normal carbohydrate regimen with a high fibre and protein content. In infancy thickening the feeds with Nestargel or Carobel (hemicellulose) can be useful.

Soya formulae which lack carnitine (Borum et al, 1979) are contraindicated in systemic carnitine deficiency, an inherited lipid-storage disease associated with hypoglycaemia, in which carnitine becomes an essential nutrient (Chapoy et al, 1980); indeed it may be an essential nutrient in newborns (Slonim et al, 1981).

GLYCOGEN STORAGE DISEASE TYPE I (GLUCOSE-6-PHOSPHATASE DEFICIENCY)

The diagnosis, manifestations and classification of the various glycogen storage diseases are fully described by Cornblath and Schwartz (1976), and Hug (1980) and Stanbury et al. (1983). A definite diagnosis is usually possible in most patients although the condition may not be readily recognized in infants, with the result that the diagnosis is delayed (Hufton & Wharton 1982).

Glycogen consists of glucose molecules linked together into a branched chain, and is the body's major carbohydrate reserve. Glycogen is synthesized in the liver from glucose. Plasma glucose normostasis is maintained by the release of glucose from the liver (Fig. 14.1) and is dependent on adequate glucose-6-phosphatase activity whether the glucose-6-phosphate is derived from glycogen degradation, or synthesized

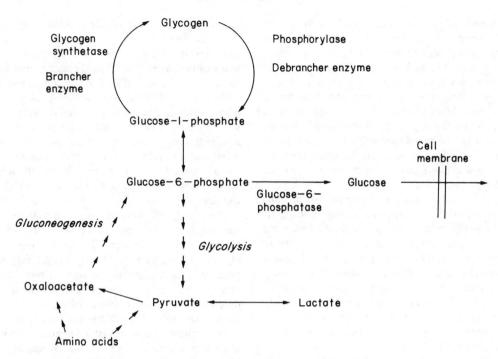

Fig. 14.1 Schematic glucose and glycogen metabolism in the liver. From Leonard *et al.* (1979).

from galactose, fructose, glycerol or amino acids (gluconeogenesis). Available glucose on a continuous basis, in amounts equal to that produced by the normal liver in the fasted state, is essential for the normal growth and development of human beings.

In glycogen storage disease type I there is a deficiency of glucose-6-phosphatase enzyme, and hypoglycaemia results unless blood glucose is maintained by a regular intake of dietary carbohydrate (Crigler & Folkman 1978). Growth retardation, hyperlipidaemia, and increased plasma uric acid occur (Crigler & Folkman 1978, Kinmonth & Baum 1982).

Management of type I glycogen storage disease is directed at maintaining the blood glucose within the normal range (4 to 6 mmol/l) throughout the 24 hours by regular carbohydrate administration. This largely corrects the secondary biochemical features of metabolic acidosis, hyperlipidaemia and raised uric acid levels and improves growth velocity (Leonard *et al*, 1979, Chen *et al.* 1984, Smit *et al*, 1984).

CARBOHYDRATE SUPPLEMENT

Continuous intravenous glucose effectively maintains normoglycaemia but is impractical for long-term treatment. Oral carbohydrate supplements such as glucose (or glucose polymers) are therefore prescribed

to provide 0·5 g carbohydrate/kg per hour in infancy, decreasing to 0·1 g carbohydrate/kg per hour by the teens in patients with type I glycogen storage disease. The prescribed carbohydrate is given as the calculated volume of a 15 to 25% solution of glucose polymer as appropriate for the child's age. Oral glucose supplements given as a continuous nasogastric feed provide optimal control and growth rate is normal. A more practical regimen is the use of overnight continuous nasogastric feed with one to two-hourly glucose drinks by day (Greene *et al.* 1976, Leonard *et al.* 1979). The latter is the author's regimen of choice, at least in the prepubertal patient with severe disease, and agrees with the recommendation of Smit *et al.* (1984).

Children adapt extremely well to overnight continuous nasogastric drip-feeding regimen. The volume of feed must be controlled accurately by a (paediatric) enteral pump, and great care must be taken to avoid accidental withdrawal of the continuous carbohydrate intake, e.g. by tube displacement, power failure, leaks at the connecting site of the nasogastric tubing, etc., as these patients become very carbohydrate-dependent and severe symptoms of hypoglycaemia may occur at blood glucose concentrations which have previously been well-tolerated (Leonard & Dunger 1978).

Parents need precise and careful teaching. An initial demonstration, followed by supervision in passing the nasogastric tube, using the equipment and preparing the feed, is essential. A number of children from school age onwards learn to pass their own nasogastric tube. An alarm watch is useful to remind the children when the next oral drink is needed during the day, and a 'baby alarm' between the child's bedroom and parents', allows them to listen for the child at night. Extra carbohydrate is recommended before games, as exercise increases the risk of hypoglycaemia.

Hypoglycaemia is often asymptomatic in patients with untreated type I glycogen storage disease, as hypoglycaemia adaptation is acquired. Treatment with continuous glucose may restore sensitivity to hypoglycaemia. If the supply of exogenous glucose is interrupted severe symptomatic hypoglycaemia may develop with potentially fatal consequences (Leonard & Dunger 1978). A moderate hyperlacticacidaemia should be maintained, as lactate appears to be a fuel for the brain, as is glucose (Fernandes *et al.* 1984), and may suppress this effect.

In patients in whom nasogastric continuous feeds are not practical, glucose drinks given one- to two-hourly by day and two- to three-hourly nocturnally can be used, but this is very demanding on the patient and his family.

A mixed meal with starch as the primary carbohydrate is preferable if the interval between feeds is extended even to two or three hours because of the slower absorption rate (Fernandes *et al.* 1979). Adequate carbohydrate must be given to maintain normal blood glucose levels and prevent excess lactate accumulation. The diet prescription and time schedule is adjusted according to serial blood glucose levels. Bicarbonate supplements may be required initially and during illness to correct metabolic acidosis.

Recently the effect of ingested uncooked cornstarch (2 g/kg body weight) in water has been studied in patients with glycogen storage disease type I and compared with uncooked starch (1 g/kg) added to a meal and thirdly glucose (2 g/kg) in water (Smit *et al.* 1984). Blood glucose levels remained in the normal range during approximately 6·5 to 9 hours, 3·5 to 6·5 hours, and 2·25 to 4 hours, respectively, during the three tolerance tests. Post-prandial blood glucose and insulin peak levels after starch administration were markedly lower than those after glucose. Different patients gave variable responses of blood lactate concentration with starch ingestion. The effect of various starches differed according to their physical state (size of granules, presence of fibre, gelatinizing due to cooking). The best results have been obtained with uncooked cornstarch mixed with tap water at room temperature. Smit *et al.* (1984) suggest than an optimal dose of 1 to 2 g/kg body weight given twice daily, at the end of the nocturnal continuous glucose administration and at lunch, would permit a less strict regimen of glucose ingestion by day. Due to the insulinogenic effect of mono- and disaccharides when given with the uncooked cornstarch, and their effect on the steady state of blood glucose induced by starch, these sugars should be avoided or limited in the diet.

Chen *et al.* (1984) have suggested that uncooked cornstarch can be used as an alternative effective therapy, except in infants. They recommend a dose of 1·75 to 2·5 g/kg of ideal body weight, which can produce a relatively constant state of normoglycaemia for as long as six hours in most patients. The dose needed by each patient must be assessed individually. The side-effects of the uncooked cornstarch were minimal and transient (diarrhoea, abdominal distension and flatulence). Cornstarch was less effective if given when the blood glucose concentration was low.

Pancreatic amylase and intestinal glucoamylase are required to hydrolyse starch. By the age of one month glucoamylase and disaccharidase levels are similar to those of adults. However, the pancreatic amylase necessary to digest raw starch is negligible in the newborn and only reaches adult levels at 2 to 4 years of age, but it can be induced by starch feeding (Chen *et al.* 1984). The latter concluded that, at least in infants, continuous glucose, by nocturnal infusion and frequent feeds, is the therapy of choice. For the majority of young children the author would agree with Smit *et al.* (1984) that it is wise to postpone the uncooked cornstarch regimen until the pubertal growth spurt of the child has been completed. However, such a regimen has many advantages for teenagers who wish to be weaned off nocturnal continuous drip-feeds, or for those in whom such a regimen is impractical.

During intercurrent infections continuous glucose must be maintained either orally, as a continuous nasogastric feed of glucose or glucose polymer, or from intravenous glucose. Fasts must be avoided. Infections should be treated rigorously and acid–base disturbances corrected.

As galactose and fructose cannot be converted to glucose they are metabolized to lactate (Fernandes 1975), thus increasing the risk of metabolic acidosis; however, mild hyperlacticacidaemia is advantageous, as discussed above. Large quantities of lactose and sucrose, from which galactose and fructose are most commonly derived, should be avoided in young children (Table 14·1). The continuous supply of carbohydrate, however, largely eliminates the need for strict diet, and thus only the avoidance of milk to drink and added sugar is required, except in infants, or if continuous carbohydrate is not possible. Sorbitol,

Table 14.1 Glycogen storage disease type I: dietary regimen for a young child.

(a) *0·5 g carbohydrate/kg per h should be prescribed in one- to two-hourly drinks by day and as an overnight continuous nasogastric drip feed.

(b) In infancy and if continuous carbohydrate is not possible a reduction of dietary galactose, fructose, lactose and sucrose, and avoidance of sorbitol, is advised. The diet can be based on the minimal lactose and sucrose diet (Table 1.9) with the following modifications:

(i)   The milk substitute selected should contain glucose, glucose polymer or starch as carbohydrate, e.g. S Formula (Cow & Gate), and Prosobee (Mead Johnson) are suitable.
Contraindicated
Lactase-treated milks, e.g. Digestelact (Sharpe).
Soya milks with sucrose, e.g. Wysoy, Granolac Infant.

(ii)   Vegetable oils and PUFA margarine are preferable to saturated fats.

(iii)   Honey contains large quantities of fructose and should be avoided.

(iv)   Avoid diabetic products containing fructose or sorbitol, including artificial sweeteners and diabetic chocolate.

(v)   Fruit contains fructose, but small to normal quantities (without added sugar) can be included in the diet from the age of weaning.

(vi)   Vegetables are permitted and the range increased from the toddler age onwards to include all vegetables.

(vii)   Cereals without added sugar can be included, e.g. Cornflakes, muesli, Shreddies, Weetabix, Farex weaning cereal.

(viii)   Hard cheeses and PUFA margarines and butter are permitted.

(ix)   Medicine containing sorbitol, lactose or sucrose should be replaced with carbohydrate-free alternatives as, particularly during intercurrent infections, metabolic acidosis can occur which is exacerbated by galactose and fructose.

*Decreases with age: see text.

which is contraindicated in patients with liver disease, should also be avoided.

A diet in which polyunsaturated fat largely replaces ordinary fat has been suggested (Fernandes 1975) to improve the hyperlipidaemia associated with glycogen storage disease type I, but this is less important than a continuous glucose intake (to maintain glucose homeostasis) which improves the blood lipid picture (Leonard *et al.* 1979).

In addition to the carbohydrate supplement the child is permitted to eat to appetite. The diet should contain the child's normal requirement of energy, protein and other nutrients for growth needs. Excess energy intake leads to increased glycogen accumulation and obesity, when general advice regarding the energy intake of the diet should be given appropriately. Inadequate energy intake will inhibit growth. In the latter case, a dietary supplement, milk substitute or enteral feed (lactose- and sucrose-free) can be given simultaneously with the prescribed carbohydrate supplements in drinks or in the nocturnal continuous nasogastric feed. For example, in infants a regimen based on Cow & Gate S formula can be devised (Table 14·2).

Careful dietary management with continuous carbohydrate intake improves all metabolic parameters, including linear growth. Catch-up growth has occurred even in older previously untreated children. Hepatic adenomas and hepatic carcinomas have developed in some older patients (Howell *et al*, 1976, Miller *et al*, 1978). Treatment may cause pre-existing lesions to regress and prevent new tumours developing (Roe *et al*, 1979).

GLYCOGEN STORAGE DISEASE TYPES III AND VI AND DEBRANCHER ENZYME DEFICIENCY

These types of glycogen storage disease cause milder clinical pictures compared to type I, but hypoglycaemia, growth failure, hepatomegaly and hyperlipidaemia occur. Glucose cannot be released by breakdown of glycogen, and hypoglycaemia is associated particularly with starvation. Plasma glucose levels can be maintained by utilizing other pathways. Amino acids, galactose and fructose are all metabolized normally to release glucose from the liver. All dietary carbohydrates are suitable, especially starch because of the slower absorption rate. A high-protein diet, with frequent meals and/or drinks to avoid fasts, is indicated to maintain normal blood glucose levels (Fernandes 1975, Aynsley-Green *et al.* 1977). The protein intake

Table 14.2   Examples of suitable feeding regime for an infant with glycogen storage disease type I.

	Energy		Carbohydrate (g)	Protein (g)	Fat (g)
	kJ	kcal			
Based on 100 ml S Formula Soya* (normal 12·7% dilution)	280	67	6·7	1·8	3·6
Aim for 0·5 g carbohydrate/kg per h					
(A) 3·5 kg infant requires 170 ml/kg per day					
600 ml S Formula, normal dilution	1680	402	40·2	10·8	21·6
Divide into 24 hourly feeds of 25 ml orally and/or by continuous nasogastric drip					
This provides (per kg)	480	115	11·5 (=0·5 g/kg per h)	3·1	6·2

(B)   7 kg infant with some weaning solids and feeds to
     provide 0·5 g carbohydrate/kg per h

8 a.m.	Farex weaning cereal (no added sugar) S Formula, normal dilution	Offer average serve and feed to appetite
10 a.m.	50 ml 15% solution glucose polymer	= 3·75 g carbohydrate (0·5 g/kg per h)
12 noon	Mince meat and gravy Milk-free potato Green vegetables, cauliflower or other vegetable	May be puréed. Offer an average serve and serve to appetite
2 p.m.	100 ml S Formula, normal dilution	= 3·35 g carbohydrate (0·5 g/kg per h)
4 p.m.	50 ml 15% solution glucose polymer	= 3·75 g carbohydrate (0·5 g/kg per h)
6 p.m.	Egg, boiled poached or scrambled (no milk) Bread and margarine and/or S Formula Custard sweetened with glucose	Offer an average serve, and feed to appetite

		Energy		Carbohydrate (g)	Protein (g)	Fat (g)
7 p.m. to 8 a.m.	Overnight nasogastric continuous drip feed, i.e. 13 hours					
	41 g S Formula Powder	910	218	21·8	5·9	11·7
	22 g glucose polymer	352	88	22		
	Water to 325 ml					
	Divide into hourly feeds of 25 ml by continuous drip					
	Total	1262	306	43·8	5·9	11·7
	Overnight feed = 3·5 g/h			= 3·4 g/h = 0·5 g/kg per h		

* New formula 1986.

may need to be as high as twice the normal intake for age. A moderate carbohydrate and normal energy intake is indicated. A snack containing both starch and a high-protein intake last thing at night usually avoids the necessity for frequent feeds during the night. The effect of the diet on blood glucose and secondary metabolic abnormalities should be monitored, and the diet and meal frequency adjusted accordingly. Continuous or very frequent glucose drinks are rarely necessary. The patient can have normal meals without restriction, but the fat intake should preferably be of polyunsaturated type. The differences in the dietary regimens used in hepatic glycogen storage disease are summarized in Table 14·3.

Good dietetic control of blood sugars improves growth and well-being. The outlook for physical and mental development has now improved in all forms of hepatic glycogen storage disease.

LEUCINE-SENSITIVE HYPOGLYCAEMIA

This condition is now thought to be very rare, and leucine sensitivity may be a mode of presentation of an islet-cell adenoma or mesidioblastosis, rather than a separate metabolic disorder (Kinmonth & Baum 1982).

Leucine, and in some patients isoleucine, causes a marked fall in blood sugars in certain infants and young children (Cornblath & Schwartz 1976). Characteristically the onset of hypoglycaemia occurs early in the first year of life, although diagnosis may be delayed, with subsequent mental retardation and neurological symptoms. Symptoms frequently occur

after a high-protein feed or meal, or after fasting, possibly due to endogenous leucine accumulation. Leucine metabolism is normal although there is excess insulin production.

Treatment of the hypoglycaemia requires immediate administration of glucose for brain metabolism either orally or intravenously; adrenaline or glucagon may be used to release glucose from glycogen. Longer term treatment in patients in whom there is no diagnosable primary cause is with a low-protein, low-leucine, high-carbohydrate diet (Roth & Segal 1964), avoiding long fasts. Drugs, e.g. diazoxide, with or without diet, may be effective in controlling the hypoglycaemia. The length of time that treatment is required is unknown, although the severity tends to decrease with age, often subsiding by 4 to 6 years of age (Cornblath & Schwartz 1976).

Dietary treatment of leucine-sensitive hypoglycaemia necessitates a moderate restriction of leucine by selection of a suitable modified infant formula with a low protein content, counterbalanced by increased carbohydrate or a low-protein high-carbohydrate diet in children (*see* Chapter 8 for low-protein diets), to give adequate blood sugar control. Supplementary leucine-free amino acids are usually unnecessary. Symptoms of hypoglycaemia can be corrected with oral glucose and prevented by a frequent feeding schedule. Parents are taught to observe the early symtoms of hypoglycaemia and to take the necessary action. Severe hypoglycaemia requires intravenous glucose and/or glucagon.

Leucine is an essential amino acid and the requirement should be supplied by natural protein. Table 10·10 gives details of the leucine content of

Table 14.3 Summary of diets required in hepatic glycogen storage disease.

	Type I (glucose-6-phosphatase deficiency)	Types III and VI, debrancher enzyme deficiency
Carbohydrate	Glucose, glucose polymers and starch to provide 50 to 70% energy Limit galactose, fructose, lactose and sucrose in young children Avoid sorbitol	All carbohydrates are suitable, especially starch
Protein	Normal intake for age	High protein intake up to twice normal intake for age
Fat	Preferably polyunsaturated type	Preferably polyunsaturated type
Frequency	Young children—overnight glucose as continuous nasogastric drip and one- to two-hourly drinks by day Children and teenagers—uncooked cornstarch	Late-night protein-rich carbohydrate supper or overnight drinks Frequent meals and drinks

Table 14.4   Examples of low-leucine high-carbohydrate feeds.

	Leucine (mg)	Protein (g)	Carbohydrate (g)	kJ	kcal
1 13 g SMA powder*	166	1·5	7·2	275	65
5 g glucose polymer			5·0	80	20
Water to > 100 ml					
Total	166	1·5	12·2	355	85

Approximately 13·6 mg leucine to each 1 g
   carbohydrate

	Leucine (mg)	Protein (g)	Carbohydrate (g)	kJ	kcal
2 13 g Aptamil Powder*	156	1·5	7·2	273	65
24 g glucose polymer			24·0	384	96
Water to (a) 150 ml total volume					
200 ml total volume					
Total	156	105	31·2	657	161
(a) Each 100 ml (diluted to 150 ml)	104	1·0	21·0	438	107
(b) Each 100 ml (diluted to 200ml)	78	0·75	15·8	328	80

Approximately 5 mg leucine to each 1 g
   carbohydrate

	Leucine (mg)	Protein (g)	Carbohydrate (g)	kJ	kcal
3 12·5 g Premium*	123	1·5	7·2	284	68
20 g glucose polymer			20·0	320	80
Water to 150 ml					
Total	123	1·5	27°2	604	148
Each 100 ml	82	1·0	18°0	403	100

Approximately 4·6 mg leucine to each 1 g
   carbohydrate

	Leucine (mg)	Protein (g)	Carbohydrate (g)	kJ	kcal
4 1 g MSUD Aid	Nil	1·0 amino acids	Nil	17	4
Isoleucine and valine as required					
0·3 g Metabolic/Aminogran Mineral Mixture					
65 ml Premium, normal dilution	80	1·0	4·9	185	44
10 g glucose polymer			10·0	160	40
Water to > 100 ml					
Total	80	2·0	14·9	362	88

Approximately 5·4 mg leucine to each 1 g
   carbohydrate

*Equivalent to 100 ml nomal dilution.
An appropriate volume per kg per day should be given to provide dietary requirements.
Supplements of 6–12 Cow & Gate Supplementary Vitamin Tablets plus 5 ml Ketovite Liquid are recommended.

different foods. In infants the requirement of leucine varies from 76 to 229 mg leucine per kg actual weight per day, although most infants do not require more than 150 mg/kg per day (Holt 1967). The requirement decreases with age and varies from one individual to another. The leucine intake, if severely restricted, must be monitored by frequent blood leucine determinations to avoid deficiency, and the diet constructed using the principles for amino acid-restricted diets in Chapter 10. Supplementary leucine-free amino acids, vitamins and minerals may be ad-vised in order to ensure adequate growth. MSUD Aid, an amino acid mixture free of leucine, isoleucine and valine, can be utilized with supplements of valine and isoleucine as necessary.

Carbohydrate is given with the feeds and/or two hours after meals, when the lowest blood sugars are predicted. Protein, leucine and carbohydrate should be distributed between the meals, and long fasts (even overnight) should be avoided. The regimen is assessed by measuring blood sugars throughout the 24 hours, and adjustments to the diet are made as appropriate.

In extreme cases as much as 1 g carbohydrate for each 5 mg leucine may be necessary to prevent hypoglycaemia. Some infants and young children require either evenly divided feeds, e.g. four-hourly × 6 feeds daily, or carbohydrate boosts during the night or a sugary drink at bedtime and on waking. Example feeds are given in Table 14·4. Refused foods and meals should be replaced with a carbohydrate-containing drink. During illness drinks of 15 to 20% solution of glucose polymer should be offered at frequent intervals.

KETOTIC HYPOGLYCAEMIA

Previously included in the syndrome of cyclic vomiting, ketotic hypoglycaemia usually presents during the later half of the first year or in the toddler age group, and is characterized by good health between episodes and control of symptoms with diet alone. Symptoms most frequently occur in the early morning or following prolonged food deprivation (Cornblath & Schwartz 1976), with increased blood ketones and a reduction in blood alanine (Kinmonth & Baum 1982).

This type of hypoglycaemia occurs more frequently in males, and the child may be underweight for height. Symptoms, which include apathy, listlessness, convulsion and coma, are usually transient and clear spontaneously with food. At the time of hypoglycaemia the urine contains ketones (Cornblath & Schwartz 1976). A diagnostic test using a ketogenic diet or fat-loading test is described in Chapter 15.

Therapy is to give glucose either orally or intravenously at the first symptoms of hypoglycaemia. Long-term treatment is to increase dietary carbohydrate intake. Relatively frequent meals spaced throughout the day are recommended, including snacks and carbohydrate drinks on waking and at bedtime, so as to avoid long fasts. Uneaten meals should be replaced with a carbohydrate drink; sodium bicarbonate may be advantageous in conjunction with carbohydrate. This type of hypoglycaemia tends to disappear by mid-childhood (Cornblath & Schwartz 1976). In the past a reduction in fat intake was advised, though this is probably unnecessary (Pagliara *et al*, 1973), apart from the necessity to counterbalance the increased energy intake from the extra carbohydrate recommended.

Ketotic hypoglycaemia should be managed as follows:

(i) Encourage carbohydrate-rich meals and snacks at relatively frequent intervals.

(ii) Avoid excess fried and fatty foods, visible fat, oil, cream. Use butter/margarine sparingly.

(iii) Replace refused meals with a drink containing carbohydrate, e.g. 20 g carbohydrate in toddlers, increasing to 40 to 50 g carbohydrate at five years of age. Some drinks containing 20 g carbohydrate are listed in Table 14·5. Sodium bicarbonate, if necessary, may be prescribed or given less formally with carbohydrate as Lucozade, soda water, Coke, etc.

(iv) When the child is unwell and not eating, two- to three-hourly carbohydrate drinks, as outlined in Table 14·5, should be given throughout the 24 hours to avoid long fasts. Fruit juice or additional drinks may be given in addition to prevent thirst.

(v) The parents can be taught to test the urine for ketones, and sodium bicarbonate can be prescribed as necessary, together with carbohydrate-containing drinks as described above.

Table 14.5 Drinks containing 20 g carbohydrate.

(a)	20 g glucose polymer, sugar or glucose. Add flavouring and water to at least 100 ml (3½ oz).
(b)	20 g glucose polymer, glucose or sugar or 28 g honey. Dissolve in 1 glass soda water.
(c)	100 ml (3½ oz) CocaCola (sweetened) plus 10 g glucose polymer, sugar or glucose.
(d)	120 ml Lucozade.
(e)	180 ml Lemonade plus 10 g glucose polymer, glucose or sugar.
(f)	120 ml orange juice plus 10 g glucose polymer, glucose or sugar.

REFERENCES

AYNSLEY-GREEN A., WILLIAMSON D.H. & GITZELMAN R. (1977) The dietary treatment of hepatic glycogen synthetase deficiency. *Helvet. paediat, Acta* **32**, 71.

BORUM P.R., YORK C.M. & BROQUIST H.P. (1979) Carnitine content of liquid formula, and special diets. *Amer. J. clin. Nutr.* **32**, 2272.

BURMAN D., HOLTON J.B. & PENNOCK C.A. (1980) *Inherited Disorders of Carbohydrate Metabolism.* Lancaster: MTP Press Ltd.

CHAPOY P.R., ANGELINI C., BROWN W.J., STIFF J.E., SHUG A.L. & CADERBAUN S.D. (1980) Systemic carnitine deficiency—a treatable inherited lipid-storage disease presenting as Reye's syndrome. *New Engl. J. Med.* **303**, 1389.

CHEN Y.T., CORNBLATH M. & SIDBURY J.B. (1984) Cornstarch

therapy in type I glycogen-storage disease. *New Engl. J. Med.* Vol. **310**, No. 3, 171–5.

CORNBLATH M, & SCHWARTZ R (1976) In *Disorders of Carbohydrate Metabolism in Infancy* (Vol. III in the series *Major Problems of Clinic Paediatrics*), 2nd Edition (ed. Schaffer A.I.), pp. 231–93. Philadelphia: W.B. Saunders.

CRIGLER J.F. & FOLKMAN J (1978) Glycogen storage disease: new approaches to therapy. *Hepatotrophic Factors, CIBA Foundation Symposium, No.55* (new series) Amsterdam: North Holland, Elsevier, Exerpta Medica.

FERNANDES J.L. (1975) Hepatic glycogen storage disease. In *The Treatment of Metabolic Disease* (ed. Raine D.N.), pp. 115–49. Lancaster: MTP Press Ltd.

FERNANDES J.L., JANSEN H. & JANSEN T.C. (1979) Nocturnal gastric drip feeding glucose-6-phosphatase deficient children. *Paediat. Res.* **13**, (4 Pt 1) 225–9.

FERNANDES J., BERGER R. & SMIT G.P.A. (1984) Lactate as a cerebral metabolic fuel for glucose-6-phosphatase deficient children. *Paediat. Res.* **18**, 335.

GREENE H.L., SLONIM A.E., O'NEILL J.A. JR & BURR J.M. (1976) Continuous nocturnal intragastric feeding for management of type I glycogen storage disease. *New Engl. J. Med.* **294**, 1125, 423–5.

HOLT L.E. JR (1967) Amino-acid requirements of infants. *Curr. ther. Res.* **9**, Suppl. 149–56.

HOWELL R.R., STEVENSON R.E., BEN-MENACHEM Y., PHYLIKY R.L. & BERRY D.H. (1976) Hepatic adenomata with type I glycogen storage disease. *J. Amer. med. Ass.* **236**, 1481.

HUFTON B.R. & WHARTON B.A. (1982) Glycogen storage disease (type I) presenting in the neonatal period. *Arch. Dis. Childh.* **57**, 309–19.

HUG G. (1980) Pre and post natal diagnosis of glycogen storage disease. In *Inherited Disorders of Carbohydrate Metabolism* (eds. Burman D. Holton J.B. & Pennock C.A.), pp. 327–67. Lancaster: MTP Press Ltd.

KINMONTH A.L. & BAUM J.D. (1982) Disorders of carbohydrate metabolism. In *Paediatric Nutrition*, 2nd Edition (eds. McLaren D. & Burman D.), pp. 281–3 Edinburgh: Churchill Livingstone.

LEONARD J.V. & DUNGER D.B. (1978) Hypoglycaemia complicating feeding regimes for glycogen-storage disease. *Lancet* **2**, 1203–4.

LEONARD J.V., FRANCIS D.E.M. & DUNGER D.B. (1979) The dietary management of hepatic glycogen storage disease. *Proc. Nutr. Soc.* **38**, 321–4.

MEYER S., DECKELBAUM R.J., LAX E. & SCHILLER M. (1981) Infant dumping syndrome after gastroesophageal reflux surgery. *J. Pediat.* Vol. **99**, No. 2, 235–7.

MILLER J.H., GATES G.F., LANDING B.H., KOGUT M.D. & ROE T.F. (1978) Scintigraphic abnormalities in glycogen storage disease. *J. nucl. Med.* **19**(4) 354–8.

PAGLIARA A.S., KARL I.E., HAYMOND M. & KIPNIS D.M. (1973) Hypoglycaemia in infancy and childhood. *J. Pediat.* Parts I and II. **82**, 365–558.

ROE T.F., KOGUT M.D., BUCKINGHAM B.A., MILLER J.H. & GATES G.F. (1979) Esophageal motility and gastric emptying in infants with rumination syndrome. *Pediat. Res.* **13**, 481.

ROTH H. & SEGAL S. (1964) The dietary management of leucine-sensitive hypoglycaemia, with report of a case. *Paediatrics* **34**, 831–8.

SLONIM A.E., BORUM P.R., TANAKA K. *et al.* (1981) Dietary-dependent carnitine deficiency as a cause of non-ketotic hypoglycaemia in an infant. *J. Pediat.* Vol. **99**, No 4, 551–6.

SMIT G.P.A., BERGER R., POTASNICK R., MOSES S.W. & FERNANDES J. (1984) The treatment of children with type I glycogen storage disease with slow release carbohydrate. *Pediat. Res.* Vol. **18**, No. 9, 879–81.

STANBURY J.B., WYNGAARDEN J.B., FREDRICKSON D.S., GOLDSTEIN J.L. & BROWN M.S. (eds.) (1983) *The Metabolic Basis of Inherited Disease*, 5th Edition. New York: McGraw-Hill.

CHAPTER 15

Diets for special tests

Apart from balance studies (Chapter 16) and a diet with a constant intake of one or more nutrients, some other investigatory tests require dietary involvement. Details of the test and diet required should be confirmed with the laboratory concerned with the investigation.

FAT LOAD FOR LIPID STUDIES, ABSORPTION TESTS AND CHOLECYSTOGRAMS

The appropriate quantity of fat for the age of the child must be given after an overnight fast, e.g. 1 g fat/kg actual weight. The type of fat may be significant and normally medium-chain triglyceride (MCT) is inappropriate. Carbohydrate and protein are not normally contraindicated. The appropriate volume of one or of a combination of the following is given according to the child's weight:

30 ml cow's milk	
1 ml vegetable oil	Each = 1 g fat
2 ml Prosparol or Calogen	
2 ml double cream	

Additional fluid or carbohydrate can be added. For example, a 10 kg child could be offered:

(a) 300 ml cow's milk *or*
(b) 90 ml cow's milk plus
14 ml double cream, Prosparol or Calogen *or*
(c) 10 ml vegetable oil

Table 15.1 Fatty meal given as fluid for a school-age child.

	Carbo-hydrate (g)	Protein (g)	Fat (g)
100 ml cow's milk (full-fat)	4·7	3·3	3·8
100 ml double cream	2·0	1·5	48·2
20 g skimmed milk powder	10·6	7·3	0·3
Sugar and flavouring	*		
Water to ⩾ 200 ml			
Total	17·3	12·1	52·3

* Additional fluid and carbohydrate may be added.

Cholecystogram studies are rarely performed in children. A fatty meal may be required to stimulate bile salt release. A fatty meal for a school-age child is given in Table 15.1.

TEST DIET FOR THE DIAGNOSIS OF KETOTIC HYPOGLYCAEMIA

This diet is used as a means of detecting patients with ketotic hypoglycaemia (Cornblath & Schwartz 1976) and is not to be confused with the ketogenic diet used for the treatment of epilepsy (*see* Chapter 11). An adequate normal diet containing at least 50% energy from carbohydrate is necessary for several days prior to this test.

The ketogenic test diet is made up of 66% energy from fat, 16% energy from carbohydrate and 17% energy from protein, i.e. each 1000 kJ is made up of 18 g fat, 10 g carbohydrate and 10 g protein. (Each 100 kcal is made up of 7·5 g fat, 4 g carbohydrate and 4 g protein.)

A normal energy intake for age is offered. The diet is only continued until ketosis and/or hypoglycaemia is detected, either clinically, or biochemically by urine and blood level findings for ketones, acidosis and blood glucose. The diet is continued for a maximum of three days and may be started after a 12-hour overnight fast. However, the latter often means that ketosis and hypoglycaemia occur during the second night, and therefore to avoid this the diet can be started as an overnight tube feed, after a day's normal meals, in order to precipitate ketosis and symptoms during the following day. The fluid regimen suggested in Table 15.2 is a convenient means of providing such a test diet. An appropriate volume for energy requirement should be given as bolus feeds two- to three-hourly throughout the test period.

In infants the larger volume of fluid should be used, and for children the smaller volume is more appropriate. Alternatively, the prescribed fat, protein and carbohydrate can be given from a variety of foods.

Table 15.2   Example test diet for detection of ketotic hypoglycaemia.

Each 1000 kJ, 240 kcal, is divided into:
    66% energy as fat = 18 g fat.
    17% energy as protein = 10 g protein.
    16% energy as carbohydrate = 10 g carbohydrate.

	Energy		Carbo-hydrate (g)	Protein (g)	Fat (g)
	kJ	kcal			
36 ml Calogen, double cream or Prosparol	660	162	Trace	0 to 1	18
10 g Casilan or Maxipro HBV	154	36	Trace	9	Trace
10 g sugar, glucose polymer or Nesquik	160	40	10	0	0
Water, 240 to 360 ml					
Total	980	238	10	9 to 10	18

Give an appropriate volume to provide energy needs as two- to three-hourly bolus feeds.

PROTEIN STRESS TEST

An oral load of protein, followed by estimation of plasma levels of amino acids and their metabolites, will help detect abnormalities of amino acid metabolism or transport in parents and siblings of patients. It is also used as a stress test to detect abnormalities of the urea cycle. For this purpose the amount of carbohydrate and fat should be kept to a minimum to prevent any stimulation of insulin, which would increase tissue uptake of amino acids and protein synthesis. Rossiter *et al.* (1974) showed that the levels of amino acids and urea are higher in children following a casein load (minimal carbohydrate and fat) than after an equivalent protein intake from milk. The absence of carbohydrate increases the utilization of amino acids by the liver for gluconeogenesis, thereby diverting the amine group via glutamic acid to the urea cycle for conversion into urea.

After an overnight fast in children and adults, or a six hour fast in infants, protein is given as Casilan (90% calcium caseinate) or Maxipro HBV (88% whey protein) or, where permitted, from a variety of other foods to provide:

    Infants 1·2 g protein/kg actual weight.
    Adults 0·65 to 0·85 g protein/kg weight or an average of 50 g protein.
    Children approximately 1 g protein/kg weight.

Sufficient water is given to dilute the Casilan or Maxipro HBV to at least a 10% solution in infants, and a 15 to 20% solution in older children (Table 15.3). A suitable flavouring, e.g. low-calorie dietetic squash, decaffeinated coffee, or food flavourings such as almond or peppermint essence, may be added, provided their ingredients will not interfere with the biochemical analysis (caffeine, vanilla, sorbitol, fructose and aspartame may be contraindicated). Additional water is given throughout the test to maintain an adequate urine flow.

Baseline blood and urine samples are compared with those from blood collected at 2 to 2½ hours, and urine collected over eight hours, after the protein load.

LEUCINE SENSITIVITY TEST FOR HYPOGLYCAEMIA AND GLUCAGON TEST

Children with hypoglycaemia of unknown cause may require either a leucine sensitivity test or a glucagon test. Prior to the test, in order to prevent a dangerously low blood sugar, a controlled carbohydrate but protein-free meal is given to some patients.

The amount of carbohydrate in the pre-test meal is based on age, except in infants, where an equivalent amount of carbohydrate to that contained in the infant's usual feed and/or weaning solids is appropriate. Half the carbohydrate of the pre-test meal is

Table 15.3   Example of a protein load for infants and children.

Infant
    10 g Casilan or Maxipro HBV = approximately 9 g protein
    Boiled water to 100 ml
    Give 13·5 ml/kg weight plus additional water or 5% dextrose if permitted throughout the test

Children
    15 g Casilan or Maxipro HBV = approximately 13·5 g protein
    Permitted flavouring, e.g. dietetic low-calorie squash
    Water to 100 ml
    Give 7·5 ml/kg weight plus additional water or fruit juice if permitted throughout the test

given from more slowly absorbed starch, and the re-mainder as sugar(s), in order to avoid a rapid rise of blood glucose which stimulates insulin production and subsequently produces a rapid fall in blood glucose. The ingredients can vary, but low-protein biscuits are very suitable, either as a rusk, crushed and mixed with boiled water into a porridge in tod-dlers, or given from a feeding bottle in infants.

Table 15.4 gives two suggestions to provide the carbohydrate required for different ages. Water is per-mitted in addition.

LOW-PHOSPHORUS DIETS

A low-phosphorus diet is sometimes prescribed prior to a test for ability to respond to injected parathyroid hormone. It may also be used in the treatment of hypoparathyroidism and some reduction in phos-phorus intake is now advised in chronic renal failure (*see* Chapter 8).

Reduction of dietary phosphorus to 8 mmol ($\simeq 250$ mg) per day (Table 15.5) can only be used for a few days because of the low protein content of the diet. Moderate restriction of phosphorus for long-term use must provide adequate nutrients for growth. All low-phosphorus diets require calcium supplementa-tion, and if required for an extended period vitamin and trace mineral supplements are recommended.

In infants a low-phosphorus diet can only be pro-vided adequately by using human milk or, less effi-ciently, by using a modified formula such as Aptamil, Gold Cap SMA, Premium or Osterfeed.

Moderately restricted phosphorus diet

In the construction of a phosphorus-restricted diet for long-term use, adequate nutrients, including protein for growth, must be included, as well as maintaining the required restriction of phosphorus. Calcium sup-plements continue to be necessary. Limited quantities of the foods listed in Table 15.6 can be incorporated as appropriate for the diet prescription in conjunction with the minimal phosphorus foods. Foods high in phosphorus should be omitted.

Minimal phosphorus foods which together contribute an average of $\leqslant 3 \cdot 2$ mmol (100 mg) phosphorus per day in a child's diet include:

Glucose polymers: Calonutrin, Caloreen, Maxijul, Polycal, Hycal.
Sugar, glucose.
Butter, cream, margarine, oil, fats.
Calogen, Prosparol.
Jelly, ice-lollies, boiled sweets, honey, jam, marmalade, syrup, cornflour, custard powder.
Tea, coffee, fruit juice, squash, lemonade, Ribena.
Fruit—stewed, fresh or canned (no banana and not more than one orange daily).

Foods which are high in phosphorus:

Protein foods: cheese, liver, kidney, heart, brain, sweetbread, pork, veal, game, fatty fish, e.g. kippers, sardine, fish roes.
Cereals: Bemax, porridge, Weetabix, Puffed Wheat.

Table 15.4 Controlled carbohydrate, minimal protein meals used for leucine sensitivity and/or glucagon test.

Age (years)	Carbohydrate content of pre-test meal (g)	A		B	
		Aminex biscuits (number)	+ Sugar (g)	Rice cereal (g)	+ Blackcurrant concentrate (ml)
Under 1 year	Depends on feeds	←————— Calculate individually —————→			
1	30	1½	10	20	25
2	40	2	15	25	35
3 and 4	50	2½	20	30	45
5	60	2½	30	30	55
6	65	3½	30	40	55
7 plus	75	3½	30	40	70

Select either A or B as appropriate. Additional water is permitted throughout the test.
  (i) Aminex biscuits contain approximately 10 g starch and 2 g glucose.
 (ii) 10 g rice cereal, e.g. Robinson's Baby Rice, Milupa Plain Rice or Rice Krispies, contains approximately 8·5 g carbohydrate.
(iii) 100 ml blackcurrant concentrate = 60 g glucose and/or sucrose.

Table 15.5 Example of an 8 mmol (250 mg) phosphorus diet‡.

		Calcium (mg)	Phosphorus (mg)
Breakfast	20 g (¾ oz) Cornflakes	0·6	9·4
	30 g (1 oz) milk (and water)	36	28·5
	Sugar		
	30 g (1 oz) white bread	30	29
	Glucose polymer and water	Trace	Trace
	Butter or margarine, jam, marmalade	Trace	Trace
Mid-morning	200 ml orange juice (sweetened)	9	14
	Glucose polymer and water	Trace	Trace
Dinner and supper	100 g (3½ oz) potato	4	29
	Butter or margarine		
	100 g (3½ oz) vegetables*	34	27
	180 g (6 oz) fruit (not banana)	24	20
	100 g jelly made with water	14	2
Tea	20 g biscuits, Marie type	24	16·8
	30 g sweets, peppermints or pastilles	7	Trace
	Glucose polymer and water	Trace	Trace
Supper	As dinner	76†	78‡
	Glucose polymer and water	Trace	Trace
	Sub-total	260 = 6·5 mmol	253·7 = 8·2 mmol
Supplements	(i) Calcium supplements	400 = 10 mmol	Nil
	Vitamins and trace minerals		
	(ii) Glucose polymer supplement to energy requirement		
	Daily total	658·6 mg = 16.5 mmol	253·7 = 8·2 mmol

* Vegetables low in phosphorus: greens, cauliflower, carrot, cabbage, tomato, green beans, marrow, lettuce, salad.

† Average value.

‡ The basic diet without supplements contains approximately 10 g protein and has an energy content of approximately 4200 kJ (1000 kcal). Such a diet should only be used for a *temporary* period.

Fruit: dried fruit, nuts, prunes, banana.
Vegetables: peas, beans, lentils, parsley, spinach, mushrooms, potato crisps and chips.
Bovril, Marmite, Oxo, Virol, Horlicks, Ovaltine, Bournvita.
Chocolate, toffee, ice-cream.

DRY DIET FOR WATER DEPRIVATION TESTS

temporary diet (Table 15.7) may be needed during ater deprivation tests, although frequently this test

continues for only 12 to 18 hours and not longer than 24 hours. Salty foods should be avoided as they will aggravate the child's thirst.

TEST MEAL FOR ASSESSING INTRALUMINAL PHASE OF ABSORPTION IN CHILDHOOD

In clinical practice it is sometimes necessary to assess the function of a digestive organ by stimulation with intraluminal nutrients in a physiological form. A test meal devised for this purpose was first described by

Table 15.6 Phosphorus and protein content of foods.

		Protein (g)	Phosphorus mg	Phosphorus mmol
Milk	100 ml (3½ oz)	3·3	95	3·1
Meat	100 g (3½ oz) lean	28*	200*	6·5*
Egg	One only (50 g)	6	110	3·5
Bread, white	100 g (3½ oz)	7·8	97	3·1
Potato, boiled	100 g (3½ oz)	1·5	30	1·0
Vegetables	100 g (3½ oz) low-phosphorus type (see Table 18.5)	Trace	30	1·0
Cereals	1 serve Rice Krispies, Cornflakes	0·6	10	0·3
Chips	100 g	2·2	61	2·0
Crisps	20 g	1·3	26	0·8

* Average value.

Table 15.7 Example menu for a 'dry' diet.

Foods allowed	Food forbidden
Roast and grilled meats, fried fish or fish fingers.	All drinks.
Cheese, hard-boiled egg.	Milk, tea, coffee, cocoa, squashes, juices.
Dry breakfast cereals.	Porridge.
Plain sponge cakes, biscuits. Crispbreads, cream crackers.	Ice-cream, milk puddings.
	Jellies, junkets, blancmanges.
Bread and butter.	Soups, sauces, gravies, casseroles, and stews.
Chips or potato crisps.	Fruit, vegetables.
	Jam, honey, syrup.
	Sweets, toffees, chocolates, ice-lollies.

Breakfast	Dry breakfast cereal and sugar, e.g. Cornflakes, Coco Pops, Rice Krispies, Sugar Puffs, Weetabix, *no* milk Hard-boiled egg or bacon* or ham* Bread and butter or toast and butter—*no* jam, honey, etc.
Mid-morning	Sweet biscuits
Dinner	Roast meat or chicken or fried liver or fried fish—*no* gravy, sauces, stews, etc. Chips or potato crisps—*no* boiled, mashed, roast potatoes and *no* vegetables Plain sponge pudding—*no* fruit, jam, custard Crispbread and cheese, or sweet biscuits
Tea	Bread and butter and ham*, cheese, Marmite* Plain sponge cake or biscuits
Supper	Fish fingers or cold meats or fried fish Chips or crisps or bread and butter Sweet biscuits or plain cake or cheese and biscuits

* These foods are very salty and may best be avoided as they will aggravate the child's thirst.

Table 15.8 Test meal for assessing intraluminal phase of absorption (modified Lundh test meal).

	Carbohydrate (g)	Protein (g)	Fat (g)
125 g Comminuted Chicken	0	9 to 10	3·9 to 5·5
10 g glucose	10	Nil	Nil
5 ml corn oil	Nil	Nil	5
Water to 250 ml			
Total	10	9 to 10	8·9 to 10·5
Each 100 ml contains	4	3·8 to 4	3·6 to 4·2

Homogenize to a fine suspension in an electric blender.

Give 30 ml per kg weight in infants to a full dose of 240 ml as a single feed in children.

Lundh (1962) and a variation of this test was validated by McCollum *et al.* (1977). The test meal contains 4% (w/v) of carbohydrate, protein and fat in the form of glucose, Comminuted Chicken, and corn oil (Table 15.8). This formula can be administered to children who are sensitive to cow's milk protein and/or gluten, as well as to those intolerant of disaccharides, without danger of precipitating gastrointestinal symptoms. The feed is administered by nasogastric tube after an overnight fast in older children, a four-hour fast in young infants, or a fast appropriate to the interval between feeds in very sick infants. Samples of gastric juice are collected and analysed for pancreatic enzymes and bile salts.

PURINE METABOLIC STUDIES

Caffeine interferes with the analysis of the metabolites of purines. During their investigation not only has the diet to exclude major sources of purines (Table 10.19), but caffeine should also be avoided. Therefore, tea, coffee, Coke, cola drinks and Lucozade are omitted as well as purines from the diet for the duration of the tests.

GLUCOSE TOLERANCE TEST

As a preliminary before a glucose tolerance test the child should have a nutritionally adequate diet, in-cluding a normal carbohydrate intake. Usually a dietary assessment is all that is required.

DISACCHARIDE (SUGAR) LOADING TESTS IN PATIENTS WITH MALABSORPTION AND SUSPECTED DISACCHARIDE INTOLERANCE

This test is useful in distinguishing lactose intolerance from cow's milk protein intolerance. A test dose of the appropriate sugar (lactose or sucrose) is given after an appropriate fast as a 7% (w/v) solution in infants to provide 2 g of the specific carbohydrate/kg weight up to a maximum of 24 g in 200 ml in children. A rise of blood glucose of 1·6 mmol/l (30 mg/100 ml) or more from the fasting level is considered normal; a rise of 1 to 1·6 mmol/l (20 to 30 mg/100 ml) is doubtful, and a rise of less than 1 mmol/l (20 mg/100 ml) is considered abnormal (Walker-Smith, 1979). Stool sugars are also investigated, ideally by sugar chromatography.

REFERENCES

CORNBLATH M. & SCHWARTZ R. (1976) *Disorders of Carbohydrate Metabolism in Infancy*, Vol. III, *Major Problems in Clinical Paediatrics*, 2nd Edition, (ed. Schaffer A.). Philadelphia: W.B. Saunders & Co.

LUNDH G. (1962) Pancreatic exocrine function in neoplastic and inflammatory disease: a simple and reliable new text. *Gastroenterology* **42**, 275–80.

McCOLLUM J.P.K., MULLER D.P.R. & HARRIES J.T. (1977) Test meal for assessing intraluminal phase of absorption in childhood. *Arch. Dis. Childh.* **52**, 887–9.

ROSSITER M.A., PALMER T. & EVANS K. (1974) The short-term response to a drink of milk, lactose or casein in children with apparently normal gastrointestinal tracts. *Brit. J. Nutr.* **32**, 605–13.

WALKER-SMITH J.A. (1979) *Diseases of the Small Intestine in Children*, 2nd Edition. London: Pitman Medical.

CHAPTER 16

Balance studies

The aim of balance studies is to determine how much of a given nutrient or nutrients the patient is retaining in his body, in order to assess whether they are metabolized normally. Also, the effect of specific drugs and treatment on the loss or retention of the nutrients can be studied. Other studies are to see the effect of a dietary change on the body, e.g. lipid levels in blood.

Metabolic balance studies are expensive and time-consuming for both patients and staff. Their continued usefulness is in nutritional research (Beisel 1979), for example in trace metal investigations (Aggett & Davies 1983). Modern techniques permit alternative methods of clinical assessment which have largely replaced the need for metabolic balance for diagnostic purposes. The use of jejunal biopsy in the diagnosis of coeliac disease has largely outmoded faecal fat estimations; labelled chromium studies are a more appropriate means of determining protein-losing enteropathy than a nitrogen balance. *The Handbook of Metabolic Dietetics* outlines the principles of balance studies.

There are two main types of balances:

(i) Metabolic balance with a high degree of accuracy for calcium, sodium, nitrogen, potassium or trace mineral nutrients which require analysis of a duplicate sample of the food given to the patient.
(ii) Constant calculated intakes of various nutrients from weighed diets and fat balances with 1 to 5% accuracy.

METABOLIC BALANCES

General instructions   A request for a balance requires that the following details should be established:

1   Reason for balance.
2   Length of study.
3   Accuracy and type of balance; determine whether food is to be duplicated for analysis.

4   Nutrients to be studied; need for constant menu or nutrient intake.
5   Confirm that a stool culture from the patient is negative for pathogens (to cut down risk of cross-infection).
6   Age and condition of patient, e.g. toilet-trained, incontinent, or mentally slow.
7   Meal pattern of the patient and eating habits, e.g. drinks from a teacher beaker or bottle.
8   Arrange suitable dates for trial, run-in, and actual balance with ward, parents, laboratory and dietitian.
9   The laboratory and nursing staff need to arrange the most suitable means of collecting urine and faeces during the balance. It is important that the child's activity is not inhibited because of these collections, as altered activity or immobilization may affect the handling of nutrients.

MENU ARRANGEMENTS

According to the above information, discussed with the ward staff, parents and child, plan suitable menus. Balances of more than five days requiring a constant intake should have alternating menus to reduce boredom. On a constant diet for one or two nutrients only, variation in the other nutrients may be given. In other balances no limitation on menu selection is required, but an exact duplicate of every item of food or drink, including medicines, consumed by the child must be kept for analysis in the laboratory.

Normally the child should have a diet suitable for the type of balance and the age of the child, and which contains a nutrient intake similar to the meal pattern of the child at home or just prior to the balance, unless other dietary instructions are given, e.g. normal calcium for one balance period, followed by a low-calcium diet. Adequate fluid must be supplied as fruit juice or de-ionized water if tap water is not permitted. No other food apart from that which is specially prepared should be consumed during the balance periods.

DAY-PERIODS

Balances are usually for three- or five-day periods, each 24 hours commencing at a stated time, e.g. 10 a.m. Different coloured markers are given at the beginning and end of each three or five days to colour the stools when faecal collection is required.

Menus should be planned starting with the first meal of the balance day, e.g. 10 a.m. snack. It is preferable to overestimate the child's appetite slightly rather than allow the child to be hungry or to lose weight. Allow the child to eat by appetite; any rejected food should be analysed and its content subtracted from the offered intake.

CALCULATION

The nutrients are calculated from tables in *McCance & Widdowson's The Composition of Food* (Paul & Southgate 1978), or appropriate analysis of proprietary foods given by the manufacturer. If alternating menus are used for constant-intake diets they should be equal within the balance accuracy for each nutrient under consideration. For metabolic balances where an exact duplicate of food intake is to be analysed a calculation of the diet nutrients gives a guide to the analyst, but the analytical figures are used in the final calculations. The diet sheet should be marked with instructions as to foods for duplication, samples required and method of cooking. Great care must be taken to provide an exact replica of the patient's food for analysis and to prevent contamination of the food and duplicates with trace metals from the air, the hands (sweat) or from cooking utensils, especially metals, e.g. aluminium saucepans.

Constant-intake studies

Each menu should be tried for at least 24 hours and adjusted in quantity as necessary before starting the actual balance. This trial menu is prepared from non-balance supplies of food, cooked and weighed in similar manner to the balance, but less accuracy is required at this stage.

RUN-IN PERIOD

For constant-intake metabolic balances and some other studies, a run-in period of 48 hours or longer is essential before the balance commences. Collections need not be made, nor duplicates and samples prepared, at this stage. Run-in periods are not possible with newborn infants or post-surgical follow-up studies.

Food supplies

In very accurate balances it may be necessary to use the same source or batch of foods throughout the balance and run-in period.

All food required for the total balance should be ordered from the same source or batch, e.g. tinned foods should have the same batch number, meat should come from the same animal carcass, fish fillets from the same fish, cereals and dry goods from the same packet or batch.

To estimate the quantity of food for a five-day metabolic balance, order food for 10 days; for a 10-day metabolic balance, order food for 18 days; for 20-day metabolic balance, order food for 30 days. Where alternating menus are used order food supplies for each menu. These quantities ensure there is adequate food for the run-in period, spilling or spoilage of food, or unforeseen extension of the balance, and an aliquot for analysis. If analysis of an exact duplicate of all food and drink is required, double the quantities will be required, plus extra for unforeseen accidents.

SUITABLE FOODS FOR METABOLIC BALANCES; BASIC DIET

To ensure accurate duplicates of the food consumed are analysed, each individual item of food must be weighed separately. The same batch, bottle or tin should be used for both patient and duplicate, for example:

Trimmed lean roast meat or chicken breasts from the same animal or batch. Edible portion only should be used (remove gristle and bone). Use the same part of the animal for both the patient and analysis duplicate.

Minced trimmed roast meat or lean minced steak.

Raw steak trimmed edible portions.

Frozen vegetables from the same batch.

Instant potato made to a standard recipe.

Tinned fruit, milk puddings, baby foods.

Dry cereals, sugar, crisps, jam chocolate, biscuits, salt, tea, drinking chocolate, squash, fruit juice, instant coffee, instant tea.

Gravy or milk puddings made to standard recipes in bulk and frozen in individual portions.

Bread and plain-type cakes from the same loaf or batch and frozen. Bread may be toasted to the same colour after weighing.

Salt-free butter for sodium balances. Butter or margarine for other balances.

Evaporated milk, dried powdered milks.

Ice-cream from the same batch.

Jelly made to a standard recipe then weighed in duplicate.

Sweets from the same batch must also be matched for colour as well as weight and batch.

FOODS WHICH NEED DAILY DUPLICATION OR SAMPLING

Mashed or boiled potato.

Fresh fruit and vegetables including salad (core, peel and dice weighing each item separately).

Scrambled egg made to a set recipe then weighed in duplicate.

Fish from the same fillet, grilled or baked (without batter or breadcrumbs)

Homogenized milk.

Infant feeds and milk substitutes made to a standard recipe (weighed powder made to measured or weighed total volume).

FOODS UNSUITABLE FOR METABOLIC BALANCES

Boiled, poached or fried egg.

Sausage, pies and made-up dishes such as stews and casseroles.

Fish fingers, hamburgers.

Fruit cake, chocolate rolls, pastry and pies.

Tea and coffee (brewed type).

Salted butter on sodium balances.

Tap water on sodium, calcium, nitrogen balances, and trace mineral balances.

Mixed vegetables.

Preparation of food in advance

Food can be prepared in advance from the specially ordered batch of food and suitably stored. The duplicate for analysis is prepared identically to the food intended for the patient.

Food that can be frozen; cook, trim, weigh to necessary accuracy and store in polythene or wax cartons, label and deep-freeze quickly.

Dry foods are weighed into polythene bags or cartons, sealed, labelled and stored.

Label all supplies clearly, to ensure they are not accidentally used for other patients, and store them separately.

Weighing of food for balances

Weigh the food on accurate electronic or metabolic balance scales. Counterbalance and test the scale before use. Weigh the food directly into polythene bags or cartons when preparing servings for storage. For food prepared each day, weigh directly into the plates, glasses and other dishes from which the child will eat. Counterbalance the weight of the plate with the tare on the scales. For metabolic balances weigh food and fluid to an appropriate accuracy, e.g. ± 0.05 g.

Always 'lock' the scale mechanism when the scales are not in use to prevent wear. Rinse the scale-pan in de-ionized water and dry in the air if food is to be weighed directly onto the scale-pan. The scales and all equipment must be kept spotlessly clean.

Cooking and individual preparation required for different foods

Cook and prepare food with de-ionized water for metabolic balances.

Add weighed salt after cooking and weighing for sodium balances. Use salt in cooking only on instruction. For sodium balances pure sodium chloride may be necessary, as table salt contains magnesium. Weigh salt or sodium chloride into tubes, seal and store in a dry place.

Fry chips in clean deep oil, preheated before adding the food. Renew oil each balance period of 3 to 5 days. Dry fry in a clean (non-stick) pan.

Heat cooked meat on the serving plate with weighed gravy, covered with a plate cover. A microwave oven is ideal, or heat over boiling water or in the oven.

For baked beans, spaghetti, milk puddings, either heat in a double saucepan then weigh into serving plate *or* weigh onto serving plate, cover and heat.

Use a fresh tin of canned food each day.

Toast.   Weighed frozen bread is thawed then toasted to the same colour.

Jelly.   Make to specific recipe from the same batch of crystals or jelly cubes. Weigh into moulds previously rinsed in de-ionized water and dried in the air. Refrigerate. Turn out carefully onto serving plate. Remake to the same recipe at least every balance period of 3 to 5 days.

Scrambled egg.   Beat two or three eggs together, weigh in duplicate into two separate serving dishes. Weigh butter or margarine in duplicate for each dish. Cook together over boiling water. Serve one to the child, the other is used for the duplicate.

Drinks

(a) *Tea and coffee*. Place weighed instant powder into serving cup. Pour on boiling de-ionized water to required weight. Add weighed milk and sugar. Take to the patient immediately. In some balances only the milk has to be taken into account.

(b) *Milk*. Homogenized or skimmed milk should be used, weighed directly into cups or glasses. A sample from the daily batch should be kept for analysis.

(c) *Fruit drinks*. Weigh juice or concentrate into glass in duplicate. Add de-ionized water to final total weight.

(d) *Extra de-ionized water* should be sent daily with a glass, if tap water is unsuitable, for extra drinks and to give with medicines.

A dropper or syringe, previously rinsed in de-ionized water and dried, can be used to obtain more easily the final accurate weighing of fluids.

Puddings and gravy. Make to a standard recipe and store frozen unweighed. Thaw, weigh onto plate or serving dish. Cover. Heat as for tinned foods.

Potatoes

(a) Reconstitute *instant potato* to a given recipe.

(b) *Crisps* can be weighed as dry foods.

(c) Avoid *roast potato*, or duplicate daily; pieces should be matched for size and colour.

(d) *Boiled*. Cook in de-ionized water, with salt only if instruction allows. Weigh or mash and weigh in duplicate. Weighed salt or butter can be added.

(e) *Chips*. Use frozen from the same batch. Fry in preheated oil until a golden brown constant colour. Drain well, weigh in duplicate.

Fruit

(a) *Tinned*. Weigh juice and drained fruit separately as indicated on the diet sheet, e.g. $\frac{2}{3}$ fruit, $\frac{1}{3}$ juice.

(b) *Fresh*. Double the quantity required should be peeled, cored, diced or sliced and mixed. Weigh for the child and duplicate.

Prepare fresh fruit immediately before the meal to prevent discolouration and vitamin losses.

Fish. Weigh two samples from the same fillet of fish and freeze in pairs. On the day required thaw the pair, cook identically. Serve one to child, use the other for the duplicate.

Dry goods such as biscuits, cereal and sugar should be weighed from the same batch.

Butter or margarine should be weighed directly onto the bread and spread carefully using a knife which has been rinsed in de-ionized water and air-dried.

EQUIPMENT

All equipment should be scrupulously clean and kept separately, rinsed in de-ionized water and allowed to drain and air dry. Ideally, separate easily identified serving dishes should be used. De-ionized water for rinsing equipment should be changed frequently. Trays, plates and cutlery returned from the patient should be checked for rejects, washed, then sterilized before finally rinsing in de-ionized water. Trays are washed then sprayed with disinfectant before re-use.

LABELLING

Clearly identify all balance food and individual food items, plates and trays.

SERVICE OF MEALS

Meals are served on a tray, with suitable de-ionized cutlery, glasses, salt, and sugar as permitted. The completed tray is delivered to the child, or nurse who is to supervise or feed the child on the ward. Toddlers and infants should wear a suitable de-ionized plastic 'pelican' type feeding bib to allow spilt food to be saved as rejects. The complete tray is collected back after each meal.

Daily remove the foods required from the deep-freeze and thaw in the refrigerator. When alternating menus are used the correct menu should be checked and recorded to prevent the same menu on two successive days.

Prepare, cook, serve and duplicate the food as already described according to the menu.

REJECTS

Depending on the type of study, these are weighed and recorded, or saved for analysis in a labelled de-ionized container. Saved rejects must be scraped into the rejects container and the plates rinsed with a little de-ionized water. The volume of de-ionized water should be kept to a minimum. De-ionized water in a squeeze bottle is useful for this purpose. Rejected sweets should be attached to the outside of the carton in a polythene bag as they have to be dissolved before analysis. At the end of each 24 hours it is important to check that all rejects have been collected, then close, label and date the container. Deep-freeze in a separate freezer or send direct to the laboratory, to avoid rejects being placed near food which is to be used for patients.

If a constant intake is essential it is ideal that the child eats all offered food. Encouragement and variations such as pictures or flowers on the trays or even small toys will help overcome the inevitable boredom of long-term studies.

When fat is included in the nutrients under consideration rejected food is both weighed back and saved for analysis; the fat intake is calculated, whereas the other nutrients are analysed.

Some balances only require a calculated intake. Rejected food is weighed back and calculated for the appropriate nutrients by the dietitian. The intake minus the rejects equals the daily food consumed, provided no loss or spillage has occurred. Any spillage or losses must be reported immediately. An assessment of the loss is made and reported to the person in charge who must decide if the balance can continue or should be recommenced or even abandoned.

DUPLICATE OF BASIC DIET

Metabolic balances usually require analysis of the nutrients being studied in the food.

A duplicate of all food, drinks and medicines offered to the child should be analysed. Weigh each item in duplicate, one for the child, the other for analysis. Rejected food and drink are also analysed for the nutrient concerned, the difference being the consumed intake.

Alternatively, a duplicate or aliquot of the basic diet food is prepared from the same batch and in the usual way, e.g. bread is toasted and/or buttered; meat thawed, gravy added and heated, etc. A list of each food in the basic diet is written and checked as the foods are duplicated. The duplicated food is placed in a suitable de-ionized container supplied by the laboratory ready for the analysis. Preservative is added only as directed. Sweets are attached to the outside of the container in a polythene bag as they must be dissolved before analysis. The laboratory should be notified as soon as the duplicate is pre-

pared. The basic diet foods may either be duplicated daily or prepared from the same batch of foods only once in each balance period.

Daily duplicates are essential for foods which are not prepared from the same batch, and the calculated proportion is added to the basic diet food for analysis. Care must be taken when alternating menus are used. Both basic diets must be analysed. Any five-day period has three days of menu A and two days of menu B, so careful calculation of the appropriate total five-day intake must be made.

Metabolic balances in infants

The procedure is similar to other metabolic balances, except that the feeds should be made using a specific recipe, from the same batch of ingredients. Each 24-hour feed is made in bulk, bottled, labelled and pasteurized. Ready-to-feed commercial formulae from the same batch may be used if appropriate. An aliquot is kept for analysis. Each bottle is weighed without the cover, but with the teat on the bottle, at the beginning and end of the feed. The difference is the weight of the feed consumed by the infant. The sum of the weight of feeds consumed in 24 hours is recorded and from the analysis of the feed sample the nutrients consumed can be calculated.

De-ionized disposable nappies are the most appropriate means of collecting urine, faeces, vomitus and regurgitated food in this age group.

WEANING DIET

The feeds are prepared as described for the infant, and the solids as for the older child, using, where possible, tins of the ready-prepared baby foods from the same batch.

FAT BALANCES AND CONSTANT DIETS

The general instructions are similar to those described for metabolic balances. However, a set menu, constant sources of food and duplicates for analysis are not required. The offered food is weighed to appropriate accuracy. Rejects are weighed back and the actual intake calculated. Any food can be used, provided the composition is known and is suitable for the type of diet required. Tap water can be used unless calcium and/or sodium intake is severely restricted. A direct tray service is not essential provided all foods for the child are labelled. Cutlery and glasses can be used from the ward as they do not require pre-rinsing in de-ionized water.

REFERENCES

AGGETT P.J. & DAVIES N.T. (1983) Some nutritional aspects of trace metals. *J. Inher. metab.Dis.* **6**, Suppl. 1, 22–30.

BEISEL W.R. (1979) Metabolic balance studies—their continuing usefulness in nutritional research. *Amer. J. clin. Nutr.* **32**, 271–4.

PAUL A.A., & SOUTHGATE D.A.T. (1978) *McCance & Widdowson's The Composition of Foods*, 4th Edition. London: HMSO.

THE METABOLIC GROUP OF THE BRITISH DIETIC ASSOCIATION has prepared an instruction booklet on balance studies, *The Handbook of Metabolic Dietetics* (1984) (ed. Austin E.I.). Birmingham: British Dietetic Association.

CHAPTER 17

Products used in dietetics

Details regarding the use of products are described in the appropriate chapters. Compositional details should be obtained from the manufacturer.

ALPHABETICAL LIST OF PRODUCTS, MANUFACTURER AND GENERAL CHARACTERISTICS

Name of product	Manufacturer or U.K. distributor	General characteristics
Abidec	Parke, Davis & Co. Usk Road Pontypool Gwent NP4 8YH	Multivitamin preparation
Acacia gum	Macarthys Ltd Chesham House Chesham Close Romford RM1 4JX	Emulsifying gum for preparing edible oil emulsions
Addamel	KabiVitrum Ltd Bilton House Uxbridge Road London W5 2TH	Mineral supplement for adult parenteral nutrition
Adexolin	Farley Health Products Ltd Torr Lane Plymouth PL3 5UA	Vitamin A, D, C drops
Agluttella pasta—macaroni, noodles, spaghetti, rings	GF Dietary Supplies Ltd 494–6 Honey Pot Lane Stanmore Middx HA7 1JH	Low-protein, gluten-free pasta
Aglutella Azeta Low-Protein Sweet-Filled Wafer	GF Dietary Supplies Ltd	Low-protein wafer biscuit
Albumaid Complete	Scientific Hospital Supplies Ltd 38 Queensland Street Liverpool L7 3JG	Beef serum hydrolysate with some vitamins and minerals. Carbohydrate- and fat-free
Albumaid Histidine Low	Scientific Hospital Supplies Ltd ⎫	Beef serum hydrolysates low in amino acid specified
Albumaid Methionine Low	Scientific Hospital Supplies Ltd ⎭	

Name of product	Manufacturer or U.K. distributor	General characteristics
Albumaid Phenylalanine/Tyrosine Low	Scientific Hospital Supplies Ltd	Beef serum hydrolysates low in amino acid specified
Albumaid Phenylalanine/Tyrosine/ Methionine Low	Scientific Hospital Supplies Ltd	
Albumaid RVHB Methionine Free	Scientific Hospital Supplies Ltd	
Albumaid XP Phenylalanine Low	Scientific Hospital Supplies Ltd	
Albumaid XP Concentrate Phenylalanine Low	Scientific Hospital Supplies Ltd	
Alembicol D	E J R Lovelock Alembic Products Oaklands House Oaklands Drive Sale Manchester M33 1WS	MCT oil
Alfaré	The Nestlé Co. Ltd St George's House Croydon Surrey CR9 1NR	Hydrolysed casein infant formula. Low-lactose, sucrose-free
Alprem (not available in U.K.)	The Nestlé Co. Ltd	Low-birthweight infant formula
Alsoy (not available in U.K.)	The Nestlé Co. Ltd	Soya formula
AL 110 (not available in U.K.)	The Nestlé Co. Ltd	Low-lactose formula; contains casein
Aminex (Liga)	Cow & Gate Babyfoods Ltd Trowbridge Wilts BA14 8YX	Low-protein biscuit; lactose-and sucrose-free; not gluten-free
Amino acids	*Various* East Anglian Chemicals Ltd Hadleigh, Ipswich Suffolk 1PY 68Q Cambrian Chemicals Ltd Beddington Farm Road Croydon CR0 4XB Scientific Hospitals Supplies Ltd 38 Queensland Street Liverpool L7 3JG	Pure L-amino acids
Aminogran Food Supplement	Allen & Hanbury Ltd Bethnal Green London E2 6LA	Phenylalanine-free amino acid supplement
Aminogran Mineral Mixture	Allen & Hanbury Ltd	Comprehensive mineral supplement for synthetic diets
Aproten biscuits (Carlo Erba)	Ultrapharm Ltd 5 Beaconfield Road Royal Leamington Spa Warwickshire CV31 1DH	Low-protein biscuits. Also gluten-free
Aproten crispbread (Carlo Erba)	Ultrapharm Ltd	

Name of product	Manufacturer or U.K. distributor	General characteristics
Aproten flour (Carlo Erba)	Ultrapharm Ltd	Low-protein flour and pasta Also gluten-free
Aproten pasta: anellini, ditalini, rigatini, tagliatelle (Carlo Erba)	Ultrapharm Ltd	
Aptamil	Milupa Ltd Milupa House Hercies Road Hillingdon Middx UB10 9NA	Whey-based modified infant formula
Aspartame (brand names Canderel, Nutrasweet)	Searle Laboratories Division of G.D. Searle Co. Ltd PO Box 53 Lane End Road High Wycombe Bucks HP12 4HL	Dipeptide of aspartic acid and phenylalanine
Babymilk Plus	Cow & Gate Babyfoods Ltd Trowbridge Wilts BA14 8YX	Modified infant formula
Baby Rice (plain)	Robinson & Co. Reckitt Coleman Food Division Carrow, Norwich Norfolk	Pre-cooked rice cereal for infants
Baby Rice (plain)	Milupa Ltd Milupa House Hercies Road Hillingdon Middx UB10 9NA	Pre-cooked rice cereal for infants
Bengers	Fisons Ltd Pharmaceuticals Division 12 Derby Road Loughborough LE11 0BB	Amylase and trypsin enzymes in a wheat base with sodium bicarbonate. Used to partially pre-digest milk
Bi-Aglut Biscuits	Ultrapharm Ltd 5 Beaconfield Road Royal Leamington Spa Warwickshire CV31 1DH	Gluten-free biscuit
Breads for specific diets (a) Allinson's	Various bakers Allinson Heathways House 45 Station Approach West Byfleet Surrey	100% wholemeal bread using Allinson's flour; high-fibre, lower in calcium than white bread and flour. *See* Table 12.4

Name of product	Manufacturer or U.K. distributor	General characteristics
(b) Rite-Diet Salt-Free	Various Welfare Foods (Stockport) Ltd 63 London Road South Poynton Stockport Cheshire SK12 1LA	Salt-free bread
(c) Rite-Diet Gluten-Free Low-Protein (canned) and Pre-baked	Welfare Foods (Stockport) Ltd	Gluten-free bread which is also low-protein
(d) Rite-Diet Gluten-Free with soya bran (canned) and Pre-baked	Welfare Foods (Stockport) Ltd	High-fibre gluten-free bread
(e) Rite-Diet Gluten-Free Low-Protein Salt-Free (canned)	Welfare Foods (Stockport) Ltd	Gluten-free low-protein and salt-free bread
(f) Juvela Gluten-Free Pre-baked Loaf	GF Dietary Supplies 494–6 Honey Pot Lane Stanmore Middx HA7 1JH	Gluten-free bread
(g) Juvela Low-Protein Pre-baked Loaf	GF Dietary Supplies Ltd	Low-protein bread, also gluten- and milk-free
Build-Up	Carnation Foods Co. Carnation House 11 High Road London N2 8AW	High-protein milk supplement, low in fat
Calcium-Free Mineral Mixture	Scientific Hospital Supplies Ltd 38 Queensland Street Liverpool L7 3JG	Calcium-free mineral supplement
Calogen	Scientific Hospital Supplies Ltd	50% arachis (peanut) oil emulsion
Calonutrin	Geistlich Sons Ltd PO Box 37 Newton Bank Long Lane Chester CH2 3QZ	Glucose polymer powder. Recently discontinued
Caloreen	Roussel Laboratories Ltd Broadwater Park North Orbital Road Denham Uxbridge UB9 5HP	Glucose polymer powder
Canderel	Searle Laboratories Division of G.D. Searle Co. Ltd PO Box 53 Lane End Road High Wycombe Bucks HP12 4HL	Artificial sweetener containing aspartame

Name of product	Manufacturer or U.K. distributor	General characteristics
Carobel—Instant	Cow & Gate Babyfoods Ltd Trowbridge Wilts BA14 8YX	Hemicellulose gelling agent derived from carob seeds used for thickening infant feeds. Pre-cooked
Casilan	Farley Health Products Ltd Torr Lane Plymouth PL3 5UA	Calcium caseinate protein supplement
Celacol	British Celanese Ltd PO Box 5 Spondon Derby DE2 7BP	Cellulose powder used in low-protein cooking
Ceres Margarine (not available in U.K.)	GMBH 2000 Hamburg 50 Postfach 1020 Germany	Margarine with predominantly MCT fat, vitamins A, D and E and milk solids
CF 1 (not available in U.K.)	The Nestlé Co. Ltd St George's House Croydon Surrey CR9 1NR	Carbohydrate-free formula, contains milk protein
Children's Vitamin Drops	Department of Health issue available from health clinics	Vitamins A, D and C
Clinifeed (Isovanilla, 400 vanilla, Favour neutral/coffee, Protein-rich vanilla, Select beef & carrot)	Roussel Laboratories Ltd Broadwater Park North Orbital Road Denham Uxbridge UB9 5HP	Adult enteral feeds with different flavours and protein contents
Cholestyramine (Questran)	Mead Johnson Laboratories Division of Bristol Myers Co. Ltd Stamford House Station Road Langley Slough SL3 6EB	Cholesterol-lowering drug
Coffee-mate	Carnation Foods Co. Carnation House 11 High Road London N2 8AW	Coffee creamer contains caseinate; lactose-free, low calcium
Cologel	Eli, Lilly & Co. Ltd Kingsclere Road Basingstoke Hants RG21 2XA	Methylcellulose medicinal liquid
Comminuted Chicken	Cow & Gate Babyfoods Ltd Trowbridge Wilts BA14 8YX	Puréed chicken meat in water, carbohydrate-free, used as the basis of a module infant feed
Complan	Farley Health Products Ltd Torr Lane Plymouth P13 5UA	Adult enteral feed or high-protein milk supplement

Name of product	Manufacturer or U.K. distributor	General characteristics
Compliment	Cadbury Ltd Bournville Birmingham B30 2LU	Coffee creamer
Cotazym	Organon Laboratories Ltd Crown House London Road Morden Surrey SM4 5DZ	Pancreatic enzymes
Cow & Gate Supplementary Vitamin Tablets	Cow & Gate Babyfoods Ltd Trowbridge Wilts BA14 8YX	Tablets containing a comprehensive range of water-soluble vitamins and trace minerals
Creon	Duphar Laboratories Ltd Gaters Hill West End Southampton SO3 3JD	Pancreatic enzymes with enteric-coated microspheres coating in gelatin capsules
Creon	Duphar Laboratories Ltd Gaters Hill West End Southampton SO3 3JD	Pancreatic enzymes with enteric-coated microspheres in gelatin capsules
Dalivit	Paines & Byrne Ltd Pabryn Laboratories Bilton Road Perivale Greenford Middx UB6 7HG	Multivitamin supplement
Dextrolyte	Cow & Gate Babyfoods Ltd Trowbridge Wilts BA14 8YX	Oral rehydration solution in ready-to-feed bottles
Dialamine	Scientific Hospital Supplies Ltd 38 Queensland Street Liverpool L7 3JG	Essential amino acid supplements with orange flavouring
Digestelact (not available in U.K.)	Hunter Valley Pty Ltd 168 Willoughby Road Crows Nest NSW 2065 Australia	Lactase-treated milk
Dioralyte	Armour Pharmaceutical Co. Ltd Hampden Park Eastbourne East Sussex BN22 9AG	Glucose electrolyte sachets for use as oral rehydration solution. Flavoured variety also available
dp Low-Protein Chocolate-Flavoured Chip Cookies (also Butterscotch-Flavour)	GF Dietary Supplies Ltd 494–6 Honey Pot Lane Stanmore Middx HA7 1JH	Low-protein biscuits

Name of product	Manufacturer or U.K. distributor	General characteristics
Edifas A	Imperial Chemical Industries Ltd Pharmaceuticals Division Alderley Park Macclesfield Cheshire SK10 4TF Bow Products Ltd 64 York Road Cheam Surrey SM2 2NJ	Cellulose compound used in low-protein cooking
Elemental 028	Scientific Hospital Supplies Ltd 38 Queensland Street Liverpool L7 3JG	Amino acid-based elemental formula with orange flavouring or unflavoured
En-De-Kay	Produced for Stamford Miller Ltd Hatfield Herts by Westone Products Ltd London W1M 5FU	Fluoride drops and tablets
Ensure (liquid and powder)	Abbott Laboratories Ltd Distributors (Ross Laboratories U.S.A.) Queenborough Kent ME11 5EL	Adult enteral feeds
Ensure Plus	Abbott Laboratories Ltd	Adult enteral feed high in protein
Enteral 400	Scientific Hospital Supplies Ltd 38 Queensland Street Liverpool L7 3JG	Adult enteral diet formula
Farex Weaning Food	Farley Health Products Ltd Torr Lane Plymouth P13 5UA	Gluten- and milk-free infant cereal based on rice
Farley's Breakfast Cereal	Farley Health Products Ltd	High-protein cereal for infants
Farley's Gluten-Free Biscuits	Farley Health Products Ltd	Gluten-free biscuit
Farley's Rusk		Infant rusks containing wheat and gluten
Original	Farley Health Products Ltd	Milk-free
Low-Sugar	Farley Health Products Ltd	Contain milk solids lower in sugar
Granulated Rusk	Farley Health Products Ltd	Granulated lower sugar rusk with milk solids
Wholemeal	Farley Health Products Ltd	Wholemeal high-fibre rusk containing wheat and milk solids
Flexical	Mead Johnson Nutritionals Division of Bristol Myers Co. Ltd Station Road Langley Slough SL3 6EB	Adult elemental diet formula

Name of product	Manufacturer or U.K. distributor	General characteristics
Flora margarine	Van den Bergh Sussex House Burgess Hill West Sussex RH15 9AW	Trade name of a margarine high in polyunsaturated fatty acids
Forceval Capsules	Unigreg Ltd Spa House 15/17 Worple Road Wimbledon London SW19 4JS	Vitamin–mineral capsules (junior and adult formulae available)
Forceval Protein	Unigreg Ltd	Protein supplement
Formula S	Cow & Gate Babyfoods Ltd Trowbridge Wilts BA14 8YX	Soy-isolate modified infant formula
Fortison Standard	Cow & Gate Ltd	Adult enteral feed with milk protein
Fortison Soya	Cow & Gate Ltd	Adult enteral feed with soya protein (milk protein- and lactose-free)
Fortical	Cow & Gate Ltd	Maltodextrin drink with flavourings; low-electrolyte, protein-free
Fortisip	Cow & Gate Ltd	Nutritionally balanced supplement drink
Fortimol	Cow & Gate Babyfoods Ltd	High-protein concentrated drink
Galactomin Formula 17	Cow & Gate Babyfoods Ltd Trowbridge Wilts BA14 8YX	Lactose-free formula; contains casein. Reformulation due 1986
Fructose Formula 19	Cow & Gate Baby Foods Ltd	Lactose-free formula with fructose as the carbohydrate. Contains casein. Reformulation 1987.
Gaviscon—infant	Reckitt & Coleman Pharmaceutical Division Dansom Lane Hull HU8 7DS	Medicinal thickener for treatment of vomiting; contains sodium bicarbonate and 4 mmol sodium per 2 g dose
GDL	Pfizer Ltd Sandwich Kent CT13 9NJ	Glucona delta lactone chemical raising agent
GF Crackers GF Thin Wafer Bread GF Crispbread	GF Dietary Supplies 494–6 Honey Pot Lane Stanmore Middx HA7 1JH	Gluten-free savoury biscuits, crispbreads

Name of product	Manufacturer or U.K. distributor	General characteristics
Glucagon	Eli, Lilley & Co. Ltd Kingsclere Road Basingstoke Hants RG21 2XA	Injection for rapid release of glucose from liver glycogen
Glucodin	Farley Health Products Ltd Torr Lane Plymouth PL3 5UA	Dextrose (glucose) plus vitamin C
Gluten	British Drug Houses Pharmaceuticals Ltd Lenten House Lenten Street Alton Hants GU34 1JD	Vital wheat protein powder
Glutenex (Liga)	Cow & Gate Babyfoods Ltd Trowbridge Wilts BA14 8YX	Gluten-free biscuits
Gold Cap SMA	J Wyeth & Bro. Ltd Huntercombe Lane South Taplow Maidenhead Berks SC6 0PH	Whey-based modified infant formula (known as S_{26} outside U.K.)
Granolac Infant	Granose Food Ltd Watford Herts	Infant soya milk entirely of vegetable origin for older infants
Granogen	Granose Food Ltd	Adult soya drink of vegetable origin
Hepatamine	Scientific Hospital Supplies Ltd 38 Queensland Street Liverpool L7 3JG	Essential amino acid supplement for liver failure patients
Haliborange	Farley Health Products Ltd Torr Lane Plymouth P13 5UA	Vitamins A, D, C supplement in orange chewable tablet
HOM 1 & 2	Milupa Ltd Milupa House Hercies Road Hillingdon Middx UB10 9NA	Methionine-free protein substitute for use in treatment of homocystinuria
HIST 1 & 2	Milupa Ltd	Histidine-free protein substitute for use in treatment of histidinaemia

Name of product	Manufacturer or U.K. distributor	General characteristics
Hycal	Beecham Foods Ltd Beecham House Great West Road Brentford Middx TW8 9BD	Liquid glucose with flavourings, low-electrolyte, protein-free
Intal	Fisons Ltd Pharmaceuticals Division 12 Derby Road Loughborough LE11 0BB	Sodium cromoglycate for inhalation
Intralipid	KabiVitrum Ltd Bilton House Uxbridge Road London W5 2TH	Soya oil emulsion for parenteral nutrition
Isocal	Mead Johnson Nutritionals Division of Bristol Myers Co. Ltd Station Road Langley Slough SL3 6EB	Adult enteral feed
Juvela Gluten-Free Bread Mix	GF Dietary Supplies Ltd 494–6 Honey Pot Lane Stanmore Middx HA7 1JH	Gluten-free flour for baking (pre-baked loaf also available)
Low-Protein Bread Mix	GF Dietary Supplies Ltd	Low-protein flour for baking (pre-baked loaf also available)
Kay-Cee-L	Geistlich Sons Ltd PO Box 37 Newton Bank Long Lane Chester CH2 3QZ	Potassium chloride in flavoured solution with sorbitol and colour
Kerulac	Gist-Brocades NV Delft Holland	Lactase enzyme
Keto-amino acid analogues Specification 022 or 122	Scientific Hospital Supplies Ltd 38 Queensland Street Liverpool L7 3JG	Keto-amino acid analogues and essential amino acids
Ketovite Tablets and Liquid	Paines & Byrne Ltd Pabryn Laboratories Bilton Road Perivale Greenford Middx UB6 7HG	Comprehensive vitamin preparation. Tablets = water-soluble vitamins. Liquid = vitamins A, D, B_{12} and choline chloride

Name of product	Manufacturer or U.K. distributor	General characteristics
Lactalac (not available in U.K.)	Cooperative Condensfabriek 'Friesland' Leeuwarden Holland	Lactase-treated milk—low in lactose, contains galactose and glucose
Liga Rusk	Cow & Gate Babyfoods Ltd Trowbridge Wilts BA14 8YX	Rusks for infants
Liquigen	Scientific Hospital Supplies Ltd 38 Queensland Street Liverpool L7 3JG	52% MCT emulsion
Locasol	Cow & Gate Babyfoods Ltd Trowbridge Wilts BA14 8YX	Low-calcium milk substitute. Reformulated 1985
Lofenalac	Mead Johnson Nutritionals Division of Bristol Myers Co. Ltd Station Road Langley Slough SL3 6EB	Low-phenylalanine formula
Lonalac (not available in U.K.)	Mead Johnson Nutritionals	Low-sodium formula
Low Birthweight SMA	J Wyeth & Bro. Ltd Huntercombe Lane South Taplow Maidenhead Berks SC6 0PH	Low-birthweight infant formula
LYS 1 and 2	Milupa Ltd Milupa House Hercies Road Hillingdon Middx UB10 9NA	Lysine-free amino acid protein substitute
Maxilact	Gist-Brocades NV Industrial Foods Division Delft Holland	Lactase enzyme
Maxamaid Complete	Scientific Hospital Supplies Ltd 38 Queensland Street Liverpool L7 3JG	Amino acid supplement, orange-flavoured; contains vitamins and minerals
Maxamaid XP low phenylalanine	Scientific Hospital Supplies Ltd	Amino acid supplements low in the amino acids specified; contain vitamins and minerals; orange-flavoured
Maxamaid XP Concentrate low phenylalanine	Scientific Hospital Supplies Ltd	
Maxamaid XP, XT low phenylalanine and tyrosine	Scientific Hospital Supplies Ltd	
Maxamaid XT, XP, XM low phenylalanine, tyrosine and methionine	Scientific Hospital Supplies Ltd	

Name of product	Manufacturer or U.K. distributor	General characteristics
Maxijul	Scientific Hospital Supplies Ltd	Glucose polymer powder and liquid
Maxijul LE	Scientific Hospital Supplies Ltd	Low-electrolyte glucose polymer powder
Maxipro HBV	Scientific Hospital Supplies Ltd	High biological whey protein
MCT 1 Milk	Cow & Gate Babyfoods Ltd Trowbridge Wilts BA14 8YX	Low-lactose milk substitutes with predominantly MCT in place of fat; contains casein
MCT 2 Milk	Cow & Gate Babyfoods Ltd	
MCT oil	*Various* Cow & Gate Babyfoods Ltd Trowbridge Wilts BA14 8YX Mead Johnson Nutritionals Division of Bristol Myers Co. Ltd Station Road Langley Slough SL3 6EB Scientific Hospital Supplies Ltd 38 Queensland Street Liverpool L7 3JG EJR Lovelock Alembic Products (Alembicol D) Oaklands House Oaklands Drive Sale Manchester M33 1WS	Medium-chain triglycerides; predominantly C_8 and C_{10} saturated fatty acids
MCT Pepdite 0–2	Scientific Hospital Supplies Ltd 38 Queensland Street Liverpool L7 3JG	Peptide-based elemental infant feed with MCT
MCT Pepdite 2 +	Scientific Hospital Supplies Ltd	Peptide-based elemental feed with MCT for children
Metabolic Mineral Mixture	Scientific Hospital Supplies Ltd	Comprehensive mineral supplement for synthetic diets
Milumil	Milupa Ltd Milups House Hercies Road Hillingdon Middx UB10 9NA	Modified infant formula
Minafen	Cow & Gate Babyfoods Ltd Trowbridge Wilts BA14 3HZ	Low-phenylalanine formula
MSUD Aid	Scientific Hospital Supplies Ltd 38 Queensland Street Liverpool L7 3JG	Amino acid supplements free of leucine, isoleucine and valine

Name of product	Manufacturer or U.K. distributor	General characteristics
MSUD 1 and 2	Milupa Ltd Milupa House Hercies Road Hillingdon Middx UB10 9NA	Amino acid supplements free of leucine, isoleucine and valine
Multibionta infusion	British Drug Houses Pharmaceuticals Ltd Lenten House Lenten Street Alton Hants GU34 1JD	Multivitamin injection
Nan	The Nestlé Co. Ltd St George's House Croydon Surrey CR9 1NR	Whey-based modified infant formula
Nalcrom	Fisons Ltd Pharmaceuticals Division 12 Derby Road Loughborough LE11 0BB	Sodium cromoglycate tablets
Nefranutrin	Geistlich Sons Ltd PO Box 37 Newton Bank Long Lane Chester CH2 3QZ	Essential amono acid supplement
Nenatal	Cow & Gate Babyfoods Ltd Trowbridge Wilts BA14 8YX	Low-birthweight infant formula
Neocate Neonatal Elemental Diets (amino acid-based)	Scientific Hospital Supplies Ltd 38 Queensland Street Liverpool L7 3JG	Elemental diet for infants
Nestargel	The Nestlé Co. Ltd St George's House Croydon Surrey CR9 1NR	Hemicellulose gelling agent derived from carob seeds used for thickening infant feeds. Requires cooking
Nutramigen	Mead Johnson Nutritionals Division of Bristol Myers Co. Ltd Station Road Langley Slough S13 6EB	Casein hydrolysate formula for older infants; contains sucrose; lactose-free
Nutranel	Roussel Laboratories Ltd Broadwater Park North Orbital Road Denham Uxbridge UB9 5HP	Adult elemental feed

Name of product	Manufacturer or U.K. distributor	General characteristics
Nutrasweet	Searle Laboratories Division of G. D. Searle Co. Ltd PO Box 53 Lane End Road High Wycombe Bucks HP12 4HL	Artificial sweetener based on aspartame
Nutrauxil	KabiVitrum Ltd Bilton House Uxbridge Road London W5 2TH	Adult enteral feed
Nutrizym	British Drug Houses Pharmaceuticals Ltd Lenten House Lenten Street Alton Hants GU34 1JD	Pancreatic enzymes with ox bile and bromelains
Osterfeed	Farley Health Products Ltd Torr Lane Plymouth PL3 5UA	Whey-based modified infant formulae
Ostermilk Complete Ostermilk 2	Farley Health Products Ltd Farley Health Products Ltd	Modified infant formulae
Osterprem	Farley Health Products Ltd	Pre-term and low birthweight infant formula
Oster rusks	Farley Health Products Ltd	Infant weaning rusk
OS 1 and 2	Milupa Ltd Milupa House Hercies Road Hillingdon Middx UB10 9NA	Amino acid supplement free of isoleucine, valine, threonine and methionine for treatment of certain organic acidaemias
Pancrease	Ortho-Cilag Pharmaceutical Ltd PO Box 79 Saunderton High Wycombe Bucks HP14 4HJ	Pancreatic enzymes in enteric-coated microspheres in gelatin capsules
Pancreax	Paines & Byrne Ltd Pabryn Laboratories Bilton Road Perivale Greenford Middx UB6 7HG	Pancreatic enzymes in various strengths and formats

Name of product	Manufacturer or U.K. distributor	General characteristics
Pareve-mate	Carnation Foods Co. Carnation House 11 High Road London N2 8AW	Kosher coffee creamer, protein-free
Ped-El	KabiVitrum Ltd Bilton House Uxbridge Road London W5 2TH	Paediatric mineral supplement for parenteral nutrition
Pepdite 0–2	Scientific Hospital Supplies Ltd 38 Queensland Street Liverpool L7 3JG	Peptide-based elemental infant feed
Pepdite 2 +	Scientific Hospital Supplies Ltd	Peptide-based elemental feed for children
Pepdite MCT 0–2	Scientific Hospital Supplies Ltd	Peptide-based elemental infant feed with MCT
Pepdite MCT 2 +	Scientific Hospital Supplies Ltd	Peptide-based elemental feed with MCT for children.
Peptisorbin	E Merck Ltd Winchester Road Four Marks Alton Hants GU34 5HG	Peptide-based adult elemental formula with MCT
PK Aid	Scientific Hospital Supplies Ltd	Phenylalanine-free amino acids
PKU 1 and 2	Milupa Ltd Milupa House Hercies Road Hillingdon Middx UB10 9NA	Phenylalanine-free supplement
Plamil	Plantmilk Ltd Bowles Well Gardens Dover Road Folkestone Kent	Soya drink of entirely vegetable origin. Not a nutritional replacement of milk
Plamil—sugar-free	Plantmilk Ltd	Soya liquid concentrate with only a trace of carbohydrate
Polycal	Cow & Gate Babyfoods Ltd Trowbridge Wilts BA14 8YX	Glucose polymer/maltodextrin powder
Portagen	Mead Johnson Nutritionals Ltd Division of Bristol Myers Co. Ltd Station Road Langley Slough SL3 6EB	Lactose-free milk substitute with predominantly MCT in place of fat; contains sodium caseinate, fortified with vitamins and minerals, particularly vitamin A

Name of product	Manufacturer or U.K. distributor	General characteristics
Preaptamil	Milupa Ltd Milupa House Hercies Road Hillingdon Middx UB10 9NA	Low-birthweight infant formula
Pregestimil	Mead Johnson Nutritionals Ltd Division of Bristol Myers Co. Ltd Station Road Langley Slough SL3 6EB	Hydrolysed casein modified infant formula with added cystine, tyrosine and tryptophan; lactose-, sucrose-free. Partial MCT fat
Prematalac	Cow & Gate Babyfoods Ltd Trowbridge Wilts BA14 8YX	High-protein, high-sodium, low-birthweight infant formula
Premium	Cow & Gate Babyfoods Ltd	Whey-based modified infant formula
Progress	J Wyeth & Bro. Ltd Huntercombe Lane South Taplow Maidenhead Berks SC6 0PH	'Follow-on' milk drink for infants over six months of age
Prosobee (powder and liquid concentrate)	Mead Johnson Nutritionals Division of Bristol Myers Co. Ltd Station Road Langley Slough SL3 6ED	Soy-isolate modified infant formula with added methionine
Prosparol	Duncan, Flockhart & Co. Ltd 700 Oldfield Lane North Greenford Middx UB6 0HB	50% arachis (peanut) oil emulsion
Questran	Mead Johnson Nutritionals Division of Bristol Myers Co. Ltd Station Road Langley Slough SL3 6EB	Cholestyramine powder in sachets
Rehidrat	Searle Laboratories Division of GD Searle Co. Ltd PO Box 53 Lane End Road High Wycombe Bucks HP12 4HL	Glucose and sucrose electrolyte sachets for use as oral rehydration solution; contains colour and flavouring
Rite-Diet gluten-free biscuits, bread, bread mix, flour, fruit cake	Welfare Foods (Stockport) Ltd 63 London Road South Poynton Stockport Cheshire SK12 1LA	Various gluten-free baked goods

Name of product	Manufacturer or U.K. distributor	General characteristics
Rite-Diet low-protein biscuits, bread, bread mix	Welfare Foods (Stockport) Ltd	Various low-protein baked goods
Rite-Diet Salt-Free Bread	Welfare Foods (Stockport) Ltd	Salt-free bread
Rite-Diet Low-Protein Salt-Free Bread	Welfare Foods (Stockport) Ltd	Low-protein salt-free bread
Rite-Diet Gluten-Free Low-Protein Bread with Soya Bran	Welfare Foods (Stockport) Ltd	Gluten-free, low-protein, high-fibre bread
Rite-Diet Gluten-Free Low-Protein Baking Powder	Welfare Foods (Stockport) Ltd	Gluten-free baking powder
Sandocal	Sandoz Products Ltd Pharmaceuticals Division Sandoz House 98 The Centre Feltham Middx TW13 4EP	Calcium tablets or liquid
Seravit	Scientific Hospital Supplies Ltd 38 Queensland Street Liverpool L7 3JG	Supplementary vitamin–mineral mixtures for different ages and types of diet
Modified Seravit RD 079 or 79	Scientific Hospital Supplies Ltd	
Paediatric Seravit RD 222	Scientific Hospital Supplies Ltd	
S Formula	Cow & Gate Babyfoods Ltd Trowbridge Wilts BA14 8YX	Soy-isolate modified infant formula with methionine
Skimmed milk powder (separated milk, non-milk fat solids)	*Various*	Powdered milk from which fat has been removed
SMA (Gold Cap, Low Birthweight, White Cap)	J Wyeth & Bro. Ltd Huntercombe Lane South Taplow Maidenhead Berks SC6 0PH	Modified infant formulae and low-birthweight infant feed
Sodium cromoglycate (Nalcrom; Intal)	Fisons Ltd Pharmaceuticals Division 12 Derby Road Loughborough LE11 0BB	Drug used in various types of allergy
Solivito	KabiVitrum Ltd Bilton House Uxbridge Road London W5 2TH	Water-soluble vitamin preparation for parenteral nutrition

Name of product	Manufacturer or U.K. distributor	General characteristics
Soy Bean Milk (concentrate)	Golden Archer Itona Health Food Itona Products Ltd Wigan Lancs	Soya drink. Not a nutritional replacement of milk
Soya Milk (liquid)	Granose Food Ltd Watford Herts	Soya drink. Not a nutritional replacement of milk
Supplementary Vitamin Tablets	Cow & Gate Babyfoods Ltd Trowbridge Wilts BA14 8YX	Tablets containing a comprehensive range of water-soluble vitamins and trace minerals
Telma margarine	Israel Edible Products Ltd POB 707 Haifa Israel 31 000	Trade names of kosher margarines which are milk-free
Tomor margarine	Van den Bergh Sussex House Burgess Hill West Sussex RH15 9AW	
Triosorbin	E Merck Ltd Winchester Road Four Marks Alton Hants GU34 5HG	Adult enteral feed containing MCT
Tritamyl gluten-free flour	Procea Ltd Alexandra Road Dublin 1 Eire	Gluten-free flour (self-raising)
Tritamyl PK	Procea Ltd	Low-protein flour (self-raising)
Trufree gluten-free wheat-free flours 1 to 7	Larkhall Laboratories 225 Putney Bridge Road London SW15 2PY	Various gluten-free and wheat-free flours
TYR 1 and 2	Milupa Ltd Milupa House Hercies Road Hillingdon Middx UB10 9NA	Phenylalanine-, tyrosine-free amino acid supplement for use in the treatment of tyrosinaemia
UCD	Milupa Ltd Milupa House Hercies Road Hillingdon Middx UB10 9NA	Amino acid supplement for treatment of certain urea cycle defects

Name of product	Manufacturer or U.K. distributor	General characteristics
Vamin (various)	KabiVitrum Ltd Bilton House Uxbridge Road London W5 2TH	Comprehensive mixture of 18 L-amino acids in solutions for paediatric parenteral nutrition; contains cysteine/cystine but free of taurine
Vegetarian Jelly	Snowcrest Ltd 8 White's Row Commercial Road London E2	Protein-free vegetarian jelly; gelatin-free
Verkade Gluten-Free Biscuits	GF Dietary Supplies Ltd 494–6 Honey Pot Lane Stanmore Middx HA7 1JH	Gluten-free biscuits
Vipep	Tuta Laboratories Lane Cove Australia	Peptide-based elemental diet containing MCT
Vit-lipid (adult and infant)	KabiVitrum Ltd Bilton House Uxbridge Road London W5 2TH	Vitamins A, D_2 and K_1 for use in parenteral nutrition
Vital Wheat Protein	British Drug Houses Pharmaceuticals Ltd Lenten House Lenten Street Alton Hants GU34 1JD	Source of gluten powder
Viokase	A H Robins Co. Ltd Redkiln Way Horsham West Sussex RH13 5QP	Pancreatic enzyme
Vivonex	Eaton Laboratories Regent House The Broadway Woking Surrey GU21 5AP	Adult elemental diet formula based on amino acids. Cystine- and taurine-free
Vivonex HN	Eaton Laboratories	High-protein, high osmolar, adult elemental diet formula based on amino acids
White Cap SMA	J Wyeth & Bro. Ltd Huntercombe Lane South Taplow Maidenhead Berks SC6 0PH	Modified infant formula

Name of product	Manufacturer or U.K. distributor	General characteristics
Wysoy	J Wyeth & Bro. Ltd	Soy-isolate and methionine modified infant formula
Zincomed Capsules	Medo-Chemicals Ltd Unit 3 Jackson Industrial Park Wessex Road Bourne End Bucks HP5 1EF	220 mg zinc sulphate tablet = 50 mg elemental zinc
Zymafluor	Zyma (UK) Ltd Huddersfield Industrial Estate Macclesfield Cheshire SK10 2LY	Sodium fluoride, 0·25 mg fluoride per tablet.

APPENDIX I

Borderline substances

In the U.K. a number of proprietary foods used in treatment are classified as drugs for certain conditions. The Secretary of State for Social Services has appointed a committee to advise where particular preparations should be regarded as drugs and their recommendations are published as an appendix in each edition of the *British National Formulary*, *Drug Tariff* and *MIMS*. Prescription form FC 10, used for prescribing such products, should be marked ACBS where the item prescribed is listed for the condition concerned.

REFERENCES

British National Formulary. British Medical Association and The Pharmaceutical Society of Great Britain, Pitman Press, Bath.
Drug Tariff. Prepared under Regulation 28 of the National Health Service (General Medical and Pharmaceutical Services) Regulation 1974, Family Practitioner Services Division 2C1, Elephant and Castle, London.
MIMS. Medical Publications Ltd, London.

APPENDIX II

SI units used in nutrition

Conversion of kilojoules (kJ) to kilocalories (kcal)

kJ	kcal
9000	2151
8000	1912
7000	1673
6000	1434
5000	1195
4000	956
3500	837
3000	717
2500	600
2000	478
1500	359
1000*	239
500	120
100	24
1	0·239

* 1 megajoule (MJ).
1 kcal = 4·184 kJ.

Units of energy (approx.) from different food types

	kJ	kcal
1 g Protein	17	4
1 g Fat	37	9
1 g Carbohydrate	16	4
1 g Alcohol	29	7

CONVERSION FOR MINERALS

Calcium $\dfrac{mg}{40\cdot0}$

Chloride $\dfrac{mg}{35\cdot5}$

Copper $\dfrac{mg}{63\cdot6}$

Iodine $\dfrac{mg}{126\cdot9}$

Iron $\dfrac{mg}{55\cdot8}$

Magnesium $\dfrac{mg}{24\cdot0}$

Phosphorus $\dfrac{mg}{31\cdot0}$

Potassium $\dfrac{mg}{39\cdot0}$

Sodium $\dfrac{mg}{23\cdot0}$

Zinc $\dfrac{mg}{65\cdot4}$

$\left.\right\} = $ millimole (mmol)

VITAMINS

Vitamin D_3 $1\,\mu g = 40\cdot0\,\text{i.u.}$
             $1\,\text{i.u.} = 0\cdot025\,\mu g$

Vitamin A $1\,\mu g = 3\cdot3\,\text{i.u.}$ retinol (vitamin A_1 alcohol)
            $1\,\text{i.u.} = 0\cdot30\,\mu g$ retinol (vitamin A_1 alcohol)
            $1\,\text{i.u.} = 0\cdot60\,\mu g$ carotene

APPENDIX III

Conversion for general measurements

Approximate metric conversion

---

1 ounce (oz) = 28·4 gram (g) or millilitre (ml) or cubic centimetre (cc)
1 pound (lb) = 450 g
2·2 lb = 1000 g = 1 kilogram (kg)
1 pint = 20 ounces = 560 millilitres (ml)

100 g or ml = 3½ oz
200 g or ml = 7 oz
30 g or ml approximately = 1 oz
1000 g or ml approximately = 35 oz

2·54 centimetres (cm) = 1 inch
100 cm = 1 metre = 39"
12" = 30·5 cm

Volumetric measurements

---

	ml
Standard 8 oz cup	240
Standard teaspoon	5
Standard tablespoon	15

APPENDIX IV

Scales for use with weighed diets

A simple accurate diet scale which is robust and easy to use with digital reading or a clear dial is now easier to obtain. I have found the clock dial or digital scale with 5 g and ¼ oz increments satisfactory for home use, as even children can manage this type, and the accuracy is satisfactory for diets such as described in this book.

For hospital kitchens, there are many types of metric scales available covering a wide range of accuracy and cost. Increments of 1 g are suitable for most purposes. Those with a tare mechanism enable the weight of the container in which the food is weighed to be counteracted. The ingredients of special infant feeds may need to be weighed, but because of the need for aseptic preparation the scale pans should be sterilizable or the ingredients weighed into sterilized jugs on scales with a tare mechanism.

Index